Psychotherapy for Families after Brain Injury

Pamela S. Klonoff

Psychotherapy for Families after Brain Injury

Springer

Pamela S. Klonoff
Barrow Neurological Institute
Phoenix
Arizona
USA

ISBN 978-1-4899-7818-9 ISBN 978-1-4899-8083-0 (eBook)
DOI 10.1007/978-1-4899-8083-0
Springer New York Heidelberg Dordrecht London

Printed on acid-free paper

Springer is part of Springer Science+Business Media (www.springer.com)

To Bessy and Sam Altman and all families who have endured with grace, and through love, devotion, and kindness of spirit, ultimately triumphed over suffering.

Preface

This book emanates from a wholehearted desire to describe and validate the journey of family members with a loved one who has suffered a brain injury. It is a compilation of many years of clinical experience, research, dialogue, and self-reflection about the phenomenological perspective of families. Albeit, a therapist can never truly “know” the myriad of emotions and occurrences a family member traverses, I hope this book captures a beginning essence. The book is written with much admiration, reverence, and gratitude to families and their injured loved ones, who have shared their losses, vulnerabilities, and victories with such aplomb and dignity. Their courage has inspired the content and the therapeutic process within me.

The principles depicted have been coveted and nurtured within a therapeutic milieu designed to rebuild patients’ lives through empathic responsiveness, psychoeducation, and a healing group process built on the fundamentals of awareness, acceptance, and realism. As is hopefully gleaned throughout the book, psychotherapy is most effective when in partnership with other neurorehabilitation therapies designed to meet the holistic needs of the loved one and his or her family and support network. This represents the “tiers of support” within the provision of care; a psychotherapist who interrelates with other medical personnel and rehabilitation therapists, interconnected with a broader community who typify the mission of care. Together, these three tiers of support unite on behalf of the therapeutic process to reintegrate and ultimately uplift the loved one and family unit. Key healthcare players include, but are not limited to, “tier 1” neuropsychologists, clinical psychologists, rehabilitation psychologists, and social workers in the psychotherapist role; their specialties should be considered interchangeable and equally viable for the title of “psychotherapist” or “therapist” within the text. Within this model, “tier 2” treatment supports contain physiatrists, neurologists, psychiatrists, nurses, speech-language pathologists, occupational therapists, physical therapists, recreational therapists, dieticians, rehabilitation technicians, and undoubtedly others dedicated to the treatment of families (and their loved ones). Vital “tier 3” supports include hospitals, healthcare clinics, schools, worksites, religious institutions, and many other community-based resources.

Several provisos are deemed necessary. Although this book is intended to be user-friendly, it is not considered a “self-help” text. Ideally, it is to be used in partnership with a guiding therapist to explore, converse, and even debate about key principles. I readily acknowledge shortfalls due to the limits of my expertise and clinical exposures in combination with the natural constraints of one textbook. The vantage point primarily emphasizes the post-acute time frame, with sometimes only minimal reference to the ICU and early days postinjury. The content also does not do justice to the multiplicity of hardships and needs of children and younger adolescents. In this context, when feasible, some content applicable to these younger age groups is included. The seasoned clinician and astute family member may also recognize the "idealized" viewpoints enacted in the case studies. Albeit somewhat simplistic, these are designed to portray fundamental principles embodied in the text. I humbly admit that the "real world" of families' angst and the therapeutic work may have much more intricacies and detours.

Although a milieu-oriented approach is available and optimal for some, the constructs and lessons are meant to be adaptable to whichever formats and venues are accessible and chosen by the therapist, family system, loved one, and community resources. Here within, both individual psychotherapeutic modalities and two types of family groups are provided. The audience is invited and encouraged to use this book as a springboard for further therapeutic investigation and enrichment.

Acknowledgments

This project is a labor of love and would never have birthed without the patience, cheering, and caring suggestions of my own personal "tiers of support." First and foremost, I want to thank my "tier 1" family (my husband, Irwin, and sons, Zachary, Aharon Tzvi Jeremy, and Aaron) for indulging my long absences and preoccupations inherent in the book's creation. Innumerable "tier 1" patients, families, and their supporters have furnished 28 years of heart-felt input, information, wisdom, and content for this collaborative journey. Many "tier 2" "outside readers" offered thoughtful advice and supportive commentary. A hearty thank you goes to: Dr. Kavitha Perumparaichallai, Dr. Kristi Husk, Dr. Irwin Altman, Dr. Susan Rumble, Dr. Brian Kelley, Dr. Stephen Myles, Ms. Alicia Blank, Ms. Maura Rynn, Ms. Jennifer Hunsaker, Ms. Debbie Fuchigami, Ms. Laurene Flitner, Ms. Patty Briody, Ms. Beth Heick, Ms. Lori Lindman, Ms. Pamela McNamara, Ms. Jennifer Lutton, Ms. Denise Parker-Gutierrez, Ms. Marie Reichert, and Ms. Franne Wilk. Mr. Edward Koberstein has been a sustaining, inspirational muse throughout this sometimes daunting undertaking. A special debt of gratitude goes to Mr. Koberstein and Dr. Rumble for their co-authorships. Their experience, insights, and companionship enriched the content. My professional passions are buoyed by other "tier 3" believers, most particularly, Laya Braemer, and my fellow teammates at the Center for Transitional NeuroRehabilitation, as well as extended family and friends. My writing journey requires the ideal ambience to stimulate the creative juices. I thank all of the musicians whose melodies and lyrics catalyzed and deepened the emotive and cathartic process intrinsic to this endeavor. Beyond this world, Dr. Gustavo Lage's brilliance, resonating empathy, and heartfelt encouragement continue to reverberate through my daily toils and life values; for that I remain forever indebted. Thank you all for "companioning" with me in this life-affirming venture.

Contents

Chapter 1
Introduction and Overview

1.1 Introduction

Clinicians, physicians, and researchers have come to realize the preeminence of family members' commitment, participation, education, coping, and adjustment in order for their loved ones to maximize their recovery after an acquired brain injury (Klonoff et al. 2001; Patterson and Staton 2009; Sachs 1991). Likewise, patients mostly recognize the benefit of their family's involvement, even though they cannot generally acknowledge, communicate, or express gratitude during their earlier stages of recovery. A working definition of *caregiving* is unpaid provision of care to a loved one, including his or her self-care, activities of daily living, transportation, and overall emotional support. Often this is provided by family members, although friends also function as caregivers (Collins and Swartz 2011). For the purposes of this book, reference to "family caregivers" also pertains to close friends who assume this laudable function.

Early pioneers in the exploration of the family's feelings during the emotional aftermath of their loved one's acquired brain injury include Lezak (1978, 1988). She insightfully identified the emotional distress (including depression and anxiety), family disruptions (social isolation), and adjustment difficulties (including feeling unable to mourn, trapped, and burdened). Others, such as Romano (1974), Thomsen (1974), Oddy and colleagues (Oddy et al. 1978), McKinlay and colleagues (McKinlay et al. 1981), as well as Bond (1988) have contributed formative research and clinical observations on patients' postinjury personality and behavioral changes, family reaction patterns, sources of stress, and the subjective burden of patients' brain injuries on their relatives. Additional founding contributors include Brooks (1984) and Sachs (1991) who edited/wrote early books delineating assessment considerations, injury consequences, and treatment techniques for families of brain injury survivors. Brooks (1984) and Kreutzer and associates (Kreutzer et al. 1992) provided cogent overviews of the psychosocial aspects of patients' disabilities after a brain injury, illuminating that most disturbing to the families are changes in temperament, including rage reactions, irritability, lability, aspontaneity, restlessness, and childlike behavior.

P. S. Klonoff, *Psychotherapy for Families after Brain Injury*,
DOI 10.1007/978-1-4899-8083-0_1, © Springer Science+Business Media New York 2014

More recent research has confirmed that the severity and chronicity of the injury, as well as the physical sequelae are less related to caregiver distress (see Ergh et al. 2002, for a review). Instead, it is the neurobehavioral consequences of the brain injury on cognition, behavior, and emotions, which relate to the family's emotional distress, unhealthy functioning, and overall burden (Carnes and Quinn 2005; Ergh et al. 2002; see Klonoff and Prigatano 1987, for a review; Ponsford et al. 2003; Verhaeghe et al. 2005). In addition, poorer community reintegration in patients correlates with their relatives' distress, especially anxiety (Klonoff and Prigatano 1987; Winstanley et al. 2006). Of note, relatives' subjective burden increases, not decreases over time (Kay and Cavallo 1994). There is now a growing interest in the effects of loved ones' brain injuries on family functioning, with respect to both the causes and nature of the family's reactions as well as treatment approaches.

1.2 Formats and Theoretical Frameworks Applicable for Family Therapy After Brain Injury

Treatment of the family after brain injury can be conducted in a number of formats, including individual therapy for a specific relative (e.g., the primary caregiver); marital therapy; the family unit involving multiple family members (with and without the patient); and group therapy for multiple families (Florian and Katz 1991; Klonoff and Koberstein 2010; Kreutzer et al. 2002; Rosenthal and Young 1988).

Family therapy after brain injury is often an amalgamation of a number of theoretical schools of thought. These include psychodynamic, self-psychology, behavior modification, family systems, cognitive–behavioral/family schemas, family group interventions, psychoeducation/skills training, assistive technology, mindfulness and positive psychology, as well as existential and family autobiographical approaches. All of these target the caregivers and broader family entities so as to enhance their coping capacities and skill sets. The following sections summarize pertinent constructs and approaches to family therapy after a brain injury.

1.2.1 Psychoanalytic Contributions

Psychoanalytic concepts refer to intrapsychic and intrapersonal processes; these can integrate with the interpersonal process of family systems therapy (Flaskas 2005), which are also applicable to family therapy after brain injury. For example, family dynamics implies that the family operates as a complex psychosocial unit, including its own adaptive and developmental characteristics (Schwartz 2007). An individual within the family unit can express unconscious dynamics which interfere with his or her ability to develop a sense of authority or agency (Schwartz 2007). The identified patient and his or her family also share common defenses that manifest as treatment resistance, usually based on inflexible and nonadaptive defenses, which in turn mar reality testing and distort the perception of self and other (Schwartz 2007). Therefore, by working with the family, the therapist finds and interprets the meaning of shared family defenses, so that the patient and family can emerge from a "stuck" or therapy-resistant position (Schwartz 2007).

Other germane contributions of psychoanalysis to family therapy are the unconscious influences and experiences in families, also including the parents' own experiences of attachment (Flaskas 2005). For instance, Fraiberg et al. (1975) refer to "ghosts in the nursery" as damaged infant–mother relationships which are founded on "unconscious intruders" from the parental past, or repetition of tragedies of the parent's past childhood with his or her baby in the present. The pain and suffering in the individual are repressed and undergo an unconscious alliance with the formidable past figures, which are then inflicted upon the child. Through psychotherapy, the individual accesses his or her childhood pain, which becomes a powerful deterrent against repetition when parenting (Fraiberg et al. 1975).

In addition, *transference* (i.e., the patient's unconscious patterns of relating within the therapeutic relationship, or any relationship), *countertransference* (i.e., the therapist's emotions, attitudes, and patterns of relating which are enacted within the therapeutic relationship), and *projective identification* (i.e., unconscious projection of unbearable impasses of emotion and meaning within the therapeutic and other relationships) all affect family therapy, sometimes producing therapeutic breakdowns and impasses (Flaskas 2005, 2007). Again, in the context of family treatment after brain injury, the psychotherapist must be vigilant of the contribution of these underlying psychodynamics. This requires a multidimensional awareness of complex family dynamics when introducing treatment approaches relevant to the effects of the brain injury.

1.2.2 Self-Psychology

Self-psychology, as espoused by Kohut, is the psychoanalytic study of the psychological structure, the self (Wolf 1988). Fundamental to self-psychological constructs is that the emergence of the self requires the presence of others, or *selfobject* experiences. These constitute the people who provide particular experiences which evoke the emergence, maintenance, and completion of the self (Wolf 1988). Most often, these selfobjects are provided by the parents and other significant family members. The self-psychology construct of selfobjects is related to family therapy after brain injury, as it provides a context to assess the basic preinjury psychological health in the patient. Postinjury, these altered selfobject relations with key family members either evolve or splinter the patient's emotional cohesiveness. This is especially the case for younger patients interacting with primary parental figures postinjury.

Appropriate selfobject experiences perform soothing and calming functions and promote structural cohesion, well-being, and the energized vigor of the self (Klonoff and Lage 1991; Wolf 1988). On the other hand, faulty selfobject experiences produce fragmentation (or instability, emptiness, and disintegration) of the self (Klonoff and Lage 1991; Wolf 1988). The infant requires the concrete physical presence of the caregiver object as the supplier of good selfobject experiences. However, over time, the mature individual uses reliable, consistent, endopsychic, symbolic representations of the original selfobject experiences to maintain his or her structural integrity (Baker and Baker 1987; Kohut 1984a; Wolf 1988). Another central tenet of self-psychology is the indispensable role of the parents' empathic relatedness to their children. *Empathy* is the ability to intrinsically connect to the experience of others, based on their own unique perspectives (Baker and Baker 1987).

Also, significant for the individual's preinjury psychic development are selfobject transference relationships (Baker and Baker 1987; Klonoff and Lage 1991; Kohut 1984b; Wolf 1988). These include *mirroring transferences,* which are the confirming and approving responses by the parent that validate the child's sense of self-worth (e.g., the mother's pleasure in witnessing her child's achievements). *Idealizing transferences* relate to the merging of the child with images of calmness, safety, and strength after emotional letdowns. *Twinship (or alter ego) transferences* refer to the comforting experience of alikeness with others (e.g., when engaged in similar endeavors). Early and pervasive failures in these transferences result in developmental arrests and a predisposition to more severe psychiatric dysfunction in the individual. Nonetheless, all individuals experience "optimal failures" within a "good enough" responsive parental environment. This requires the child, through a process of "transmuting internalization" or optimal frustrations, to create the internal capacity to tolerate unavoidable failures, develop inner resiliency and self-worth, and pursue suitable ambitions (Baker and Baker 1987; Kohut 1984b; Wolf 1988). Again, to the extent that there are serious developmental failures in parent–child interactions preinjury, the child becomes unable to develop and regulate self-esteem. This problem becomes compounded after the brain injury, when internal regulation and self-esteem are even more fragile. Overall, this serves to further destabilize an already precarious postinjury family unit.

In conjunction with this, after the brain injury, the loved one can be hurled into *narcissistic rage,* or an assault on self-esteem manifested by fury toward himself or herself and/or others (Baker and Baker 1987). Underlying this self-hatred are feelings of shame, vulnerability, powerlessness, emptiness, and hopelessness (Klonoff 2010). This "disintegration" anxiety is manifested as a loss of sense of self, humanness, and inner wholeness (Kohut 1984c). Similarly, "narcissistic rage" reactions can emanate from the caregiver and/or other tier supports, due to their feelings of helplessness and ineptness in preventing the brain injury and/or curing the devastating and horrifying sequelae.

1.2.3 Behavior Modification

Behavior modification techniques have been used with patients with acquired brain injury, who generally have either severe positive behavioral disorders (e.g., aggression, inappropriate sexual behavior, and disruptive behavior) or negative behavior disorders (e.g., decreased arousal or drive; see Smith and Godfrey 1995, for a review; Wood 1984). These interventions help eliminate unwanted social behaviors and shape these into more appropriate forms. The goal is to reduce behaviors that limit independence or compromise safety and increase behaviors which will empower the patient, so that he or she can function in an environment that is least restrictive (Persel and Persel 2010). Conditions are thereby created which reinforce appropriate behaviors and skills, so as to encourage motivation and success (Alderman 2004). This encompasses cuing and feedback techniques provided in a structured environment to reduce challenging behaviors and increase physical and functional independence (Alderman 2004).

Behavior modification procedures involve careful assessment, monitoring, and functional analysis of the troublesome behavior (based on the injury, the patient, and the environmental context), followed by application of behavioral interventions (Ponsford 2013). These include differential reinforcement, time-out, contingent punishment, overcorrection, and massed practice (see Smith and Godfrey 1995, for a review; Wood 1984). The overall training model for families focuses on: problem identification; problem selection; resource assessment; behavioral assessment; intervention; evaluation; and maintenance/generalization (Jacobs 1991; Persel and Persel 2010; Wilson et al. 2003). Using a team approach to train family members in these techniques can be helpful in generalizing desirable behaviors into the home and community environments (Persel and Persel 2010), although it is generally very taxing on family members to learn and successfully implement these strategies consistently (see Smith and Godfrey 1995, for a review).

1.2.4 Family Systems

The family systems theory presupposes that the family (not the individual) is the primary unit and is comprised of the functioning and interaction of structural elements, including positions, norms, and roles (Maitz 1991). This theory also espouses the principles of *non-summativity,* or the necessity of assessing the system as a whole, not just individual members; *wholeness,* whereby a change in one part of a family system affects all of the other parts; and *homeostasis,* in which families strive to maintain a fluid balance (Maitz 1991). Within the family systems framework, there are seven broad categories of family functions: economic, daily care, recreation, socialization, affection, self-definition, and educational/vocational (see Turnbull and Turnbull 1991). Other main components of the family systems perspective include: family interaction patterns affect how the members are arranged into subsystems, which in turn carry out family functions; members have multiple and sometimes competing responsibilities with respect to individual and collective needs; and the family has a dynamic organization and progresses through a number of different lifestyle stages during the developmental process (Maitz and Sachs 1995; Turnbull and Turnbull 1991; Verhaeghe et al. 2005).

Several authors have espoused that the family systems approach plays a significant role in the treatment of families with a loved one who has sustained a brain injury (Gan and Schuller 2002; Kay and Cavallo 1994; Lansky 1990; Laroi 2003;

Rosenthal and Young 1988; Yeates 2009). Therefore, injury to the loved one affects all other family members with reverberations of stress throughout (David 1998). This implicates the entire family as affected by the injury, not just the primary caregiver (Gan and Schuller 2002; Judd 1999; Kay and Cavallo 1994). Family systems are also affected differently, based on their diversity, complexity, and social context (Yeates 2009). The injury results in a breakdown in the operation of the entire family system, characterized by distress in the whole family, as well as shame and catastrophic reactions (see Chap. 4, Sect. 4.6) in the loved one, thereby affecting communication, problem solving, norms, needs, cohesiveness, and role performance (Gan et al. 2006; Judd 1999; Kay and Cavallo 1994; Lansky 1990). A *role* is defined as an integrated and socially determined set of beliefs, values, and expectations related to how the individual should behave (Maitz and Sachs 1995).

Laroi (2003) references the factors associated with the transition of the patient into a new role within the family structure and hierarchy, as well as assisting other family members in adjusting to this altered role. Laroi (2003) and Maitz and Sachs (1995) posit that the brain injury can result in either a reestablishment of preinjury roles (e.g., restoring the parent's authority) or a redistribution of postinjury roles (e.g., the power and authority when the individual with the brain injury can no longer assume the same degree of responsibilities as preinjury). Interventions should take into account different configurations of family members and provide varying resources, based on the needs of the particular family (Yeates 2009). Ultimately, incorporation of the conceptual and practical aspects of the family systems approach will enhance therapeutic endeavors (Laroi 2003).

1.2.5 Cognitive–Behavioral and Family Schema Approaches

The ingrained and shared beliefs of families about their functioning, based on interaction patterns, are referred to as family schemas (Dattilio 2005). *Schemas* are a cornerstone of modern cognitive–behavior therapy and represent a template for the person's life experiences. They are central to thought and perception, also influencing emotions and behavior (Dattilio 2005). Therefore, family members both influence and are influenced by one another's thoughts, emotions, and behaviors. Assumptions are then formed which develop into relatively stable schemas or "cognitive structures" (Dattilio 2005).

Kosciulek (1997) indicated that the family schemas after brain injuries (including their mutual beliefs, values, goals, priorities, and expectations) affect their interrelationships, as well as community and social system affiliations. After a brain injury, the family's self-appraisal and coping paradigm (e.g., adaptability) are shaped by their family schema. Specifically, Kosciulek (1997) found that the family's higher manageability or controllability of the brain injury challenges positively influenced their adaptation. In addition, those families who could ascribe meaningfulness through redefinition of traumatic events adapted better. Kreutzer et al. (2009) utilized a structured treatment, which incorporated cognitive–behavioral techniques, including education about common injury sequelae; psychological support to recognize inner feelings and improve emotional wellness; and skills training to improve families' problem solving, communication, and emotional control.

1.2.6 Family Group Interventions

An effective methodology for family therapy is group settings. Therapist-guided and self-guided family group interventions are potent antidotes to families' pervasive feelings of anguish, helplessness, and isolation (Dell Orto and Power 2000). In these environments, families can share their predicaments; interface about resources; and learn from one another's angst, disappointments, and accomplishments (Dell Orto and Power 2000; Klonoff and Koberstein 2010). Support groups can be effective even in the acute phase of the injury (Norup et al. 2011). They can also emanate from several post-acute settings, including community support groups, as well as family groups either during or after traditional or holistic treatment for patients with acquired brain injuries (Degeneffe 2001; Klonoff and Koberstein 2010; Klonoff et al. 2008; Klonoff and Prigatano 1987; Rosenthal and Hutchins 1991; Rosenthal and Young 1988). Group treatment prioritizes education and can draw from the techniques of instructional lectures or discussions; written materials; multimedia (e.g., videotapes, DVDs); and treatment observations (Armengol 1999; Klonoff and Koberstein 2010; Klonoff and Prigatano 1987; Rosenthal and Hutchins 1991).

Backhaus et al. (2010) have successfully devised a coping skills group; a 12-session manualized cognitive–behavioral treatment group providing psychoeducation, support, and coping skills training for caregivers and their loved ones simultaneously. Other outlets for families after a brain injury are social support groups, including family mentoring programs whereby "seasoned" families provide experiential input and support to families of newly injured loved ones; self-help groups; family outreach and advocacy efforts; as well as community networking for mobilization of resources and self-directed long-term supports (Klonoff 2010; Sachs 1991; Williams 1991).

Family groups within my holistic treatment milieu focus on a combination of education, emotional support, and peer mentorship (Klonoff and Koberstein 2010; Klonoff and Prigatano 1987). This also includes periodic guided lectures by relatives of patient graduates, who can share perspectives on their (and their loved ones') posttreatment psychological health and community reintegration. A family aftercare group enables continued professional and peer support and education for the long haul (Klonoff and Koberstein 2010). See Chap. 9 for a detailed rendition of a family group and Chap. 11 for a description of an aftercare group.

1.2.7 Psychoeducation and Skills Training

Integral to the coping and adjustment process for family members of patients with acquired brain injuries are psychoeducation and skills training (Collins and Swartz 2011; Gan et al. 2010; Kay and Cavallo 1994; Klonoff 2010; Klonoff and Prigatano

1987; Kreutzer et al. 2009; Lefebvre et al. 2008; McLaughlin and Carey 1993; Miller 1993; Shaw and McMahon 1990; Smith and Godfrey 1995). Holistic milieu-oriented therapy enables a multidisciplinary and interdisciplinary treatment approach for the loved one, and by extension, the necessary breadth and depth of education and guidance for the caregiver, family, and support network (Klonoff 2010). The psychotherapist functions as the "trail blazer" for these new insights by unearthing and tackling queries and concerns and coordinating interventions and training with other rehabilitation specialists (Klonoff 2010). Being part of a healing therapeutic community enables the relatives to feel a sense of safety, nurturance, empathy, and unified purpose. This translates to greater mastery and self-confidence.

Psychoeducation can be accomplished within the context of individual family meetings (with and without the patient); written informational booklets; Internet-based resources; structured, manualized curriculum training systems; or, as part of didactic lectures (with handouts) during family and aftercare groups (Collins and Swartz 2011; Gan et al. 2010; Klonoff and Koberstein 2010; Morris 2001). In my setting, topics center on the nature of the brain injury, as well as the expected aftermath for the family. Typical psychoeducational topics which affect the family are the patients' array of physical, cognitive, language, psychological, and interpersonal sequelae of the brain injury and their anatomical correlates, as well as patients' functional challenges within the family unit and community. Representative topics to enhance the family members' coping and adjustment include remedies for sources of upheaval and concomitant self-care techniques. Skills training techniques focus primarily on educating the relatives and support network about the patients' essential compensations, as well as helpful methods to simplify and organize their own lifestyles, given the additional tasks foisted upon them (Klonoff 2010).

1.2.8 Assistive Technology

Assistive technology devices (ATDs) are items, equipment, or product systems which improve the functional capabilities of the individual with a brain injury (Scherer 2012). Currently, there is an abundance of products with an assortment of features and accessories (Scherer 2012). ATDs can enhance the loved one's vision, communication, mobility, daily living and housekeeping skills, computer usage, and functionality with transportation, leisure, school, and work activities (Scherer 2012). One recent resource for ATDs is *Assistive Technologies and Other Supports for People with Brain Impairment* by Scherer (2012). It includes various current databases in the form of accessible websites.

1.2.9 Mindfulness and Positive Psychology

Using the constructs of mindfulness and self-psychology, the psychotherapist can assist the support network in recalibrating their coping stances and outlook for the future. *Mindfulness* has been defined as "nonjudgmental awareness" of one's current emotions and experiences in the present, with an attitude of kindness, openness, and curiosity (see Gambrel and Keeling 2010, for a review). Mindful practices yield tolerance for discomfort, development of emotional regulation, and insight into defenses (Siegel and Germer 2012). In relationships, mindfulness can promote communication, acceptance, attunement, perspective taking, and ultimately relationship well-being (see Gambrel and Keeling 2010, for a review; Siegel and Germer 2012). This phenomenon is also relevant to the practice of the psychotherapist, who should take a similar stance of self-understanding (i.e., wisdom) and self-compassion, so as to create a healing presence within the therapeutic relationship (Siegel 2010; Siegel and Germer 2012).

Mindful living promotes positivity, resiliency, and gratitude (Aniskiewicz 2007). Positive psychology is the study of happiness and well-being with an emphasis on developing positive experiences, traits, and institutions (Evans 2011). Seligman, as the founder of this worthy branch of psychology, has proposed a cutting-edge conceptualization of the elements of well-being as positive emotion, engagement, relationships, meaning, and achievement (Seligman 2011). The goal of positive psychology is to increase human flourishing (Seligman 2011). To date, the application of positive psychology, including posttraumatic growth, has focused on the loved one with a brain injury (Collicutt McGrath and Linley 2006; Evans 2011; Hawley and Joseph 2008). However, the principles are readily applied to the support network. To this end, psychotherapy should focus on helping in the attainment of positive mental health and life satisfaction by building inner strengths and virtues as well as learning optimism (Evans 2011; Seligman and Peterson 2003). This includes thriving through positive or posttraumatic growth (Evans 2011; Joseph 2011; see Peterson et al. 2008, for a review). Herein, positive psychological changes emerge from traumatic events, including a changed sense of self, improved relationships, openness to novel possibilities, enhanced appreciation of life, greater personal strength, and spiritual development (Calhoun and Tedeschi 2013; see Peterson et al. 2008, for a review). Techniques include personal participation in working toward valued goals and identifying and adopting specific actions based on character strengths (Evans 2011; Peterson et al. 2008). The premise is to "build what is strong, rather than fix what is wrong" (Evans 2011). For more information about mindfulness, see the resource *The Mindfulness Revolution,* edited by Boyce and the editors of the *Shambhala Sun* (2011).

1.2.10 Existential Psychotherapy

It is incumbent on the psychotherapist to incorporate existential psychotherapy when assisting patients' family members in their quest for meaning and fulfillment, especially given the life-altering disruptions to their daily routine, interpersonal relationships, as well as short and long-term ambitions. Existential considerations include the individual's freedom, control (versus vulnerability), sense of belonging (versus isolation), justice, meaning, responsibility, and mortality (Roos 2002; Strang et al. 2001; Yalom 1980). Yalom (2009) simplifies the definition of existentialism to dealing with the individual's existence. Existentialism includes spirituality, which is defined as the convictions and guiding principles, values, and core beliefs which imbue meaning to life, illness, and death (Strang et al. 2001). Spirituality encompasses positive emotions (e.g., compassion, trust, gratitude, awe, love, hope, joy, and forgiveness); social connection; and the need for solace and revelation (Vaillant 2008). Existential psychotherapy also provides an overarching interpretive framework to assist relatives in recalibrating their perception of their personal existence in the context of the realities of their loved ones' injuries. There is a transformation of feelings of loss, hopelessness, and despair into a reconfigured assumptive world, coherence, renewed hope, personal growth, refashioned purpose, and futuristic planning (Attig 2002; Klonoff and Koberstein 2010; Roos 2002; Strang et al. 2001).

1.2.11 Family Autobiographical Books and Articles

Family-authored articles and books provide the personalized, phenomenological journey of the family members whose loved ones have sustained a brain injury. Examples include: *Someone Stole Yesterday* by Wright (2000); *Where is the Mango Princess* by Crimmins (2001); *Smile and Jump High* by Lloyd and Kehoe (2001); "Traumatic brain injury: Help for the family" by Bond (2002); *Being with Rachel* by Brennan (2002); *In an Instant* by Woodruff and Woodruff (2008); *Successfully Surviving a Brain Injury: A Family Guidebook* by Prowe (2010); and *Gabby: A Story of Courage and Hope* by Giffords et al. (2011). These writings provide the "insider's viewpoint" of the relatives' woes, as well as a portrayal of the anticipated steps in the recovery process, with a focus on practical advice for caregiving, reducing stressors, and accessing proper resources for themselves and their loved ones. Based on their vantage points, the family members are also able to educate treating professionals about what approaches will be most efficacious and compassionate for the families (and their loved ones).

There are other informative books by caregivers who are also sometimes patients themselves and/or medical professionals. They describe the general venture and stresses of caregiving which are not specific to a brain injury. Nonetheless, these publications provide insightful and practical advice in a user-friendly manner and should be considered as valuable therapeutic adjuncts. Resources include *Caregiving Without Regrets: 3 Steps to Avoid Burnout and Manage Disappointment, Guilt, and Anger* by Dr. Rackner (2009); *Caring for the Caregiver* by Harris (2009); *Passages in Caregiving: Turning Chaos into Confidence* by Sheehy (2010); *The Caregiver's Guide to Self Care: Help for Your Caregiving Journey* by Hamilton (2011); and *Leaning into Sharp Points* by Dr. Goldberg (2012). There are also various caregiver websites which constitute rich resources. Table 1.1 contains relevant self-help books and websites on the topic of caregiving.

Table 1.1 Resources on the topic of caregiving

Caregiver material specific to brain injury
Head Injury: A Family Matter (Williams and Kay 1991)
Head Injury: Information and Answers to Commonly Asked Questions (Sturm et al. 1998)
Confronting Traumatic Brain Injury: Devastation, Hope, and Healing (Winslade 1998)
Living with Brain Injury: A Guide for Families and Caregivers (Acorn and Offer 1998)
Someone Stole Yesterday (Wright 2000)
Brain Injury and the Family: A Life and Living Perspective (2nd ed.) (Dell Orto and Power 2000)
Living with Brain Injury: A Guide for Families (2nd ed.) (Senelick and Dougherty 2001)
Where Is the Mango Princess (Crimmins 2001)
Smile and Jump High (Lloyd and Kehoe 2001)
"Traumatic brain injury: Help for the family" (Bond 2002)
Being with Rachel: A Story of Memory and Survival (Brennan 2002)
Stroke and the Family: A New Guide (Stein 2004)
Coping with Brain Injury: How to Help After Accidents, Stroke and Illness (Rich 2005)
Living with a Brain Tumor: Dr. Peter Black's Guide to Taking Control of Your Treatment (Black and Hogan 2006)
Brain Injury Survivor's Guide: Welcome to Our World (Jameson and Jameson 2007)
In an Instant: A Family's Journey of Love and Healing (Woodruff and Woodruff 2008)
Climbing the Mountain: Stories of Hope and Healing After Stroke and Brain Injury (Fancher et al. 2008)
Mindstorms: The Complete Guide for Families Living with Traumatic Brain Injury (Cassidy 2009)
Successfully Surviving a Brain Injury a Family Guidebook: From the Emergency Room to Selecting a Rehabilitation Facility (Prowe 2010)
Living with Stroke: A Guide for Families (4th ed.) (Senelick 2010)
Navigating Through a Strange Land: A Book for Brain Tumor Patients & Their Families (Roloff 2010)
Connecting Through Compassion: Guidance for Family and Friends of a Brain Cancer Patient (Aldrich and Peterson 2010)
Stroke Diaries: A Guide for Survivors and Their Families (Williams 2010)
When Your Spouse Has a Stroke: Caring for Your Partner, Yourself, and Your Relationship (Palmer and Palmer 2011)
Gabby: A Story of Courage and Hope (Giffords et al. 2011)
One Hundred Names for Love: A Stroke, a Marriage, and the Language of Healing (Ackerman 2011)
General caregiver material
Families Living with Chronic Illness and Disability: Interventions, Challenges, and Opportunities (Power and Dell Orto 2004)
Caregiving Without Regrets: 3 Steps to Avoid Burnout and Manage Disappointment, Guilt, and Anger (Rackner 2009)
Caring for the Caregiver (Harris 2009)
Passages in Caregiving: Turning Chaos into Confidence (Sheehy 2010)
The Caregiver's Guide to Self-care: Help for Your Caregiving Journey (Hamilton 2011)
Leaning into Sharp Points: Practical Guidance and Nurturing Support for Caregivers (Goldberg 2012)
Website: American Psychological Association: Caregiver briefcase http://www.apa.org/pi/about/publications/caregivers/index.aspx
Website: FCA: Family Caregiver Alliance http://www.caregiver.org/caregiver/jsp/home.jsp
Website: Caregiving.com http://www.caregiving.com
Website: Caregiver Action Network http://caregiveraction.org
Website: Strength for Caring a Place for Caregivers http://www.strengthforcaring.com
Website: National Alliance for Caregiving http://www.caregiving.org
Website: Today's Caregiver http://www.caregiver.com
Website: Well Spouse http://www.wellspouse.org

Table 1.1 (continued)

General caregiver material
Website: CaregivingHelp http://www.caregivinghelp.org
Website: Young Carers (Australia) http://www.youngcarers.net.au
Website: American Association of Caregiving Youth http://www.aacy.org
Website: Caring From a Distance http://www.cfad.org
Website: Family Caregivers' Network Society (Canada) http://www.fcns-caregiving.org
Website: Canadian Caregiver Coalition http://www.ccc-ccan.ca
Website: Resources for Caregivers and Caregiving http://kspope.com/payton/caregiving.php

Of note, regardless of the psychotherapist's preferred theoretical basis, including eclecticism, he or she must establish a plausible therapeutic rationale and incorporate activities and goals accordingly (Truscott 2010). The family must also trust the competency of the therapist and experience a collaborative relationship (Sohlberg et al. 2001; Truscott 2010).

1.3 An Interactive Model of Psychotherapy After Brain Injury and the Role of Three Tiers of Support

An earlier publication by this author defined the process of psychotherapy with the patient (loved one) after a brain injury as "the collaborative working relationship between a psychotherapist and a brain-injured patient, with the goals of increasing the patient's awareness of, acceptance of, and realism about his or her predicament. At the same time, the psychotherapist educates and supports the patient's family and community connections, so as to facilitate the patient's renewed sense of identity, hope, and meaning" (Klonoff 2010, p. 2).

Figure 1.1 depicts how the loved one, caregiver, family, and community support network are resolutely interrelated in the psychotherapeutic process after the brain injury. *Tier 1* is defined as the primary caregiver(s), for instance, a spouse, significant other, parent(s), adult child, sibling, or close friend who takes the main responsibility for addressing the multiple needs of the loved one. *Tier 2* is the next level of support, often comprised of members of the immediate or extended family, or close friends. These individuals are the "second string" and devote genuine energies toward the practical and preferably the emotional needs of the loved one as well as the tier 1 caregiver(s). *Tier 3* is the outer ring of integral sustenance for the loved one as well as tiers 1 and 2. Tier 3 includes any individual or entity that is committed to enhancing everyone's quality of life, for instance, more distant relatives, friends, employers, coworkers, or community resources. Figure 1.2 is an artist's rendition of the concept of tiers of support (Rynn 2013).

All parties within these three tiers have a myriad of contexts or "spheres of influence," in which they interpret their realities and relate to one another and the psychotherapist. For the loved one, this pertains to his or her history, culture, psychodynamics, environment, social context, personality, motivations, cognitions, emotions, behavior, values, spirituality, and aspirations. These external influences

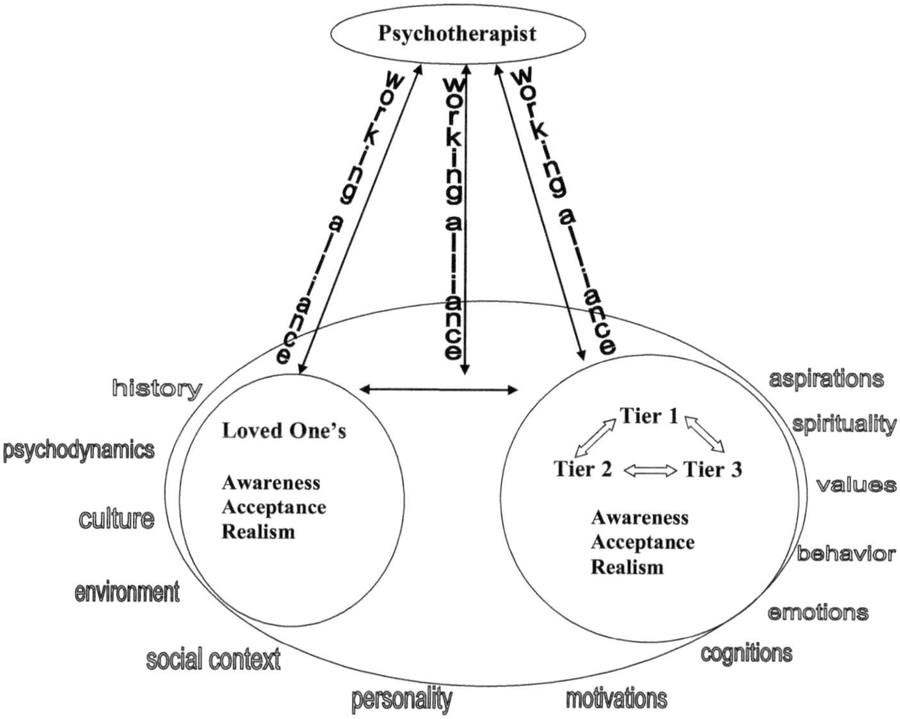

Fig. 1.1 An interactive model of psychotherapy after brain injury and the role of three tiers of support. Psychotherapy after Brain Injury: Principles and Techniques, Pamela S. Klonoff. 2010. Copyright Guilford Press. Modified with permission of the Guilford Press

and inner aspects are modified intrinsically in the loved one, in part, according to the nature and severity of the brain injury, as well as his or her position in the family/societal frameworks. The second and third tiers have the same contributions to their own contextual realities—their history, culture, psychodynamics, environment, social context, personality, motivations, cognitions, emotions, behavior, values, spirituality, and aspirations. All of these impact the loved one and primary caregiver(s), including their overall physical and psychological health.

The therapist needs to create a "culture-friendly" environment (Uomoto and Wong 2000). Such distinguishing characteristics as age, race, socioeconomic status, income, community involvements, cohesiveness, identity, and values will determine how the family (tiers 1–3) chooses to render care to their loved ones (Armengol 1999; Degeneffe 2001). For example, Sander et al. (2007) reported that race and ethnicity differences between whites and blacks/Hispanics affected caregiving behaviors. The latter group more often incorporated emotion-focused coping strategies (e.g., managing emotional distress) and a more traditional ideology, including a greater sense of obligation and familial duty. Watanabe et al. (2001) evaluated cultural differences between family members in the UK and Japan, whose loved ones sustained a traumatic brain injury, and found that Japanese relatives were more susceptible to social

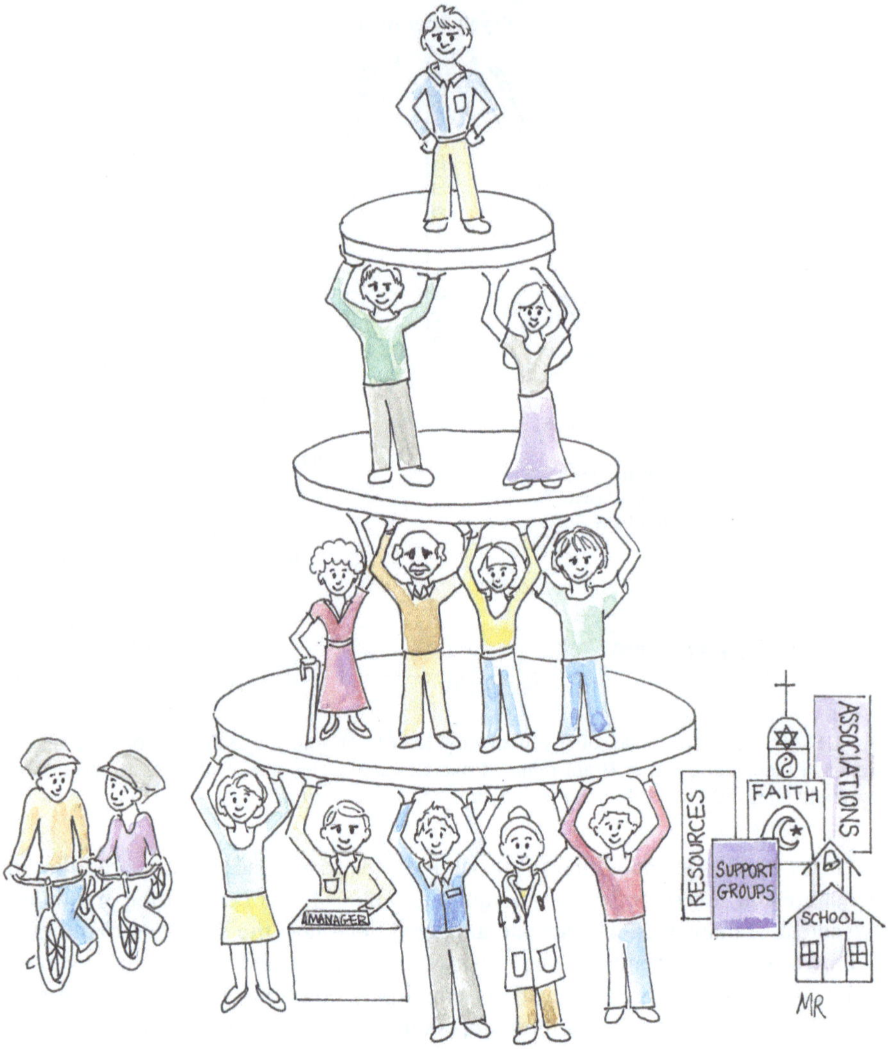

Fig. 1.2 Artist's rendition of the three tiers of support

embarrassment, with reliance on others considered a personal disgrace. Asian Americans may be uncomfortable in group settings and various cultures communicate and demonstrate mood changes differently (Umoto and Wong 2000). It therefore behooves the psychotherapist to gain a detailed understanding of all of these influences on the family, as their worldviews, values, beliefs, and practices will shape their intra- and extra-family communications, coping, and adjustment, and ultimately the success of the intervention approaches (Uomoto and Wong 2000).

Of note, the possible changes from a preinjury lifestyle to postinjury existence in the above domains for families are second order, that is, they are the direct consequence of the generalized effects of their loved one's brain injury on the family's circumstances and are not organically mediated per se, as they are for the patient. Overall, these underlying factors shape the family member's inner and external constitutions, which in turn mold the patient's treatment and recovery process.

Of course, the family unit is synergistic with a broader social context of the community (i.e., tier 3), which greatly influences the loved one's neurorehabilitation, recovery, and outcome (Judd and DeBoard 2009). Mutual participation, goal setting, and collaboration between the individual with the brain injury and support network (or natural helpers, including community supports and resources) enhance reacquisition of meaningful life roles (Judd 2003; Judd and DeBoard 2009). This reciprocal relationship between the loved one and social context will inevitably be affected by cultural diversities where there may be a multitude of values, beliefs, and attitudes (Judd 2003; Judd and DeBoard 2009). Interestingly, some research suggests that despite cultural and ethnic differences, families with a loved one with a brain injury in combination with caregiving itself can be considered its "own culture," with common traditions, customs, beliefs, and behaviors (Ayalong 2004; Sherwin and O'Shanick 2000). The clinical experience of this author supports this contention, as so often family members speak of their "unique commonality," regardless of their background.

Within the domain of psychotherapy, the bridge of communication and life change is embedded within the working alliance which exists between the psychotherapist and the loved one, his or her primary caregiver(s), the broader family unit, and ideally the global support network. All have a common mission of commitment to the loved one's recovery and should collaborate with the psychotherapist. The working alliance is contingent on the psychotherapist's capacity to convey understanding, interpretations, and education, which in turn produces change, adjustment, and goal attainment (Klonoff 2010). In fact, the outcome of the loved one is usually predicated on the caregiver/family's (i.e., tier 1 and 2) abilities to first develop a strong working alliance with the therapist. Often, the therapeutic bond between the psychotherapist and family augurs the growth of trust and partnership between the loved one and therapist, as he or she is often much more skeptical of the apparent benefit of treatment, secondary to organic unawareness and/or the overall level of emotional pain (Klonoff 2010). Paramount to this process is how tiers 1 and 2 evolve in their degree of awareness, acceptance, and realism, independent of, yet interconnected with, the analogous process in their loved one. By extension, when the psychotherapist advocates for the needs of the loved one with the extended family, friends, and community supports (i.e., tier 3), the loved one's reintegration into society is optimized.

Therefore, psychotherapy with the family/support network of a patient with a brain injury can be defined as: three-tiered, multi-person, collaborative, and dynamic working relationships between the psychotherapist, the primary caregiver(s), and other committed relatives and community individuals (including and on behalf of their loved one with the brain injury) to increase the whole support network's internal awareness, acceptance, and realism about their own as well as the loved one's postinjury existence, while at the same time creating renewed personal adjustment, meaning, and quality of life, within an external nourishing community.

1.4 Characteristics of Psychotherapists and Families

1.4.1 Educational Background of Psychotherapists Treating Relatives of Patients with a Brain Injury

Psychotherapists providing family therapy after acquired brain injuries require eclectic training venues and skill sets. First, the therapist requires a strong background in brain and behavior relationships, in order to understand the multifaceted sequelae of a brain injury in the patient. This includes both diagnostic skills (e.g., neuropsychological and personality testing) as well as treatment interventions (e.g., interview and consultation skills, psychotherapy, cognitive rehabilitation, and compensation training; Klonoff 2010). In the USA and Canada, this knowledge base is usually derived as part of either the postgraduate and residency training as a neuropsychologist or, alternatively, as a clinical psychologist, who develops a subspecialty in neuropsychology. Board certification is also available as a form of higher specialization in the field of brain–behavior relationships and/or rehabilitation, through the American Board of Professional Psychology or the American Academy of Neuropsychology.

Secondly, the psychotherapist needs concentrated training in family therapy, so as to have an armamentarium of conceptual frameworks and techniques in which to treat the patient's contextual system (e.g., the family and overall support system). Sometimes, other mental health professionals amalgamate their training and interest in family work with the unique challenges associated with an individual with an acquired brain injury. This includes family therapists, marriage and family counselors, rehabilitation psychologists, psychiatrists, behavioral/mental health counselors, and clinical social workers. There is a dearth of integrated educational opportunities where the psychotherapist can attain the breadth of expertise required to effectively treat both the patient with the brain injury and his or her relatives. Often, this requires a piecemeal approach of training and mentoring relationships during formal university training, or more likely after formal university training is completed. Some have argued for educational settings with dual training as a "neurobehavioral family specialist" (Johnson and McCown 1997).

1.4.2 Psychotherapist Qualities

Previous publications have identified the ideal qualities for the psychotherapist treating patients with acquired brain injuries (Klonoff 2010, 2013). These have in part been conceptualized as the internal, or "within" attributes, across the spectrum of "personality traits"; "cognitive capabilities"; "narcissistic/ego structures"; "relational behaviors"; and "existential qualities." Review of the cohort of qualities suggests that ideally, when working with family members of patients with acquired brain injuries, the psychotherapist needs to be able to wear many hats to address multiple needs (Klonoff 2010). To this end, he or she must shift communication styles from those most beneficial for the patient (e.g., more concrete, directive, solution focused), to more open inquiry, reflective listening, and process oriented for his or her relatives and support network.

The psychotherapist working with diverse treatment populations also requires the capability for perceptiveness and empathic relatedness to two often disparate realities. Oftentimes, the patient and family members are at different (or even opposite) places emotionally and existentially as they grapple with the ill effects of the brain injury. The psychotherapist must be attuned and adaptable to the shifting needs of his or her clients, while at the same time maintaining a nonjudgmental stance, so as not to appear to "take sides" unfairly. Therefore, the psychotherapist requires the capacity to be patient with and validate incongruent perspectives, while at the same time having the ability to build a bridge of communication and collaboration between the parties.

The psychotherapist's ability to devise creative treatment techniques which are sensitive to the family's needs, yet in the best interest of the patient, are also vital for progress within the psychotherapeutic relationship and overall recovery process. However, this is predicated on sophisticated and accommodating communication skills, whereby the psychotherapist actively involves family members in the dialogue process, in the "spirit of partnership" (Sohlberg et al. 2001). This is especially salient, given the multiplicity of modern day family structures, also including varying intergenerational, cultural, and societal considerations (Dell Orto and Power 2000; Judd 2003).

The depth and compounding nature of the patients' and relatives' guilt, self-blame, despair, and aggravation draw on the psychotherapist's capacity for tolerance of painful inner feelings, as well as his or her access to reserves of emotional resiliency (Dell Orto and Power 2000; Klonoff 2013). This is especially critical when patients and family members may simultaneously or alternately unleash their emotional torment upon the psychotherapist, related to their inner battles with acceptance and realism. The psychotherapist's existential qualities form the archetype for vision and hope that the family (and patient) is blinded to, at least temporarily.

Psychotherapists working in a team setting must develop the proficiency to collaborate with different medical and therapeutic specialties (e.g., physiatrists, neurologists, speech–language pathologists, physical therapists, occupational therapists, etc.) to collectively evolve treatment techniques which are most efficacious for the family (as well as the patient) and which then generalize clinic-based accomplishments to the home and community (Klonoff 2011, 2013). This involves a concerted willingness to prioritize the family members' psychological and general well-being through a holistic or multimodal approach, as well as when necessary, personal and team self-scrutiny about treatment shortfalls and even breakdowns. The team effort will enable the working alliance with all parties to flourish and will empower the family to cope with and adjust in the long term to their loved one's predicament.

1.4.3 Family Characteristics

One approach to identifying core family characteristics to enhance their own and their loved one's coping and adjustment is to examine possible parallel traits and family patterns through the premises of marriage and family counseling for the non-brain injured population. In this case, there are considerable research and clinical formulations. However, there are two paradigms to consider in this regard: the first represents what defines or constitutes a healthy family unit; the second represents the factors associated with an individual family member's psychological health within the unit, especially for the primary caregiver(s). (More of this is addressed in Chap. 3, Sect. 3.1).

With respect to healthy family characteristics in general, Krysan et al. (1990) as well as Smith and Stevens-Smith (1992) have provided an overview of the literature, with the following qualities identified: flexibility; clear boundaries and rules; balanced cohesion and adaptability; individual autonomy; appropriate assertiveness and the ability to negotiate; mutual commitment; social connectedness; the ability to spend time and work together; communicative; nurturing, caring, trusting, tender, and warm; capacity for intimacy; possessing humor; the ability to express spontaneity, appreciation, and encouragement; and a religious/spiritual orientation.

The family system also has various "family tasks," so that the members grow and develop through the family life cycle. These include care for children; form bonds of affection; help create an identity to both belong and individuate from the family; assist members to recognize and accept limits in life; help them be educated and adjust to different stages of life; prepare them for meaningful and purposive community activities; and foster the capacity for creativity and happiness (Schwartz 2007). Brodie and Wright (2002) also note the importance of the family's ability to learn from experience.

Conversely, "dysfunctional" families are depicted as rigid and dogmatic; chaotic, inconsistent, and unruly; enmeshed; in flux; prone to power struggles; disengaged; lacking in communication; distrusting, pessimistic, humorless, and cold; as well as lacking in intimacy and spontaneity (see Smith and Stevens-Smith 1992, for a review). However, the authors note that these characteristics are not dichotomous and instead are hypothetical, abstract, subjective, and therefore difficult to measure. Wilcoxon (1992) reminds clinicians that family relationships are interrelated, pluralistic, and multidimensional, and that their referral basis is usually based on "transitional crises," which are stressful even for "healthy" families (see Wilcoxon 1992, for a review).

White et al. (1997) provided research findings on specific client characteristics which facilitate a positive therapeutic outcome in marriage and family counseling. These include commitment to participate in therapy, personal resources of the client (e.g., empathy, trust, creativity, and a self-view as competent), and commitment to others, including positive attitudes about other family members and interest in others.

Review of the literature indicates few references to the characteristics of family members which will maximize their investment and benefits from family therapy after brain injury. Bishop and Miller (1988) reviewed a number of family assessments for relatives of loved ones with brain injuries, including self-report questionnaires, semi-structured interviews, and observational measures. These evaluate a number of family dimensions, including adaptability; cohesion; structure (e.g., power, coalitions, and closeness); autonomy; problem solving and task efficiency; communication; roles; affective responsiveness and involvement (including empathy and conflict); behavioral control; and general functioning.

Some authors have identified problems with communication breakdowns between the family and medical professionals and/or prolonged denial after a brain injury as creating adversarial working alliances and threatening the progress of family therapy (see Brooks 1984 for a review; McLaughlin and Carey 1993; Romano 1974; Rosenthal and Young 1988). A recent study by Sady et al. (2010) indicates that caregivers with low preinjury social support, higher emotional distress, and overall unhealthy family functioning negatively impacted the outcome of the loved ones with acquired brain injuries at 1 year postinjury.

Conversely, Turnbull and Turnbull (1991) identified a larger family size (who share caretaking), positive coping styles (e.g., proactivity, seeking social and spiritual support), as well as family cohesion and adaptability as positive indicators for benefits from family therapy. Social support for caregivers has been found to be an important moderator of caregiver psychological distress after a traumatic brain injury, directly impacting the outcome of their loved ones (Ergh et al. 2002).

1.5 Understanding the Family's Experience after Brain Injury

As depicted in Fig. 1.1, similar to patients with an acquired brain injury, relatives are also struggling with their own internal process of awareness, acceptance, and realism, which in many ways is akin to the challenges their loved ones are facing, albeit from a different vantage point. Family therapy assists the relatives in their strivings. An overview of a clinical, conceptual model depicting this process for family members of patients with moderate to severe acquired brain injuries is depicted in Fig. 1.3. The Family Experiential Model (FEM) of Recovery after a brain injury has been described previously in its complete form (Klonoff et al. 2008) and in a shortened version (Klonoff and Koberstein 2010). Figure 1.3 recapitulates the full version and is applicable to family members of patients who participate in holistic milieu-oriented therapies and/or insight-oriented family treatment in any other treatment setting. I use this as a major resource, as it graphically depicts the emotional toils of family members as a "road map," starting at the time immediately prior to the injury (phase 0), through the completion of the treatment process, back to the "real world" (phase 7; Klonoff and Koberstein 2010; Klonoff et al. 2008). Dotted lines between phases 3 and 7 represent the fluid successions through the phases in that families often cycle back through the earlier phase of awareness through to later phases of realism and a transformed future, as they gain new insights and life experiences. The column "loved one's condition" with the arrows at the left connotes the integral interconnections and interdependency between the family's emotional state and the patient's medical, psychological, and functional status.

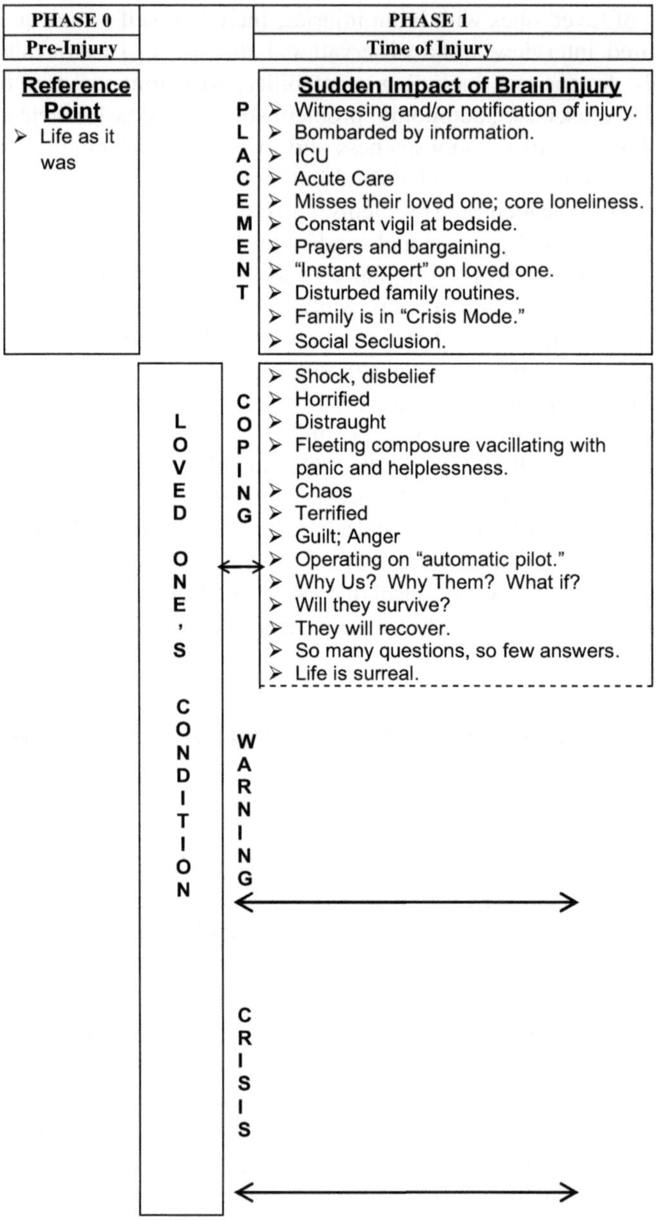

Fig. 1.3 A Family Experiential Model of Recovery after Brain Injury, Klonoff et al. 2008. Copyright Guilford Press. Reprinted with permission of the Guilford Press

PHASE 2 Early Adjustment	PHASE 3 Seeks Help	PHASE 4 Holistic Treatment Starts *AWARENESS*
Initial Problems ➢ Inpatient Neuro-rehabilitation/Home/Out-Patient Neurorehabilitation. ➢ Meandering in a foggy reality. ➢ Undertakes "insurance trauma." ➢ Family begins to believe that the injury occurred. ➢ Orchestrate and facilitate their loved one's medical and self care needs. ➢ Family wants their loved one to "beat the odds" and expects instant results.	**How to Cope** ➢ "24/7" ➢ What will happen now? ➢ Financial setbacks hit. ➢ Schedule and life upheaval. ➢ Family receives the brunt of their loved one's dependency and negativity. ➢ Family member feels segregated with loved one within the family system. ➢ Physical, mental, and emotional exhaustion. ➢ Looking for treatment resources.	**Confronting Reality** ➢ Holistic assessment and documentation of the patient's neurological condition. ➢ Learns appropriate vocabulary and terminology about the injury sequelae ("c.r. by proxy"). ➢ Unpredictability about the future. ➢ Family recognizes they need help and are not alone. ➢ Realizes the patient may think he/she doesn't need therapy, or will experience a "honeymoon period."
➢ Sacrifices personal needs in favor of patient's care. ➢ Family succumbs to intense emotions, with islands of resiliency. ➢ Family is frightened but begins to ask questions and hear information about the prognosis. ➢ Nervous about patient's progression through the hospital but gradually tolerates. ➢ Worries that something else "bad" could happen, but trusts that the professionals will do their best. ➢ Family lovingly encourages their loved one.	➢ Parent / spousal role switches to caregiver / advocate. ➢ Family is reluctant but allows a select few to get involved. ➢ Transforms feelings of helplessness into proactive behavior. ➢ Family realizes they can't manage the "injury aftermath" without further treatment.	➢ Tentative yet hopeful. ➢ Family increases their awareness of the effects of the injury. ➢ Family constructively manages grief, sadness, worry, and protectiveness; becomes less overwhelmed and recognizes these feelings are universal. ➢ May feel a sense of relief or respite while the patient attends therapy.
↕	↕	↕
➢ Deprives oneself of any enjoyment because the patient is suffering. ➢ Family is too anxious and afraid to ask questions. ➢ Too overwhelmed to digest feedback and suggestions. ➢ Family may feel the doctors and others are not doing enough. ➢ Family overtaxes or overindulges their loved one. ➢ Do not want to discuss and/or believe the seriousness of the injury. ➢ Family is lost in regret and / or avoidance and denial.	➢ Family wishes the injury had never happened. ➢ Family feels hopeless, bitter, and resentful. ➢ Becomes overprotective or overly controlling of their predicament. ➢ Won't accept outside help; pushes others away. ➢ Family feels inadequate and helpless; lapses into a passive state. ➢ Feels depressed, overwhelmed and alone; oppressed by sole responsibility for the patient. ➢ Develops disruptive stress-induced ailments. ➢ "Second tier" of family and outside help dwindle.	➢ Family uses prolonged denial, disavowal, resistance, anger, or blaming to avoid facing the effects of the injury. ➢ Are overprotective or under-involved. ➢ Family's intense emotions interfere with their own and their loved one's progress in the program. ➢ Feels misunderstood, dissatisfied, and mistrustful towards the therapists and the treatment process. ➢ Becomes detached from others.
↕	↕	↕

Period of Disintegration
Absence of critical therapeutic interventions or premature and abrupt abandonment of treatment. Life implodes. Refusal to become aware and acceptant; negation of reality (cont'd).

Fig. 1.3 (continued)

		Discharge
PHASE 5	**PHASE 6**	**PHASE 7**
Re-training	**Transition from Therapy**	**Future ∞**
ACCEPTANCE	***REALISM***	
Compensations ➢ Mourn the losses. ➢ Expectations are adjusted. ➢ "Things Take Time." ➢ Family learns compensations for themselves and patient. ➢ Accepts patient for who he/she is now. ➢ New relationships are formed. ➢ Family gains perspective.	**Approaching Discharge** ➢ Observes patient's new freedoms and independence. ➢ Family prepares themselves to assume more post-program responsibility for their loved one. ➢ Family juggles work schedule, finances and care giving.	**The Real World** ➢ The new reality sets in. ➢ Family and loved one maintain collaborative dialogue about the injury effects and compensations. ➢ Things aren't the same, but everyone can live a meaningful and productive life. ➢ Life is ever-changing and evolving.
➢ Family learns to cope with their own emotional reactions. ➢ Motivated to learn, monitor and support their loved one's use of compensations. ➢ Actively interacts with the therapists and participates in goal setting. ➢ Family feels a sense of emotional bonding and camaraderie in Relatives' Group. ➢ Family resolves to "count their blessings."	➢ Family collaborates with the patient and the therapists towards community reintegration. ➢ Supportive yet realistic about their loved one's level of independence, productivity, and socialization skills. ➢ Constructively manages fears and trepidations about discharge. ➢ Develops self-confidence in their skill attainment. ➢ Family expands their support system. ➢ Family finds inner strength and courage through facing adversity.	➢ Family more intuitively evolves the strategies and tools learned in rehab to accommodate and enhance their loved one's quality of life. ➢ "Door is always open" for further help and support if needed. ➢ Over time family finds a balance between different roles and has a healthy social network for support. ➢ Regularly schedules respite time.
➢ Family becomes disgruntled with the complexities and limitations of the recovery process. ➢ Family is passively engaged and lacks follow through with support of compensations; inconsistent or no attendance at Relatives' Groups or family meetings. ➢ May become locked in a "power struggle" with therapists and wants to "prove the experts wrong." ➢ Family's essential emotional, mental, and physical energies are sapped. ➢ Struggles to fulfill multiple roles of caregiver, family life, and work.	➢ Insufficient knowledge negatively impacts the patient's progress and goal attainment. ➢ Family under- or over-estimates ("Flight into Health") the effects of the injury on independence, productivity, and/or relationships. ➢ Exhibits self-doubts, anxieties, and inadequate coping techniques. ➢ Unable to focus on personal needs and aspirations. ➢ Unwilling or unable to develop a social network. ➢ Sets unrealistic goals. ➢ Unprepared functionally and emotionally for the discharge and transition process because their loved one isn't 100%.	➢ Family observes their loved one's slippage in his/her use of compensations, but is ill-equipped to provide constructive feedback or assistance. ➢ Less likely to seek help or support for themselves. ➢ Unresolved skewed roles. ➢ Becomes burned out, disengaged, and socially isolated.

Period of Disintegration
(cont'd).Overcome with rage, anguish, despair, and helplessness. Apathy and self-defeating behavior. Work failure and financial ruin. Social alienation. Neglect, fragmentation, and/or dissolution of family life.

Fig. 1.3 (continued)

As described previously, the FEM captured the phenomenological experiences of 87 relatives of patients with acquired brain injuries, using their heartfelt descriptions and terminology (Klonoff and Koberstein 2010; Klonoff et al. 2008). It embodies the experiential journey of the relatives, focusing on the specific undertakings of where the families are in the course of psychological recovery (e.g., placement phases), as well as their emotions and coping styles (coping, warning, and crisis zones). These latter portions are modeled after a "stoplight," with the "coping" zone, or "green" light, representing a better adaptation and adjustment. The "warning" zone, or "yellow" light, indicates potentially detrimental and self-defeating coping approaches, which undermine the family's overall adaptation to their loved one's injury. The "crisis" zone, or "red" light, illustrates the "period of disintegration," in which the family's overall functioning and coping skills collapse. Regardless of the zone, the family is traversing; the overall chart normalizes their meandering progression. Arrows between the coping zones indicate the inevitable oscillations families undergo in their coping capacity, adaptability, and overall adjustment (Klonoff and Koberstein 2010).

Phase 0 is the reference point of the model and signifies "life as it was." This comes to represent the idyllic and idealized past, which families yearn for longingly.

Phase 1 represents the sudden impact of the injury, characterized by either witnessing or being notified about their loved one's neurological injury/event. The family is catapulted into a new and usually overwhelming "crisis mode," with a constant bedside vigil, disconnected from external routines and relationships. Family members are typically inundated by many emotions, including shock, horror, helplessness, panic, guilt, and/or anger. To make matters worse, the loved one is neurologically compromised and cannot fathom his or her predicament. Therefore, the family must trudge ahead unaided by their cherished loved one. Their life feels surreal and they are consumed with many practical and existential questions—why us? why them? what if?—with a dearth of answers. The gamut of these feelings are considered typical and adaptive, hence they are not differentiated from the "yellow warning" or "red crisis" zones.

In phase 2, the patient traverses through the stages of acute hospitalization and neurorehabilitation, often in a foggy reality. The family is saddled with insurance quandaries and is in charge of the totality of their loved one's medical and self-care needs. The relatives begin to acknowledge the injury, but are convinced their loved ones will surpass the physicians' seemingly pessimistic prognosis. Family members who are coping adaptively are committed to their loved one and encourage him or her in the recovery process. Although sometimes overwhelmed by the magnitude of the stresses, they begin to trust the professionals. Families in the "yellow warning" zone are self-depriving and are overcome with anxiety and fear. Seeds of distrust in the professionals are sewn and the family misunderstands and mismanages their loved one's situation. Avoidance, regret, and denial are prevalent.

In phase 3, the family is consumed with care of their loved one "24/7." Financial and schedule upheavals abound. The family is the scapegoat for the patient's negativity and dependency, producing physical, mental, and emotional exhaustion. They come to realize that they need to seek further treatment for their loved one. Relatives who are coping well have embraced the caregiver and advocate role. They are proactive and willing to delegate to others and consult with medical specialists. Family members who are in the "yellow warning" zone are lost in regret, hopelessness, and resentment. Despite the oppressiveness of fulltime caregiving, they are unwilling to accept outside support. The family plummets into helplessness, inadequacy, and passivity. To make matters worse, the support network fades.

Phase 4 represents the family's awareness training. Through therapeutic assessment and education, they confront the reality of their loved one's rehabilitation needs. They witness their loved one's resistance to therapy, or in better scenarios, they see their loved one in the "honeymoon phase." They also recognize the uncertainty of their own situation and appreciate the efforts of treating professionals in guiding them along. When coping well, the family feels tentatively hopeful. With enhanced awareness, they are able to better manage their understandable emotional suffering. By sharing their journey with other relatives, they come to appreciate the universality of their predicament. Relatives who are struggling to cope in the "yellow warning" zone tend to resort to denial, disavowal, resistance, antagonism, or external blaming, rather than face the agonizing effects of the injury. Their intense emotions interfere with their own adaptation as well as that of their loved one and they detach from others who are trying to help. Oftentimes, they feel misunderstood and disgruntled, with a growing distrust for the therapists.

In phase 5, the relatives are immersed in the acceptance process, which involves mourning their losses and eventually adjusting their expectations, with an altered, more reasonable perspective. Compensatory strategies must be learned, which take time and patience. Family members who are coping adaptively actively participate in the compensation training. Their spirits are bolstered by the camaraderie of support groups with other family members. Gradually, they begin to count their blessings. Relatives who are in the "yellow warning" zone are coping poorly; their defenses are up, and they are peeved with the therapists. They engage in power struggles and are determined to prove the professionals wrong. Their attempts to juggle multiple duties are faltering, sapping their energies.

In phase 6, family members are embracing a realistic outlook and rebalancing their daily activities. Although they see their loved one's improved independence, they also realize they will be acquiring more responsibility for their loved one as he or she approaches the completion of the rehabilitation process. Relatives who cope adaptively, collaborate closely with their loved one and the therapists toward community reintegration. The relatives are now more confident with their skill sets and are able to handle normal trepidations about discharge. They develop and nurture support systems. Their grapples with adversity have imbued them with inner strength and courage. Family members who are in the "yellow warning" zone have not integrated sufficient knowledge about the recovery process. They miss the mark with respect to their loved one's level of functioning, which leads to their own qualms and worries. They are unsuccessful in building a healthy social network. They are unrealistic and are unprepared practically and psychologically for their loved one's treatment termination, hankering for a 100% recovery.

In phase 7, the family is in the "real world" for the foreseeable future, which is a new, yet meaningful and productive existence. The family and patient continue to collaborate, realizing that life is ever changing and evolving. Relatives who are coping constructively have mastered the necessary compensations and can accommodate new life developments. They are receptive to seeking more professional help, if needed. They have a balance in their personal and caregiving responsibilities, including taking care of their own needs. Families struggling to cope in the "yellow warning" zone detect suboptimal functioning in their loved ones, but are ill equipped to truly assist them. They remain resistant to outside help. Their social roles are skewed, and they become burned out, disengaged, and socially isolated.

The "red" or "crisis" zone depicts a period of disintegration and can occur anytime between phases 2 and 7. It results from either an absence of critical therapeutic interventions or the family's and/or patient's premature and abrupt abandonment of treatment. The family is clearly unable or unwilling to improve their awareness, acceptance, or realism about the injury aftermath. They are overcome with intense rage, and profound anguish, despair, and helplessness, descending deeper into apathy and ennui. Life implodes, with work calamities and financial destitution. The family is socially alienated and the family experiences neglect, fragmentation, and likely dissolution.

1.6 Overview of Chapters

The remainder of this book describes in detail family therapy techniques for families of patients with varying etiologies and severities of brain injuries ranging from the acute postinjury phases (e.g., several weeks or months) to many years later. The author's experience is mainly with adult patients and their support systems in a larger metropolitan area, and the book material emulates this. The unique role, needs, and challenges of the primary caregiver(s), other involved relatives, and the broader support network are delineated. Conceptual models and elements of the FEM are interwoven into the chapters, with particular emphasis on the constructs of awareness, acceptance, and realism within the three tiers of patients' supports. The book is rife with sample verbalizations and experiences from the perspective of the support network. Chapters contain "helpful hints" and psychoeducation. Multimodal techniques are described, with a pragmatic emphasis. Case study and multimedia material are incorporated throughout to illustrate key principles.

Chapter 2 provides theoretical and practical considerations for initial and early sessions with family members after brain injuries, including an overview of salient forms of emotional and psychosocial distress, with concomitant general treatment considerations. Chapter 3 encompasses a deeper inquiry into the family system, including a model of their psychological health and exploration of four configurations of spousal, parental, son or daughter, and sibling relationships with the loved one. Selected chapters target specific populations and their relevant factors for family therapy. These include moderate to severe traumatic brain injuries (Chap. 4);

the spectrum of milder brain injuries, also including the postconcussive syndrome (Chap. 5); cerebrovascular accidents and anoxia (Chap. 6); brain tumors (Chap. 7); and seizure disorders (Chap. 8). Chapter 9 outlines a flexible 9-week structured format for family group therapy during active treatment. Chapter 10 explores end-of-life and existential considerations using brain tumors as a prototype. Positive aspects of caregiving will be appraised. Ideas for enhancing the family's commitment, adjustment, hope, and longevity are also supplied in this chapter. Chapter 11 presents a semi-structured six-theme curriculum for an aftercare group to address the support network's longer range needs. Techniques for the tiers of support to maintain self-care are interwoven throughout the book, including resources for navigating complex medical and social systems.

References

Ackerman, D. (2011). *One hundred names for love: A stroke, a marriage, and the language of healing*. New York: W. W. Norton.

Acorn, S., & Offer, P. (Eds.). (1998). *Living with brain injury: A guide for families and caregivers*. Toronto: University of Toronto Press.

Alderman, N. (2004). Disorders of behavior. In J. Ponsford (Ed.), *Cognitive and behavioral rehabilitation: From neurobiology to clinical practice* (pp. 269–298). New York: Guilford Press.

Aldrich, J. J., & Peterson, N. M. (2010). *Connecting through compassion: Guidance for family and friends of a brain cancer patient*. United States of America: Cancer Lifeline Publications.

Aniskiewicz, A. S. (2007). *Psychotherapy for neuropsychological challenges*. Lanham: Jason Aronson.

Armengol, C. G. (1999). A multimodal support group with Hispanic traumatic brain injury survivors. *Journal of Head Trauma Rehabilitation, 4*(3), 233–246.

Attig, T. (2002). Questionable assumptions about assumptive worlds. In J. Kauffman (Ed.), *Loss of the assumptive world: A theory of traumatic loss* (pp. 55–68). New York: Brunner-Routledge.

Ayalong, L. (2004). Cultural variants of caregiving or the culture of caregiving. *Journal of Cultural Diversity, 11*(4), 131–138.

Backhaus, S. L., Ibarra, S. L., Klyce, D., Trexler, L. E., & Malec, J. F. (2010). Brain injury coping skills group: A preventative intervention for patients with brain injury and their caregivers. *Archives of Physical Medicine and Rehabilitation, 91,* 840–848.

Baker, H. S., & Baker, M. N. (1987). Heinz Kohut's self psychology: An overview. *American Journal of Psychiatry, 144*(1), 1–9.

Bishop, D. S., & Miller, I. W. (1988). Traumatic brain injury: Empirical family assessment techniques. *Journal of Head Trauma Rehabilitation, 3*(4), 16–30.

Black, P., & Hogan, S. C. (2006). *Living with a brain tumor: Dr. Peter Black's guide to taking control of your treatment*. New York: Henry Holt and Company.

Bond, C. (2002). Traumatic brain injury: Help for the family. *RN, 65*(11), 60–66.

Bond, M. R. (Ed.). (1988). Families of the brain injured (Special issue, J2712). *Journal of Head Trauma Rehabilitation, 3*(4).

Boyce, B., & the editors of the Shambhala Sun. (Eds.). (2011). *The mindfulness revolution: Leading psychologists, scientists, artists, and meditation teachers on the power of mindfulness in daily life*. Boston: Shambhala Hall.

Brennan, K. (2002). *Being with Rachel: A story of memory and survival*. New York: W. W. Norton.

Brodie, F., & Wright, J. (2002). Minding the gap not bridging the gap: Family therapy from a psychoanalytic perspective. *Journal of Family Therapy, 24*(2), 205–221.

Brooks, N. (1984). Head injury and the family. In N. Brooks (Ed.), *Closed head injury: Psychological, social, and family consequences* (pp. 123–147). Oxford: Oxford University Press.

Calhoun, L. G., & Tedeschi, R. G. (2013). *Posttraumatic growth in clinical practice*. New York: Routledge.

Carnes, S. L., & Quinn, W. H. (2005). Family adaptation to brain injury: Coping and psychological distress. *Families, Systems, & Health, 23*(2), 186–203.

Cassidy, J. W. (2009). *Mindstorms: The complete guide for families living with traumatic brain injury*. Philadelphia: Da Capo Press.

Collicutt McGrath, J., & Linley, P. A. (2006). Post-traumatic growth in acquired brain injury: A preliminary small scale study. *Brain Injury, 20*(7), 767–773.

Collins, L. G., & Swartz, K. (2011). Caregiver care. *American Academy of Family Physicians, 83*(11), 1309–1317.

Crimmins, C. (2001). *Where is the mango princess? A journey back from brain injury*. New York: Vintage.

Dattilio, F. M. (2005). The restructuring of family schemas: A cognitive-behavior perspective. *Journal of Marital and Family Therapy, 31*(1), 15–30.

David, C. O. (1998). Brain injury and the family system. In S. Acorn & P. Offer (Eds.), *Living with brain injury: A guide for families and caregivers* (pp. 111–125). Toronto: University of Toronto Press.

Degeneffe, C. E. (2001). Family caregiving and traumatic brain injury. *Health and Social Work, 26*(4), 257–268.

Dell Orto, A. E., & Power, P. W. (2000). *Brain injury and the family: A life and living perspective* (2nd ed.). Boca Raton: CRC Press.

Ergh, T. C., Rapport, L. J., Coleman, R. D., & Hanks, R. A. (2002). Predictors of caregiver and family functioning following traumatic brain injury: Social support moderates caregiver distress. *Journal of Head Trauma Rehabilitation, 17*(2), 155–174.

Evans, J. J. (2011). Positive psychology and brain injury rehabilitation. *Brain Impairment, 12*(2), 117–127.

Fancher, C., McDivitt, L., & Fletcher, J. B. (Eds.). (2008). *Climbing the mountain: Stories of hope and healing after stroke and brain injury*. Minneapolis: Fairview Press.

Flaskas, C. (2005). Psychoanalytic ideas and systemic family therapy: Revisiting the question "why bother?" *Australian & New Zealand Journal of Family Therapy, 26*(3), 125–134.

Flaskas, C. (2007). Systemic and psychoanalytic ideas: Using knowledges in social work. *Journal of Social Work Practice, 21*(2), 131–147.

Florian, V., & Katz, S. (1991). The other victims of traumatic brain injury: Consequences for family members. *Neuropsychology, 5*(4), 267–279.

Fraiberg, S., Adelson, E., & Shapiro, V. (1975). Ghosts in the nursery: A psychoanalytic approach to the problems of impaired infant-mother relationships. *Journal of the American Academy of Child Psychiatry, 14*(3), 387–421.

Gambrel, L. E., & Keeling, M. L. (2010). Relational aspects of mindfulness: Implications for the practice of marriage and family therapy. *Contemporary Family Therapy: An International Journal, 32*(4), 412–426.

Gan, C., & Schuller, R. (2002). Family system outcome following acquired brain injury: Clinical and research perspectives. *Brain Injury, 16*(4), 311–322.

Gan, C., Campbell, K. A., Gemeinhardt, M., & McFadden, G. T. (2006). Predictors of family system functioning after brain injury. *Brain Injury, 20*(6), 587–600.

Gan, C., Gargaro, J., Kreutzer, J. S., Boschen, K. A., & Wright, F. V. (2010). Development and preliminary evaluation of a structured family system intervention for adolescents with brain injury and their families. *Brain Injury, 24*(4), 651–663.

Giffords, G., Kelly, M., & Zaslow, J. (2011). *Gabby: A story of courage and hope*. New York: Scribner.

Goldberg, S. (2012). *Leaning into sharp points: Practical guidance and nurturing support for caregivers*. Novato: New World Library.
Hamilton, J. M. (2011). *The caregiver's guide to self-care: Help for your caregiving journey*. West Conshohocken: Infinity Publishing.
Harris, R. W. (2009). *Caring for the caregiver*. Mustang: Tate Publishing.
Hawley, C. A., & Joseph, S. (2008). Predictors of positive growth after traumatic brain injury: A longitudinal study. *Brain Injury, 22*(5), 427–435.
Jacobs, H. E. (1991). Family and behavioral issues. In J. M. Williams & T. Kay (Eds.), *Head injury: A family matter* (pp. 239–251). Baltimore: Brookes Publishing.
Jameson, L., & Jameson, B. (2007). *Brain injury survivor's guide: Welcome to our world*. Denver: Outskirts Press.
Johnson, J., & McCown, W. (1997). *Family therapy of neurobehavioral disorders: Integrating neuropsychology and family therapy*. New York: Haworth Press.
Joseph, S. (2011). *What doesn't kill us: The new psychology of posttraumatic growth*. New York: Basic Books.
Judd, T. (1999). *Neuropsychotherapy and community integration: Brain illness, emotions and behavior*. New York: Kluwer Academic/Plenum Publishers.
Judd, T. (2003). Rehabilitation of the emotional problems of brain disorders in developing countries. *Neuropsychological Rehabilitation, 13*(1/2), 307–325.
Judd, T., & DeBoard, R. (2009). Community-based neuropsychological rehabilitation in the cosmopolitan setting. *Neuropsychological Rehabilitation, 19*(6), 841–866.
Kay, T., & Cavallo, M. M. (1994). The family system: Impact, assessment, and intervention. In J. M. Siver, S. C. Yudofsky, & R. E. Hales (Eds.), *Neuropsychiatry of traumatic brain injury* (pp. 533–567). Washington, D. C.: American Psychiatric Press.
Klonoff, P. S. (2010). *Psychotherapy after brain injury: Principles and techniques*. New York: Guilford Press.
Klonoff, P. S. (2011). A therapist experiential model of treatment for brain injury. *Bulletin of the Menninger Clinic, 75*(1), 21–42.
Klonoff, P. S. (2013). Internal and team attributes for effective psychotherapy after brain injury. In C. A. Noggle & R. S. Dean (Eds.), *Neuropsychological rehabilitation*. New York: Springer.
Klonoff, P. S., & Koberstein, E. J. (2010). Family life. In P. S. Klonoff (Ed.), *Psychotherapy after brain injury: Principles and techniques* (pp. 150–170). New York: Guilford Press.
Klonoff, P. S., & Lage, G. A. (1991). Narcissistic injury in patients with traumatic brain injury. *Journal of Head Trauma Rehabilitation, 6*(4), 11–21.
Klonoff, P. S., & Prigatano, G. P. (1987). Reactions of family members and clinical intervention after traumatic brain injury. In M. Ylvisaker & E. M. R. Gobble (Eds.), *Community re-entry for head injured adults* (pp. 381–402). Boston: College-Hill Press.
Klonoff, P. S., Lamb, D. G., & Henderson, S. W. (2001). Outcomes from milieu-based neurorehabilitation at up to 11 years post-discharge. *Brain Injury, 15*(5), 413–428.
Klonoff, P. S., Koberstein, E. J., Talley, M. C., & Dawson, L. K. (2008). A family experiential model of recovery after brain injury. *Bulletin of the Menninger Clinic, 72*(2), 109–129.
Kohut, H. (1984a). Self-selfobject relationships reconsidered. In A. Goldberg & P. E. Stepansky (Eds.), *How does analysis cure?* (pp. 49–63). Chicago: University of Chicago Press.
Kohut, H. (1984b). The curative effect of analysis: A preliminary statement based on the findings of self psychology. In A. Goldberg & P. E. Stepansky (Eds.), *How does analysis cure?* (pp. 64–79). Chicago: University of Chicago Press.
Kohut, H. (1984c). A re-examination of castration anxiety. In A. Goldberg & P. E. Stepansky (Eds.), *How does analysis cure?* (pp. 13–33). Chicago: University of Chicago Press.
Kosciulek, J. F. (1997). Relationship of family schema to family adaptation to brain injury. *Brain Injury, 11*(11), 821–830.
Kreutzer, J. S., Marwitz, J. H., & Kepler, K. (1992). Truamatic brain injury: Family response and outcome. *Archives of Physical Medicine and Rehabilitation, 73,* 771–778.

Kreutzer, J. S., Kolakowsky-Hayner, S. A., Demm, S. R., & Meade, M. A. (2002). A structured approach to family intervention after brain injury. *Journal of Head Trauma Rehabilitation, 17*(4), 349–367.

Kreutzer, J. S., Stejskal, T. M., Ketchum, J. M., Marwitz, J. H., Taylor, L. A., & Menzel, J. C. (2009). A preliminary investigation of the brain injury family intervention: Impact on family members. *Brain Injury, 23*(6), 535–547.

Krysan, M., Moore, K. A., & Zill, N. (1990). *Research on successful families* (Contract # HHS-100-89-0041). Prepared for office of the assistant secretary for planning and evaluation U.S. Department of Health and Human Services. Washington, D. C.: U. S. Department of Health and Human Services.

Lansky, M. R. (1990). Escalation of trauma in the family of the patient with organic brain disease. *Family Systems Medicine, 8*(3), 231–240.

Laroi, F. (2003). The family systems approach to treating families of persons with brain injury: A potential collaboration between family therapist and brain injury professional. *Brain Injury, 17*(2), 175–187.

Lefebvre, H., Levert, M. J., Pelchat, D., & Lepage, J. G. (2008). Nature, sources, and impact of information on the adjustment of family caregivers: A pilot project. *Canadian Journal of Nursing Research, 40*(1), 143–160.

Lezak, M. D. (1978). Living with the characterologically altered brain injured patient. *Journal of Clinical Psychiatry, 39*, 592–598.

Lezak, M. D. (1988). Brain damage is a family affair. *Journal of Clinical and Experimental Neuropsychology, 10*(1), 111–123.

Lloyd, D. J., & Kehoe, S. L. (2001). *Smile and jump high!: The true story of overcoming a traumatic brain injury*. Monroe: Starlight Press.

Maitz, E. A. (1991). Family systems theory applied to head injury. In J. M. Williams & T. Kay (Eds.), *Head injury: A family matter* (pp. 65–79). Baltimore: Brookes Publishing.

Maitz, E. A., & Sachs, P. R. (1995). Treating families of individuals with traumatic brain injury from a family systems perspective. *Journal of Head Trauma Rehabilitation, 10*(2), 1–11.

McKinlay, W. W., Brooks, D. N., Bond, M. R., Martinage, D. P., & Marshall, M. M. (1981). The short-term outcome of severe blunt head injury as reported by relatives of the injured persons. *Journal of Neurology, Neurosurgery & Psychiatry, 44*(6), 527–533.

McLaughlin, A. M., & Carey, J. L. (1993). The adversarial alliance: Developing therapeutic relationships between families and the team in brain injury rehabilitation. *Brain Injury, 7*(1), 45–51.

Miller, L. (1993). Family therapy of brain injury: Syndromes, strategies, and solutions. *American Journal of Family Therapy, 21*(2), 111–121.

Morris, K. C. (2001). Psychological distress in carers of head injured individuals: The provision of written information. *Brain Injury, 15*(3), 239–254.

Norup, A., Kristensen, K. S., Siert, L., Poulsen, I., & Mortensen, E. L. (2011). Neuropsychological support to relatives of patients with severe traumatic brain injury in the sub-acute phase. *Neuropsychological Rehabilitation, 21*(3), 306–321.

Oddy, M., Humphrey, M., & Uttley, D. (1978). Stresses upon the relatives of head-injured patients. *British Journal of Psychiatry: The Journal of Mental Science, 133*, 507–513.

Palmer, S., & Palmer, J. B. (2011). *When your spouse has a stroke: Caring for your partner, yourself, and your relationship*. Baltimore: The Johns Hopkins University Press.

Patterson, F. L., & Staton, A. R. (2009). Adult-acquired traumatic brain injury: Existential implications and clinical considerations. *Journal of Mental Health Counseling, 31*(2), 149–163.

Persel, C. S., & Persel, C. H. (2010). The use of applied behaviour analysis in traumatic brain injury rehabilitation. In M. J. Ashley (Ed.), *Traumatic brain injury: Rehabilitation, treatment, and case management* (3rd ed., pp. 621–674). New York: CRC Press.

Peterson, C., Park, N., Pole, N., D'Andrea, W., & Seligman, M. E. (2008). Strengths of character and posttraumatic growth. *Journal of Traumatic Stress, 21*(2), 214–217.

Ponsford, J. (2013). Assessment and management of behaviour problems. In J. Ponsford, S. Sloan, & P. Snow (Eds.), *Traumatic brain injury: Rehabilitation for everyday adaptive living* (2nd ed., pp. 164–191). New York: Psychology Press.

Ponsford, J., Olver, J., Ponsford, M., & Nelms, R. (2003). Long-term adjustment of families following traumatic brain injury where comprehensive rehabilitation has been provided. *Brain Injury, 17*(6), 453–468.

Power, P. W., & Dell Orto, A. E. (2004). *Families living with chronic illness and disability: Interventions, challenges, and opportunities*. New York: Springer.

Prowe, G. (2010). *Successfully surviving a brain injury a family guidebook: From the emergency room to selecting a rehabilitation facility*. Gainesville: Brain Injury Success Books.

Rackner, V. (2009). *Caregiving without regrets: 3 steps to avoid burnout and manage disappointment, guilt, and anger*. Seattle: Medical Bridges.

Rich, M. (2005). *Coping with brain injury: How to help after accidents, stroke and illness*. London: Sheldon Press.

Roloff, T. A. (Ed.). (2010). *Navigating through a strange land: A book for brain tumor patients & their families*. Tucson: Indigo Press.

Romano, M. D. (1974). Family response to traumatic head injury. *Scandinavian Journal of Rehabilitation Medicine, 6*(1), 1–4.

Roos, S. (2002). *Chronic sorrow: A living loss*. New York: Brunner-Routledge.

Rosenthal, M., & Hutchins, B. (1991). Interdisciplinary family education in head injury rehabilitation. In J. M. Williams & T. Kay (Eds.), *Head injury: A family matter* (pp. 273–282). Baltimore: Brookes Publishing.

Rosenthal, M., & Young, T. (1988). Effective family intervention after traumatic brain injury: Theory and practice. *Journal of Head Trauma Rehabilitation, 3*(4), 42–50.

Rynn, M. (2013). Three tiers of support after brain injury [Drawing]. Arizona.

Sachs, P. R. (1991). *Treating families of brain injury survivors*. New York: Springer.

Sady, M. D., Sander, A. M., Clark, A. N., Sherer, M., Nakase-Richardson, R., & Malec, J. F. (2010). Relationship of preinjury caregiver and family functioning to community integration in adults with traumatic brain injury. *Archives of Physical Medicine and Rehabilitation, 91,* 1542–1550.

Sander, A. M., Davis, L. C., Struchen, M. A., Atchison, T., Sherer, M., Malec, J. F., et al. (2007). Relationship of race/ethnicity to caregivers' coping, appraisals, and distress after traumatic brain injury. *NeuroRehabilitation, 22*(1), 9–17.

Scherer, M. J. (2012). *Assistive technologies and other supports for people with brain impairment*. New York: Springer.

Schwartz, A. (2007). A view for Riggs: Treatment resistance and patient authority—VI. Working with family resistance to treatment. *Journal of the American Academy of Psychoanalysis and Dynamic Psychiatry, 35*(4), 607–625.

Seligman, M. E. P. (2011). *Flourish: A visionary new understanding of happiness and well-being*. New York: Atria.

Seligman, M. E. P., & Peterson, C. (2003). Positive clinical psychology. In L. G. Aspinwall & U. M. Staudinger (Eds.), *A psychology of human strengths: Fundamental questions and future directions for a positive psychology* (pp. 305–317). Washington, D. C.: American Psychological Association.

Senelick, R. C. (2010). *Living with stroke: A guide for families* (4th ed.). Birmingham: HealthSouth Press.

Senelick, R., & Dougherty, K. (2001). *Living with brain injury: A guide for families* (2nd ed.). Birmingham: HealthSouth Press.

Shaw, L. R., & McMahon, B. T. (1990). Family-staff conflict in the rehabilitation setting: Causes, consequences, and implications. *Brain Injury, 4*(1), 87–93.

Sheehy, G. (2010). *Passages in caregiving: Turning chaos into confidence*. New York: William Morrow.

Sherwin, E. D., & O'Shanick, G. J. (2000). The trauma of paediatric and adolescent brain injury: Issues and implications for rehabilitation specialists. *Brain Injury, 14*(3), 267–284.

Siegel, D. J. (2010). *The mindful therapist: A clinician's guide to mindsight and neural integration*. New York: W. W. Norton.

Siegel, R. D., & Germer, C. K. (2012). Wisdom and compassion: Two wings of a bird. In C. K. Germer & R. D. Siegel (Eds.), *Wisdom and compassion in psychotherapy: Deepening mindfulness in clinical practice* (pp. 7–34). New York: Guilford Press.

Smith, L. M., & Godfrey, H. P. D. (1995). *Family support programs and rehabilitation: A cognitive-behavioral approach to traumatic brain injury*. New York: Plenum Press.

Smith, R. L., & Stevens-Smith, P. (1992). A critique of healthy family functioning. In R. L. Smith & P. Stevens-Smith (Eds.), *Family counseling and therapy: Major issues and topics* (pp. 3–13). Ann Arbor: ERIC Counseling and Personnel Services Clearinghouse.

Sohlberg, M. M., McLaughlin, K. A., Todis, B., Larsen, J., & Glang, A. (2001). What does it take to collaborate with families affected by brain injury? A preliminary model. *Journal of Head Trauma Rehabilitation, 16*(5), 498–511.

Strang, S., Strang, P., & Ternestedt, B. M. (2001). Existential support in brain tumour patients and their spouses. *Supportive Care in Cancer: Official Journal of the Multinational Association of Supportive Care in Cancer, 9*(8), 625–633.

Stein, J. (2004). *Stroke and the family: A new guide*. Cambridge: Harvard University Press.

Sturm, C. D., Forget, T. R. Jr., & Sturm, J. L. (1998). *Head injury: Information and answers to commonly asked questions*. St. Louis: Quality Medical Publishing.

Thomsen, I. V. (1974). The patient with severe head injury and his family. *Scandinavian Journal of Rehabilitation Medicine, 6*(4), 180–183.

Turnbull, A. P., & Turnbull, H. R. III. (1991). Understanding families from a systems perspective. In J. M. Williams & T. Kay (Eds.), *Head injury: A family matter* (pp. 37–63). Baltimore: Brookes Publishing.

Truscott, D. (2010). *Becoming an effective psychotherapist: Adopting a theory of psychotherapy that's right for you and your client*. Washington, D. C.: American Psychological Association.

Uomoto, J. M., & Wong, T. M. (2000). Multicultural perspectives on the neuropsychology of brain injury assessment and rehabilitation. In E. Fletcher-Janzen, T. L. Strickland, & C. R. Reynolds (Eds.), *Handbook of cross-cultural neuropsychology* (pp. 169–184). New York: Kluwer Academic/Plenum Publishers.

Vaillant, G. E. (2008). Positive emotions, spirituality and the practice of psychiatry. *Medicine, Mental Health, Science, Religion, and Well-being, MSM, 6*, 48–62.

Verhaeghe, S., Defloor, T., & Grypdonck, M. (2005). Stress and coping among families of patients with traumatic brain injury: A review of the literature. *Journal of Clinical Nursing, 14*(8), 1004–1012.

Watanabe, Y., Shiel, A., McLellan, D. L., Kurihara, M., & Hayashi, K. (2001). The impact of traumatic brain injury on family members living with patients: A preliminary study in Japan and the UK. *Disability and Rehabilitation, 23*(9), 370–378.

White, M. B., Edwards, S. A., & Russell, C. S. (1997). The essential elements of successful marriage and family therapy: A modified Delphi study. *American Journal of Family Therapy, 25*(3), 213–231.

Wilcoxon, S. A. (1992). Healthy family functioning: The other side of family pathology. In R. L. Smith & P. Stevens-Smith (Eds.), *Family counseling and therapy: Major issues and topics* (pp. 14–26). Ann Arbor: ERIC Counseling and Personnel Services Clearinghouse.

Williams, J. M. (1991). Family support. In J. M. Williams & T. Kay (Eds.), *Head injury: A family matter* (pp. 299–312). Baltimore: Brookes Publishing.

Williams, J. M., & Kay, T. (Eds.). (1991). *Head injury: A family matter*. Baltimore: Brookes Publishing.

Williams, O. (2010). *Stroke diaries: A guide for survivors and their families*. New York: Oxford University Press.

Wilson, B. A., Herbert, C. M., & Shiel, A. (2003). *Behavioural approaches in neuropsychological rehabilitation: Optimising rehabilitation procedures*. New York: Psychology Press.

Winslade, W. J. (1998). *Confronting traumatic brain injury: Devastation, hope, and healing*. New Haven: Yale University Press.

Winstanley, J., Simpson, G., Tate, R., & Myles, B. (2006). Early indicators and contributors to psychological distress in relatives during rehabilitation following severe traumatic brain injury: Findings from the brain injury outcomes study. *Journal of Head Trauma Rehabilitation, 21*(6), 453–466.

Wolf, E. S. (1988). *Treating the self: Elements of clinical self psychology*. New York: Guilford Press.

Wood, R. L. (1984). Behaviour disorders following severe brain injury: Their presentation and psychological management. In N. Brooks (Ed.), *Closed head injury: Psychological, social, and family consequences* (pp. 195–219). Oxford: Oxford University Press.

Woodruff, L., & Woodruff, B. (2008). *In an instant: A family's journey of love and healing*. New York: Random House.

Wright, H. (2000). *Someone stole yesterday*. Franklin: Providence House Publishers.

Yalom, I. D. (1980). *Existential psychotherapy*. New York: Basic Books.

Yalom, I. D. (2009). *Staring at the sun: Overcoming the terror of death*. San Francisco: Jossey-Bass.

Yeates, G. (2009). Working with families in neuropsychological rehabilitation. In B. A. Wilson, F. Gracey, J. J. Evans, & A. Bateman (Eds.), *Neuropsychological rehabilitation: Theory, models, therapy and outcome* (pp. 138–156). New York: Cambridge University Press.

Chapter 2
Families' Early Sessions, Emotional Status, and Treatment Themes

2.1 The Initial Consultation

Emotional support for family members is usually the by-product of the provision of neurorehabilitation therapies for their loved ones, especially in the acute aftermath of the injury, while the patient is hospitalized. As depicted in phases 1 through 3 of the Family Experiential Model (FEM) of Recovery, the primary caregiver's and close relatives', as well as the support networks' total preoccupation is with the crisis of the patient's injury, especially given the gravity of the news and the uncertainty of his or her survival (see Chap. 1, Sect. 1.5; Klonoff and Koberstein 2010; Klonoff et al. 2008; Turner et al. 2007). Understandably, the relatives want the emphasis to be on the best care for their loved one; they ignore and may even resent any emphasis by the health-care professionals on their own psychological needs. Although the primary caregiver and overall family may initially rebuff support, once the patient is discharged home, they begin to glean some appreciation of the magnitude of their responsibilities. They now may gain an inkling of how overwhelmed and grief-stricken they are, whether by their own self-appraisal or through input from others around them. Their feelings of helplessness and dismay may then propel them to seek at least some level of professional input and support. However, their principal motivation to do so is most often because they are seeking more help for their loved one.

In an outpatient treatment environment, it often comes as a surprise to the patient and caregivers that the family will be so central to the neurorehabilitation process. Typically, the first contact with family members is the joint interview with the psychotherapist, with their loved one present. Usually, it is the primary caregiver who attends the appointment and the patient (if capable) signs the appropriate medical release form to allow the family member to participate in the appointment. Components of the initial consultation with patients have been reviewed previously (Klonoff 2010). This includes the necessary physician referral, appropriate medical records and neuropsychological test results, as well as domains of inquiry (demographics, social history, medical history, injury-related data, patients' subjective reports of postinjury status, and current medical treatment; Klonoff 2010). Here, the primary emphasis is on the patient; the family member's function is to provide other associated history and input, especially if the patient is unable to recall relevant pre- and/or

P. S. Klonoff, *Psychotherapy for Families after Brain Injury*,

DOI 10.1007/978-1-4899-8083-0_2,

postinjury information. Although the family may feel their role is perfunctory, the astute clinician will use the consultation as an opportunity to introduce the integral role and importance of the caregiver (i.e., tier 1), second-order family members or friends (i.e., tier 2), and broader support network (i.e., tier 3) for the loved one and each other. The therapist can also gather meaningful early observations about the primary caregiver's mood, demeanor, and psychological health through his or her clinical presentation, as well as the interaction patterns between the family member and the loved one (Klonoff 2010).

A fundamental aspect of the first session is to clarify the role of the psychotherapist in treating the family. The therapist needs to clarify who the identified patient is; in outpatient neurorehabilitation settings, it is the individual who has suffered the brain injury. The family members represent the concerned third parties in a collateral relationship, who are present to receive emotional support and education in order to maximize the harmony in the family relationships, so as to facilitate the best recovery for their loved one. They do not have a patient–doctor relationship; therefore, the information they share is not considered private or privileged. Outside of the neurorehabilitation setting for the patient with the brain injury (e.g., a separate private practice setting or clinic), family members may seek psychotherapy for themselves; in this case, they are the identified patient and their communications are considered privileged between themselves and their identified treater. In this latter scenario, the family members' overall psychological needs and interests are paramount and they may or may not coincide with the requirements and goals for the individual with the brain injury. In fact, the patient may not even be a participant in the sessions. Oftentimes, this type of therapy is undertaken when the relative (e.g., spouse) has some ambivalence about the future of the relationship or would benefit from his or her own psychotherapeutic relationship, secondary to the level of distress or other psychological needs. Therefore, it is imperative to obtain the family member's expectations of the therapy process, both for himself or herself and his or her loved one. If the boundaries of the therapeutic relationships involving the patient and family members are not clear, the psychotherapist has the ethical obligation to take the necessary time to define this, so that all parties are aware of the intent of the psychotherapeutic process.

In addition, written materials which describe the treatment process should be available at the commencement of psychotherapy. These should clearly delineate how family members are integrated into the treatment setting, including a review of the expected types of documentation related to the family's involvement and treatment. Figure 2.1 provides a sample explanation whereby the family members are receiving support and education as part of a holistic approach, but where the identified patient is the loved one who has sustained a brain injury.

2.2 Early Sessions

Once a mutual decision is made by the psychotherapist, patient, and family members to continue the psychotherapy process, a more in-depth assessment of the relatives' knowledge base, subjective impressions, emotional status, challenges, and needs

Neurorehabilitation Program Requirements:

Family Members:

Our clinical experience and program research indicates that the recovery and rehabilitation of your loved one is strongly related to the working alliance and education we provide to you. In addition, your experience and input is vital to our team efforts to understand and effectively treat your loved one.

Of note, your loved one is considered the identified patient in this setting. We will, of course, obtain the necessary medical releases from him or her to enable us to have open dialogue with you. Our role in working with you is to provide emotional support and instruction to enhance your loved one's adjustment, as well as his or her family relationships and community reintegration. As part of our documentation about your loved one's rehabilitation progress and challenges, you should expect that there will be content related to the treatment interventions being provided to you, as family members, also including relevant recommendations to support and educate you. Of note, as you are not the identified patient, there is no expectation of a patient-doctor relationship. Nonetheless, your involvement and focus on improving your awareness, acceptance, and realism about your loved one's brain injury is of paramount importance to the therapists in this setting and to your loved one.

Fig. 2.1 Sample explanation of the family members' role in holistic treatment

can be obtained through a separate follow-up meeting without the patient present. This form of inquiry is appropriate for both the primary caregiver(s) and the second tier of family supports, although generally it is the primary caregiver(s) who attends the first and early sessions. The patient is aware of this process and he/she has given written permission for this follow-up dialogue. As referenced in Chap. 1 (see Fig. 1.1), the family members' personality, emotions, and behavior "set the stage" for their interventions, and of course, a parallel process unfolds with their loved one. Table 2.1 depicts a list of important and common emotional and behavioral observations, which the psychotherapist can garner based on these initial interactions with the caregiver(s). Based on these first impressions, the psychotherapist can then formulate early working hypotheses, which are later refined based on follow-up contact. Of note, the family members' emotions and behaviors are fluid and can oscillate between many or all of these within one or more early sessions.

With respect to other salient factors, some clinicians prefer to utilize questionnaires or structured interviews to amass pertinent historical and practical information about the patient/family unit, based on the family member(s)' self-report(s), including caregiver burden (Nabors et al. 2002; see Saban et al. 2010, for a review; see Visser-Meily et al. 2004, for a review). However, I prefer a semi-structured approach, which covers topics using open-ended questions. Deviation from a scripted approach facilitates dialogue and is a more fluid outlet for family members to describe their

Table 2.1 Family members' presenting behaviors and the therapist's working hypotheses

Behaviors	Working hypotheses
Tearful, pessimistic, overwhelmed	Is the caregiver depressed and/or burned out?
Frustrated, angry, blaming, demanding	Has the caregiver had negative experiences with the health-care system prior to this interaction? Is the caregiver in the "yellow warning" zone of coping?
Anxious, passive, helpless	Does the caregiver have any of the necessary tools and/or psychoeducation to help himself/herself and the loved one?
Lonely, resentful, aloof	Does the caregiver have a wider support system helping himself/herself?
Composed, inquisitive, caring, attuned	Has this family member already had access to helpful resources? Does this family member have a "green adaptive" coping style?

unique perspectives and experiences. Again, the questions are applicable to the primary caregiver(s) and the broader family support system, based on whoever attends the beginning sessions. The topics and sample questions are presented in Table 2.2 and include germane aspects of their social history prior to their loved one's injuries. Many of these subject domains relate to the relatives' contextual realities, as defined in Fig. 1.1, namely their history, culture, environment, social context, psychodynamics, values, spirituality, and accomplishments.

As illustrated in Table 2.2, the interview also affords the opportunity for the psychotherapist to appraise the family members' current functional and psychological status (based on their personal account of the injury-related events); perception of their loved one's injury consequences and course of recovery; the relatives' current daily activities, stressors, and coping paradigms; the relatives' priorities, goals, and aspirations for their loved one and themselves; and the family's support system. This last factor is noteworthy, as it begins to frame the overall support system, based on the tier 1 (i.e., main caregiver(s)), tier 2 (family and friends who are actively involved), and tier 3 (relatives, friends, and community contacts with adjunct roles). With all of this input and material, the psychotherapist can now better collaborate with the patient and family to devise the next steps in the psychotherapy process, namely to ascertain their baseline level of awareness, acceptance, and realism.

2.2.1 A Baseline Determination of the Family's Awareness, Acceptance, and Realism

As a gauge of the direction of psychotherapy, the psychotherapist should obtain an overview of the family members' beginning level of awareness, acceptance, and realism about: (a) their loved one's injury sequelae and (b) their own situation, challenges, and needs. *Self-awareness* has been defined as "the understanding and acknowledgement of postinjury neurological strengths and difficulties, as well as their functional implications" (Klonoff 2010, p. 46). *Acceptance* is the individual's "ability and willingness to cope with his or her new reality and identity" (Klonoff 2010,

Table 2.2 Relatives' history and current functioning

Social history	
Topics:	*Sample inquiries*
Birthplace, family structure, and childhood development	Where were you born? Describe your childhood and family structure
Educational history	How much education do you have? Where were you trained?
Marital status (and prior marriages)	How long have you been married? How many times have you been married? Do you have children from your current marriage? Do you have children from your prior marriage(s)? How much contact did you have with your children prior to the injury?
Preinjury living situation	What was your preinjury living situation? Who was in charge of various household chores and responsibilities?
Preinjury occupational history	What type of work did you do prior to your loved one's injury? Was it full- or part-time? Did you enjoy your work? Was it stressful?
Preinjury financial status	What was your preinjury financial status? Were there any stressors?
Preinjury psychiatric history and treatment	Have you ever seen a psychologist or psychiatrist? For what purpose(s)? Did the treatment help? If so, how?
Preinjury substance use/abuse	Did you drink, smoke, or use street drugs prior to your loved one's injury? Have you ever had a problem with addiction to alcohol or drugs? Did you pursue treatment for this problem? Was the treatment successful?
Preinjury challenges and "traumas"	Have you ever experienced any prior challenges, or life "traumas?" How did you deal with these?
Preinjury relationship with your loved one with the brain injury	What was your preinjury relationship with your loved one who has the brain injury?
Preinjury supports	What values are most essential to you? What was the role of spirituality and faith in your life preinjury?
Subjective report of postinjury status:	
Topics:	*Sample inquiries*
More detailed exploration of the family's injury-related experiences	Describe the circumstances of your loved one's injury How were you notified and by whom? How would you describe his/her acute care? How has it been since he/she came home?
More detailed exploration of the family member(s)' perception(s) of injury-related sequelae and interface with health professionals	How have you acquired information about your loved one? How has the experience been in interacting with health professionals thus far? Describe the physical, cognitive, emotional, and functional challenges of your loved one

Table 2.2 (continued)

	How have these affected you and your relationship with your loved one? Which problem(s) affect(s) you the most and why?
Perception of their loved one's course of recovery	What is your sense of your loved one's recovery—is he/she improving, or not?
Current daily activities (i.e., work, hobbies, and leisure) and finances	How do you spend your day? Are you working? If yes, how has your work been affected? If not working, how is your family supporting itself? Do you have time for hobbies or leisure and what are they? Do you have time to see friends and socialize?
Overall stressors and coping paradigms	What are your current emotions? What is going well for you right now? What are your main stressors? Are you experiencing changes in your appetite, sleep patterns, or energy level? What do you miss the most? How are your other family members doing? How have you and your other family members coped with the stressors?
Priorities, goals, and aspirations for their loved one	What are your priorities for your loved one? What are your aspirations for your loved one? Where do you see your loved one in 6 months?
Priorities, goals, and aspirations for themselves	What are your own priorities? What are your aspirations? Where do you see yourself in 6 months?
More detailed exploration of current supports	How many relatives and friends are involved with the care of your loved one who sustained the injury? What types of assistance do they provide? Do you feel you are getting sufficient help?

p. 100), typified by embracing and implementing compensations (Klonoff 2010). *Realism* represents the "integration of accumulated internal perceptions and external life experiences to produce healthy judgments and attainable objectives for the future" (Klonoff 2010, p. 198). Table 2.3 contains baseline determinants of the family members' degree of awareness, acceptance, and realism. These are divided according to "limited" versus "good" indicators. This prototype is helpful, as it can be used with multiple members of the support system, including the primary caregiver(s) as well as associated relatives and friends. It captures the initial breadth and depth of the overall support network's degree of attunement with the complexities of the injury and its impact on themselves.

2.2.1.1 Awareness

Table 2.3 describes two broad categories of the baseline determinants of awareness in the family members after brain injury. The first grouping relates to questions about the patient, that is, the relatives' loved one. This pertains to how well the caregiver/family initially understands and acknowledges to the therapist, the nature and extent of

Table 2.3 Baseline determinant of family members' awareness, acceptance, and realism

Limited awareness	*Good awareness*
Patient-related inquiries:	
1. Spontaneous acknowledgment of physical injury-related changes only, without recognition of cognitive, mood, or psychosocial sequelae based on open-ended questions (what changes have you observed in your loved one?)	1. Spontaneous identification of a broader range of physical, emotional, cognitive, and psychosocial difficulties, based on open-ended questions (e.g., what changes have you observed in your loved one?)
2. Ability to identify one or two rudimentary nonphysical, postinjury difficulties with direct questions (e.g., what thinking changes have you noticed? or how has your loved one's memory/personality changed?)	2. Ability to recognize the saliency of cognitive, personality/mood, and interpersonal difficulties (compared with physical problems) for the loved one's overall adjustment
3. Significant underestimation of the severity of possible deficits based on a rating scale (see Table 2.4: no problem; small, medium, or large problem) compared with objective data (e.g., medical/neuropsychological data) and/or their loved one's subjective self-ratings	3. Deficit ratings on Table 2.4 are "in the ball park" based on collateral objective data (e.g., medical/neuropsychological records) and/or subjective ratings by their loved one
4. Inability to generalize possible injury-related difficulties to community environments (e.g., school or work)	4. Ability to generalize how the injury-related difficulties affect home and community independence as well as productivity
Caregiver/support network topics:	
1. Reluctance or unwillingness to acknowledge possible deleterious or stressful effects of their loved one's neurological event	1. Ability to acknowledge that the neurological event in their loved one has had a life-altering effect, including certain stressors
2. Lack of insight into the need for outside treatment for themselves and therefore reject help	2. Recognize and communicate openly the need for outside professional interventions for themselves
Limited acceptance	*Good acceptance*
Patient-related inquiries:	
1. Lack of "buy in" into the potential value of compensations for their loved one and unwilling to participate in the training process	1. Receptive to the idea of compensations for their loved one and interested/coachable in the training process
2. "Yeah buts" and rejection of available objective feedback from collateral sources (e.g., school grades and work-performance evaluations)	2. Receptive to the meaningful contribution of existing postinjury objective external data to their loved one's symptom picture
3. Expect a full recovery in the patient "no matter what"	3. Open to the idea that a full recovery may not be feasible
4. Want instant results for their loved one	4. Realize that "things take time" and that the recovery process is slow and arduous
Caregiver/support network topics:	
1. Present with a defensive, demanding, or argumentative stance about how they are coping with their circumstances	1. Are cooperative and amenable to inquiry about how they are coping
2. Are distrustful of the motives of the psychotherapist regarding providing the family with assistance and relief	2. Are trusting that the psychotherapist will have the family's best interest at heart

Table 2.3 (continued)

3. Are unwilling to commit to and engage in the therapy process for themselves, thinking it is superfluous	3. Are eager to immerse themselves in the therapy process
Limited realism	*Good realism*
Patient-related inquiries:	
1. Overly idealistic, with the "shoot for the stars" and "prove the doctors wrong" mindset about their loved one	1. Practical and "down to earth" approach, yet hopeful about their loved one
2. Overshooting school/work goals, based on their loved one's neurological limitations	2. Reasonable fit between their loved one's neurological limitations and their work/school aspirations
3. Overreliance on community supports at school and work to ensure their loved one's success	3. Appropriate level of community supports at work and school to ensure their loved one's bona fide accomplishments
Caregiver/support network topics:	
1. Insufficient planning for the realities of the changes in their own circumstances, resulting in "being spread too thin"	1. Initial steps taken to accommodate their complex circumstances, so as to aptly juggle multiple responsibilities
2. Resentful of others who suggest the need for reconfiguration of schedules and priorities, at least temporarily	2. Appreciative of others who suggest or actively volunteer to provide assistance so as to reduce strains

his or her loved one's injury consequences. In this regard, there are gradations of awareness, as oftentimes, the physical compromises are at first more obvious to the family, while the cognitive, emotional, and interpersonal factors seem more elusive (Smith and Godfrey 1995). Therefore, when the psychotherapist asks general questions (i.e., what changes have you observed in your loved one?), the family with "limited" baseline awareness may spontaneously identify only one or two obvious physical difficulties (e.g., balance or vision changes), yet be unable to identify other cognitive, mood, or psychosocial challenges. Even with direct questions (e.g., what thinking changes have you noticed? or, how has your loved one's memory/personality changed?), relatives with "limited" awareness will show a dearth of insight, with a tendency either to negate any other difficulties or acknowledge only one or two rudimentary changes (e.g., forgetfulness). Conversely, when the psychotherapist asks open-ended questions about the family's perception of injury-related changes, those with "good" beginning awareness are able to spontaneously identify a broader range of physical, emotional, cognitive, and psychosocial difficulties. With further inquiry, they recognize the saliency of cognitive, mood, and psychosocial problems as impediments to their loved one's level of adjustment.

Emotional and behavioral symptoms are crucial to evaluate (Jackson et al. 2009). Therefore, another mechanism to abstract the family's early perceptions is to ask direct questions about specific injury effects based on multiple domains. Table 2.4 is a family checklist which contains severity ratings of a number of common neurologically based physical, cognitive, language, emotional, behavioral, and psychosocial deficits which may be negatively impacting the family. Ratings can be based on numerical values (e.g., 0 = no problem; 1 = small problem; 10 = large problem) or descriptive terminology of none, small, medium, or large problems. This represents a more extensive overview of possible patient characteristics which could be most troubling to and cumbersome for the family. Depending on the preference of the psychotherapist, he or she can either obtain verbal ratings from the family or, alternatively, have the family members provide written ratings. Families with more "limited" baseline awareness will provide ratings which are at the lower, less impaired end of the spectrum, relative to what other medical and neuropsychological records indicate. For example, if a family member rates memory and attentional problems in his or her loved one as a small problem, while neuropsychological test data suggest large (or severe) deficits, the psychotherapist can hypothesize that the family is underestimating the severity of the deficits, suggesting that they may not be fully aware of the seriousness of the injury. A hallmark of limited awareness in family members are less severe ratings of injury deficits compared to those of their loved one, especially when collateral data are also contradictory to the family's ratings. However, the scores on the Deficit Rating Scale by families with "good" preliminary awareness are "in the ballpark," based on good concordance with collateral objective data (e.g., medical and neuropsychological test data). Generally, the family's perception of the severity of problem areas are higher than the perception of their loved one, secondary to his or her organic unawareness.

As depicted in Table 2.3, another mechanism for assessing the family members' initial awareness of their loved one's injury sequelae is their ability to generalize possible deficits to the "real world." This includes whether or not the relatives recognize that certain deficits would hinder community activities. For instance, if the family endorses big problems with memory, speed of thinking, and attentional skills, but then suggests that their loved one is capable of returning to graduate-level coursework in a university or highly cognitively based occupations (e.g., law, medicine, engineering, etc.), the psychotherapist may begin to surmise that the family members do not fully understand or are not able to acknowledge how their loved one's challenges are translating to functional difficulties.

As indicated in Table 2.3, the other index of family members' baseline level of awareness is their insight into their own predicament. For the more aware family, this includes their realization that the neurological event in their loved one has had a substantial and enduring effect on their own existence. The relatives also perceive that they need assistance from outside professionals (phase 3 of the FEM), as there is a limit to their own knowledge and experience with the effects of brain injury in a loved one. In contrast, the family with "limited" early awareness communicates a reluctance or unwillingness to acknowledge the deleterious and/or stressful aspects of their new lifestyle. Due to their poor grasp of the complexities of their situation, they also discount the need for outside professional interventions.

2.2.1.2 Acceptance

Examples of markers of the family's baseline acceptance are also presented in Table 2.3. As with the conceptualization of awareness, the acceptance considerations

Table 2.4 Family member's deficit rating scale. (Have the family member provide ratings of patient deficit domains. Use the following scale: No problem; Small problem; Medium problem; Large problem)

Domain:	No problem	Small	Medium	Large
Physical:				
Vision				
Headaches				
Dizziness				
Weakness/hemiparesis				
Overall coordination				
Tremors				
Balance				
Fatigue				
Cognitive/Language:				
Confusion				
Memory				
Attention and concentration				
Speed of thinking				
Reasoning and problem solving				
Decision making				
Organization				
Multitasking				
Impulsivity				
Initiation (getting tasks started)				
Perseveration (fixated)				
Understanding language				
Expressing himself/herself				
Reading				
Writing				
Spelling				
Arithmetic				
Emotional/Behavioral:				
Frustration				
Depression				
Anxiety				
Mood swings				
Feeling overwhelmed				
Irritability/anger				
Aggression/rage reactions				
Distrust				
Apathy				
Poor insight				
Childlike				
Restless				
Irresponsible				

Table 2.4 (continued)

Domain:	No problem	Small	Medium	Large
Psychosocial:				
Dependency				
Hyperverbal (talkative)				
Tangential (wanders off topic)				
Blunt				
Self-centered				
Disinhibited (speaks before thinking)				
Snarky/argumentative				
Flat affect				
Reduced initiation				
Judgment				
Lonely				

are divided into the categories of patient-related inquiries and caregiver/support network topics. Relatives with "limited" initial acceptance will communicate a lack of "buy in" into the potential value of compensations for their loved one. They will express reticence about participating in the strategy training process, usually citing having too many other responsibilities and insufficient time. When the idea that they may also benefit from exposure to new tools (e.g., their own datebook or an electronic system) is proposed, they will negate the value. Overall, they seem set in their ways, feeling that new systems will be too confusing or burdensome. In comparison, the family with "good" beginning acceptance is receptive to the idea of compensations and looks forward to the training process. They are curious about new compensations or adaptations to enable them to function better personally, and on behalf of their loved one, and therefore, they convey a coachable attitude.

Family members with "limited" baseline acceptance tend to reject outside objective data (e.g., from work or school), especially if it is perceived as negative or critical of their loved one. Their responses are characterized by "yeah buts" (Klonoff 2010) and they resort to external blame, finding fault in others, thereby dismissing the role of their loved one's brain injury. In conjunction with this, they are adamant about a full recovery in their loved one and want the recovery process to move quickly and smoothly. Then again, relatives with "good" early acceptance have assimilated some of the postinjury life experiences they and their loved one have experienced and have begun to adjust their expectations. This translates to the recognition that a full recovery may not be possible and that the recovery process will be gradual and sometimes grueling. They are open to the mantra that "things take time" (Hein 2003).

Another important factor in the psychotherapist's baseline understanding of the family's acceptance is their coping strategies for their own challenges. When the therapist initiates gentle inquiries, the family with "limited" acceptance becomes defensive or even argumentative, deflecting their emotions onto other topics (e.g., their loved one or the medical system at large). They have not yet developed enough trust in the therapist to feel comfortable sharing inner worries and sorrows and may assume the psychotherapeutic process for themselves is superfluous. Alternatively, relatives who have "good" initial acceptance are cooperative and amenable to inquiries about how they are coping, recognizing that the psychotherapist has their best interest at heart. They are relieved and, in fact, eager to immerse themselves in the therapy process and are welcoming of the care and support.

2.2.1.3 Realism

Table 2.3 reviews psychotherapeutic considerations when assessing the family members' preliminary degree of realism about their loved one, as well as their own situation. Relatives with "limited" realism are hopeful, but overly idealistic, and espouse the "shoot for the stars" or "anything is possible" approach. Often, they have perceived prior medical professionals as overly pessimistic and unempathic and are determined to "prove the experts wrong" (Klonoff et al. 2008). Their initial perception of their loved one usually overshoots his or her actual capabilities and the relatives expect the community to make many accommodations or even allowances so that their loved one will succeed. Conversely, the family with better baseline realism takes the more "down to earth" practical approach, yet remains hopeful about the future. They want their loved one to succeed in their community endeavors, so they focus on a path that matches their loved one's capabilities (and limitations). Their expectations of community supports are reasonable and they want their loved one to succeed based on his or her own merit.

Caregivers and family members with limited realism also underestimate the realities of their own state of affairs. They are "spread too thin" because they refuse to reconfigure their current responsibilities, especially their new emotional and practical needs. They are resentful and even rejecting of others who suggest changes and are usually too prideful or uncomfortable accepting help from other external supporters. The family with better realism has taken initial steps to accommodate their complex predicament. They realize the stresses created by juggling multiple responsibilities, not only for their loved one, but for themselves and other family members. They are appreciative of others who give pertinent suggestions and they invitingly accept outside help.

Of note, the above baseline determinants of awareness, acceptance, and realism are on a continuum and family members will usually oscillate between limited and better insight, coping, and adaptation, based on a myriad of factors. These factors are unique to the family constellation and brain-injury effects and should be explored as part of unfolding sessions. As will be discussed in later chapters, evolving acceptance is predicated on a foundation of awareness; similarly, eventual realism emerges from enhanced awareness and acceptance.

2.3 Prominent Emotional Reactions and Psychosocial Changes in Families After Brain Injury

Clinical experience and the research literature have identified a series of prominent emotional changes after brain injury. These include depression, anxiety, and demoralization; anger and frustration; grief and loss; denial; and guilt. Also, relatives report significant burdens, because of the major shifts in their identity, family, and societal roles, as well the assault on their sense of self. The following is an overview of these constructs, which will be revisited throughout the book.

2.3.1 Depression, Anxiety, and Demoralization

Caregivers experience elevated levels of depression and anxiety after a neurological event in their loved ones (see Blake 2008, for a review; Collins and Swartz 2011; Harris et al. 2001; Hoofien et al. 2001; Judd 1999; Kreutzer et al. 1994; Lezak 1986; Marsh et al. 1998, 2002; Schonberger et al. 2010; Turner et al. 2010). As identified in phase 1 of the FEM, relatives react with panic upon notification of their loved one's injury, in combination with dread that their loved one may not survive (Klonoff et al. 2008; McAlaster et al. 2004). The family feels powerless (Testani-Dufour et al. 1992); they live in constant trepidation of "what ifs," related to possible medical complications.

Later sources of depression and anxiety are the challenges emerging from the transition from the hospital setting to the home environment, at least for the first few months. This is consistent with the increase in practical responsibilities, with fears and worries about future unknowns, including incomplete recovery, and/or other accidents or misfortunes (Inzaghi et al. 2005; Stebbins and Pakenham 2001; Turner et al. 2010; Williams 1991). Also, heightened depression and anxiety in the primary caregiver have been linked to greater and long-lasting cognitive, behavioral, and emotional changes in his or her loved ones; physical symptomatology in the caregiver; less social support and social isolation; and ineffective problem-solving techniques (Harris et al. 2001; Ponsford et al. 2003; Riley 2007; Rivera et al. 2007; Schonberger et al. 2010; Williams 1991).

Sometimes, depression dissipates into sadness, which is the capacity to integrate neurological and functional progress as "good news" and develop a more positive life view (Prigatano et al. 1986). Other times, family members bear "soul sickness" or demoralization (Perakis 2010). Demoralization is characterized by feelings of hopelessness, helplessness, incompetence, alienation, and existential despair brought on by suffering and insufficient coping skills for external stresses (Clarke and Kissane 2002; Perakis 2010). It has been linked to the frame of mind of psychological impotence, or the "giving up–given up" complex (Engel 1968).

To treat depression, anxiety, and "soul sickness," the psychotherapist should help the caregiver restore his or her morale by learning coping skills (Perakis 2010). This will embody self-soothing techniques, self-management skills, and improved self-esteem through empathic responsiveness, psychoeducation, goal setting, and cognitive behavioral techniques (Clarke and Kissane 2002; Klonoff and Koberstein 2010; Perakis 2010). This recreates empowerment, hope, purpose, and meaning in life (Buchholz 1990; Clarke and Kissane 2002; Klonoff and Koberstein 2010; Perakis 2010).

2.3.2 *Anger and Frustration*

Anger and frustration often erupt from the family's feelings of helplessness, caused by their abrupt expulsion from their familiar routine into the foreign medical setting (Sachs 1991). The slowness and unpredictable nature of the recovery also amplifies the family's aggravation (McAlaster et al. 2004). A dearth of instructive information and/or medical/rehabilitation resources compounds the families' vexations. Crucial to the psychotherapy process is ameliorating the caregivers' and tier supports' anger and frustrations.

2.3.3 *Grief and Loss*

Relatives of patients with acquired brain injuries are justifiably grief-stricken. Grief and loss reactions after brain injury have been differentiated into personal sacrifice burden; heartfelt sadness; longing and worry; and isolation (Marwit and Kaye 2006; Testani-Dufour et al. 1992). Pertinent concepts are "ambiguous loss" and "chronic sorrow" (Boss 2006; Boss et al. 2011; Olshansky 1962, as cited in Roos 2002) depicting the misery about the permanency of the life-altering circumstances. As depicted in phase 4 of the FEM, this anguish is an unavoidable by-product of budding awareness of the seriousness and complexity of the injury effects (see Chap. 1, Sect. 1.5; Klonoff and Koberstein 2010; Klonoff et al. 2008). This includes the replacement of the familiar loved one with a new person whose attributes may be quite different and foreign to the family member (Williams 1991). The family is thrust into acknowledging "what is" versus "what was" with respect to their lifestyle and family relationships (Dell Orto and Power 2000).

Intense feelings of loss in the family members precipitate "catastrophic reactions by proxy" (CRs by proxy; see Sect. 2.4.2.1; Klonoff and Koberstein 2010; Klonoff et al. 2008). Williams (1991) has described "episodic loss reactions," in which families reexperience profound sorrow, which is usually precipitated by reminders of the preinjury person, or historical events, and/or inherent disappointments in the recovery process. The process of adjustment implies a lessening of grieving and a gradual process of adaptation (Klonoff 2010; Williams 1991).

2.3.4 *Denial*

A working definition of *denial* in the support network is an enduring psychological disbelief in the seriousness of the effects of the loved one's brain injury, despite objective evidence to the contrary. Manifestations can span a spectrum from outright rejection of any aftereffects to denunciation, minimization, or excuse making about selected deficit arenas. Denial is a coping strategy employed by family members after brain injury in a loved one. The adaptive benefit of denial is controversial and is based on when and how long it occurs after the injury. In the immediate upheaval of the brain injury, denial functions as a protective defense mechanism or a buffer against intense and debilitating emotional distress (see Klonoff 2010, for a review; Verhaeghe et al. 2005). Denial can also be considered a necessary stepping stone in the family's acceptance process (Klonoff 2010). They should not be forced to "accept the unacceptable" (Novack and Richards 1991). Conversely, pervasive denial can be counterproductive, if it prevents an accurate appraisal of the patient's injury deficits through avoidance and/or negation, hinders the family's involvement in the rehabilitation process, and/or impedes the patient's rehabilitation progress (e.g., creating danger for the loved one or caregiver; Klonoff et al. 2008; Novack and Richards 1991; Romano 1974; Rosenthal and Young 1988; Sachs 1991). Family members who are more removed from daily caregiving may fall folly to denial (Johnson and McCown 1997).

2.3.5 Guilt

Family members' guilt is a natural reaction, which often emanates from seeing a loved one hurt and not being able to relieve his or her suffering (Kreutzer et al. 2002; Lezak 1986; Zinner et al. 1997). Sometimes, family members blame themselves for their loved one's injury (McKinlay and Hickox 1988), adopting a "hindsight is 20/20" mentality. This can evolve into survivor's guilt, which in a severe form, culminates in the family's inability for gratifying pursuits, due to a belief system predicated on self-punishment and self-deprivation (Klonoff and Koberstein 2010; Zinner et al. 1997). In the post-acute phase of recovery, the family's guilt feelings also emanate from negative feelings about the loved one, which although inevitable in the context of the tumultuous injury-related changes, are still perceived by the family member as unjustifiable (Knight et al. 1998). Alternatively, forced absenteeism, related to outside responsibilities, feeds the uninvolved relatives' guilt (Johnson and McCown 1997). Addressing guilt reactions in psychotherapy is fundamental to the relatives' self-forgiveness and evolving psychological well-being.

2.3.6 Identity and Social Role Changes

Identity has been described as "the person's subjective characterization of his or her individuality in the social context" (Klonoff and Myles 2010, p. 76); *social roles* have been defined as "the individual's societal position and responsibilities as perceived and defined by both the person himself or herself and members of the social network" (Klonoff and Myles 2010, p. 76). The relative's identity often shifts, secondary to the injury disruptions and transformed priorities. Role changes postinjury affect the family's equilibrium and manifest as either gains or losses (Frosch et al. 1997). These dramatic role alterations affect personal responsibilities and patterns of living within the home and community, as well as those roles specific to the care of and relationship with their loved one postinjury, compared with those prior to the injury (Degeneffe 2001). Sometimes, this translates into an overwhelming number of roles (Frosch et al. 1997). Also, spouses, siblings, and children may now be thrust into the role of caregiving for an individual who previously was self-sufficient (Degeneffe 2001; Gan et al. 2006). Some studies have reported greater role changes in partners, compared with parents (Leathem et al. 1996). Other sacrifices include alteration in living arrangements (with the loved one living at home) and/or temporary or permanent changes in employment, with a concomitant increase in time and energy regarding their loved one (Degeneffe 2001; Frosch et al. 1997). Psychotherapeutic tools for coping with the impact of brain injuries on family roles are inherent to a recalibration of the family system.

2.3.7 Subjective Caregiver Burden

Caregiver burden has a multiplicity of definitions and subcomponents, including the perceived level of stress (Chwalisz and Kisler 1995); personal and role strain (Siegert et al. 2010); relationship disruptions (Marsh et al. 1998); and perceived level of mastery (Hanks et al. 2007). Care needs after brain injury usually arise out of necessity, rather than choice (Degeneffe 2001), and some individuals thrust into this role do not have the requisite disposition. Many caregivers feel inadequately trained for their duties and have not received formal education (Collins and Swartz 2011). In fact, caregivers have been described as the "hidden patients" (Fengler and Goodrich 1979). Overall, burden evolves over time when the caregiving situation exceeds the caregiver's coping resources (Chwalisz 1992).

Patient factors which exacerbate caregiver burden include their emotional and behavioral challenges (e.g., anger, impulsivity, apathy, lack of empathy) and their dependency needs (see Blake 2008, for a review; Knight et al. 1998; Machamer et al. 2002; Marsh et al. 1998; Wells et al. 2005). Reduced social support for their loved one and themselves also intensifies caregiver burden (Hanks et al. 2007). Other stressors include monitoring the loved one's safety and helping to occupy his or her time productively (Collins and Swartz 2011). Caregiver variables associated with increased burden include lower household income, employment changes, younger age, lower education, less time for themselves, and greater unmet needs (Marsh et al. 2002; Nabors et al. 2002).

Tier 1 primary caregivers are perhaps at the greatest risk of subjective burden, especially given their holistic responsibilities for their loved one after a brain injury. This creates an emotional, physical, and financial toll, destabilizing the primary caregiver's well-being and quality of life (Collins and Swartz 2011; Marsh et al. 2002; Turner et al. 2010). Gradually, family life may become inextricably altered, with often permanent postinjury trajectories and overall reduced life satisfaction (Livingston et al. 2010; Wongvatunyu and Porter 2008). Conversely, mitigating factors for caregiver burden include the feeling of personal reward, the capacity to reframe or positively appraise challenging conditions, clear personal expectations, inner resiliency, self-reliance, flexibility to adjust life goals, satisfaction with coping techniques, sufficient respite, and community-based information and services (see Blake 2008, for a review; Machamer et al. 2002; Man 2002; Perlesz et al. 1999; Wells et al. 2005). For further discussion of the positive aspects of caregiving, see Chap. 10, Sect. 10.2.

2.3.8 *Shattering of the Assumptive World and Loss of Sense of Self*

A neglected consequence of brain injury with respect to acknowledgment and treatment is the shattering of the assumptive world in the family (Klonoff and Koberstein 2010), with a concomitant loss of sense of self. Trauma forces the family to confront mortality and recognize the fragility and uncertainties of life, and it often ruins their underlying and consoling life assumptions and convictions (Corr 2002; Kao and Stuifbergen 2004). In cases of accidental injury, the family is terrified about the randomness and powerlessness of their predicament, especially when an unscathed survivor (Corr 2002).

The aftermath of the brain injury for some families is like a never-ending crisis, with a precarious homeostasis, alternating with periodic and unpredictable imbalances (Davis et al. 2003). In essence, the family is experiencing a "transcrisis state" or situational crises, with inadequate resolution due to ongoing reverberations from the injury embedded in an ambiguous future (Davis et al. 2003). Other families experience a roller coaster of emotions, mirroring their loved one's experience of dashed expectations alternating with renewed hopes (Williams 1991).

Often, relatives suffer a "crisis of meaning" emanating from ordinary factors, including safety, control, and justice, as well as existential meaning, encompassing how to redefine purpose in life (Landsman 2002). In an attempt to understand the devastating event (e.g., "How did this happen?"), the family strives to form a coherent account of how the incident happened (Landsman 2002). Sometimes, as a way to enhance a sense of control of their state, family members resort to self-blame or blame of others (Landsman 2002). Other techniques to address the shattering of assumptive worlds in family members include for them to revise their personal schemas and themes about how they interrelate with the world, so as to eventually reengage in life and their future (Landsman 2002).

In order for the family to recalibrate their personal- and worldview, they must tackle the loss of their sense of self. Figure 2.2 is a useful tool to help the family explore possible alterations in their sense of self. This questionnaire is derived from a Sentence Completion Task for patients after brain injury (Myles 2007; see Klonoff and Myles 2010, for a review). This tool helps the caregiver and family identify changes in their core sense of self, especially in the domains of their emotions and overall self-perception, connection and roles with others, and central life themes and priorities, as well as their contemplations for the future.

2.4 General Treatment Considerations

In the context of the aforementioned emotional challenges, the following general treatment considerations represent global factors in working effectively with family members after brain injury. They include the fundamentals and techniques

Instructions: Complete the following sentences any way you want.

1: Since my loved one's injury, my sense of who I am…
2: Since my loved one's injury, I feel…
3: Since my loved one's injury, the way I see myself…
4: Since my loved one's injury, my sense of connection with other people…
5: Since the injury, when I think about the future, I feel…
6: Since the injury, when I think about my role in my family…
7: When I think about life before my loved one's injury, I feel…
8: Since my loved one's injury, what matters to me…
9: Since my loved one's injury, when I think about work…
10: Compared to before my loved one's injury, my emotions…
11: Since my loved one's injury, my role in life…
12: Compared to before the injury, my level of stress...
13: Since the injury, my place in the world…
14: Compared to before my loved one's injury, I get upset...
15: Since my loved one's injury, my sense of purpose…
16: Since my loved one's injury, when I compare myself to my friends…
17: Compared to before my loved one's injury, I feel sad…
18: Since my loved one's injury, the things that are important to me…
19: When I compare myself to how my life was before the injury…
20: Compared to before my loved one's injury, I worry…
21: Since my loved one's injury, my relationships with the people close to me…
22: Compared to before my loved one's injury, I feel anxious…
23: Since my loved one's injury, my life is...
24: Since my loved one's injury, my ability to deal with problems…
25: Compared to before my loved one's injury, I get frustrated …
26: Since my loved one's injury, when I think about my life…
27: Since my loved one's injury, my ability to cope with stress…
28: Compared to before my loved one's injury, I feel angry…

Fig. 2.2 Family's sense of self following brain injury: sentence completion task

for a positive working alliance, as well as pervasive themes which arise in the psychotherapeutic process with the primary caregiver and other tier supports.

2.4.1 How to Build a Positive Working Alliance

Forging a positive working alliance requires the psychotherapist to have keen perceptiveness and sensitivity to the multiplicity of factors impinging on the family members. As stated in Chap. 1 (Sect. 1.3), it behooves the psychotherapist to gain an appreciation of the contextual background of the family, including their history, culture, psychodynamics, environment, aspirations, values, and spirituality, in order to glean a more accurate appraisal of the family unit's uniqueness. Some clinicians have espoused the "whole family approach," based on holistic treatment and consideration of the roles, customs, and traditions within the family system (Clark et al. 2009). Without this information, the psychotherapist can easily misinterpret the behavior of the family. This fragments the working alliance, as the family will react by feeling misunderstood and possibly mistreated.

The relatives' current emotions and behaviors are also often shaped by prior experiences with health-care professionals, which then either bolster or contaminate the current relationship. For example, sometimes health-care professionals feel threatened addressing complex issues about the patient's health issues. They can then inadvertently avoid, dismiss, or exclude the family (Jackson and Manchester 2001). The family then feels that the advice they have received is inadequate, incorrect, or withheld (Jackson and Manchester 2001). Alternatively, the family's chaotic schedules may preclude the time or benefits from training (Jackson and Manchester 2001), which taints the working alliance.

Another major challenge to the development of a positive working alliance with families after brain injury is the psychotherapist or rehabilitation staff functioning as the "bearer of bad news" (Lefebvre and Levert 2006; Simpson et al. 2000). It can be awkward, burdensome, and anxiety provoking for the professional to disclose upsetting news, especially when there is such uncertainty and initial shock value to the information (Lefebvre and Levert 2006; Lefebvre et al. 2005). Health-care professionals and psychotherapists can be unprepared and overwhelmed by the families' reactions, which are often unpredictable and laden with grief and/or anger (Jackson and Manchester 2001; Lefebvre and Levert 2006).

Clearly, the psychotherapist must share feedback in "bite-sized pieces," which can be digested by highly distressed family members. The psychotherapist must be savvy in this realm of uncertainty, and at the same time, provide comfort and validate the family's myriad of emotions. The relatives' vulnerable state should predispose the psychotherapist to avoid conflicts, which will add unnecessary stress (Verhaeghe et al. 2005).

Unfortunately, sometimes adverse circumstances preempt the attempts of the psychotherapist to establish a positive working alliance with the family. One example is significant disharmony within key family relationships, including married partners. The therapist's careful inquiry often reveals preexisting marital and/or broader family friction, which is now markedly exacerbated by the effects of the brain injury. This level of turmoil can greatly strain the development and maintenance of a stable working relationship with the dissenting spouse or relatives, who may feel ambivalent about their loved one with the injury, as well as the overall therapeutic process. To cultivate the working alliance, the therapist will need to be attuned to the complex entity of an unstable family, with many "moving parts," specifically, uncertainty in the support system, fluctuating goals, and polarized perceptions between various family members (Webster et al. 1999; see Chap. 3, Sect. 3.1.1 for more discussion).

Lefebvre and colleagues (Lefebvre and Levert 2006; Lefebvre et al. 2005, 2007) and Sohlberg and others (Sohlberg et al. 2001) have emphasized the importance of mutual exchange and respect, as well as a partnership approach in fostering a collaborative relationship with family members. The treating therapist must remember that the family has the "upper hand" in historical knowledge about the loved one (Sherwin and O'Shanick 2000) and must be watchful not to fall folly to a power struggle centered on "who knows best." This means the psychotherapist (and interdisciplinary team) "join" the support network and create a climate of trust, concern, respect, candor, reflective listening, and teamwork using nonjudgmental and sophisticated communication skills (Klonoff 2010, 2013; Kreutzer et al. 2010). This promotes empathy for the emotional upheaval which families are thrust into (Lefebvre et al. 2007) and validates their distress as understandable to their predicament, rather than their shortcomings (Kreutzer et al. 2010).

The therapist should proffer information which explains treatment interventions and is applicable to the family's immediate concerns about the impact of the injury on daily life and longer-term prognosis. Also, strategies for caregivers, review of possible financial repercussions, and available community resources in the context of an upbeat positive focus will contribute maximally to a collaborative working relationship (Lefebvre et al. 2008). Incorporating families as "co-therapists" also maximizes the likelihood that patients will adopt compensations and achieve therapeutic goals (McKinlay and Hickox 1988). Ultimately, through a consensus approach (also including the patient), the family is assisted in the quest for solutions, as well as in rebuilding their confidence and autonomy to manage their daily lives and determine their own future life goals (Lefebvre et al. 2007).

McLaughlin and Carey (1993) have developed a number of guidelines to further nurture a positive working alliance between the treatment team and family members, including prioritizing families' interests and needs; providing support and education in the context of the family's readiness; adherence to realism (versus extreme pessimism or optimism); regular communication, including clarification of outcome expectations; and recognition of the same mutual goals between all parties, namely the rehabilitation of the patient. In addition, the treatment staff's realization that adversarial relationships are at times inevitable (especially in the highly stressed families with more damaged loved ones) will sustain the sometimes precarious working alliance. Overall, to the extent that intervention approaches are flexible, proactive, health- and prevention-oriented, as well as responsive to the families' needs, the working alliance will be bolstered (Kay and Cavallo 1994).

2.4.1.1 Believe in and Trust the Process

Understandably, family members usually find the psychotherapy and neurorehabilitation process confusing and daunting. Their sense of helplessness is exacerbated by the bombardment of ever-changing phases of the recovery and rehabilitation process for themselves and their loved one, including new therapists in each stage of the treatment process (e.g., acute hospital, inpatient rehabilitation, outpatient therapies, etc.). To the extent that the psychotherapist and interdisciplinary team provide written materials which depict the expectations for family members and an overview of the treatment philosophy, family members will feel more "grounded" in the unfolding process. Figure 2.3 is an example of a "Welcome Letter" which can be shared with family members (and patients) to help acquaint them with the holistic milieu-oriented therapy process they are about to embark upon.

To quell some of the family's dismay and perturbation, I share the mantra to "trust the process" (R. Robles, personal communication, n.d.) and couch this in a small clinical vignette: A few years back, this patient's mother entered the rehabilitation and psychotherapy process with much skepticism and angst. With time, she came to see the value of the holistic treatment and appreciated the many facets of the rehabilitation process for her son and herself. She coined the phrase "trust the process" to illustrate how her belief in the therapy practices evolved and also spearheaded its inclusion as part of the treatment program's vernacular. This included frequent visits to family groups as a "program graduate" to encourage new members in their meandering rehabilitation journey.

Similarly, the adage "patience, trust, and collaboration" (Klonoff 2010) anchors family members and sets the stage for an often extended, intensive, and convoluted therapeutic process, steeped in dialogue, cooperation, and persistence for all parties. The film, *The King's Speech* (Brett et al. 2010) eloquently depicts these principles and is an excellent therapeutic tool.

2.4.1.2 Content, Timing, Pacing, and Documentation of Psychotherapeutic Interpretations

Given the adverse and disturbing nature of some of the feedback to family members about the aftereffects of brain injury, it is vital for the therapist to carefully monitor the content, pacing, and timing of information, feedback, and interpretations, especially early on in the working alliance or when family members are feeling overwhelmed, irate, or vulnerable. The shared knowledge should: be informative and pragmatic; match the relatives' needs and concerns (Lefebvre et al. 2008; Yeates et al. 2007); and be predicated on a comprehensive analysis of the demeanor, knowledge base, and emotional readiness of the relatives, so as to be consonant with their sensitivities.

The psychotherapist should be wary of the timing of upsetting information that is perceived by the relatives as overly critical or gloomy; conversely, the disclosures need to occur in an opportune fashion so that the concerned parties can make educated and realistic decisions (Kay and Cavallo 1994; Klonoff 2010). This includes addressing possible misconceptions (based on insufficient input from professionals, misleading depictions in the media, or the relatives' difficulties processing complex material during crises), which will derail the family (and their loved one) in their rehabilitation process (Smith and Godfrey 1995; Springer et al. 1997). Common caregiver misperceptions include: lack of appreciation of the long-term effects of brain injury; unawareness of the diversity of cognitive and behavioral problems; visible or invisible disabilities causing unrealistic expectations; and misidentification of the behavioral problems after brain injury as indicative of a mental health problem

To Our New CTN Patients and Families February 18, 2013

Welcome to the Center for Transitional NeuroRehabilitation (CTN)! The following information will acquaint you with the approach and philosophy of treatment at the CTN.

1. You will be participating in a "milieu" setting. This is a French term for "community." The CTN operates as a small therapeutic community, where social reintegration and mutual support are emphasized. As a participant, you will receive not only individual therapies, but group-oriented therapies that simulate productive functioning in the family, community, and work/school environments.

2. The therapy approach at CTN is holistic; all aspects of your recovery will be addressed, including the cognitive, physical, language, emotional, and interpersonal domains. Your treatment needs will be determined (with input from you and your family) based on the evaluations you will go through during the first 2-3 weeks of program participation. You will undergo evaluations in the areas of Neuropsychology, Speech-Language Therapy (ST), Physical Therapy (PT), and Occupational Therapy (OT), including the area of work. The Recreational Therapist (RT) will meet with you and conduct an interview about your hobbies and leisure interests. You may also be seen by the dietician and/or psychiatrist, based on your needs.

   During the evaluation phase, the number of treatment sessions is less until the testing is completed. Essential therapies to prevent neurological decline will be incorporated to continue to facilitate the healing process.

3. When the treatment phase intensifies, you can generally expect 2-4 individual treatment sessions in each discipline (e.g., Psychotherapy, OT, PT, ST, RT) per week. Individual treatment needs will be supported by group-oriented therapies (e.g., Current Events, Cognitive Group, Motor Group, Therapeutic Balance and Stretching Groups, Upper Extremity Group, Vocational Group, and Community Outings). The specifics of your treatment (e.g., the frequency of individual sessions and group therapies) are evaluated on an ongoing basis and will also incorporate your and your family's input.

4. The program emphasizes functionality: every activity you do enhances recovery. Like in the movie, *The Karate Kid* (Weintraub et al. 1984), day to day activities (e.g., dressing, laundry, and kitchen chores) stimulate brain function and recovery. The more you do to enhance your independence with functional tasks, the better your recovery and quality of life will be. To help improve your functioning in the home and community, the OT will do a home visit with you and a family member within the first 2-3 weeks of the program. Additional home visits will occur on a regular basis (usually weekly) if you are in the Home Independence Program. Of note, you and your family should meet with the PT and OT to determine the type and extent of activities you do in and outside of the program that might lead to over- or under-exertion.

5. To improve your level of independent functioning, the CTN program emphasizes the use of compensatory strategies, such as a datebook or electronic system. The OT and/or ST will help you implement this system. Do not buy a system until the therapist provides you with the best resource. Procedural checklists at home, and likely at work, will also be incorporated as part of your treatment at CTN.

6. Program research has shown that the role of family in your recovery is integral in the recovery and rehabilitation process. Family members are required to participate in the milieu treatment approach. The best and most efficient mode of communication with family members is the weekly Family Group. During this group, family members will receive education, emotional support (in the form of a support group), and weekly updates from specific therapists. If family members cannot attend this group, they need to notify the Clinical Director, Dr. Klonoff. Individual meetings with the family

Fig. 2.3 Sample welcome letter about holistic treatment

members (also involving you in conjoint meetings) and attendance at Relatives' Day are other valuable resources. Lack of attendance or fragmented communication between the therapists and family can result in probation or termination of treatment.

7. Clinical experience and CTN research has shown that a positive working alliance with you and your family is integral for the best rehabilitation experience and ultimate outcome (e.g., return to school and/or work). We define the working alliance as a positive relationship with the staff (trust; acceptance; mutual respect; and open, honest communication); the use of rehabilitation tools (e.g., scores from follow through with memory assignments; Home Independence Checklist scores; homework follow through); and the setting and accomplishment of realistic, attainable goals (e.g., living alone; driving; medication management; appropriate school courses and/or career/work placement) (Bordin, 1979). Your Clinical Neuropsychologist will take the lead in communicating how the working alliance with you and your family is perceived. At the time of the Initial Program Summary and every month thereafter, all parties will rate their perceptions of the working alliance. Of note, significant and/or chronic problems with the working alliance which affect your progress, or positive interactions with family, or a disruptive milieu experience for others will be grounds for probationary status and for discharge. This includes two consecutive months of a staff rating of "needs work" for you and/or your family.

8. Confidentiality:

   At the time of your admission, you reviewed and signed paperwork related to the federal government's Health Information Privacy Acknowledgement Act (HIPAA). The information you share with the program will not be released to outside personnel or agencies without a written release (other than HIPAA allowed entities).

   Part of the efficacy and efficiency of the milieu treatment environment is the regular staffing meetings (five per week) held by the team. At these meetings, your progress, challenges, and goals are reviewed to be sure all staff therapists are working in a synchronized manner regarding the rehabilitation goals. This means that there needs to be an open exchange of information between team members. The same principle applies to communication with your family members. Of note, personal information shared with your psychotherapist that does not influence your treatment or recovery will not be shared with the team without your permission.

   If you are uncomfortable with this process of information exchange within this setting, the milieu approach is not a therapeutic "fit" for you. If this is the case, the CTN staff will coordinate efforts to find an alternative, more compatible treatment environment for you.

Feel free to talk with me or your Clinical Neuropsychologist if there are any questions or concerns during your participation at CTN.

Sincerely,

Pamela S. Klonoff, PhD, ABPP
Clinical Director
Center for Transitional NeuroRehabilitation

Received:

Patient:____________________ Family:____________________

(Signature) *(Signature)*

Date: ____________________ Date: ____________________

Fig. 2.3 (continued)

or learning disability (Swift and Wilson 2001). Concrete techniques include presentation of material in user-friendly language (versus technical jargon) and avoiding emotionally alarming feedback at the end of the week, over the telephone, or between intermittent appointments (Klonoff 2010). Encouraging family members to take notes during psychoeducational sessions and at doctors' appointments helps them keep a coherent written record of salient events which they can consult as needed.

2.4.1.3 Empathy for the "No Win" Situation

The psychotherapist fosters a climate of empathy by validating the primary caregiver's torment when forced into the seemingly thankless role of a "pseudotherapist." The caregiver is unwontedly catapulted from a position of mutual sharing into the role of an authoritative figure who feels compelled to provide endless constructive feedback to a loved one, who because of his or her own suffering, reacts with hostility. This can escalate into the loved one expressing resentment or rage toward the family member, eroding these crucial relationships. The psychotherapist should validate the family member's predicament by volunteering to shoulder the responsibility of voicing hard-to-hear feedback and ideas. This provides relief to the family member, who can more comfortably recede into the role of the supportive ally to their loved one. To this end, I often encourage family members to use the therapist as the "bad guy" when constructive feedback is shared in the home or community environment. A case in point, when the patient is fuming about restrictions related to supervision in the home and/or driving, the caregiver can take the position of "only following the doctor's orders." This allows the caregiver to join in the understandable frustrations of the situation, so as not to be scapegoated by the patient.

A second scenario is the family's consternation when the patient enthusiastically embraces a suggestion from the therapist and expresses rapture at his or her extraordinary talent and expertise, when in fact the family member has made the identical recommendations countless times previously, but to no avail. This adds to the family's feelings of hurt, helplessness, and ineptness and can breed annoyance with the therapist. It is paramount for the therapist to validate the family efforts and insights and empathically convey the reality that "it is only a matter of time" until the tide turns and the patient reacts just as negatively to the therapist. This helps the family avoid personalizing unpleasant or dismissive behavior, thereby bolstering their self-esteem and bond with the psychotherapeutic process.

2.4.1.4 "Red Flags"

Certain behaviors in the caregiver and/or families serve to undermine the development of a healthy working alliance with the psychotherapist and other treating staff (see Chap. 3, Sect. 3.1.1 for more discussion). One example is the tendency on the part of some family members to want to "keep secrets" from their loved one or from other family members. This can result in a splitting phenomenon, whereby certain team members are put in the position of "taking sides," based on the tumult and conflict within the family. This is likely to happen when there are quarrels or communication impasses within the family system or when there is a family breakdown (e.g., separation or divorce; Webster et al. 1999). The psychotherapist and treating therapists should be wary in this regard, especially if withholding information is detrimental to the primary patient's overall needs and progress.

Another problematic scenario is interaction patterns between the psychotherapist and family members which are characterized by intense animosity or provoking behavior. Often, this acrimony is targeted toward a specific member(s) of the therapy team, which can further fragment team efforts. Rage reactions toward therapists can also represent scapegoating behavior secondary to extremely high levels of emotional anguish or disturbance in the relatives (Klonoff and Koberstein 2010).

The psychotherapist and overall treatment team should create an ambience of containment of these forceful emotions and counterproductive behaviors, also including healthy constraints and limit setting (Book et al. 1978; Henry 2010). For the "secret keeper," the parameters and expectations for dialogue and confidentiality should be reviewed in written form to protect the working alliance (see Sect. 2.1 and Figs. 2.1 and 2.3). This will clarify for the instigator the importance of open and inclusive exchanges, so as to maintain the integrity of collaborative efforts. Similarly, the psychotherapist and other therapists should set requirements for two-way interactions that are respectful and cooperative versus aggressive or destructive to the therapeutic process. If necessary, the psychotherapist and treatment team may need to discontinue services based on their ethical obligation to not compromise their professional judgment and capacity to do their job, based on a relative's abusive or disruptive behavior (W. Sammons, personal communication, n.d.). These agreed-upon "rules," in combination with setting clear boundaries and conditions with which to work with the family, minimize ruptures in the working alliance and maximize accomplishment of treatment goals for all parties (Klonoff 2011; Webster et al. 1999).

2.4.1.5 Multimedia Techniques

The psychotherapist should integrate all possible "tools in the tool kit." This constitutes eclectic and creative intervention techniques to best reach the diverse population of family members and their overall support networks, thereby solidifying the working alliance. This is especially critical, given varying levels of life experience, education, and cultural backgrounds. Helpful techniques include simplified graphs and diagrams. For instance, a depiction of the bell curve, with labeled deficits according to impairment levels, is worthwhile when reviewing neuropsychological testing, to help families (and their loved ones) assimilate this complex data (Klonoff 2010; see Chap. 4, Sect. 4.2.1). Similarly, brain models (Smith and Godfrey 1995) and computerized three-dimensional renditions of the brain are effective for education about brain anatomy.

The therapist can refer to relevant and personalized metaphors, slogans, mantras, proverbs, and autobiographical writings by other families combating the repercussions of a brain injury. These provide refreshing and palatable input, which can function as "transitional objects" during taxing times. Pie charts and lists of pros and cons help families with complicated decisions (Klonoff 2010). Other multimedia outlets, including YouTube videos, fables, literature, movies, and short films are alternate meaningful, nontechnical vehicles for the psychotherapist to illustrate essential principles for the caregiver and other tier supports.

2.4.2 *Pervasive Themes*

The following constructs represent common themes conveyed by family members after brain injury, regardless of injury etiology, chronicity, or symptomatology.

2.4.2.1 Catastrophic Reactions by Proxy

A preponderant by-product of increased awareness in relatives after brain injury is catastrophic reactions (CRs) by proxy (Klonoff and Koberstein 2010; Klonoff et al. 2008). These are the counterpart to CRs in the loved one and they are precipitated when the caregiver or any member of the support network witnesses irrefutable evidence of injury-produced ineptitudes in his or her loved one (Klonoff and Koberstein 2010). These may or may not occur concurrently with CRs in the loved one; in fact, often the family becomes agonizingly aware of the disabilities before their loved one does. The similarity emanates from the starkly shared realization of a profound sense of loss (Klonoff et al. 2008). A primary focus of psychotherapy is to provide the necessary empathic support, as well as psychoeducation and coping techniques, to assist the family members in recognizing and dealing with these intense emotions. This is best accomplished in both individual and group-oriented settings, given the universality of the experience (Klonoff and Koberstein 2010).

2.4.2.2 You Always Hurt the One(s) You Love

Families often express chagrin that their family members are on their "best behavior" in the therapy setting, but then come home and unleash negative verbal torrents. Similarly, apathetic patients in the home may be more stimulable in the structured treatment environment, while depressed patients may display a more cheerful demeanor in front of therapists or visitors (Lezak 1988). One way to reassure families is for the psychotherapist to place this discrepancy in the context that because their loved ones feel most comfortable with them, they forfeit possible (and often necessary) internal censors and regulators. This translates to the old saying, "you always hurt the one(s) you love." Also, psychoeducation about the impact of their loved one's physical, emotional, and mental exhaustion at the end of a long treatment day eroding their frustration tolerance and self-control helps the family avoid personalizing the behavior. To the extent that the therapists validate the sometimes disparate descriptions by the family compared with their own clinical observations, relatives will feel heard and affirmed.

2.4.2.3 "Shifting Sands" and "Picking Battles"

Given the totality of the family's responsibilities for the loved one, especially the primary caregiver(s), it is crucial for the therapist to help them establish healthy boundaries when supervising and guiding their loved one. This is a fluid and complicated process, as the role of the family shifts depending on the overall condition and recovery of the loved one and the internal constellation of the family. Certainly in the acute phases of recovery, when the loved one is sickest and most vulnerable, the family's involvement can be pervasive, even including doing basic self-care (e.g., feeding, dressing, bathing, etc.) for their loved one. However, over time, as the patient's functional abilities improve, the family must adapt their style and amount of supervision. Family members can feel overwrought about how to recalibrate their efforts, in the context of rapid health changes in their loved one. Given his or her ever-changing multiple needs, this can feel like "shifting sands" to the relatives. Working closely with treating therapists will be key to helping the family better comprehend and anticipate their loved one's needs, so that they do not become overly protective or meddling.

Similarly, when giving corrective feedback, the family should be encouraged to "pick their battles," so as to best maintain harmony in the relationship and preserve the psychological well-being and emotional resources of all parties. In general, the guiding principle regarding when the family should intervene is the physical and psychological safety of the patient (and others). Postponing input based on the patient's mood, alertness, and receptivity is advisable. Favorable outcomes are most likely when the patient is feeling calm and well rested.

2.4.2.4 Every Cloud Has a Silver Lining

This proverb, when used judiciously by the psychotherapist, helps the primary caregiver and overall support network cogitate about the possible constructive, practical, and existential outgrowths from the suffering induced by the brain injury. Early on, the caregiver and family at large may reframe their traumatic situation as being hugely grateful that their loved one has survived (Wells et al. 2005). This can metamorphose into feeling positive about their competence as caregivers and sharing other positive life experiences through interfacing with caring relatives and friends (Wells et al. 2005). Another manifestation of the "silver lining" maxim is the redefinition of the injury as a "wake-up call" for their loved ones, and even themselves. Subsequently, they translate their current circumstances to a "second chance" for personal betterment (Klonoff 2010). Literally and figuratively speaking, the short film, *Partly Cloudy* (Reher and Sohn 2009) poignantly illustrates this principle, exemplifying the need for adaptability and perseverance.

2.4.2.5 Faith, Hope, and Love

This therapeutic mantra acts as a sustaining thought for family members in the midst of the disarray of life. Faith is a valuable coping mechanism for many families, whereby they find emotional rest and lightening of their emotional load through the belief that God is watching over them (Verhaeghe et al. 2005). Faith has also been defined as the fighting spirit or the will and courage to improve (Linge 1990). An attitude of hope is crucial for the long journey families (and their loved ones) must undertake, especially given the inevitable disappointments and downturns (Linge 1990). Love conquers the feeling of aloneness and nurtures hope (Linge 1990). In our setting, we have a carved wooden plaque of this mantra posted over the entrance doorway to a group treatment room where the family group meets, as a constant uplifting visual reminder.

The next chapter builds upon many of these concepts through an investigation into the impact of brain injuries on various configurations within the family system.

References

Blake, H. (2008). Caregiver stress in traumatic brain injury. *International Journal of Therapy & Rehabilitation, 15*(6), 263–271.

Book, H. E., Sadavoy, J., & Silver, D. (1978). Staff countertransference to borderline patients on an inpatient unit. *American Journal of Psychotherapy, 32*(4), 521–532.

Bordin, E. S. (1979). The generalizability of the psychoanalytic concept of the working alliance. *Psychotherapy: Theory, Research & Practice, 16*(3), 252–260.

Boss, P. (2006). *Loss, trauma, and resilience: Therapeutic work with ambiguous loss*. New York: W. W. Norton.

Boss, P., Roos, S., & Harris, D. L. (2011). Grief in the midst of ambiguity and uncertainty: An exploration of ambiguous loss and chronic sorrow. In R. A. Neimeyer, D. L. Harris, H. R. Winokuer, & G. F. Thornton (Eds.), *Grief and bereavement in contemporary society: Bridging research and practice* (pp. 163–175). New York: Routledge.

Brett, P., Canning, I., Dorfman, C., Egan, S., Foligno, M., Heslop, P., et al. (Producers), & Hooper, T. (Director). (2010). *The king's speech* [Motion picture]. United States: The Weinstein Company.

Buchholz, W. M. (1990). A piece of my mind: Hope. *JAMA: The Journal of the American Medical Association, 263*(17), 2357–2358.

Chwalisz, K. (1992). Perceived stress and caregiver burden after brain injury: A theoretical integration. *Rehabilitation Psychology, 37*(3), 189–203.

Chwalisz, K., & Kisler, V. (1995). Perceived stress: A better measure of caregiver burden. *Measurement & Evaluation in Counseling & Development, 28*(2), 88–98.

Clark, C., Brown, J., Bailey, C., & Hutchinson, P. (2009). Supporting families in the context of adult traumatic brain injury. *British Journal of Neuroscience Nursing, 5*(5), 216–220.

Clarke, D. M., & Kissane, D. W. (2002). Demoralization: Its phenomenology and importance. *Australian & New Zealand Journal of Psychiatry, 36*(6), 733–742.

Collins, L. G., & Swartz, K. (2011). Caregiver care. *American Academy of Family Physicians, 83*(11), 1309–1317.

Corr, C. A. (2002). Coping with challenges to assumptive worlds. In J. Kauffman (Ed.), *Loss of the assumptive world: A theory of traumatic loss* (pp. 127–138). New York: Brunner-Routledge.

Davis, J. R., Gemeinhardt, M., Gan, C., Anstey, K., & Gargaro, J. (2003). Crisis and its assessment after brain injury. *Brain Injury, 17*(5), 359–376.

Degeneffe, C. E. (2001). Family caregiving and traumatic brain injury. *Health and Social Work, 26*(4), 257–268.

Dell Orto, A. E., & Power, P. W. (2000). *Brain injury and the family: A life and living perspective* (2nd ed.). Boca Raton: CRC Press.

Engel, G. L. (1968). A life setting conducive to illness. *Annals of Internal Medicine, 69*(2), 293–300.

Fengler, A. P., & Goodrich, N. (1979). Wives of elderly disabled men: The hidden patients. *The Gerontologist, 19*(2), 175–183.

Frosch, S., Gruber, A., Jones, C., Myers, S., Noel, E., Westerlund, A., & Zavisin, T. (1997). The long term effects of traumatic brain injury on the roles of caregivers. *Brain Injury, 11*(12), 891–906.

Gan, C., Campbell, K. A., Gemeinhardt, M., & McFadden, G. T. (2006). Predictors of family system functioning after brain injury. *Brain Injury, 20*(6), 587–600.

Hanks, R. A., Rapport, L. J., & Vangel, S. (2007). Caregiving appraisal after traumatic brain injury: The effects of functional status, coping style, social support and family functioning. *NeuroRehabilitation, 22*(1), 43–52.

Harris, J. K. J., Godfrey, H. P. D., Partridge, F. M., & Knight, R. G. (2001). Caregiver depression following traumatic brain injury (TBI): A consequence of adverse effects on family members? *Brain Injury, 15*(3), 223–238.

Hein, P. (2003). T. T. T. In *PoemHunter.com*, poems by Piet Hein. http://www.poemhunter.com/poem/t-t-t/. Accessed 3 July 2011.

Henry, C. (2010). Aggression, containment, and treatment enactments in the psychodynamics of limit setting. *Journal of the American Academy of Psychoanalysis and Dynamic Psychiatry, 38*(2), 341–356.

Hoofien, D., Gilboa, A., Vakil, E., & Donovick, P. J. (2001). Traumatic brain injury (TBI) 10–20 years later: A comprehensive outcome study of psychiatric symptomatology, cognitive abilities and psychosocial functioning. *Brain Injury, 15*(3), 189–209.

Inzaghi, M. G., De Tanti, A., & Sozzi, M. (2005). The effects of traumatic brain injury on patients and their families: A follow-up study. *Europa Medicophysica, 41*(4), 265–273.

Jackson, D., Turner-Stokes, L., Murray, J., Leese, M., & McPherson, K. M. (2009). Acquired brain injury and dementia: A comparison of carer experiences. *Brain Injury, 23*(5), 433–444.

Jackson, H., & Manchester, D. (2001). Towards the development of brain injury specialists. *NeuroRehabilitation, 16*(1), 27–40.

Johnson, J., & McCown, W. (1997). *Family therapy of neurobehavioral disorders: Integrating neuropsychology and family therapy*. New York: Haworth Press.

Judd, T. (1999). *Neuropsychotherapy and community integration: Brain illness, emotions and behavior*. New York: Kluwer Academic/Plenum Publishers.

Kao, H. F. S., & Stuifbergen, A. K. (2004). Love and load-the lived experience of the mother-child relationship among young adult traumatic brain-injured survivors. *Journal of Neuroscience Nursing, 36*(2), 73–81.

Kay, T., & Cavallo, M. M. (1994). The family system: Impact, assessment, and intervention. In J. M. Siver, S. C. Yudofsky, & R. E. Hales (Eds.), *Neuropsychiatry of traumatic brain injury* (pp. 533–567). Washington, D. C.: American Psychiatric Press.

Klonoff, P. S. (2010). *Psychotherapy after brain injury: Principles and techniques*. New York: Guilford Press.

Klonoff, P. S. (2011). A therapist experiential model of treatment for brain injury. *Bulletin of the Menninger Clinic, 75*(1), 21–45.

Klonoff, P. S. (2013). Internal and team attributes for effective psychotherapy after brain injury. In C. A. Noggle & R. S. Dean (Eds.), *Neuropsychological Rehabilitation*. New York: Springer.

Klonoff, P. S., & Koberstein, E. J. (2010). Family life. In P. S. Klonoff (Ed.), *Psychotherapy after brain injury: Principles and techniques* (pp. 150–170). New York: Guilford Press.

Klonoff, P. S., & Myles, S. M. (2010). Sense of self and identity. In P. S. Klonoff (Ed.), *Psychotherapy after brain injury: Principles and techniques* (pp. 75–99). New York: Guilford Press.

Klonoff, P. S., Koberstein, E. J., Talley, M. C., & Dawson, L. K. (2008). A family experiential model of recovery after brain injury. *Bulletin of the Menninger Clinic, 72*(2), 109–129.

Knight, R. G., Devereux, R., & Godfrey, H. P. D. (1998). Caring for a family member with a traumatic brain injury. *Brain Injury, 12*(6), 467–481.

Kreutzer, J. S., Gervasio, A. H., & Camplair, P. S. (1994). Primary caregivers' psychological status and family functioning after traumatic brain injury. *Brain Injury, 8*(3), 197–210.

Kreutzer, J. S., Kolakowsky-Hayner, S. A., Demm, S. R., & Meade, M. A. (2002). A structured approach to family intervention after brain injury. *Journal of Head Trauma Rehabilitation, 17*(4), 349–367.

Kreutzer, J. S., Marwitz, J. H., Godwin, E. E., & Arango-Lasprilla, J. C. (2010). Practical approaches to effective family intervention after brain injury. *Journal of Head Trauma Rehabilitation, 25*(2), 113–120.

Landsman, I. S. (2002). Crises of meaning in trauma and loss. In J. Kauffman (Ed.), *Loss of the assumptive world: A theory of traumatic loss* (pp. 13–30). New York: Brunner-Routledge.

Leathem, J., Heath, E., & Woolley, C. (1996). Relatives' perceptions of role change, social support and stress after traumatic brain injury. *Brain Injury, 10*(1), 27–38.

Lefebvre, H., & Levert, M. J. (2006). Breaking the news of traumatic brain injury and incapacities. *Brain Injury, 20*(7), 711–718.

Lefebvre, H., Pelchat, D., Swaine, B., Gelinas, I., & Levert, M. J. (2005). The experiences of individuals with a traumatic brain injury, families, physicians and health professionals regarding care provided throughout the continuum. *Brain Injury, 19*(8), 585–597.

Lefebvre, H., Pelchat, D., & Levert, M. J. (2007). Interdisciplinary family intervention program: A partnership among health professionals, traumatic brain injury patients, and caregiving relatives. *Journal of Trauma Nursing, 14*(2), 100–113.

Lefebvre, H., Levert, M. J., Pelchat, D., & Lepage, J. G. (2008). Nature, sources, and impact of information on the adjustment of family caregivers: A pilot project. *Canadian Journal of Nursing Research, 40*(1), 143–160.

Lezak, M. D. (1986). Psychological implications of traumatic brain damage for the patient's family. *Rehabilitation Psychology, 31*(4), 241–250.

Lezak, M. D. (1988). Brain damage is a family affair. *Journal of Clinical and Experimental Neuropsychology, 10*(1), 111–123.

Linge, F. R. (1990). Faith, hope, and love: Nontraditional therapy in recovery from serious head injury, a personal account. *Canadian Journal of Psychology, 44*(2), 116–129.

Livingston, L. A., Kennedy, R. E., Marwitz, J. H., Arango-Lasprilla, J. C., Rapport, L. J., Bushnik, T., & Gary, K. W. (2010). Predictors of family caregivers' caregivers' life satisfaction after traumatic brain injury at one and two years post-injury: A longitudinal multi-center investigation. *NeuroRehabilitation, 27*(1), 73–81.

Machamer, J., Temkin, N., & Dikmen, S. (2002). Significant other burden and factors related to it in traumatic brain injury. *Journal of Clinical and Experimental Neuropsychology, 24*(4), 420–433.

Man, D. W. K. (2002). Family caregivers' caregivers' reactions and coping for persons with brain injury. *Brain Injury, 16*(12), 1025–1037.

Marsh, N. V., Kersel, D. A., Havill, J. H., & Sleigh, J. W. (1998). Caregiver burden at 1 year following severe traumatic brain injury. *Brain Injury, 12*(12), 1045–1059.

Marsh, N. V., Kersel, D. A., Havill, J. H., & Sleigh, J. W. (2002). Caregiver burden during the year following severe traumatic brain injury. *Journal of Clinical and Experimental Neuropsychology, 24*(4), 434–447.

Marwit, S. J., & Kaye, P. N. (2006). Measuring grief in caregivers of persons with acquired brain injury. *Brain Injury, 20*(13–14), 1419–1429.

McAlaster, R., Lundgren, G., & Higa, C. (2004). *Brain injury: A guide for families* (2nd ed.). Houston: HDI Publishers.

McKinlay, W. W., & Hickox, A. (1988). How can families help in the rehabilitation of the head injured? *Journal of Head Trauma Rehabilitation, 3*(4), 64–72.

McLaughlin, A. M., & Carey, J. L. (1993). The adversarial alliance: Developing therapeutic relationships between families and the team in brain injury rehabilitation. *Brian Injury, 7*(1), 45–51.

Myles, S. M. (2007, Feb). Changes to sense-of-self post-brain injury: Research and treatment. Paper presented at the 35th Annual Meeting of the International Neuropsychological Society (Continuing Education Program), Portland, OR.

Nabors, N., Seacat, J., & Rosenthal, M. (2002). Predictors of caregiver burden following traumatic brain injury. *Brain Injury, 16*(12), 1039–1050.

Novack, T. A., & Richards, J. S. (1991). Coping with denial among family members. *Archives of Physical Medicine and Rehabilitation, 72*(7), 521.

Perakis, C. R. (2010). Soul sickness: A frequently missed diagnosis. *Journal of the American Osteopathic Association, 110*(6), 347–349.

Perlesz, A., Kinsella, G., & Crowe, S. (1999). Impact of traumatic brain injury on the family: A critical review. *Rehabilitation Psychology, 44*(1), 6–35.

Ponsford, J., Olver, J., Ponsford, M., & Nelms, R. (2003). Long-term adjustment of families following traumatic brain injury where comprehensive rehabilitation has been provided. *Brain Injury, 17*(6), 453–468.

Prigatano, G. P., Fordyce, D. J., Zeiner, H. K., Roueche, J. R., Pepping, M., & Wood, B. C. (1986). *Neuropsychological rehabilitation after brain injury*. Baltimore: The Johns Hopkins University Press.

Reher, K. (Producer), & Sohn, P. (Director). (2009). *Partly cloudy* [Short motion picture]. United States: Pixar Animation Studios.

Riley, G. A. (2007). Stress and depression in family carers following traumatic brain injury: The influence of beliefs about difficult behaviours. *Clinical Rehabilitation, 21*(1), 82–88.

Rivera, P., Elliott, T. R., Berry, J. W., Grant, J. S., & Oswald, K. (2007). Predictors of caregiver depression among community-residing families living with traumatic brain injury. *NeuroRehabilitation, 22*(1), 3–8.

Romano, M. D. (1974). Family response to traumatic head injury. *Scandinavian Journal of Rehabilitation Medicine, 6*(1), 1–4.

Roos, S. (2002). *Chronic sorrow: A living loss*. New York: Brunner-Routledge.

Rosenthal, M., & Young, T. (1988). Effective family intervention after traumatic brain injury: Theory and practice. *Journal of Head Trauma Rehabilitation, 3*(4), 42–50.

Saban, K. L., Sherwood, P. R., DeVon, H. A., & Hynes, D. M. (2010). Measures of psychological stress and physical health in family caregivers of stroke survivors: A literature review. *Journal of Neuroscience Nursing, 42*(3), 128–138.

Sachs, P. R. (1991). *Treating families of brain injury survivors*. New York: Springer.

Schonberger, M., Ponsford, J., Olver, J., & Ponsford, M. (2010). A longitudinal study of family functioning after TBI and relatives' relatives' emotional status. *Neuropsychological Rehabilitation, 20*(6), 813–829.

Sherwin, E. D., & O'Shanick, G. J. (2000). The trauma of paediatric and adolescent brain injury: Issues and implications for rehabilitation specialists. *Brain Injury, 14*(3), 267–284.

Siegert, R. J., Jackson, D. M., Tennant, A., & Turner-Stokes, L. (2010). Factor analysis and Rasch analysis of the Zarit Burden Interview for acquired brain injury carer research. *Journal of Rehabilitative Medicine, 42*(4), 302–309.

Simpson, G., Mohr, R., & Redman, A. (2000). Cultural variations in the understanding of traumatic brain injury and brain injury rehabilitation. *Brain Injury, 14*(2), 125–140.

Smith, L. M., & Godfrey, H. P. D. (1995). *Family support programs and rehabilitation: A cognitive-behavioral approach to traumatic brain injury*. New York: Plenum Press.

Sohlberg, M. K. M., McLaughlin, K. A. M., Todis, B., Larsen, J., & Glang, A. (2001). What does it take to collaborate with families affected by brain injury? A preliminary model. *Journal of Head Trauma Rehabilitation, 16*(5), 498–511.

Springer, J. A., Farmer, J. E., & Bouman, D. E. (1997). Common misconceptions about traumatic brain injury among family members of rehabilitation patients. *Journal of Head Trauma Rehabilitation, 12*(3), 41–50.

Stebbins, P., & Pakenham, K. I. (2001). Irrational schematic beliefs and psychological distress in caregivers of people with traumatic brain injury. *Rehabilitation Psychology, 46*(2), 178–194.

Swift, T. L., & Wilson, S. L. (2001). Misconceptions about brain injury among the general public and non-expert health professionals: An exploratory study. *Brain Injury, 15*(2), 149–165.

Testani-Dufour, L., Chappel-Aiken, L., & Gueldner, S. (1992). Traumatic brain injury: A family experience. *Journal of Neuroscience Nursing, 24*(6), 317–323.

Turner, B., Fleming, J., Cornwell, P., Worrall, L., Ownsworth, T., Haines, T., et al. (2007). A qualitative study of the transition from hospital to home for individuals with acquired brain injury and their family caregivers. *Brain Injury, 21*(11), 1119–1130.

Turner, B., Fleming, J., Parry, J., Vromans, M., Cornwell, P., Gordon, C., & Ownsworth, T. (2010). Caregivers of adults with traumatic brain injury: The emotional impact of transition from hospital to home. *Brain Impairment, 11*(3), 281–292.

Verhaeghe, S., Defloor, T., & Grypdonck, M. (2005). Stress and coping among families of patients with traumatic brain injury: A review of the literature. *Journal of Clinical Nursing, 14*(8), 1004–1012.

Visser-Meily, J. M. A., Post, M. W. M., Riphagen, I. I., & Lindeman, E. (2004). Measures used to assess burden among caregivers of stroke patients: A review. *Clinical Rehabilitation, 18*(6), 601–623.

Webster, G., Daisley, A., & King, N. (1999). Relationship and family breakdown following acquired brain injury: The role of the rehabilitation team. *Brain Injury, 13*(8), 593–603.

Weintraub, J., Louis, R., Smith, B., (Producers), & Avildsen, J. (Director). (1984). *The karate kid* [Motion picture]. United States: Columbia Pictures.

Wells, R., Dywan, J., & Dumas, J. (2005). Life satisfaction and distress in family caregivers as related to specific behavioural changes after traumatic brain injury. *Brain Injury, 19*(13), 1105–1115.

Williams, J. M. (1991). Family support. In J. M. Williams & T. Kay (Eds.), *Head injury: A family matter* (pp. 299–312). Baltimore: Brookes Publishing.

Wongvatunyu, S., & Porter, E. J. (2008). Changes in family life perceived by mothers of young adult TBI survivors. *Journal of Family Nursing, 14*(3), 314–332.

Yeates, G., Henwood, K., Gracey, F., & Evans, J. (2007). Awareness of disability after acquired brain injury and the family context. *Neuropsychological Rehabilitation, 17*(2), 151–173.

Zinner, E. S., Ball, J. D., Stutts, M. L., & Philput, C. (1997). Grief reactions of mothers of adolescents and young adults with traumatic brain injury. *Archives of Clinical Neuropsychology, 12*(5), 435–447.

Chapter 3
The Impact of Brain Injury on Different Family Members

3.1 Scenario: General Considerations about the Impact of Brain Injury on the Family System

Brain injury in a loved one causes profound reverberations, crises, and upheaval throughout the entire family unit, affecting often the immediate (i.e., tier 1) and extended (i.e., tiers 2 and 3) family (Cavallo and Kay 2011; David 1998; Klonoff and Koberstein 2010; Perlesz et al. 2000; Verhaeghe et al. 2005). Emotional distress manifests as depression, anxiety, anger, and loneliness (see Klonoff and Koberstein 2010, for a review; Norup et al. 2010; Perlesz et al. 2000). Relatives may ask questions such as: *What has happened to our family? Why are things so different? When will life get "back to normal?"*

3.1.1 Addressing the Needs of Families Based on their Psychological Health

It is a safe conclusion that all families struggle mightily with the aftermath of a brain injury in a loved one. However, the process varies according to the family's overall psychological health. Figure 3.1 depicts a proposed model of the family/support network's psychological health when a loved one has sustained a brain injury. This can be conceptualized on a continuum ranging from "healthy" to "difficult" to "dysfunctional" patterns. Salient attributes within both the family system itself and the psychotherapy/treatment process (e.g., the working alliance) also span a spectrum. One category is personality or *structural components:* trust/distrust; compassionate/egocentric; agreeable/disagreeable; good/poor boundaries; cohesive/fragmented; and resilient/fragile. The other is *therapeutic process components*: engaged/disconnected; receptive/resistant; patient/impatient; flexible/rigid; collaborative/adversarial; and realistic/unrealistic. Table 3.1 describes some examples of manifestations of these qualities within both the family dynamics and the therapeutic arena, based on sample verbalizations.

P. S. Klonoff, S. Rumble, *Psychotherapy for Families after Brain Injury*,
DOI 10.1007/978-1-4899-8083-0_3, © Springer Science+Business Media New York 2014

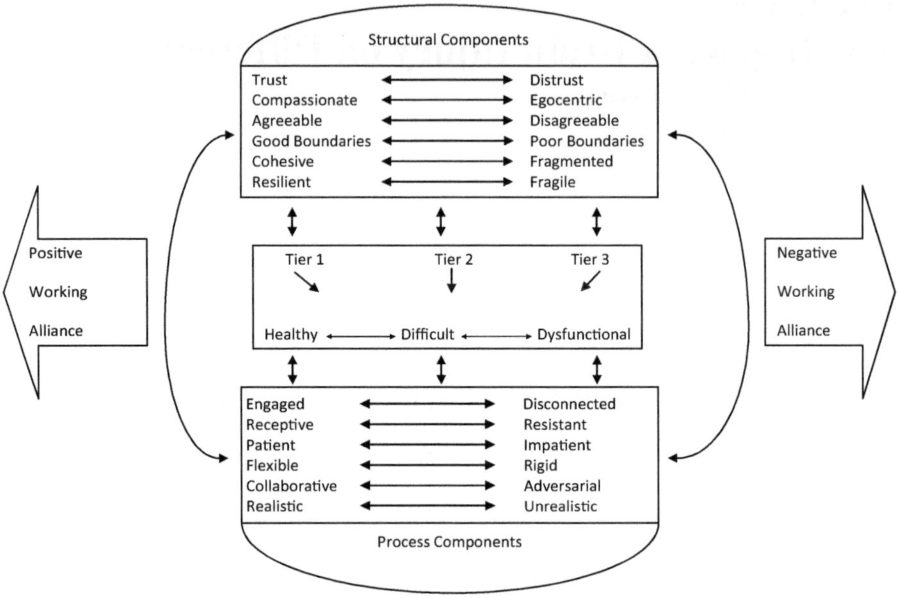

Fig. 3.1 Model of the family/support network's psychological health after brain injury

The degree of overall family health versus dysfunction is based on the relative amount of vigor in each contributing attribute within each family member, which then fuses to impact and shape the family system. This fashions a global and distinctive family constellation of strengths and difficulties. The model emphasizes plasticity rather than compartmentalization into rigid categories. Noteworthy is that the condition of each contributing variable can shift based on the circumstances of the relatives within the system, which in turn affects the overall mental health of the family unit at any given time, including everyone's adjustment to the brain injury.

As touched upon in Chap. 1 (see Sect. 1.4.3), healthy families are characterized by qualities of flexibility and the ability to accommodate changing states; a preponderance of cohesion, cooperation, and adaptability; clear boundaries and rules; commitment, attachment, and interconnectedness; warmth, tenderness, and intimacy; and fortitude and dignity (Kay and Cavallo 1994; Krysan et al. 1990; Minuchin 1974; Sachs 1991; Smith and Stevens-Smith 1992; Zarski et al. 1988). Adaptation also ensues when the family has an outlet to express their feelings and adopts the "one day at a time" mindset (Klonoff and Koberstein 2010; Lefebvre et al. 2005). Although healthy families experience considerable disruptiveness, the process of developing a positive working alliance with them tends to be more trouble-free (Klonoff 2011; Sachs 1991), even though the psychotherapist may find himself or herself wearing "multiple hats" of intervention, including those of "a detective, trailblazer, guide, pragmatist, educator, coach, "external conscience," advocate, witness, protector, companion, and mediator" (Klonoff 2010, p. 235).

Table 3.1 Sample verbalizations about the family and therapy indicative of the family's psychological health

Structural components
Trust
Family: We're confident our family will help and support us
Therapy: We believe the therapists have our best interests at heart
Distrust
Family: Our relatives don't believe what we are telling them
Therapy: The therapists are just doing this for the money
Compassionate
Family: We love our son/daughter with the injury and we'll do anything for him/her and the rest of the family
Therapy: We see how much those therapists are trying to help
Egocentric
Family: This accident is a huge inconvenience and it's messing up our lives
Therapy: All of those therapists want a piece of us and we can't take it
Agreeable
Family: We want to get along with everyone in the family and make this work
Therapy: We like the therapists and want to follow all of their suggestions
Disagreeable
Family: Our family is driving us crazy
Therapy: Why do we have to put up with all of these requirements from the therapists?
Good boundaries
Family: We need to respect each other's needs and space
Therapy: We need to let the therapists do their jobs
Poor boundaries
Family: Things would be so much better if the rest of the family would always listen to us and do it our way
Therapy: We wish the therapist could also be our friend and spend time with us
Cohesive
Family: We are such a close family
Therapy: It's great to be on the same page with the therapists
Fragmented
Family: No one gets along with each other and half of us aren't talking to the other half
Therapy: We like what the speech therapist is doing, but we can't stand the approach of the neuropsychologist
Resilient
Family: Don't worry, we'll be able to bounce back from this—we just have to hang in there
Therapy: Things are so different, but we see so much growth in ourselves and our loved one
Fragile
Family: Everything is so topsy-turvy—we don't know how we can go on like this
Therapy: We can't take the stress of all of this; our family is falling apart because of all of the therapy requirements
Process components
Engaged
Family: We are interested to learn more about our loved one's injury and how best to assist him/her
Therapy: We will make it a priority to attend therapy sessions as well as listen to and incorporate suggestions
Disconnected
Family: We are not really in touch very much with the loved one and don't feel we need to be
Therapy: There is no need for us to participate in the therapy process; other people are handling it just fine

Table 3.1 (continued)

Receptive	
Family: Whatever ideas everyone in the family has, we're "all ears"	
Therapy: These compensations and recommendations are wonderful and we know they will help our loved one AND us	
Resistant	
Family: We don't see what the point of all of these discussions is, as our loved one will be all better soon enough	
Therapy: These recommendations won't work and they seem like a waste of time	
Patient	
Family: Recovering from a brain injury is a gradual process; we all need to be patient and tolerant and let the process unfold	
Therapy: We realize that this is a "marathon, not a sprint" and we are here for the long haul to coordinate with the therapists	
Impatient	
Family: This healing process is too slow; we don't have time for this	
Therapy: Our loved one isn't improving fast enough; isn't there more you could/should be doing to speed up the process?	
Flexible	
Family: We are prepared to make whatever necessary changes within our family if they will help our loved one	
Therapy: We realize that if one approach isn't working well, we need to be open to trying something else	
Rigid:	
Family: This is the way our family operates and we're not about to change now	
Therapy: Your system won't work for us; we can't change things around the way you expect us to	
Collaborative	
Family: Our family works together and cooperates with each other to help our loved one	
Therapy: We are all part of the team to help our loved one; there is no "I" in team	
Adversarial	
Family: We don't like the caregiver's approach to things; he's/she's making the situation worse	
Therapy: We're angry at those therapists—we don't think they know what they are doing	
Realistic	
Family: We realize this process will go on indefinitely and we are ready for it	
Therapy: We realize we have to adjust our expectations. Things aren't the same, but everything will be okay	
Unrealistic	
Family: Our family needs to get back to our lives, so we expect our loved one to make a 100 % recovery and move on with his/her life	
Therapy: Our loved one will be just fine—the therapists have to get him/her to the point of living on his/her own and back to driving and work	

In contrast, there are several configurations of difficult or dysfunctional families. One conceptualization is the Family Experiential Model (FEM) of Recovery (Klonoff and Koberstein 2010; Klonoff et al. 2008), which differentiates families who are coping more adaptively at any given time (i.e., "green coping" zone) from those who are struggling with emotional stumbling blocks (i.e., "yellow warning" zone). Another approach is descriptive of family types (Sachs 1991). One example is the "overinvolved" family, who, because of underestimation or denial of either specific deficits or the totality of the impairments, may have unreasonable expectations of the loved one and the psychotherapist/treatment team (Sachs 1991). This manifests as an overinvestment of energy which precludes non-therapy activities for the loved one and themselves (Sachs 1991). The "defiant" family is dominated by distrust, anger, and fear, which can be projected onto the psychotherapist and the treatment team (Klonoff et al. 2008; Sachs 1991). "Dependant" families grapple with insecurities about decision making, which translates to hesitation in incorporating therapeutic feedback and suggestions (Sachs 1991). Neglectful, uninvolved, noncommunicative, and fragmented relatives are not engaged enough in the care or well-being of the loved one coming from either problematic and disjointed internal family dynamics or possibly an avoidance stress reaction to the repercussions of the brain injury on the loved one (Klonoff et al. 2008; Sachs 1991).

As depicted in Fig. 3.1, the greater the dysfunction in the family, the tougher it can be for the psychotherapist (and other treating therapists) to establish a positive working alliance (Klonoff 2011). This will spawn "red flags" for treating therapists (see Chap. 2, Sect. 2.4.1.4). For instance, Kay and Cavallo (1994) surmised that oftentimes, dysfunctional families were uninformed, underinvolved, and so did not have their basic needs met through the rehabilitation process. This *adversarial alliance* often emerges when the family is resistant to feedback, distrusts the team's expertise, negates the effects of the injury, experiences a "mismatch" in goals and expectations, is impatient with the pace of recovery, and is unpleasant in their interactions (e.g., angry, antagonistic, hostile, and controlling; McLaughlin and Carey 1993; Romano 1974; Sachs 1991; Shaw and McMahon 1990). Fragmented cross-communications and refusal to adopt therapeutic opinions polarize treatment objectives, with the therapists at one extreme and the family at the other (Klonoff 2011). Relatives may resort to "doctor shopping," emanating from an inability to accept painful realities (Roos 2002). The greater the family's stresses, the greater the potential for conflict with the psychotherapist and treatment team. The upshots of this are poorer coping mechanisms and outcomes for the patient and family (Klonoff 2010; McLaughlin and Carey 1993).

The clinician can adopt certain tactics which will ease tensions with difficult and dysfunctional families and strengthen the working alliance. These include: incorporating the input from the loved one with the injury into the support network's dialogue, accommodating varying realities between family members, recognizing the limits of scientific knowledge, respecting the power of motivation in recovery, adopting the principle of "dignity of risk" (see Chap. 4, Sect. 4.5.2), and using the notion of "elaborate and collaborate" to break targets into bite-sized pieces (Cavallo and Kay 2011; see Klonoff 2010, for a review). At the same time, it is critical for the psychotherapist and other neurorehabilitation staff to monitor their own negative counter-transference reactions and/or professional burnout to the "problem family"; otherwise, they may inadvertently scapegoat them; exacerbate tensions; convey a sense of futility; and impede the loved one's treatment and recovery, possibly through premature closure (David 1998; Klonoff 2010, 2011; Lansky 1990; Shaw and McMahon 1990). The fable, *The Bird, the Frog, and the Light* by Avi (1994) is symbolic of how the therapeutic process can "uncover" unhealthy misconceptions and propose new possibilities for the therapeutic relationship.

3.1.2 Impact of the Brain Injury on Family Patterns

The loved one's diminished self-awareness, impaired social perception and self-control, childlike egocentricity, emotional factors (e.g., apathy, heightened reactivity, irritability, anxiety, paranoia, depression), as well as emotional and physical dependency and the inability to learn from experience create turmoil and weariness in the caregiver (Lezak 1988). Some have described feeling "continually on standby" for the loved one (Engström and Söderberg 2011). The loved one's personality alterations can precipitate friction, discomfort, or jealousy, especially when other family members resent him or her for unfairly receiving the preponderance of attention (Wongvatunyu and Porter 2008a). Sometimes, the family entity is split apart, either by the stresses of the injury or because treatment is sought in a different locale (Wongvatunyu and Porter 2008a). This can result in cascading financial perils (Wongvatunyu and Porter 2008a), threatening the family's stability. These emotional and psychosocial problems can persist, or even build over many years postinjury, thereby eroding the relatives' quality of life (Florian and Katz 1991; Kolakowsky-Hayner et al. 2001).

By extension, the brain injury also radically alters the family's juxtaposition of the individual's and others' needs, affecting the organizational structure and communication patterns (Laroi 2003). The orderliness of specific family subsystems is also disrupted (David 1998). Research has shown that families can be fractionated especially when some relatives do not fathom the injury ramifications, leading to dissension (Wongvatunyu and Porter 2008a). Alternatively, when possible tier 2 and 3 supports are unavailable (e.g., due to distance, lack of interest, or wariness), tier 1 caregivers may experience greater pressures and segregation (Cavallo and Kay 2011).

3.1.3 "Helpful Hints" and Tools to Address Family Patterns after Brain Injury

Table 3.2 summarizes "helpful hints" and tools to address family patterns after brain injury. Psychotherapy for the family system after brain injury is akin to that for the loved one, in that everyone must adapt, "right themselves," and find a new equilibrium (Cavallo and Kay 2011; Verhaeghe et al. 2005). This entails family education and support by a psychotherapist who is well versed in both brain injury and family therapy (Laroi 2003). He or she must "join" the family unit to best forge a therapeutic dialogue and relationship (Minuchin 1974). The process can be conceptualized in three phases: (1) acutely, the focus is on the loved one's survival and medical interventions to reduce permanent damage; (2) during rehabilitation, family energies are directed toward the restoration of as much function as possible in the loved one; and (3) the community reintegration phase, in which the loved one and tier supports settle into longer-term patterns and a new balance (Cavallo and Kay 2011; Gan et al. 2010; Kay and Cavallo 1994).

Table 3.2 "Helpful Hints" and tools for families to address family patterns after brain injury

Find a psychotherapist who is well versed in both brain injury and family therapy
Therapy will help the family system adapt, "right themselves," and find a new equilibrium
Interventions are for three phases: acutely, during rehabilitation, and for community reintegration
Interventions combine psychoeducation, problem solving, ventilation, therapeutic confrontation, clinical interpretations, and emotional support
Treatment approaches should incorporate the family's social microcosm, diversity, cultural beliefs, expectations, traditions, gender roles and responsibilities, and readiness for feedback
After the brain injury, expect family disorganization or chaos at the outset
Lifelong adjustments will mirror various life-cycle transitions and will rekindle strong emotions
Families will experience destabilization and rotate back through the phases of awareness, acceptance, and realism
Family therapy will study individuals' personality structures, general attitudes, expectations of the loved one, their strengths and weaknesses, and relational patterns
Family systems therapy will reestablish a workable family composition taking into account roles, structure, routines, balance of power and authority, and communication patterns:
Functional generational boundaries must be reestablished
There needs to be fluid role assignments
The approach moves away from the loved one as "the problem" to a breakdown in the whole family system's operation and evolving adjustment
Treatment styles include using two or more clinicians, collaborative self-examination, therapeutic alliance with various subsystems, as well as reframing or reinterpreting troubling behaviors
Perspective taking, self-monitoring, and improved awareness are encouraged within all parties
Cognitive behavioral techniques help in problem solving, functional skills training, and coping mechanisms
"Milieu meetings" are helpful forums to discuss relevant family activities, needs, and challenges
Information and education are fundamental to family therapy, a positive working alliance, and the success of rehabilitation. Topics include:
What is caused by the brain injury versus a reaction to it versus unrelated life situations
How not to personalize the loved one's verbal attacks
Understanding "catastrophic reactions"
Therapy approaches will validate the families' emotional wounds and suffering, yet foster resilience, hardiness, compassion, empowerment, and flexible adaptation
Goals are to:
Address misinterpretations and misunderstandings about the loved one's behavior
Implement better interactions
Create positive-constructive behaviors in the loved one
Provide for the safety of the family
Learn life skills
Improve cohesion
Incorporate strategies for correcting misbehavior
Set good boundaries for privacy and autonomy
Utilize existential principles related to core values and quality of life
Transform the caregiving role into a mission based on love, sympathy, and solidarity
Multimedia resources
Model
The Family Experiential Model (FEM) of Recovery (Klonoff and Koberstein 2010; Klonoff et al. 2008)

Ideal psychotherapeutic interventions are an amalgamation of psychoeducation, problem solving about practical worries, an outlet for ventilation, therapeutic confrontation, clinical interpretations of family behaviors and functioning, and emotional support for individual members, germane subsystems, and the overall family unit (Cavallo and Kay 2011; Gan et al. 2010; Klonoff and Koberstein 2010; Sachs 1991). All treatments should be built on a keen awareness of the family's social microcosm, diversity, cultural beliefs, expectations, and traditions, including gender roles and responsibilities, as well as readiness for feedback, so as to not inadvertently insult or alienate the family (Bednar and Peterson 1995; Cavallo and Kay 2011; Laroi 2003; Maitz and Sachs 1995; Yeates 2009; see also Chap. 1, Sect. 1.3, and Fig. 1.1; and Chap. 2, Sect. 2.4.1.2). As one father said "I appreciate you giving us small doses of "mental medicine," rather than heaping it on" (S. Daugharty, 1-11-2013, personal communication).

The therapist will reassure the family that initial disorganization or chaos is to be expected and that it takes time for the fragmentation to abate (Roos 2002). Relatives will be updated that there will likely be lifelong adjustments which mirror various life-cycle transitions and rekindle feelings of desolation, worries, and "chronic sorrow" (see Roos 2002, for a review; see also Sect. 3.3.2 and Chap. 9, Sect. 9.5.1). This is also aptly illustrated in the seven phases of the FEM (Klonoff and Koberstein 2010; Klonoff et al. 2008; see also Chap. 1, Sect. 1.5 and Fig. 1.3). As is also depicted in the FEM, phase 7, families may experience destabilization and rotate back through the phases of awareness, acceptance, and realism at the time of new developmental transitions throughout the life cycle (Kay and Cavallo 1994; Klonoff et al. 2008).

The psychotherapist should study the caregiver's and other individual relatives' personality structure, general attitudes, expectations of the loved one, and the strengths and weaknesses they contribute to the family unit (Cavallo and Kay 2011). Family therapy should also explore relational patterns within the family, including its interconnectedness and richness (Yeates 2009). A family systems' approach is fitting, so that the family's various roles, structure, routines, balance of power and authority, and communication patterns can be modified according to the special requirements of the loved one in order to reestablish a workable family composition (Kay and Cavallo 1994; Laroi 2003; Maitz and Sachs 1995). Functional generational boundaries must be reestablished, for instance, between parents and children (Sachs 1991). This process necessitates a fluid versus rigid view of role assignments, a shift from identifying the loved one as "the problem" to a breakdown in the operation of the whole family system, and evolving adjustments (Gan et al. 2006; Kay and Cavallo 1994; Lansky 1990; Lefebvre et al. 2005).

Paradigms include interventions to reinsert the parent with the brain injury into parenting responsibilities, persuading other relatives to empathically listen to the loved one's verbalizations, redefining and relinquishing certain duties for a parent with a brain injury and outsourcing these to other family members, creating new tasks for a father with a brain injury to reestablish his position and power in the family, and lessening the strain on caregivers by redistributing some items to other supporters (Cavallo and Kay 2011; Gan et al. 2006; Laroi 2003).

Some advocate the involvement of two or more clinicians to model "reflecting conversations" and/or different configurations of family members (see Yeates 2009, for a review). Others incorporate collaborative self-examination whereby each relative shares his or her viewpoint on events and behaviors. Alliance with various subsystems (e.g., parents versus the loved one) to lend support and power as well as reframing or reinterpreting troubling behaviors or occurrences are also effective psychotherapy practices (Sachs 1991). Therefore, perspective taking, self-monitoring, and greater awareness within all parties are encouraged (Kreutzer et al. 2009). Based on cognitive–behavioral theory, families should also be taught group problem-solving techniques, functional skills training, and coping mechanisms (Gan et al. 2006; Kay and Cavallo 1994; Kreutzer et al. 2009; Shaw and McMahon 1990). This may extend to prescriptive treatment interventions outside of sessions, for example, "milieu meetings" to discuss pertinent family activities, needs, and challenges (Klonoff 2010; Sachs 1991; see also Chap. 4, Sect. 4.4.4).

Information and education are central to family therapy, a positive working alliance after brain injury, and the success of the rehabilitation process (Kay and Cavallo 1994; Klonoff 2010; McLaughlin and Carey 1993; Shaw and McMahon 1990; Springer et al. 1997). Psychoeducation will teach the family members to differentiate between: (1) the direct results of the brain injury (i.e., primary reactions); (2) reactive (or secondary) reactions related to the loved one's perceptions of the implications of the injury, including psychological factors and family dynamics; and (3) life situations separate from the brain injury (Laroi 2003). For instance, the psychotherapist will instruct the family not to personalize the loved one's problematic behaviors (e.g., "meanness") or misattribute these to purely motivational considerations that he or she has control over (Laroi 2003). Similarly, the support network's responses and reactions evolve when they appreciate the loved one's form of "catastrophic reactions" (CRs) from the exposure of deficits and underlying shameful feelings in the loved one with the brain injury (Klonoff et al. 1993; Lansky 1990; see also Chap. 4, Sect. 4.6). Grasping the etiology of mood and behavioral sequelae translates to enhanced insight, improved coping, and decreased family turbulence (Laroi 2003).

The psychotherapist may employ a treatment course which validates the families' emotional wounds and suffering, yet fosters resilience, hardiness, compassion, empowerment, and flexible adaptation (Nicoll 2011; Roos 2002). Interventions include addressing misinterpretations and misunderstandings about the loved one's behavior by implementing better interactions, which in turn create greater positive-constructive behaviors in the loved one (Nicoll 2011). Specific components include providing for the safety of family members, learning life skills, improving cohesion (e.g., a sense of belonging and connectedness), incorporating strategies for correcting misbehavior, and setting good boundaries for privacy and autonomy (Nicoll 2011). Psychotherapy will also incorporate existentialism, including helping the relatives appreciate "small things," focusing on their love for and mutual happiness with the loved one, and relying on core values as a life compass (Engström and Söderberg 2011). Over time, family members can transform their caregiving role into a mission predicated on love, sympathy, and solidarity (Engström and Söderberg 2011; see Chap. 10, Sect. 10.2, for more discussion on the positive aspects of caregiving).

3.2 Scenario: Impact of a Brain Injury on Spousal Relationships

Spouses face unique obstacles when a partner sustains a brain injury. The person, relationship, and lifestyle are usually radically altered. Both the loved one and healthy spouse encounter marital disturbances. Spouses often pose questions such as: *What happened to my life partner? How will our relationship be now? Can we still be happy together?*

3.2.1 Challenges for a Spouse with a Partner with an Acquired Brain Injury

There is much literature indicating that partners experience greater emotional upset than parents after brain injury, including more health and psychological complaints, greater depression, and more frequent crises (see Brooks 1984, for a review; Florian and Katz 1991; Kieffer-Kristensen and Teasdale 2011; Kreutzer et al. 1994; Verhaeghe et al. 2005; Zeigler 1999). The noninjured spouse is usually a wife who will assume a new caregiver role on her own and can suffer great burdens (versus as part of a parental dyad; Cavallo and Kay 2011; Hall et al. 1994; Larson et al. 2008; Zeigler 1999). This is especially onerous if the husband was the "family executive" and the wife was secondary or uninvolved in the major house decisions (Cavallo and Kay 2011). Frequently, the uninjured spouse will feel encumbered with an "extra child" instead of a mate (Bowen et al. 2010; Butler and Satz 1988; Cavallo and Kay 2011; Klonoff and Koberstein 2010).

Research is inconclusive regarding specific threats to marital stability after brain injury. Some studies implicate younger age, shorter preinjury marriages, male gender, traumatic brain injury caused by violence, and more severe injuries as contributors to marital instability (Arango-Lasprilla et al. 2008; Kreutzer et al. 2007). Aphasia and depression in the loved one can have negative consequences on the marriage (see Blonder et al. 2007, for a review). A brain tumor diagnosis places more strain on the marital dyad, which can create a vicious cycle of stress over the workload, leading to resentment and then guilt about the latter feelings (Black and Hogan 2006). This alternates with profound grief about the loved one's suffering (Black and Hogan 2006).

The uninjured partner can feel like a "married widow" or "hidden patient," suffering in loneliness and isolation with wishful thinking that the old spouse would reappear (Chwalisz and Stark-Wroblewski 1996; Fengler and Goodrich 1979; Lezak 1988; Threats 2010; Wedcliffe and Ross 2001; Zeigler 1999). Neuropsychological deficits in the areas of executive functions, memory, attention, language, emotion recognition, affective attunement, and responsiveness may negatively influence the interpersonal relationship between couples (Yeates 2013). Troubling injury-related personality changes include childlike behavior, impulsivity, self-centeredness, emotional lability, volatility, and aggression; these can create embarrassment, misery, or resentment in the spouse (Bowen et al. 2010; Florian and Katz 1991; see Gill et al.

2011, for a review; Sachs 1991; Yeates 2013). In the context of the brain injury, the loved one may struggle to decode his or her partner's mental state; this is also known as *mentalizing,* which is the capability to infer the spouse's intentions, goals, perspectives, and beliefs (Bowen et al. 2010; Yeates 2013). Social communication skills, including the capacity for empathy, are also affected (Bowen et al. 2010). Some partners feel that the injury altered their mate's personhood, creating emotional distance and disconnection (Black and Hogan 2006; Bowen et al. 2010; Gill et al. 2011; Yeates 2013).

Other elements affecting the tier 1 caregiver are loss of affection, companionship, and a confidante; feeling overloaded and overworked from lack of support from the injured spouse; and the loved one's sexual difficulties and greater dependency; all of these lead to the uninjured spouse feeling neglected, dejected, and burned out (Cavallo and Kay 2011; Chwalisz and Stark-Wroblewski 1996; Fengler and Goodrich 1979; Gill et al. 2011; Kreutzer et al. 1994; Lezak 1988). Ancillary pressures complicate the caregiver's role, including financial stresses and the pressures of making unilateral life decisions (Cavallo and Kay 2011; Chwalisz and Stark-Wroblewski 1996; Gill et al. 2011; Hammond et al. 2011; Sachs 1991; Wedcliffe and Ross 2001). Some have characterized the stress "as being on an emotional roller coaster with a lifetime pass" (Chwalisz and Stark-Wroblewski 1996, p. 36). Table 3.3 contains some sample verbalizations along these lines by spouses, based on completed Sense of Self Questionnaires (see Chap. 2, Sect. 2.3.8 and Fig. 2.2).

The spouse with the brain injury can become cantankerous when he or she feels treated like a child or an invalid (Gill et al. 2011). He or she also experiences a loss of sense of self, which can be demoralizing (Gill et al. 2011; Klonoff and Myles 2010). Overall, the marital relationship becomes unsteady and vulnerable, with the loved one feeling insecure about his or her spouse's true commitment (versus obligation) to the marriage and the uninjured spouse feeling uncertain about the loved one's authenticity or depth of feelings (versus fear of abandonment; Gill et al. 2011). Although the loved one has "vanished," the spouse may feel that it is impermissible to grieve the loss, as he or she is still alive (Lezak 1988). The uninjured spouse wrestles with the thought of divorce, consumed by guilt and/or worry of social rejection (Lezak 1988). Nonetheless, the rate of separation and divorce varies from 15 to 79 % (Arango-Lasprilla et al. 2008, see Bowen et al. 2010, for a review; Kreutzer et al. 2007; see Verhaeghe et al. 2005, for a review) and the uninjured divorcing partner may be consumed by self-recrimination and anxiety (Verhaeghe et al. 2005).

3.2.2 "Helpful Hints" and Tools for Spouses with a Partner with an Acquired Brain Injury

Table 3.4 summarizes "helpful hints" and tools for spouses to cope with a brain injury in a partner. Marital therapy will be crucial after brain injury, especially as many spouses feel transformed into the parent role when tending to the injured loved one (Klonoff and Koberstein 2010; Kreutzer et al. 1994; Tyerman and Booth 2001; Wedcliffe and Ross 2001). The psychotherapist should start with obtaining a history

Table 3.3 Examples of spouses' verbalizations

Sense of Self Questionnaire responses
Since my loved one's injury, I feel... sad, overwhelmed, stressed, anxious, and often unhappy. I feel unloved and taken for granted. I feel like more of a roommate and personal assistant than a wife
Compared to before my loved one's injury, I feel angry... about how this all could have been prevented
Since my loved one's injury, the way I see myself... has been reduced to someone who looks after someone else. I have become the sole decision maker and I don't get any help from him
Since the injury, when I think about my role in the family.... I went from a wife to caregiver and single parent overnight. I hate being in charge of everything—I have to handle finances, travel, etc.
Since my loved one's injury, my relationship with people close to me... has changed—I'm more distant, I just don't have the time
Since my loved one's injury, my sense of connection with people... has diminished—they just don't get it
Since my loved one's injury, when I compare myself to my friends ... I do a lot less comparing now—but sometimes I am envious of their freedom
Compared to before my loved one's injury, I get frustrated... with all the changes—his moods, medications, and struggles. I hate to see him grieve for the past; it breaks my heart
Compared to before my loved one's injury, I worry... about my husband's long-term outcome, his future, his job, and his sense of purpose. I worry that I will not figure out the future before it arrives
Compared to before the injury, my level of stress... has skyrocketed. It's not only his injury, but also our son with attention deficit hyperactivity disorder (ADHD) and my mother's dementia
Since my loved one's injury, when I think about work... I wish I had fewer work commitments with the same income
When I think about life before my loved one's injury, I feel... wistful
Since my loved one's injury, when I think about my life... I feel selfish—I should be focused on his recovery
Pretherapy verbalizations
I feel like I have a (another) child instead of a husband
I feel so insecure—we were a team and now it's just me
I've lost someone to talk to
I lost my partner—I miss him
Everything is on my shoulders now
All I do is worry about him and everything else
My emotions are on an endless roller coaster
I haven't worked in years... what will I do to support the kids?
Posttherapy verbalizations
It is not a "have to" but a "want to"
I've learned to live life in the slow lane—anyhow, it's better for taking in the scenery
I've realized that I should focus on the right things more and the things that don't matter less
I find myself feeling both sad and hopeful
Life is "alright;" not in the way we thought it would be... but in another way
Could the new course be better than the old?
I'm coping better—more days are good than bad
The future will be okay
I feel like we have found a new existence together and we are moving into new horizons
My role in life has more purpose, satisfaction, and meaning now

Table 3.4 "Helpful hints" and tools for spouses with a partner with an acquired brain injury

Marital therapy is crucial, especially as spouses feel transformed into the "parent" role
The therapist will obtain a history of the preinjury marital relationship, including "critical events" and the role of culture, age of partners, values, and environment
Both conjoint and separate meetings with the partners are useful
Approaches include the attachment theory and stress management techniques
Each partner must take personal responsibility, with no "finger pointing"
Psychoeducation should be provided about how the loved one's cognitive, behavioral, and social impairments affect the marriage
The goal is to improve the "give and take" in the relationship:
The loved one's executive function deficits will need to be remediated
Role playing and perspective-taking exercises will be incorporated
Adjunct speech therapy is helpful
Coping techniques will be addressed:
Increase decision making
Boost partner communication and bonding
Reduce disagreements
Reestablish emotional and sexual intimacy
Redefine roles
Homework includes "milieu meetings"
Recreate reciprocity, equality, personal autonomy, and positive interaction cycles with mutual attunement
Changes in sexual compatibility will be explored:
Obtain a sexual history and postinjury concerns from the partners
Solicit physician input (e.g., psychiatrist, physiatrist, or neurologist)
Explore and address current obstacles to sexual intimacy from the perspective of the caregiver and factors related to the loved one's injury (e.g., anatomical, hormonal, physiological, psychological, cognitive, physical, communication, perceptual, and self-esteem)
Liaison with a speech–language pathologist to retrain "psychosocial graces," also including a social skills or communication pragmatics group
Treatment approaches include sex education, relaxation strategies, cognitive–behavioral techniques, or referral to a sex therapist
Help the spouse transition from a parent/caregiver to a partner
Rekindle the romance
Plan "date nights" with a graded increase in sexual activity
The uninjured spouse needs help with "chronic sorrow" and "nonfinite loss," which can result in excessive self-sacrifice
Psychotherapy will help in recalibrating expectations and finding new ways to feel connected and happy as a couple
Utilize an occupational therapist and social worker as adjunct resources for prioritizing and handling crises
Reframe guilt about "leaving" the loved one as much needed respite and quality of life for both parties
Psychotherapy will teach mechanisms to solicit help and support from tier 2 and 3 members
For committed relationships, build on couples' preexisting relationship strengths as a foundation to cope with current stressors
Rely on journaling, finding humor, and spiritual outlets
Strive for a recalibrated and fluid balance between support and independence, mutual caring, and acceptance of losses with a hopeful outlook
If a spouse plans to divorce, recommend he/she find his/her own therapist for personalized input
Pursue leisure and social activities as a couple and individually
Utilize input from a recreational therapist and social worker for leisure ideas

Table 3.4 (continued)

For more severe brain injuries, consider a personal assistant or day-care program
Join a support group or attend "refresher" annual workshops
Multimedia resources
Books
Emotionally Focused Couple Therapy with Trauma Survivors: Strengthening Attachment Bonds (Johnson 2005)
Sexual Difficulties After Traumatic Brain Injury and Ways to Deal With It (Aloni and Katz 2003)
Successfully Surviving a Brain Injury: A Family Guidebook (Prowe 2010)
Ten Big Toes and a Prince's Nose (Gow 2010)
Website
Well Spouse Association: Support for Spousal Caregivers http://www.wellspouse.org
Song
"I'll Stand by You" (Hynde et al. 1994)

of the preinjury marital relationship, to glean an indication of the relative constancy or shakiness. In addition to the brain injury, marriages may have experienced prior "critical events" or threats, such as infidelity, work troubles, communication stalemates, and general conflicts (Layman et al. 2005). The role of culture, age of partners, values, and environment should be incorporated into any diagnostic formulation.

Therapy can incorporate the "attachment theory," whereby a wound occurs when one spouse fails to respond to the other at a critical time; the instance becomes a recurring theme and a hindrance to the relationship (Johnson et al. 2001). These negative attachment incidents (e.g., when the spouse fails to respond in a reparative, reassuring manner) disrupt marital intimacy and trust (Johnson et al. 2001). In the context of the brain injury, this may come from either spouse; the loved one's cognitive and affective challenges produced by the brain injury may impede his or her ability to connect with the noninjured spouse causing him or her to feel unaffirmed and unappreciated (Hammond et al. 2011). Alternatively, the healthy spouse may distance himself or herself from the loved one, secondary to feeling frightened, overwhelmed, inundated, or resentful about the injury effects, especially in the realm of personality (Hammond et al. 2011). The psychotherapist will aid spouses in recognizing the specific impasses and facilitate repair processes employing emotionally focused couple therapy (Johnson et al. 2001). Interactions will be restructured so that the spouses become more accessible and responsive to each other, including cultivating positive cycles of caring, comfort, and intimacy (Bowen et al. 2010; Johnson et al. 2001). For more material on this therapy, consult the resource, *Emotionally Focused Couple Therapy with Trauma Survivors: Strengthening Attachment Bonds* by Johnson (2005).

In this clinician's experience, a combination of conjoint meetings with both the spouse and the loved one, in conjunction with individual meetings with each partner, is most efficacious for providing the requisite support and education. Separate meetings can focus on furthering the awareness, acceptance, and realism process and addressing everyday, emotional, interpersonal, and existential concerns applicable to each spouse (Klonoff and Koberstein 2010). Stress management education is also advantageous (Gill et al. 2011). It is imperative for each partner to take personal accountability for change, as "finger pointing" is a threat to the integrity of the sessions and marriage (Klonoff and Koberstein 2010).

The psychotherapist will need to focus on the impact of the loved one's cognitive, behavioral, and social impairments on the marriage, as these aspects create greater psychological distress in the spouse (Anderson et al. 2009). Psychoeducation about the multitude of brain injury sequelae will be critical (Klonoff 2010; see also Chaps. 4, 5, 6, 7, 8, and 10, for more information on specific aspects after acquired brain injury). One aim of interventions should be to create more of a reciprocal "give and take" relationship. Often, this entails remediation of the loved one's executive function shortfalls (e.g., poor initiation, rigidity, impulsivity, disinhibited behavior, and black-and-white thinking) using role playing and perspective-taking exercises and speech therapy (see also Chap. 4, Sects. 4.4 and 4.6 and Figs. 4.6 and 4.9). Other topics include how to: cope with increased decision making; boost partner communication and bonding and reduce disagreements; reestablish emotional and sexual intimacy; and redefine roles (Bay et al. 2012; Kieffer-Kristensen and Teasdale 2011; Tyerman and Booth 2001). Often, homework is assigned in the form of "milieu meetings" to address specific aspects of the marriage (chores, social plans, finances). This will ameliorate the uninjured spouse's feelings of "a ceaseless juggling act" of work and home duties (Gill et al. 2011). Ultimately, both spouses need to reestablish a sense of a reciprocity, equality, and personal autonomy in the relationship.

Yeates (2013) asserts that couples counseling should focus on positive interaction cycles so that the loved one can be more "tuned in" and the uninjured spouse can feel more connected and emotionally secure. This involves improving each partner's perspectives and emotions so as to facilitate attunement, teaching potent social cues to the uninjured partner so that he or she can signal the loved one, and improving "mentalizing" to enhance positive interactions (Yeates 2013).

The psychotherapist should explore the underlying reasons for sexual incompatibility postinjury so as to provide cogent and relevant recommendations. This interview should include both spouses and will include obtaining a sexual history which addresses preinjury needs, expectations, and behaviors (Ducharme 1993; Zasler and Martelli 2011). Given the sensitive nature of the discussion, the psychotherapist may need to initiate the dialogue (Ducharme 1993). He or she should provide a private atmosphere; be nonbiased, patient, and compassionate during inquiry; and use comfortable language (Zasler and Martelli 2011). Postinjury considerations include sexuality concerns and current likings; questionnaires can be useful in this regard (Zasler and Martelli 2011). Physician input by a psychiatrist, physiatrist, or neurologist can be important to realizing possible physical and emotional barriers to sexual functioning in the loved one (Zasler and Martelli 2011). These should incorporate the role of anxiety, depression, some medications (e.g., antidepressants, antipsychotics, and anxiolytics), and other effects of the brain injury on hormones and neurotransmitters (Butler and Satz 1988; Zasler and Martelli 2011).

Postinjury, there are various obstacles to sexual intimacy. Usually, the caregiver's high stress levels, mood variations (e.g., depression), and time constraints pose strong interferences (Butler and Satz 1988; Gill et al. 2011). The loved one may experience sexual dysfunction due to the manifestations of the brain injury. Multiple brain structures subsume sexual functioning, including cortical (e.g., frontal and temporal lobes), subcortical (e.g., hippocampus, amygdala, and hypothalamus), and brainstem (e.g., reticular activating system) areas (Butler and Satz 1988; Dombrowski et al. 2000; Zasler and Martell 2011). Hormonal factors and physiological (e.g., erection difficulties, ejaculatory or orgasmic dysfunction, decreased libido) and/or psychological aspects (e.g., lack of empathic sensitivity, disinhibition, or childlike conduct attributable to personality or behavioral changes) affect the loved one's sexuality (Butler and Satz 1988; Dombrowski et al. 2000; Elbaum 2010; Gill et al. 2011; Lezak 1988; Zasler and Martelli 2011). Cognitive deficits (e.g., decreased judgment, attention, and initiation), physical limitations (e.g., neurogenic bowel or bladder dysfunction, decreased balance, sensation, or tremor), as well as communication and perceptual problems, all influence the loved one's sexual interest and capacity to forge an intimate experience (Butler and Satz 1988; Dombrowski et al. 2000; Elbaum 2010; see Zasler and Martelli 2011, for a review).

Alterations in the loved one's self-esteem, body image, self-concept, or personal view of attractiveness can also impede emotional and sexual intimacy (Ducharme 1993; Klonoff 2010; Zasler and Martelli 2011). Individual psychotherapy for the loved one to restore a positive sense of self and psychological well-being (including reducing depression and anxiety) is a prerequisite for greater interest in intimacy (Ducharme 1993; Klonoff 2010). This includes "feeling comfortable in his or her own skin" (Klonoff 2010). Psychotherapy can further the interactions between spouses, by addressing vexing personality and communication impairments in the loved one as well as guiding the healthy spouse to become more knowledgeable and tolerant about the ramifications of the brain injury. The psychotherapist can also help the couple develop better communication about their sexual relationship (Ducharme 1993).

Liaison with a speech–language pathologist to retrain "psychosocial graces" is warranted, including a social skills or communication pragmatics group (see Bowen et al. 2010, for a review; Dombrowski et al. 2000; Klonoff 2010; Zasler and Martelli 2011). Referral to a sex therapist may be necessary, depending on the marital needs and the expertise of the treating psychotherapist (Ducharme 1993; Zasler and Martelli 2011). Interventions include sex education, relaxation strategies, and cognitive–behavioral techniques to reduce anxiety (Dombrowki et al. 2000; Ducharme 1993; Medlar 1998; Simpson and Long 2004; Zasler and Martelli 2011). The healthy spouse's transition from the role of the "parent/caregiver" to "partner," will also spark more intimacy in the relationship (Ducharme 1993; Gill et al. 2011; Klonoff 2010). Devoting time to rekindling the romance is a key stepping stone, including planning and implementing "date nights," with a graded increase in intimate and sexual activities (Bowen et al. 2010). A resource on sexuality after brain injury is *Sexual Difficulties after Traumatic Brain Injury and Ways to Deal with It* by Aloni and Katz (2003).

Many spouses feel an inordinate amount of obligation toward the loved one's physical and emotional well-being and may willingly sacrifice their needs, especially if the loved one is "clingy" or there is risk of further injury or deterioration. Spouses will often verbalize that they feel they have the best expertise to assist the loved one and preserve their safety and happiness. They also do not want to overtax outsiders, who have their own busy lives. The psychotherapist should respond empathically to the spouse's ongoing grief and loss, related to the conundrum of having a partner, but losing his or her personality and day-to-day contributions. Concepts such as "chronic sorrow" (Olshansky 1962, as cited in Roos 2002) and "nonfinite loss" (Bruce and Schultz 2002; see Collings 2008, for a review) provide a vocabulary with which to promote sharing and validation in the context of a safe haven (see also Sect. 3.3.2 and Chap. 9, Sect. 9.5). It is a daunting undertaking to adjust to the many setbacks, requiring recalibrating expectations and finding new ways to feel connected and happy together (Klonoff and Koberstein 2010; Niemeier and Karol 2011a).

Discussions will undoubtedly focus on the multitude of drains on the spouse, including household management, parenting, obtaining an income, and dealing with the health-care system (Zeigler 1999). The psychotherapist will propose incorporating valuable insights from an occupational therapist and a social worker as resources. Given that the brain injury does not occur in a vacuum (Chwalisz and Stark-Wroblewski 1996), the psychotherapist can educate the spouse in prioritizing and handling havoc and identifying and fulfilling his or her personal needs (Niemeier and Karol 2011a). The psychotherapist will need to coach the caregiver to reframe guilt about being apart from the spouse to access much needed respite and quality of life for himself or herself (Niemeier and Karol 2011a). With time and practice, both the partner and loved one with the injury generally come to enjoy their separate time.

The psychotherapist may need to advise the spouse to curb his or her hesitations and request support from tier 2 and 3 members, as others may not recognize his or her handicaps (Niemeier and Karol 2011a). Requests may include transportation options (when the spouse works), meal preparation, or respite breaks (Niemeier and Karol 2011b). The noninjured spouse may also need to access resources to better identify and cope with financial threats. One possible resource is *Successfully Surviving a Brain Injury: A Family Guidebook* by Prowe (2010), as this contains a chapter on bill paying, health insurance considerations, disability pay, government programs, and utilization of attorneys. Educating the tier supports (including in-laws) provides essential support and reprieve to the spouse and loved one and also diminishes negative or inappropriate reactions due to ignorance or misinformation, which add to the consternation experienced by the spouse (Chwalisz and Stark-Wroblewski 1996; Gill et al. 2011; Zeigler 1999). An educational resource is the website, Well Spouse Association: Support for Spousal Caregivers http://www.wellspouse.org/.

There is some evidence that older couples absorb the aftereffects of brain injury more smoothly than their younger counterparts (Layman et al. 2005). This may be linked to the qualities of dedication, persistence, acceptance of one another's imperfections, and interpersonal relatedness (Layman et al. 2005). Overall, in spite of age, better adjusted caregivers perceived their own inner strength and competency in handling numerous tasks (Chwalisz and Stark-Wroblewski 1996). Other marriage-preserving qualities are: acceptance of the loved one unconditionally, bolstered by the loved one's capacity to express gratitude and love to his or her mate; a mindful decision to move forward and not dwell on the losses; commitment to optimal communication about concerns; the foundation of a strong preinjury relationship built on trust and respect; focus on the "friendship" within the marriage; and prior experience with hardships (Gill et al. 2011). Effective coping tools include journaling, finding humor, and spiritual outlets (Chwalisz and Stark-Wroblewski 1996). The book, *Ten Big Toes and a Prince's Nose* by Gow (2010) is a charming reminder that despite shortcomings (which in fact are universal), love and happiness are achievable. One wife chose the song, "I'll Stand by You" (Hynde et al. 1994) to illustrate her endless love and devotion to her husband who had sustained a stroke in his late 60s after 40 years of marriage. Hopefully, after brain injury, the marriage will be recalibrated with a fluid weighting between support and independence, care for the loved one and the uninjured spouse, and acceptance of losses with a hopeful outlook for the future (Gill et al. 2011).

Should a partner decide to divorce a loved one with a brain injury, he or she should be guided toward a different therapist to work through this complex decision. He or she will need an objective party to help with the decision-making process and to address the understandable feelings of guilt and worry (Cavallo and Kay 2011; Sachs 1991; Zeigler 1999). The psychotherapist working with the loved one can try to facilitate an amicable parting and if possible preserve some semblance of communication and mutual support, depending on the preferences of the two spouses.

Spousal life satisfaction and happiness are enriched when the couple participates together in leisure and social activities (Eriksson et al. 2005). The psychotherapist can encourage and facilitate involvement in community-based activities, some of which may be new, given the decline in the health status of the spouse. To reduce "social limbo" (Lezak 1988; Zeigler 1999), input should be obtained from a recreational therapist and social worker. Some examples of enjoyable activities are movie clubs, concerts and theater, game groups, and if feasible, travel. Each partner may also need his or her own outlets for leisure (Zeigler 1999), as these provide an eclectic mixture of pastimes and friendships to augment quality of life. With more severe brain injuries, hiring a personal assistant or enrollment in a day-care program may be suggested for the loved one to receive the requisite structure and care (see Fengler and Goodrich 1979, for a review; Gill et al. 2011). Support groups for the loved one and spouse (including separate meetings) are also beneficial adjunctive therapeutic and social avenues (Fengler and Goodrich 1979; Klonoff 2010; Zeigler 1999). Attending "refresher" annual workshops for psychoeducation and peer support, if available, is ideal (Tyerman and Booth 2001).

3.3 Scenario: Impact of a Brain Injury on Parents of Older Adolescent and Adult Individuals with an Acquired Brain Injury

Parents face particular snags when tending to an older adolescent or adult son or daughter with an acquired brain injury. As depicted in phase 1 of the FEM, parents are abruptly catapulted into a foreign territory of profound losses and often life-threatening complications (Klonoff and Koberstein 2010; Klonoff et al. 2008). This misfortune is terrifying and overwhelming to the parents, who raise questions such as: *What has happened to my semi-independent/independent and healthy son or daughter? What will become of him or her? What does this mean for my life?*

3.3.1 Challenges for Parents with a Son or Daughter with an Acquired Brain Injury

Parents will experience many emotions when confronted with a brain injury in an older adolescent or adult son or daughter. They are horrified and heartbroken when witnessing the loved one's acute confusion, disorientation, and physical incapacities, whereby he or she cannot perform even basic activities (e.g., eat, groom, or toilet himself or herself). They feel inundated with questions of "why us/why them" and "what if," with a desperate longing to turn back the clock (Klonoff et al. 2008). Often, parents are miserable and guilt-ridden about not protecting their children from befalling a brain injury in the first place, shattering their self-concept of "good parents" (Niemeier and Karol 2011a). At times, parents are angry or blaming over the circumstances of the accident, particularly if alcohol or street drugs are implicated (Minnes et al. 2010; Sherwin and O'Shanick 2000). In this latter scenario, the parents sustain a "second blow," as they may have denied, overlooked, or been oblivious to the adolescent/young adult's behavior (Sherwin and O'Shanick 2000).

Table 3.5 summarizes some representative verbalizations by parents, also based on completed Sense of Self Questionnaires. Early and postacute experiences include: extraordinary stress, events feeling out of control, pressure to make monumental decisions quickly with limited data, profound disruptions in family life, uncertainty about prognosis and lack of feedback, social estrangement and isolation, reduced leisure and hobbies, marital turbulence, family disharmony, "extended parenthood," and the fight to maintain hope (Hawley et al. 2003; Kao and Stuifbergen 2004; Klonoff and Koberstein 2010; Sachs 1991; Singer and Nixon 1993; Zinner et al. 1997).

Apprehension, sorrow, grief, guilt, anger, bewilderment, helplessness, alternating love and hatred, personal sacrifice, feeling overwhelmed and trapped because of the loved one's dependency and the totality of responsibility, loss of vigor, despondency about the slowness of recovery, and dashed hopes for the future also abound (Kao and Stuifbergen 2004; Klonoff and Koberstein 2010; Lezak 1988; Sherwin and O'Shanick 2000; Singer and Nixon 1993; Zinner et al. 1997). As one parent said, "I observe the difference between caregivers whose loved one is a "child" as opposed to a different relationship. When it's your young adult child, not only do you see the effects of the injury itself, you also see all the future losses—the things your child may never have, may never be .... It causes a heartbreaking amount of grief" (J. Cosper, personal communication, n.d.).

Parental stress builds in accordance with the severity of the brain injury (especially behavioral problems) and can worsen as the injury chronicity lengthens (Hawley et al. 2003; Zinner et al. 1997). Nonetheless, parents often feel deep love and conscientiousness in the face of the injury aftermath (Elbaum 2010). Hence, they can suffer from social isolation correlated with their total absorption both practically and emotionally in their loved one's care and recovery (Singer and Nixon 1993). This includes basic worries, for instance, transitioning the loved one back to school or work (Allen et al. 1994). They are plagued by financial drains, with respect to

Table 3.5 Examples of parents' verbalizations

Sense of Self Questionnaire responses
Compared to before my loved one's injury, my emotions... are much more on the surface. I never cried before; since his injury, I cry at the smallest things. Every time I see a bicyclist without a helmet, I just want to stop them and tell them what they could put themselves and their families through because of their arrogance and stupidity. I also get so angry at drivers who are not super careful around bicyclists
Compared to before my loved one's injury, I feel anxious... at unpredictable times. Something will trigger a memory and I go right back to that phone call and those weeks he was in the hospital. Phone calls at unusual times kill me. If I can't get a hold of him, I'm frantic. I can no longer relax and give him the space he thinks he deserves as a young adult man. What if he struggles for the rest of his life?
Compared to before my loved one's injury, I feel sad... all the time. So much loss; so much grief; so many horrible memories. So much of a disruption in what we thought would be a normal progression in his life and our lives. I despair when I see his friends moving forward with their lives in ways he cannot
Compared to before my loved one's injury, I get frustrated... when I see my daughter making a bad decision—yet I know she has her own path to lead in life
Compared to before my loved one's injury, I worry about... his quality of life and how to help his life be worth living. Also, I worry about getting sick in the future and not being able to take care of him
Since my loved one's injury, my relationships with the people close to me... are challenged, as my spouse and I have had differences of opinions about our son and other family decisions. I don't have enough time to spend with him or my other children
Since the injury, when I think about my role in my family... it makes me worry. I was already a "protective mom" and this sent me over the edge. This causes my son to see me as a "nut" sometimes. I worry more than most moms and he gets frustrated with me
Since my loved one's injury, my role in life... has changed. I am more of a nurturer, more like I was when my child was young. My role has changed back to being a caregiving parent rather than just a mentoring parent. I am out of balance—all work, no play
Since the injury, my place in the world is... unclear. I had retired only a month or two before his injury; the "good thing" is that I could help him recover as long as he needed me. The "not so good" thing is he resented my presence. It was hard on both of us
Since the injury, when I think about the future, I feel... the need to make sure my loved one is financially secure. Although I was retired for several years, I have gone back to work so as to provide economically for her
Since the injury, when I think about the future, I feel... very scared. Will he be okay long-term? What if he is ever reinjured? Will he have learning difficulties? Will he ever be happy?
Pretherapy verbalizations
I'll be doing this forever
My emotional bucket is full
The haunting reminders are endless
Others have it so easy
I want freedom
I don't know what to do with this anger
I feel so helpless
I'm so overwhelmed at holiday time, I'm "growly" and I don't want to be
How do I make emotional room for my husband, when all my energy is going to my son/daughter
I need help in widening the "fine line" of proper parenting so my loved one doesn't fall apart
Will anyone else (i.e., a future spouse) love him or her?
Posttherapy verbalizations
I feel a brand new love

Table 3.5 (continued)

I am thankful he/she is here
We've had to create a new life
I experience deeper grief and sadness, yet greater joy in his/her accomplishments
This experience taught me to love everyone more deeply and that is a gift
I'll live to fight another day

both ancillary medical costs for the loved one and lost wages (Hawley et al. 2003; Singer and Nixon 1993). Parents and their loved ones may actively or passively withdraw from the public sphere due to fear of rejection or ridicule (Kao and Stuifbergen 2004). Anxiety and reticence can translate to overprotectiveness of the loved one, and parents may inadvertently stifle his or her development, autonomy, and aspirations (Kao and Stuifbergen 2004).

Some mothers described radical ruptures in their relationship with their child, often feeling like a stranger relating to another stranger (Guerriere and McKeever 1997). Others translate the "brush with death" into extreme closeness and attunement (Guerriere and McKeever 1997). Mothers have described the bafflement of holding onto the child from before while getting to know a new child (Wongvatunyu and Porter 2008b). They often suffer from further guilt and maternal grief, feeling pulled between catering to the specialized needs of the loved one versus trying to regain a personal life (Zinner et al. 1997). As a son or daughter begins to grasp his or her predicament and limitations, he or she can alternate between clinging to and fighting against dependence on the parent; this is a pervasive theme usually well into the chronic phases of the brain injury (Cavallo and Kay 2011; Sherwin and O'Shanick 2000). Thus, some have argued that mothers carry a greater burden of caregiving (Guerriere and McKeever 1997; Zinner et al. 1997).

Multiple aggravations also cause friction between parents. Complications include incompatible coping styles; irritation and reproach of one another for ineptitudes or lack of progress in the loved one; preoccupation with the needs of the loved one, which crowds out deserved attention and affection toward the husband and other siblings; neglect of the marriage secondary to overwhelming outside obligations; and isolation from social respite with friends (Cavallo and Kay 2011; David 1998; Lezak 1988). Now and again, divorce ensues from marital and family conflict (Lezak 1988).

Elderly parents are propelled out of the pleasures of retirement into "on the spot" invasion into a young adult/adult's existence, who beforehand was self-sufficient (Elbaum 2010; Lezak 1988). Also, as parents age, the physical, social, and emotional sequelae of the loved one's brain injury, coupled with their own declining health, intensifies the toll (Minnes, et al. 2010; Ponsford 2013). For the long haul, they are petrified about the loved one's future care, including living accommodations and providing for him or her financially (Allen et al. 1994; Minnes et al. 2010). Overall, a trend in the literature is the lack of emotional support and resources for parents, especially in the postacute phases (Minnes et al. 2010).

3.3.2 *"Helpful Hints" and Tools for Parents to Cope with a Son or Daughter with an Acquired Brain Injury*

Table 3.6 summarizes "helpful hints" and tools for parents to cope with a son or daughter with an acquired brain injury. Psychotherapy and psychoeducation for parents are fundamental to their adjustment in caring for an older adolescent or adult son or daughter with an acquired brain injury, up to many years postinjury (Hawley et al. 2003; Klonoff 2010; Verhaeghe et al. 2005). This starts with a systematic and integrated discharge plan prior to the loved one leaving the hospital (Kao and Stuifbergen 2004). Constructive venues are meetings just with the parents to attend to their specific concerns as well as conjoint meetings with their son or daughter to address family matters and promote cohesive and cooperative interventions in the home (Klonoff and Koberstein 2010). Conjoint meetings are also favored for the psychotherapist to witness potentially unhealthy interactions and proffer remedies. Marital therapy is integral to address "marital menace" and restore constructive communication patterns and new life aspirations (Kao and Stuifbergen 2004). The tenets described elsewhere apply in all combinations, including the value of medical education about brain function, neurological syndromes, neurorehabilitation options (hopefully all-inclusive treatment), and compensation training (Elbaum 2010; Hawley et al. 2003; Klonoff 2010; Sherwin and O'Shanick 2000; see also Chaps. 4, 5, 6, 7, 8, and 10 for psychoeducation about specific etiologies).

When the loved one is an adolescent, the parents should seek a therapist with specialized background in developmental phases, as this will interface with the brain injury when deciding on treatment directions and goals (Sherwin and O'Shanick 2000). The psychotherapist will teach parents to recognize germane developmental factors, including the need to integrate the loved one's changing body into his or her self-image, the importance of a peer group, the fragility of the preaccident sense of self, maturation in the realms of intimacy and sexuality, as well as strivings for independence (see Sherwin and O'Shanick 2000, for a review). Zinner et al. (1997) have described a transition from a state of "partial death" of the loved one to "partial living."

The psychotherapist should review the expected consequences of *chronic sorrow,* which is enduring and episodic stress characterized by a myriad of feelings and experiences, including feeling hollow, rumination, social withdrawal, reactive guilt, anger, depression, wariness, and even posttraumatic stress disorder (PTSD; see Roos 2002, for a review). *Loss spirals* are catalyzed by new and compound reminders of the losses, which intensify the grief reactions (Roos 2002). There are seemingly constant reminders of the discrepancy between parental hopes and expectations and the harsh realities of defeats (Roos 2002). The parents feel unable to enjoy life, until the same is true for the loved one (Roos 2002).

The psychotherapist should employ empathic responsiveness to the profound and all-encompassing suffering through a model of "companioning," characterized by nonjudgmental coaching and collaboration (Roos 2002). This creates a working alliance in which there is a "calm presence in the midst of chaos" in a secure "holding environment," rather than a "fix it" or "resolve it" orientation (Roos 2002).

Table 3.6 "Helpful hints" and tools for parents to cope with a son or daughter with an acquired brain injury

Psychotherapy, psychoeducation, and compensation training are fundamental, starting with hospital discharge
Varied venues are ideal, including parents with and without the loved one
For adolescents, find a psychotherapist with training in developmental phases
Understand the concepts of "chronic sorrow" and "loss spirals" and their impact on the parents' mood and outlook
The therapist will employ various treatment interventions for "chronic sorrow":
"Companioning" with nonjudgmental coaching and collaboration
Interpersonal and cognitive–behavioral therapies to build adaptive repertoires
Allow a normal process of separation and individuation
Consider psychotropic medication if needed
Stress reduction techniques are helpful
Focus on a close and affectionate parental/child relationship
Develop self-efficacy and empowerment
Proliferate kindness, empathy, and wisdom
Update values, core beliefs, and self-views
Transform and adapt by finding meaning in suffering
Embrace the "realism" process
"Let go" and embrace the "new normal"
Examine the unique qualities and challenges of the "mother role"
Solicit assistance in coping with "ambiguous loss"
Engage in marital therapy to fortify the relationship
Explore the "intuitive" and "instrumental" grief styles
Learn how to divide attentions between the loved one, siblings, and the other spouse
Use limit-setting techniques and find time to nurture the marital relationship
Explore and resolve chronic and unproductive rage, bitterness, and self-recriminations through the concepts of "hindsight is 40/40," "what-ifs," "would-have, could-have, should-have syndrome," the "resource bucket," "good enough" parenting, "optimal frustrations," "transmuting internalizations," "catastrophic reactions," and "catastrophic reactions by proxy"
Accept pointers for dealing with outsiders who may unintentionally misstep in their communications and actions
Learn skills necessary for the loved one to achieve his or her maximal level of independence:
Include an occupational therapist to teach home independence skills
Create a shadow Home Independence Checklist and/or "Do Not Do" Checklist
Consider alternative living arrangements (e.g., casita, nearby apartment, or group home)
Find appropriate work activities for all parties to foster socialization and a sense of meaning
Obtain psychotherapeutic and adjunct resources for reducing fears and anxieties and help the loved one foray into community life:
Speech and language therapy and other group therapies to learn social skills for friendships
School personnel for school reentry
Driving evaluations by specialized therapists
Substance abuse treatment
Job seeker
Learn techniques to avoid "wearing out" as elderly caregivers
Establish healthier interactions with estranged relatives, based on duty, loyalty, and forgiveness
As aging parents, engage in "permanency planning":
Referral to local agencies and a social worker
Public awareness campaigning, networking, and partnerships
Brainstorm with other aging parents in a support group about alternative living situations
Learn problem-solving approaches as well as coping and reframing skills to reduce anguish

Table 3.6 (continued)

Replenish emotional reserves through the second and third tiers of support
Undertake the transition from "going back" to "going beyond"
Multimedia resources
Websites
www.eeoc.gov/facts/intellectual_disabilities.html
www.t-tap.org
www.caringbridge.org

Treatment interventions include interpersonal and cognitive–behavioral therapies so that the parents can identify destructive patterns of relating and build adaptive repertoires (Roos 2002). This means communicating feelings without alienating others (Roos 2002). Structured writing assignments generate choices which boost the parents' self-regulation of the strong emotions of victimization or helplessness (Roos 2002). The "stop think" method coupled with structuring time-limited "worry time" also helps the parents gain control of the tendency to become agitated or to ruminate (Roos 2002). Psychotherapy can also instruct parents to avoid "symbiotic enmeshment" so as to uphold a normal process of separation and individuation (Roos 2002). The parent(s) may benefit from psychotropic medication to address entrenched depression, anxiety, or PTSD symptoms (Roos 2002).

Gradually, the psychotherapist can gently propose other mitigating solutions, including stress reduction techniques (e.g., progressive deep muscle relaxation, diaphragmatic breathing, and meditation); focusing on a close and affectionate parental/child relationship; developing self-efficacy and empowerment (through knowledge acquisition); proliferation of kindness, empathy, and wisdom; updating values, central beliefs, and self-views; and transformation and adaptation through finding meaning in suffering (see Roos 2002, for a review). The therapist will aid the parents in relinquishing the fantasy of "how life should have been" through the "realism" process (Klonoff and Koberstein 2010; Roos 2002). There remains an acknowledgement of the cataclysmic experiences, yet "letting go," so as to adjust and hopefully embrace the "new normal" (Roos 2002).

The psychotherapist should be mindful of the uniqueness of the "mother role"; this is not necessarily a role variation, but rather role continuity with new circumstances (Wongvatunyu and Porter 2008b). Mothers serve as "first observers," given their close perspective and intuition emanating from "being a mom." Hence, their observations and input are often pivotal to the recovery of the loved one (Wongvatunyu and Porter 2008b). The psychotherapist will educate the parents that the adage of "hurting the one you love" is typified by this relationship, as the loved one both needs yet resents and resists the often extensive backing (Cavallo and Kay 2011; Sherwin and O'Shanick 2000; see Chap. 2, Sect. 2.4.2.2). Often, mothers feel especially targeted, perhaps because the son or daughter feels safe in expressing the chagrin, embarrassment, and despair about his or her dire state of affairs.

Owing to the inclination to dominate the caregiver role and maintain the loved one at home, mothers have the propensity to: make safety the top priority and prohibit risky activities; take the lead in planning ahead; act protectively toward the loved one's vulnerabilities; adopt a strong advocacy role for the foreseeable future;

and be extremely cautious about outside tier 3 resources, including other caretakers or nursing homes (Wongvatunyu and Porter 2005). They come to realize that they will be "starting over" with reraising their loved one. Frequently, they describe mothering "different children" with existential realizations of the fragility and unpredictability of life (Guerriere and McKeever 1997; Sachs 1991). Psychotherapy can assist mothers in coping with "ambiguous loss," including accepting the altered child who has survived (Boss 2006; see Guerriere and McKeever 1997, for a review; see Chap. 10, Sect. 10.4). This includes normalizing feelings of guilt and powerlessness (Guerriere and McKeever 1997). Mothers are also guided to redefine priorities; reconfigure their life tempo; appreciate the positive aspects of their devotion as a caregiver; and "reinvent the family's life," with emphasis on the loved ones' maximal outcome, in tandem with other family members' needs as well as their own (Guerriere and McKeever 1997; Wongvatunyu and Porter 2005).

Marital discord after brain injury is presumed and should be normalized by the psychotherapist. The psychotherapist will introduce parents to different forms of grieving: the *intuitive* griever experiences the affective components and the outward expression mirrors the inner feelings (Doka and Martin 2010). The intuitive griever favors lamenting about his or her anguish with others (Doka and Martin 2010). The *instrumental* griever experiences grief through the cognitions rather than emotions; he or she will be less willing to emote (Doka and Martin 2010). His or her worldview is that through the sense of control, the calamity can be mastered (Doka and Martin 2010). He or she channels thoughts into planned activity and problem solving to overcome the obstacle (Doka and Martin 2010). Often, the grieving parents blend both styles, although they may fall at different points along the continuum (Doka and Martin 2010). Although not an absolute by any means, some men fall more into instrumental grieving, while women may be intuitive grievers (Doka and Martin 2010). Cultural norms also shape expressions of grief (Doka and Martin 2010). Guiding the couple to recognize and tolerate disparate grieving approaches is paramount for the preservation of the marriage. Many parents describe a seesaw pattern of shifting back and forth between different ways of grieving, both within each griever and between the parents, depending on the phase of the loved one's recovery and the nature of the specific stressors. In the context of healthy communication, this can be seen as complementary and a "survival" mechanism.

Given the encumbrances on the marital relationship, marital therapy also enables expressing emotions and deciding how best to meet the needs of the loved one in the context of the deserved attention toward the other spouse and siblings. This requires vigilance on the part of each parent not to become excessively invested in the polarized "nurturing" role (i.e., the mother) versus the "breadwinner" role (i.e., the father) to the exclusion of time together. Otherwise, one parent becomes enmeshed with the loved one, while the other feels ostracized and peripheral (Minuchin 1974). To facilitate this, the psychotherapist will push the parents to find equilibrium in their disparate roles, including not becoming overly engrossed in the needs of the loved one or escaping a complex and unpredictable situation through safe and familiar work pursuits (Niemeier and Karol 2011a). Clear boundaries should also be set with the loved one so as to devote precious time to one another. This includes finding ways to nurture one another and taking time to be with each other with a strict agreement not to focus on or talk about the loved one (Roos 2002). Delegating to willing second and third tiers of support can also reduce the inimitable pressures.

Therapy will address the chronic and unproductive rage, bitterness, and self-recriminations that can cloak parents over their helplessness in preventing their son's or daughter's brain injury and any subsequent self-perceived inadequacies. One apropos adage is *hindsight is 40/40,* indicating that retrospective attempts at second guessing, "what ifs," and the "would-have, could-have, should-have" syndrome are nonproductive (Klonoff 2010). Another handy conceptualization is the *resource bucket,* implying that there are finite coping reserves from which these debilitating emotions siphon valuable life-affirming energies. Through cognitive restructuring, parents can make a conscious effort to contain and/or dissipate these otherwise exhausting preoccupations.

The psychotherapist will introduce parents to the concepts of "good enough" parenting (Bettelheim 1987; Winnicott 1994), "optimal frustration" (Kohut 1987), and "transmuting internalization" (Wolf 1988). Basically, this psychoanalytic and self-psychology terminology translates to the inevitable flaws and failures associated with parenting (and therapy) as stepping stones for the loved one to strengthen his or her ego structure (Wolf 1988). This reduces self-inflicted stress and guilt and breeds self-forgiveness for mistakes in the parenting role. The psychotherapist will reframe the process as actually beneficial to the loved one in learning to tolerate some degree of aggravation and imperfections (in self and others). Put another way, some frequency of CRs (Goldstein 1952) and CRs by proxy (Klonoff and Koberstein 2010) are unavoidable as the family unit traverses a tricky path to recovery. (See Chap. 4, Sect. 4.6 and Table 4.6 for more about CRs, see Chap. 2, Sect. 2.4.2.1; Chap. 4, Sect. 4.8.2 and Table 4.10; and Chap. 9, Sect. 9.4 and Tables 9.7 and 9.8 for more about CRs by proxy).

Parents may need pointers in dealing with outsiders who may unintentionally "misstep" in their feedback. One clear example is the predisposition to reinterpret the dreadful incident as a sign of the parents "being chosen" or "special," with comments such as "God doesn't give you more than you can handle." This stance can be perceived by the sorrowful parents as shallow and offensive (Roos 2002). The psychotherapist may need to reframe these comments as well-meaning (if not naïve) so that the parents do not to displace their grief or rage onto other undeserving persons.

A primary objective of rehabilitation is for loved one to achieve his or her maximal level of independence. This empowers the parents, especially overprotective mothers, to find the wherewithal to foster autonomy and "let go" of their sons or daughters (Kao and Stuifbergen 2004; see also Chap. 9, Sect. 9.6). The process usually starts in the home environment. Occupational therapy in conjunction with family therapy can steer parents (especially mothers) to transfer home chores to the loved one. In one scenario, the parent can complete a shadow Home Independence Checklist (see also Chap. 4, Sect. 4.4.4 and Fig. 4.7; Klonoff 2010), where he or she tracks which tasks the loved one does independently, as compared with cuing, or not completed. This is an awareness exercise for the parent to appreciate how much "cuing" and/or "doing" is embedded in the familial interactions at home. Another illustrative alternative is to create a "Do Not Do" checklist for parents, which reminds them what chores they should abstain from. Ultimately, psychotherapy (and adjunct therapies) should guide parents to encourage self-sufficiency in the loved one, including achieving maturational ambitions of living as independently as possible. Possible choices are a group home, casita, or nearby apartment. The psychotherapist will put forward a return to work somehow, even part-time, for the caregiver (and loved one) as crucial for socialization and a sense of meaning (Kao and Stuifbergen 2004; Klonoff and Koberstein 2010).

Psychotherapy helps fearful and anxious parents navigate the loved one's tumultuous foray into community life, which rebuilds his or her self-esteem and self-sufficiency (Elbaum 2010; Klonoff 2010). A case in point, speech and group therapies can reacquaint the loved one with appropriate social skills so as to reestablish friendships. Collateral specialists will usually be involved. This includes school personnel with whom the psychotherapist can liaison, so as to facilitate the school reentry process (Sherwin and O'Shanick 2000). Driving evaluations by therapists specialized in this domain provide for the parents' peace of mind (see Chap. 8, Sect. 8.3.1.4; Klonoff 2010). In instances of substance abuse, specialized drug and/or alcohol treatment is usually necessary (Sherwin and O'Shanick 2000).

The psychotherapist can be an advocate for these often convoluted resources to facilitate the loved one's community reintegration and to ease the parents' angst. This includes engaging a job seeker for "customized employment" which matches his or her interests, talents, injury-related limitations, accommodations, and the employer's expectations (T-Tap 2012). However, a strong partnership with the parents is imperative, as usually concerted and persistent efforts are necessary to meet the loved one's needs as he or she reintegrates into the community, especially school environments (Elbaum 2010; Singer and Nixon 1993). This should take into account the upshot of paid work on disability benefits, health-care coverage, work incentives, and The Americans with Disabilities Act (T-Tap 2012; www.eeoc.gov/facts/intellectual_disabilities.html). For more specifics relevant to parents with a loved one trying to return to the job market, see www.t-tap.org and www.eeoc.gov/facts/intellectual_disabilities.html.

The psychotherapist will be sensitive to caregivers who are aging or "wearing out" (Roos 2002). Depending on others' involvement (e.g., siblings), conflict may be reactivated, especially if there are residual feelings of shame or resentment (Roos 2002). Family therapy can facilitate working through these emotions with estranged relatives, so as to establish healthier interactions based on duty, loyalty, and forgiveness (Roos 2002). With respect to other options for "permanency planning" for aging parents (Minnes et al. 2010), the psychotherapist can also coordinate services, including referral to local agencies (e.g., the Brain Injury Alliance) and a social worker. Public awareness campaigning, networking, and partnerships also provide possible social, work, and living opportunities (Minnes et al. 2010). Family members also experience solace through brainstorming with other like-minded aging parents in a support group setting (see also Chaps. 9 and 11). Creative problem solving can unearth possibilities, including group homes, residential settings, or other shared community-living arrangements with hired caregivers (Elbaum 2010).

Psychotherapy will teach coping skills so that parents can lessen their anguish. A goal is to reframe the predicament as a manageable family hurdle instead of a hopeless catastrophe (Elbaum 2010). Techniques include advancing "aggressive determination," realistic recognition of their loved one's gains and potentials, constructive communication and proper limit setting, improving control through mastery, using adaptive outlets for frustration, as well as finding meaning in suffering (Elbaum 2010; Singer and Nixon 1993). Table 3.5 contains some examples of parents' verbalizations reflecting a transformed view of their condition through the therapeutic process.

The psychotherapist will emphasize the importance of parents replenishing their emotional reserves, including reaching out to their second and third tiers of support for emotional solace and respite care (Klonoff and Koberstein 2010; Singer and Nixon 1993). Specifically, immediate extended family, friends, coworkers, blogs (e.g., www.caringbridge.org/), faith-based contacts, family support groups, as well as community agencies and institutions (e.g., schools and youth groups) are key lifelines (Kao and Stuifbergen 2004; Klonoff and Koberstein 2010; Singer and Nixon 1993). Eventually, there is a gradual psychological transition from "going back" to "going beyond" toward meaning, core values, purpose, and joy.

3.3.3 Challenges for Reconfigured Families with a Son or Daughter with an Acquired Brain Injury

Currently, there is increasing variability in Western family structures, including single parents, divorced parents, and serial marriages (Roos 2002). In addition, identities have evolved, such as women choosing to bifurcate their lives between child rearing and work (Roos 2002). Some have argued that family patterns are more transient, roles are more flexible, and members are more often divided geographically (Roos 2002). In the context of this complexity and shift, very little is written about how "modern" redesigned family systems react and cope with a brain injury in a loved one. A detailed exploration of various family compositions is beyond the scope of this chapter; however, parents of the loved one who are in the process of divorcing, or are already divorced with possibly new partners will be addressed.

Understandably, there are impediments in meeting the everyday and emotional needs of the loved one when parents are newly or previously divorced or remarried with new partners. Unresolved marital tensions can create "difficult" or "dysfunctional" families, particularly when harmful interaction patterns are entrenched and conflict-ridden. Blaming behavior is common, with accusations of the other parent's shortfalls in providing the requisite physical, financial, or emotional support (Ackerman 1997; Pedro-Carroll 2010). All too frequently, the loved one with the brain injury is "caught in the middle" and is expected to take sides in a polarized environment (David 1998). For instance, the loved one may feel compelled to listen to a parent's venting or allegations about vexing qualities in the other parent. Given the loved one's lower frustration tolerance and emotional reactivity, these episodes can spark CRs and/or feelings of burden or worthlessness.

3.3.4 "Helpful Hints" and Tools for Reconfigured Families to Address Challenges with a Son or Daughter after Acquired Brain Injury

Table 3.7 summarizes "helpful hints" and tools for reconfigured families to address difficulties with a son or daughter after acquired brain injury. The psychotherapist can draw on general resources about the ramifications of divorce on parenting as a first step. Examples include *Parenting through Divorce* by Reynolds (2011), *Putting Children First* by Pedro-Carroll (2010), and *Does Wednesday Mean Mom's House or Dad's?* by Ackerman (1997).

Treating reconfigured families can be challenging for the therapist, especially if behavior patterns are indicative of "difficult" or "dysfunctional" coping styles. The psychotherapist may need or want to suggest family therapy to address pervasive setbacks, especially if his or her role is to primarily provide emotional support and education about the ramifications of the brain injury on the family system. Often, the divorcing/divorced parents may need their own personal counselor (separate from the rehabilitation setting), so as to continue to address their personal torment over their quandaries (Karpf and Shatz 2005).

When providing family support in the context of the loved one's brain injury, all involved parties (i.e., the divorced parents and new partners) should be invited, in order to impart consistent psychoeducation and therapeutic recommendations. This avoids misperceptions and misinterpretations which are rife with elevated emotions in various family members. All parties should be informed of the limits of the working relationship, which is for the well-being of the loved one. Suitable medical releases must be obtained before sharing information (Webster et al. 1999), with signatures from the primary guardian(s) when the loved one is a minor.

The "red crisis" zone or "Period of Disintegration" on the FEM (Klonoff et al. 2008) becomes a worthwhile therapeutic tool for family members to be vigilant about the threats to the loved one's rehabilitation and recovery if their "structural" and "process" components are detrimental (see Chap. 1, Sect. 1.5 and Fig. 1.3; and Sect. 3.1.1 and Fig. 3.1). Of note, the rehabilitation team/psychotherapist must be mindful not to become ensnared in polarized relations or parenting methods between divorcing/divorced parents or triangulated relationships between one parent and the therapist in clashes with the other partner (Becvar and Becvar 2013). This "splitting" causes "rifts" between therapists that mirrors the family's divisiveness, which then fragments care (Klonoff 2011; Webster et al. 1999).

The psychotherapist and reconfigured family will realize that many of the family therapy principles during and after a divorce are applicable to parenting after brain injury, with the "volume turned up" or intensified (Klonoff 2010). For instance, the feelings of loss, anxiety, sadness, frustration, powerlessness, insecurity, devastation, bleakness, and unpredictability that are prominent in divorce (Ackerman 1997; Pedro-Carroll 2010; Vollmer 2008) can be greatly exacerbated for the loved one trying to cope with a divorced family life together with the repercussions of the brain injury. This creates a "double whammy." To make matters worse, if the divorce

Table 3.7 "Helpful hints" and tools for reconfigured families to address challenges with a son or daughter after acquired brain injury

The psychotherapist will likely draw on general literature about divorce
Psychotherapy will define the goals and limits of family therapy, namely to provide emotional support and education about the effects of the brain injury on the family system
Adjunct family or personal therapy may be necessary for "difficult" or "dysfunctional" reconfigured families
The therapist will likely prefer to meet with all parties simultaneously to impart consistent psychoeducation and therapeutic recommendations
The limits of the working relationship and proper protocols for patient confidentiality will be reviewed
The "red crisis" zone of the Family Experiential Model (FEM) of Recovery is a helpful training tool
The therapist and treatment team will be mindful of keeping healthy boundaries with complex family systems
Principles of family therapy for reconfigured family systems are applicable to the effects of brain injury, with the "volume turned up," including the emotional distress
Put the needs of the loved one in the forefront
Develop healthy co-parenting partnerships
Maintain flexibility, good communication skills, and a willingness to share decisions and responsibilities
Parents and new partners must stay focused, use self-control, remain sensitive and selfless, and prioritize the best interests of the loved one
Collaborate with an attitude of division of labor and loyalty to the rehabilitation and recovery process
Consider living within a proximal distance of one another to reduce burdens
Reassure the loved one that he/she did not cause the divorce and is loved
Consider the age, developmental stage, and injury implications when sharing information with the loved one
In times of flux and angst, keep the psychotherapist closely informed
Shield the loved one from squabbles, dissention, disputes, and disparaging comments, so he/she is not caught in the middle or in the cross fire
Do not ask the loved one to keep secrets and do not alienate him/her from the other parent
Establish clear and consistent ground rules and boundaries for the loved one
Present a "united front" with respect to limit setting for the loved one
Don't use the loved one as a "go-between" or to spy on the other parent
Don't "bribe" or be overly lenient or indulgent with the loved one
Stick to rules, routines, and predictable schedules between the two homes
Communicate with other adults through datebook or tablet entries so as to stay in the loop
The parental figures should brainstorm beforehand, so as to present consistent messages to the loved one
Do "practice milieu meetings" with the therapist and apply the same format in the home with the loved one
Remember that no matter what the level of acrimony, all caregivers should strive to get along with each other for the benefit of the loved one
Multimedia resources
Books
Parenting Through Divorce (Reynolds 2011)
Putting Children First (Pedro-Carroll 2010)
Does Wednesday Mean Mom's House or Dad's? (Ackerman 1997)
Model
The Family Experiential Model (FEM) of Recovery (Klonoff and Koberstein 2010; Klonoff et al. 2008)

results after the loved one's brain injury, he or she may experience profound guilt and self-blame for creating enough of a millstone on the parents to cause the divorce.

In the context of family restructuring and reorganization, it is pivotal to put the needs of the loved one in the forefront (Ackerman 1997; Karpf and Shatz 2005). The aim of therapy will be to develop positive co-parenting partnerships, whereby the finest qualities and expertise of each parent are incorporated in the context of respect and trust for one another (Karpf and Shatz 2005; Vollmer 2008). Parenting styles can be *parallel,* with minimal interaction between parents and clear boundaries to reduce or prevent conflict, or *cooperative,* in which there is a high degree of teamwork, decent communication, shared decision making, and flexibility (Ackerman 1997; Pedro-Carroll 2010; Reynolds 2011). The psychotherapist will guide the parents and new partner(s) to stay focused, use self-control, and remain sensitive and selfless, so as to prioritize the best interests of the loved one (Ackerman 1997; Karpf and Shatz 2005; Pedro-Carroll 2010; Reynolds 2011; Vollmer 2008). Given the time-consuming nature of caring for the loved one after the brain injury, divorcing/divorced family units need to agree to an attitude of division of labor and loyalty to the rehabilitation and recovery process. Living within a proximal distance of one another reduces the load on the parents (Ackerman 1997), who are generally the primary mode of transportation. Technological resources (e.g., a shared Internet-based calendar) allow for communication, yet minimize contentious face-to-face interactions.

Divorcing/divorced parents must be extremely mindful of how the aftereffects of the divorce will negatively impact a son or daughter with a brain injury. The age, developmental stage, and injury implications need to be factored into the timing and delivery of information to the loved one. The loved one should be reassured that he or she did not cause the divorce and is loved by the parents (Pedro-Carroll 2010; Reynolds 2011). If the loved one's living arrangement is altering, a family meeting to review this in advance is essential in a neutral location in the home, when there is plenty of opportunity for discussion (Pedro-Carroll 2010; Reynolds 2011), taking into account the specifics of the loved one's constraints. This infuses some stability into an inherently unstable situation. The psychotherapist should be kept closely apprised (and hopefully involved) in these discussions, so as to facilitate a smoother transition.

The loved one should be shielded from all squabbles and dissension between parents/new partners so that he or she does not feel caught in the middle or in the cross fire (Ackerman 1997; Karpf and Shatz 2005; Pedro-Carroll 2010; Reynolds 2011; Vollmer 2008). Open disputes and disparaging comments can be frightening to the loved one, whose sense of self and existence are already shattered (Reynolds 2011). Caregivers should never ask the loved one to keep secrets from one another (Ackerman 1997; Vollmer 2008), as after the injury, the loved one will likely forget, precipitating heightened furor and/or may experience needless pressures and anxiety. Otherwise, alienation from one of the parents can occur through programming the loved one against the other parent (Ackerman 1997). This can be more pronounced and destructive in the context of the loved one's "black-and-white" thinking after a brain injury.

The therapist will propose that divorcing/divorced parents and new partners establish clear and consistent ground rules and boundaries for treatment of the loved one with the brain injury. A "united front" with respect to limit setting must be adhered to (Ackerman 1997), especially when the loved one suffers from memory and executive function deficits which compromise his or her adaptation to changing rules and expectations. An example is not using the loved one as a partner in which to confide (Ackerman 1997; Reynolds 2011). This becomes especially salient because the loved one is dealing with his or her own psychosocial and emotional ineptitudes and may also lack the cognitive capability to grasp the parent's complex emotional needs. Otherwise, the loved one may become overwhelmed and overtaxed.

Divorcing/divorced parents should not be using the loved one as a "go-between" or "spy" on the other parent (Ackerman 1997; Karpf and Shatz 2005; Pedro-Carroll 2010; Reynolds 2011; Vollmer 2008), as this can be unnerving to the loved one and detracts from his or her focus on recovery and treatment. Parents and new partners should be wary of being overly lenient or indulgent with the loved one as a way to "bribe" him or her for affection (Ackerman 1997; Pedro-Carroll 2010). After the injury, sticking to rules, routines, and predictable schedules between two homes is vital for the loved one (Vollmer 2008), who otherwise can become flummoxed and nonproductive. Communicating through datebook or tablet entries also keeps both parents in the loop about the loved one's rehabilitation needs and homework.

When addressing the loved one's challenges, the psychotherapist will offer the idea of all parties "brainstorming" beforehand, so as to provide consistent messages to the loved one (Ackerman 1997). This reduces the likelihood of manipulation and/or unacceptable behavior in the loved one (Ackerman 1997; Reynolds 2011), which can already be thorny, related to organic problems with judgment, impulse control, and disinhibited behavior. "Milieu meetings" are useful forums to address subjects and resolve differences. "Practice milieu meetings" with the psychotherapist present model harmonious interactions which can then be generalized to nonclinical environments. Regardless of the chosen therapy method, the guiding standard should be that no matter what the level of acrimony, all caregivers strive to get along with each other for the benefit of the loved one.

3.4 Scenario: Impact of a Brain Injury on Children of a Parent with an Acquired Brain Injury

Limitations faced by children of any age with a parent with a brain injury differ based on a multiplicity of considerations, including the nature and consequences of the brain injury, age and maturational status of the child, family system, culture, environment, psychodynamics, and other historical variables correlated with the aspect of health versus dysfunction of the family and children (Hallé et al. 2011; Urbach et al. 1994; see also Chap. 1, Sect. 1.3 and Fig. 1.1). In childhood and adolescence, the experience of undergoing a sudden and often alarming event in a previously stable parental figure can be destabilizing and traumatizing (Kieffer-Kristensen et al. 2011). There is a shattering of their assumptive world (see Chap. 2, Sect. 2.3.8; Chap. 9, Sect. 9.10.1 and Table 9.20; and Chap. 10, Sect. 10.4 and Table 10.6), with a dearth of guidance and nurturance (Cavallo and Kay 2011). Younger children may wonder or inquire: *What happened to my mom or dad? Why is he or she so different? How come everyone seems so upset?* Adult children faced with a brain injury in their parent contend with the same scenario, and they also have superimposed angst from juggling their other roles and endeavors with a newly acquired family trauma. Adult children may inquire: *What will become of my injured parent? How can I help my parents when I have so many of my own family obligations? Is my other parent able to take care of my injured parent? What is my role in caregiving and rehabilitation?*

3.4.1 Challenges for Children with a Parent with an Acquired Brain Injury

This segment will focus briefly on the barriers and treatment needs of younger children and adolescents, while Sects. 3.4.3 and 3.4.4 will address the factors for adult children whose parents have sustained a brain injury.

When a parent sustains a brain injury, minor children are exposed to diminished parental attention along with more responsibility (Cavallo and Kay 2011; Elbaum 2010; Lezak 1988; Ponsford 2013; Verhaeghe et al. 2005). This emanates from the fact that the injured parent has many more needs, translating to an upsurge of duties for the healthy parent, and consequently, crammed time for the children (Elbaum 2010; Kieffer-Kristensen and Teasdale 2011). The injured parent may demonstrate disrupted caretaking and a lack of responsiveness to the children, attributable to cognitive, personality, and physical impairments (Kieffer-Kristensen et al. 2011; Skippon 2013). The children's new developmental life phases often flummox the injured parent (Skippon 2013). This decline in parenting performance by both the injured and uninjured parent causes acting-out behaviors or posttraumatic stress symptoms in their children, as well as emotional and/or relationship problems (Kieffer-Kristensen et al. 2013; Kieffer-Kristensen and Teasdale 2011; Kieffer-Kristensen et al. 2011; Pessar et al. 1993). This has been referred to as *disrupted parenting,* defined as a reduction of support, effort, neglect, and/or absence due to chronic illness in a parent (Armistead et al. 1995). Depending on the severity of the injury, the uninjured parent becomes the "gate keeper," whereby he or she monitors the nature and amount of parenting by the injured parent, based on deficient skill sets (Kieffer-Kristensen et al. 2013). The overwhelming burdens can cause unhappiness and depression in the healthy parent, which in turn negatively impacts his or her parenting (Kieffer-Kristensen and Teasdale 2011; Pessar et al. 1993).

Strain in the parental dyad causes stress, depression, upside-down routines, and conflicts between parents or the parent and child, and thus behavior and adjustment difficulties in children (Armistead et al 1995; Visser-Meily et al. 2005a). Upheaval produces other emotions in children and adolescents, such as shame, guilt (as the cause of the parent's injury), embarrassment (about disturbing personality deviations), fear (about another injury to a loved one), frustration, sadness, anxiety, withdrawal, and anger (Butera-Prinzi and Perlesz 2004; Cavallo and Kay 2011; Elbaum 2010; Lezak 1988; Skippon 2013). Some children have described feeling left out and invisible, succumbing to devastating grief and loss (Butera-Prinzi and Perlesz 2004). They also battle to mourn when the parent is still alive (Butera-Prinzi and Perlesz 2004). Children may become socially isolated or drift away, as they are adverse to bringing peers into the home (Butera-Prinzi and Perlesz 2004; Cavallo and Kay 2011; Lezak 1988; Ponsford 2013). Conversely, children and adolescents may become "parentified," feeling the onus to take over adult realms (Skippon 2013; Urbach et al. 1994). To complicate matters, the children worry about the condition of the uninjured parent, perceiving his or her burnout (Butera-Prinzi and Perlesz 2004). To adolescents, the family system may no longer feel like a dependable or secure base (Skippon 2013). Ultimately, children are apprehensive that the family structure will disintegrate (Butera-Prinzi and Perlesz 2004).

Unfortunately, many of these children are not commonly included in the family-focused neurorehabilitation process, owing to ill attunement of the parents with the children's suffering, as well as staff issues, including a lack of training and resources, anxiety, and negative attitudes toward the necessity of including youngsters (Butera-Prinzi and Perlesz 2004; Kieffer-Kristensen et al. 2011; Webster and Daisley 2007).

3.4.2 *"Helpful Hints" and Tools for Children with a Parent with an Acquired Brain Injury*

Table 3.8 summarizes "helpful hints" and tools for minor children and adolescents with a parent with an acquired brain injury. Untreated children are considered "at risk" (Urbach and Culbert 1991). Given the seriousness of a parent's brain injury regarding children, a family-centered approach is instrumental to their adjustment (Kieffer-Kristensen et al. 2011; Visser-Meily et al. 2005a; Visser-Meily et al. 2005b). This should be a five-pronged one. First, the parent with the brain injury will require psychotherapeutic interventions to reduce the injury's aftermath on the dependent children and improve parenting competencies (Klonoff and Myles 2010; Urbach et al. 1994). This includes multidisciplinary therapies to reduce the parent's problems with disinhibition, impulsivity, rigidity, lability, hyperactivity, depression, apathy, and paranoia (Urbach et al. 1994). Psychiatric services should be considered to reduce the disruptive influence of the injured parent's significant emotional problems (see Urbach et al. 1994, for a review). As the injured parent resumes household and child-rearing tasks through the neurorehabilitation process, the child can abdicate unwarranted functions, thereby reducing his or her stress level.

Second, the uninjured parent will benefit from treatment of his or her depression and assistance in stress management and coping skills (Klonoff and Koberstein 2010). This can repair fractionated parenting behaviors (Pessar et al. 1993). He or she will also need therapeutic guidance to adequately juggle the roles of the tier 1 caregiver with respect to the spouse and the often profound parental assignments

Table 3.8 "Helpful hints" and tools for minor, adolescent, and adult children to cope with a parent after an acquired brain injury

Minor children/adolescents
Remember these children are "at risk"
A five-pronged family-centered approach is instrumental for the children's adjustment
Therapies should target the parent with the brain injury, the uninjured parent, the marriage, the youngsters, and the whole family
Interventions for the children can include:
Early screening
User-friendly psychoeducation (including that the child did not cause the brain injury)
Monitoring school performance
Liaison with school personnel and clergy
Errorless Compliance Training
Behavior therapy
Psychodynamic therapy
Support group with peer validation
Pharmacotherapy
Try to safeguard the attachment relationship with the injured parent
Focus on resiliency
For stability, try to recreate preinjury daily routines
Utilize an occupational therapist to incorporate practical compensations for the injured parent so as to enable togetherness with the children
Help the injured parent explore how to meaningfully reengage with the children
Involve the children with age-appropriate household activities
Have the healthy parent set aside time with the children
Build relationships with other tier supports, including grandparents
Encourage children to share emotions with friends and other family members
Nurture peer relationships outside of the home
Involve youngsters in social activities and sports
Allow pets for comfort
Help adolescents pursue healthy independence and identity formation
Give adolescents "permission" to seek their milestones to avoid oppression and resentment
"Keep the door open" for later treatment for the family unit as new dilemmas or crises evolve
Help the family system appreciate positive aspects of family life
Adult children
Seek psychotherapy to enlighten and sustain tier 2 adult children so as to:
Furnish respite for the primary caregiver
Prepare them for future responsibilities
Elements of therapy should include psychoeducation, compensation training, and understanding supervision needs and medical restrictions
Involve other therapy disciplines, including occupational and physical therapists, as well as speech–language pathologists
Collaborative interventions with tier 1 and tier 2 supports should target whatever is most helpful to the overall support network
Conjoint sessions involving the loved one and adult children enable:
Mutual sharing
Group sensitivity
Reestablishment of as normal routines as possible
Processing of why the injured parent shuns support
Assist adult children in experiencing joy and relief as the injured parent resumes aspects of prior roles
Learn feasible techniques to facilitate coping and time management:

Table 3.8 (continued)

Ways to balance their own family, career, and community endeavors
Access respite for the loved one, if needed
Pursue marital therapy for the adult child, if needed
Multimedia resources
Book
Love You Forever (Munsch 2013)

(see Kieffer-Kristensen and Teasdale 2011, for a review). This becomes paramount, as children may rely more on the healthy parent for support and protection from psychological distress (Kieffer-Kristensen et al. 2013). Helpful resources include respite breaks, third parties to help with outside stressors (e.g., finances), and support groups (Skippon 2013; see also Chaps. 9 and 11 for support groups).

Third, marital therapy is usually warranted to consolidate efforts to address anguish in the children and to focus on rebonding and holistically reintegrating the injured parent into the parenting role (Kieffer-Kristensen and Teasdale 2011; Urbach and Culbert 1991). As a first step, a "parental risk assessment" may need to be completed in order to identify strengths and difficulties in both parents, the children's functioning, and the overall family coping capacity, including their social context and support resources (Skippon 2013). Follow-up parental training is key and parental support groups encompassing "competent" parents coping with a brain injury are a useful resource (Skippon 2013). Psychoeducation for both parents incorporating input from the healthy parent is crucial, especially related to observations of compromised safety awareness (Skippon 2013). Both parents will need to be taught compensatory strategies (Skippon 2013).

Fourth, and importantly, children need therapeutic interventions to address their myriad of questions and complex emotions. As part of this, the minor child needs reassurance that he or she is not the cause of the parent's injury-related behaviors (Urbach et al. 1994). Given that children's early adaptation after parental brain injury is predictive of later adjustment, early screening is critical (Butera-Prinzi and Perlesz 2004; Visser-Meily et al. 2005b). Concerned parties should be aware of the fact that the upset child may try to imitate the injured parent's erratic or problematic behavior as a way to identify with him or her (Urbach et al. 1994). As part of the rehabilitation process, children (and the uninjured parent) should have access to user-friendly psychoeducation about the consequences of brain injury, family impact, and advice on how to deal with feelings (Cavallo and Kay 2011; Elbaum 2010; Skippon 2013; Urbach and Culbert 1991; Visser-Meily et al. 2005b; Webster and Daisley 2007). The psychotherapist should be mindful of academic shortfalls in children as indicative of unhappiness (Urbach et al. 1994). Tier 3 school personnel should be notified (e.g., the principal, school psychologist, and teachers), as well as clergy, so that they are privy and attentive to the children's sorrow and special needs (Elbaum 2010; Skippon 2013; Urbach and Culbert 1991; Urbach et al. 1994).

Additional professional interventions should be acquired for the youngsters, given their vulnerabilities (Kieffer-Kristensen et al. 2011; Urbach et al. 1994; Visser-Meily et al. 2005b). Interventions are fortified by adapting the focus of who is treated and shifting modalities (Urbach and Culbert 1991). One methodology to develop the parent–child interactions and the child's level of cooperation is "errorless compliance training" for parents with brain injuries and their children with oppositional or compliance-related behaviors (Ducharme et al. 2002). Other forms of treatment for affected children to facilitate long-term adjustment are: age-appropriate psychoeducation; behavior therapy; psychodynamic therapy; family therapy sessions; a children's support group incorporating peer validation; and, if necessary, pharmacotherapy (Butera-Prinzi and Perlesz 2004; Urbach and Culbert 1991; Urbach et al. 1994). Safeguarding the attachment relationship with the injured parent is ideal (Skippon 2013). Skippon (2013) proposes a "strengths-based resilience approach" which identifies and reinforces resiliency within the parents and children, family unit, and social networks.

Lastly, whole family therapy is efficacious in shifting family structures and relationships, sharing in the grief process, and defining new family adaptation systems (Urbach and Culbert 1991), especially as new developmental life phases unfold in the children (Skippon 2013). Recreating the family's preinjury daily routines, to whatever degree possible, can rekindle stability for minor children (Skippon 2013). With the help of an occupational therapist, the injured parent can be taught practical compensations (e.g., adaptive equipment and transportation alternatives to driving) to enable togetherness with his or her youngsters (Skippon 2013). Employing creativity and sensitivity, the psychotherapist can also help the injured parent explore how to meaningfully reengage with his or her children based on his or her expectations, priorities, and identity as a parent (Skippon 2013). Involving the children with age-appropriate household activities with the injured parent is satisfying and normalizing to all parties (Skippon 2013). Other positive coping tools that the psychotherapist can endorse are: setting aside special time with the healthy parent; building relationships with other tier supports (e.g., a grandparent); encouraging the children to share emotions with friends and family members; nurturing relationships outside of the home with peers; involvement in social activities and sports; and allowing pets in the home as a source of comfort (Butera-Prinzi and Perlesz 2004; Skippon 2013; Urbach et al. 1994).

Adolescents may push boundaries and struggle with the normal individuation and separation process (Skippon 2013). An appropriately trained psychotherapist can help adolescents pursue healthy independence and identity formation in the context of the altered family system (Skippon 2013). This may involve helping the family give the young person "permission" to leave home and pursue appropriate milestones, including attending university, taking a new job, moving away, etc. (Skippon 2013). This reduces the likelihood of feeling oppressed and/or resentful (Skippon 2013). Keeping the "door open" for later treatment if new dilemmas or crises evolve helps the family unit with long-term adjustment (Klonoff and Koberstein 2010; Skippon 2013). With timely interventions, families can experience posttraumatic growth, with a revitalization of family appreciation, respect, and connectedness (see Skippon 2013, for a review).

3.4.3 Challenges for Adult Children of a Parent with an Acquired Brain Injury

Although the loved one's spouse or parents more commonly provide tier 1 caregiver support, sometimes, the duties fall to the adult children (Cavallo and Kay 2011). When this happens, the adult children are often torn between the needs of their own children, spouse, work, and the illness in a parent (Cavallo and Kay 2011). They may become guilt-ridden when they are not accessible for caregiving (Cavallo and Kay 2011). There are usually strains on relationships, causing conflicts between the adult child and his or her spouse and children (Cavallo and Kay 2011). This can be intensified in a multichild family, whereby siblings clash over the aftereffects of the injury and how to adequately and fairly subdivide responsibilities (Cavallo and Kay 2011). The stress on the family system and roles may be more prominent during holidays or extended family gatherings for family members who do not engage in daily contact and who do not fathom the nature and reverberations of the brain injury.

Caregiving for a parent with a brain injury disrupts the family system, with essentially a reversal in the caregiver role from parent-to-child to child-to-injured parent. For example, an aphasic mother may be viewed as vulnerable and fragile by her daughter, translating to a desire to be protective (Hallé et al. 2011). The loved one may be reluctant to accept this role turnaround, vetoing the adult child's attempts to bestow care. Table 3.9 contains some sample verbalizations by adult children with a parent with an acquired brain injury, based on completed Sense of Self Questionnaires.

3.4.4 "Helpful Hints" and Tools for Adult Children of a Parent with an Acquired Brain Injury

Table 3.8 also summarizes "helpful hints" and tools for adult children of a parent with an acquired brain injury. Psychotherapy to enlighten and sustain tier 2 adult children is urged for several reasons. First, it furnishes crucial respite for the primary caregiver. Moreover, undertakings will likely expand once their parents age, necessitating greater allegiance. Specific elements include education about the nature and extent of the injured parent's difficulties, compensation training, as well as comprehending the loved one's supervision needs and medical restrictions to ensure that he or she is safe and well attended to (Klonoff and Koberstein 2010). Involvement with other therapists is beneficial, especially for pointers to enhance the loved one's performance in the home and community. This includes physical and occupational therapists to address self-sufficiency and speech–language pathologists to inform the family about the effect of potential language and cognitive challenges on quality of life. Combining tier 1 with tier 2 caregivers in individual or conjoint neurorehabilitation sessions is advisable. Collaborative interventions should be based on whatever is most helpful to the overall support network and, of course, the loved one (Klonoff and Koberstein 2010).

Table 3.9 Examples of adult children's verbalizations after a brain injury in a parent

Sense of Self Questionnaire responses
Since my loved one's injury, my sense of who I am ... changed from child to guardian overnight. I always need to be "on top of my game," as I'm the one who is responsible if things don't go right. I need to be a protector and advocate
Since my loved one's injury, I feel... I lost my big anchor
When I compare myself to how my life was before the injury... I felt freer and I realize how much I took for granted
Compared to before the injury, my level of stress... has exploded. I have so many "have to's" and so few "get to's"
Compared to before my loved one's injury, I feel sad... knowing she can't enjoy the things she always wanted as much; I miss the relationship we had, our talks, and her advice. I maybe could have done more to prevent the injury if I was more in tune
Compared to before my loved one's injury, I worry... all the time about someone else getting hurt or injured. I wait for the other shoe to drop. What happens if he goes downhill?
Since my loved one's injury, my relationship with people close to me... is pulled in too many directions... no matter how much I do, I feel I am letting someone down, either my injured mom, or my wife and children
Compared to before my loved one's injury, I get frustrated... because I am trying to be his "golf caddy" and he refuses to take my best advice
Since the injury, my place in the world... changed radically. I was forced to find out who I was and what I needed to accomplish "solo"
Since my loved one's injury, my sense of connection with other people... has deepened; I look for connections that are substantial, not superficial

Conjoint psychotherapy sessions with the loved one and adult children enable mutual sharing and sensitivity to varying perspectives within the family unit (Klonoff and Koberstein 2010). Recalibrating the family system is a primary purpose of psychotherapy, including reestablishing whatever level of normalcy is viable for the loved one, who yearns for self-reliance, self-worth, and meaningful contributions (Klonoff 2010). Role modifications can be explored, including reasons why the injured adult parent shuns support. Sharing reveals that this often emerges from his or her selfless desire to protect the son or daughter from stressors and/or to shield himself or herself from shame and sorrow over dependency on the adult children. The psychotherapist can normalize the fated transition of parents resorting to relying on adult children as part of the life transitions, so as to assuage the injured parent's guilt. The book, *Love You Forever* by Munsch (2013) poignantly depicts the inescapable cycle of unconditional love.

Adult children experience joy and relief when they observe tangible gains in the injured parent's functionality. This process is predicated on realistic expectations and adjustment, which can be supported through family therapy sessions. To this end, the psychotherapist can unearth reasonable prospects for the injured parent to reassume pieces of prior roles in a stepwise fashion. For instance, a loved one who feels he has lost his role as the "man of the family" may begin to be included in decision making in specified areas at home. Adult children may support their injured parents in reassuming prior roles by requesting assistance or input in similar preinjury domains.

Adult children will benefit from learning feasible techniques to facilitate coping and support time management (Elbaum 2010; Klonoff and Koberstein 2010), particularly in light of the need to counterbalance their own family, career, and community endeavors. This includes accessing respite for the loved one, such as day programs (Gan et al. 2010). For an adult child who experiences tensions in the spousal relationship from these daunting and competing demands, therapeutic interventions incorporating his or her partner's vantage point is a worthwhile way to restabilize the support system (Cavallo and Kay 2011).

3.5 Scenario: Impact of a Brain Injury on Siblings

Siblings face unique and often ignored challenges after their brother or sister sustains a brain injury. This is true whether the injury occurs during the siblings' childhood/adolescence or in adulthood, although the specifics vary based on developmental level and life occurrences (Cavallo and Kay 2011). Siblings may ask questions such as: *Why did this happen to my brother/sister? What will happen to him/her now? How is this going to affect me and our relationship? What is the expectation for me in my brother/sister's care and rehabilitation?*

3.5.1 Challenges for Siblings of a Loved One with an Acquired Brain Injury

Siblings often become the "unrecognized" and "silent victims" of family system alterations after a brain injury (Cavallo and Kay 2011; Degeneffe and Olney 2010). Often, siblings' reactions are dichotomous (i.e., to the negative or positive extreme); however, they often undergo an altered sense of self as well as major psychological distress, including depression and other life curve balls (e.g., divorce, relationship estrangement and dysfunction, health matters, altered life rhythm, and other undesirable life experiences; Degeneffe and Lynch 2006; Degeneffe and Olney 2010; Gan et al. 2006; Gill and Wells 2000; Orsillo et al. 1993). Some siblings feel like "assistant parents," thanks to their intensified hassles (see Gill and Wells 2000, for a review). Disruptions are associated with health of the sibling, the relative sturdiness and dynamics of the family unit, and the preinjury relationship between the sibling and injured loved one, which can have a "rippling effect" over time (Degeneffe and Olney 2010).

Young siblings mourn the loss of their "partner in crime" of childhood naughtiness, now replaced with overwhelming accountability for policing his or her restricted activities. Suffering the loss of one's sibling rival may spur recrimination and turmoil over being the uninjured sibling (Gill and Wells 2012). The young brother or sister may be consumed with conflicting emotions, characterized by glumness about the loved one's losses, yet jealousy and resentment because of the parents' preoccupation

Table 3.10 Examples of adult siblings' verbalizations after a brain injury in a brother or sister

Sense of Self Questionnaire responses
Since the injury, when I think about my role in my family... it is clouded... the entire focus became about the accident, my sister, and her recovery. I don't have a normal relationship with my mother, although I know she loves me, takes care of me, and is always there for me, just in a different way
Since my loved one's injury, I feel... discouraged, as it changed my whole family's future and we were never the same. Life is so uncertain. I regret my own unrealized dreams and my loved one got cheated
Since my loved one's injury, the way I see myself is... as the "back up" caretaker/"adult" figure to my sister. I am less carefree, and I have the weighty responsibility to help out and to uplift my sister. It will be even worse when my mother dies
Since my loved one's injury, what matters to me... is everything, as things can change in a second like it did when the accident happened. My "Beaver Cleaver" life was no longer a reality
Compared to before my loved one's injury, my emotions... are always near the surface.... then again I do not always express my emotions to my mother as I don't want to put additional stress on her; she has enough on her plate
Since my loved one's injury, when I compare myself to my friends... I feel completely sad. I feel jealous of my friends who have normal relationships with their siblings... it's weird because it's like I am an only child, even though that is not the case
Compared to before my loved one's injury, I feel angry... about this whole situation, that I was never allowed an adult relationship with my brother, along with feeling guilty because my parents gave up their entire life to take care of him. What did we do to deserve this? Why did God let this happen?
Since the injury, when I think about the future, I feel... more anxious that something catastrophic might happen

with his or her special needs. Other behavioral manifestations are acting out, including failing grades and misbehavior in school (Cavallo and Kay 2011). Siblings may feel blameworthy because they are not more involved in the care of their loved one (Degeneffe and Olney 2010). Of note, each sibling may experience varied reactions and behaviors, which reverberate throughout the family system (Cavallo and Kay 2011).

Adult siblings of loved ones with an acquired brain injury wonder about their future role as caregivers (Degeneffe and Olney 2008), especially as elderly parents may be unable to sustain the duties. In some cases, the adult siblings' encumbrances in their own lives and families compete against the desire to aid their injured sibling (Cavallo and Kay 2011). Regardless of the age of the brothers and sisters, loving parents may want to shield them from the grief and hardships associated with the loved one's limitations and the caregiving role. Conversely, parents who are overloaded may look to the uninjured siblings to handle the demands and may not recognize how this negatively affects their growth and development. In families with multiple siblings, the onus may fall entirely on one sibling who has historically been the tier 1 caregiver or in an authority role among the siblings. This can cause frustration and/or bitterness for this sibling as well as a sense of entitlement over other siblings for weight in decision making for the loved one. Overall, siblings' misery emanates from the loss of an equal; the continual pressures from the brain injury; and their ineptness in managing the dilemmas (Gill and Wells 2000). Table 3.10 contains some sample verbalizations by siblings with a brother or sister with an acquired brain injury, based on completed Sense of Self Questionnaires.

Table 3.11 "Helpful hints" and tools for brothers and sisters to cope with a sibling after an acquired brain injury

Invite the "deputized" sibling into the neurorehabilitation process
Encourage out-of-town siblings to observe a day of therapies
Eclectic formats are useful for involving siblings separate or together; siblings/parents without the injured loved one; and larger family meetings
Siblings should be encouraged to share their insights and historical perspectives
Provide health information to siblings using:
Psychoeducation
Strategy training
Medication management
Behavioral queries
Stress management techniques
Training to be on the "advisory board"
Monitor the adverse ramifications of the "pseudotherapist" role
Siblings close in age should be prepared for and given pointers to deal with negative feelings in the loved one when the siblings reach milestones that the injured sibling missed
Siblings can learn various types of backup support in the emotional and instrumental realms
Psychotherapy should address potential strife between uninjured siblings with an emphasis on strengthening their insight, acceptance, and hence harmony:
Facilitate open communication
Delegate responsibilities sensibly
Rotate respite
Gain support from the immediate families of each sibling
Seek external social support
Suggest reliance on faith for solace
Focus on positive benefits from caregiving and involvement in rehabilitation:
Foster a "do what it takes" attitude
Frame involvement as a way to grow closer to the loved one
Recognize the value of "paying back" childhood debts to the loved one
Realize the potential for posttraumatic growth
Multimedia resources
Website
American Association of Caregiving Youth http://www.aacy.org
Book
There's a Monster Under My Bed (Howe 1998)

3.5.2 "Helpful Hints" and Tools for Siblings with a Loved One with an Acquired Brain Injury

Interventions targeting siblings of persons with an acquired brain injury are rare (Boschen et al. 2007). This may be because of the seemingly peripheral relationship position as compared to a parent or spouse, who may more naturally be expected to take on the tier 1 caregiver role. Yet, sibling relationships can be the most elongated, given that these often begin at or near birth and continue to or near death (Degeneffe and Burcham 2008; Yeates and Daisley 2013). The healthy brother and/or sister are therefore ripe for involvement with the injured sibling. Table 3.11 contains "helpful hints" and tools for brothers and sisters coping with a brain injury in a sibling. Given that siblings may be eventually "deputized" into the caregiving role, they should be invited into the neurorehabilitation of their brother or sister (Degeneffe and Olney 2010; Gill and Wells 2000). Also, inviting out-of-town siblings to join the loved one during a day of therapies can be a great opportunity to provide in-the-moment observation and education. Family therapy will necessitate candid dialogue to fashion a new homeostasis. Session formats should be eclectic, based on the structure and needs of the family unit. Options include meeting with: siblings separately or together; the siblings with parents without the injured loved one (as long as permission is given by the loved one); and larger family meetings addressing broader issues. The savvy psychotherapist will invite the insights and historical perspectives about the family system, also from the siblings' perspectives, to guide the treatment process (Degeneffe and Lynch 2006; Degeneffe and Olney 2010).

Adult siblings rate their main need as health information (Degeneffe 2009) and have queries about how complete their loved one's recovery will be, whether he or she will be able to develop meaningful relationships with family and friends, and the prognosis for an overall level of independence (Degeneffe and Olney 2008). Targeted psychotherapeutic interventions include education to siblings about the nature of their loved one's brain injury and strategies, so as to properly support the loved one in the home and community environments. Other relevant areas include: medication management; how best to respond to behaviors (e.g., CRs); and stress management techniques (Degeneffe and Olney 2010; Klonoff and Koberstein 2010). Siblings can be integral social supports to the injured loved one and can serve as a trusted member of the "advisory board" for major decision making (Klonoff 2010). Of course, any psychoeducation should be predicated explicitly on permission by the loved one and vigilant monitoring of the potential adverse indicators of the sibling in a "pseudotherapist" role. Ideally, the sibling conveys stand-by support based on an acquired repertoire of knowledge through the psychotherapy process. To this end, another resource is the website American Association of Caregiving Youth (http://www.aacy.org/).

In the case of adolescent and young adult siblings who are close in age, the psychotherapist should prepare the family and loved one for negative feelings that may erupt when the uninjured sibling passes through new phases of life. This can be particularly agonizing if the healthy sibling is younger than the patient and reaches these milestones first, while the loved one may feel as though life is "on hold." Rites of passage and rituals such as graduations, prom, leaving for college, moving out, getting married, or having children, often trigger these feelings. Incorporating these siblings in the loved one's neurorehabilitation and psychotherapy process teaches them empathy about the predicament, gives them an outlet to pose questions, and identifies ways they can meaningfully contribute.

Psychotherapy can empower siblings to provide different types of backup, based on the loved one's needs and the siblings' skill sets, preferences, and availability. For instance, *affective* (i.e., emotional) support encompasses encouragement, companionship, and "check-ins" which can be provided long distance through text messaging, emails, telephone calls, and letters (Degeneffe and Burcham 2008). Alternatively, *instrumental* (i.e., "hands on") efforts toward transportation, errands, finances, and locating service providers are necessitated if the loved one's injury is more severe, when the uninjured sibling lives in close proximity, and is of the age to play a part (Degeneffe and Burcham 2008). There should be fairness between his or her aspirations in tandem with the requirements of the injured sibling. The children's book, *There's a Monster Under My Bed* by Howe (1998) eloquently portrays the mutuality of sibling fears, best addressed through joint pledges and can be weaved into the therapeutic dialogue.

Limited involvement (e.g., due to living circumstances) can precipitate strife between uninjured siblings, who vary in their level of awareness, acceptance, and realism about the loved one's limitations and prognosis. Involving all siblings in the psychotherapy strengthens their insight, acceptance, and hence harmony. Typical topics are "why me?" "what ifs?" "catastrophic reactions by proxy"; grief and mourning; healthy and unhealthy coping techniques; as well as catalysts for burnout and self-care techniques (Klonoff and Koberstein 2010). When several siblings are struggling or dissenting about caregiving obligations, therapy should advocate open communication among the siblings and creation of a cohesive family system based on sensible delegation of responsibilities and rotating respite to navigate complex management concerns. Support from the immediate family of each of the siblings is required so that unfettered energies can be devoted to the loved one (Cavallo and Kay 2011). Brothers and sisters fare better when they perceive external social support (Degeneffe and Lynch 2006); consequently, the psychotherapist should promote pursuit of these resources. Some siblings find solace in their religious faith (Degeneffe and Olney 2010).

The psychotherapist will facilitate longer-term adjustment through existential exploration of values and life priorities (Klonoff and Koberstein 2010). Siblings may find positive benefits from caregiving and involvement in their brothers' or sisters' rehabilitation process. This has been described as "doing what it takes" and can be envisioned as a way to grow closer to the injured sibling (Gill and Wells 2000). Siblings may also interpret involvement in their loved one's care as "pay back" for a perceived childhood debt to the now injured sibling. Their posttraumatic growth includes personal development; family bonding; a wake-up call engendering new values and priorities; pursuit of careers in health care; increased compassion, tolerance, and maturity; and a deeper grip on life's meaning (Degeneffe and Olney 2010; Gill and Wells 2000).

References

Ackerman, M. J. (1997). *"Does Wednesday mean mom's house or dad's?": Parenting together while living apart.* New York: Wiley.

Allen, K., Linn, R. T., Gutierrez, H., & Willer, B. S. (1994). Family burden following traumatic brain injury. *Rehabilitation Psychology, 39*(1), 29–48.

Aloni, R., & Katz, S. (2003). *Sexual difficulties after traumatic brain injury and ways to deal with it.* Springfield: Charles C Thomas Publisher, LTD.

Anderson, M. I., Simpson, G. K., Morey, P. J., Mok, M. M. C., Gosling, T. J., & Gillett, L. E. (2009). Differential pathways of psychological distress in spouses vs. parents of people with severe traumatic brain injury (TBI): Multi-group analysis. *Brain Injury, 23*(12), 931–943.

Arango-Lasprilla, J. C., Ketchum, J. M., Dezfulian, T., Kreutzer, J. S., O'neil-Pirozzi, T. M., Hammond, F., & Jha, A. (2008). Predictors of marital stability 2 years following traumatic brain injury. *Brain Injury, 22*(7/8), 565–574.

Armistead, L., Klein, K., & Forehand, R. (1995). Parental physical illness and child functioning. *Clinical Psychology Review, 15*(5), 409–422.

Avi. (1994). *The bird, the frog, and the light*. New York: Orchard Books.

Bay, E. H., Blow, A. J., & Yan, X. E. (2012). Interpersonal relatedness and psychological functioning following traumatic brain injury: Implications for marital and family therapists. *Journal of Marital and Family Therapy, 38*(3), 556–567.

Becvar, D. S., & Becvar, R. J. (2013). *Family therapy: A systemic integration* (8th ed.). Upper Saddle River: Pearson.

Bednar, R. L., & Peterson, S. R. (1995). Marital and family therapy: Primary and unique considerations. In R. L. Bednar & S. R. Peterson (Eds.), *Self-esteem: Paradoxes and innovations in clinical theory and practice* (pp. 271–337). Washington, D. C.: American Psychological Association.

Bettelheim, B. (1987). *A good enough parent: A book on child-rearing*. New York: Knopf.

Black, P., & Hogan, S. C. (2006). *Living with a brain tumor: Dr. Peter Black's guide to taking control of your treatment*. New York: Henry Holt and Company.

Blonder, L. X., Langer, S. L., Pettigrew, L. C., & Garrity, T. F. (2007). The effects of stroke disability on spousal caregivers. *NeuroRehabilitation, 22*(2), 85–92.

Boschen, K., Gargaro, J., Gan, C., Gerber, G., & Brandys, C. (2007). Family interventions after acquired brain injury and other chronic conditions: A critical appraisal of the quality of the evidence. *NeruoRehabilitation, 22*(1), 19–41.

Boss, P. (2006). *Loss, trauma, and resilience: Therapeutic work with ambiguous loss*. New York: W. W. Norton

Bowen, C., Yeates, G., & Plamer, S. (2010). *A relational approach to rehabilitation: Thinking about relationships after brain injury*. London: Karnac Books.

Brooks, N. (1984). Head injury and the family. In N. Brooks (Ed.), *Closed head injury: Psychological, social, and family consequences* (pp. 123–147). Oxford: Oxford University Press.

Bruce, E., & Schultz, C. (2002). Non-finite loss and challenges to communication between parents and professionals. *British Journal of Special Education, 29*(1), 9–13.

Butera-Prinzi, F., & Perlesz, A. (2004). Through children's eyes: Children's experience of living with a parent with an acquired brain injury. *Brain Injury, 18*(1), 83–101.

Butler, R. W., & Satz, P. (1988). Individual psychotherapy with head-injured adults: Clinical notes for the practitioner. *Professional Psychology: Research and Practice, 19*(5), 536–541.

Cavallo, M. M., & Kay, T. (2011). The family system. In J. M. Silver, T. W. McAllister, & S. C. Yudofsky (Eds.), *Textbook of traumatic brain injury* (2nd ed., pp. 483–504). Washington, D. C.: American Psychiatric Publishing.

Chwalisz, K., & Stark-Wroblewski, K. (1996). The subjective experiences of spouse caregivers of persons with brain injuries: A qualitative analysis. *Applied Neuropsychology, 3*(1), 28–40.

Collings, C. (2008). That's not my child anymore! Parental grief after acquired brain injury (ABI): Incidence, nature and longevity. *British Journal of Social Work, 38*(8), 1499–1517.

David, C. O. (1998). Brain injury and the family system. In S. Acorn & P. Offer (Eds.), *Living with brain injury: A guide for families and caregivers* (pp. 111–125). Toronto: University of Toronto Press.

Degeneffe, C. E. (2009). The rehabilitation needs of adult siblings of persons with traumatic brain injury: A quantitative investigation. *The Australian Journal of Rehabilitation Counselling, 15*(1), 12–27.

Degeneffe, C. E., & Burcham, C. M. (2008). Adult sibling caregiving for persons with traumatic brain injury: Predictors of affective and instrumental support. *Journal of Rehabilitation, 74*(3), 10–20.

Degeneffe, C. E., & Lynch, R. T. (2006). Correlates of depression in adult siblings of persons with traumatic brain injury. *Rehabilitation Counseling Bulletin, 49*(3), 130–142.

Degeneffe, C. E., & Olney, M. F. (2008). Future concerns of adult siblings of persons with traumatic brain injury. *Rehabilitation Counseling Bulletin, 51*(4), 240–250.
Degeneffe, C. E., & Olney, M. F. (2010). 'We are the forgotten victims': Perspectives of adult siblings of persons with traumatic brain injury. *Brain Injury, 24*(12), 1416–1427.
Doka, K. J., & Martin, T. L. (2010). *Grieving beyond gender: Understanding the ways men and women mourn* (Revised ed.). New York: Routledge.
Dombrowski, L. K., Petrick, J. D., & Strauss, D. (2000). Rehabilitation treatment of sexuality issues due to acquired brain injury. *Rehabilitation Psychology, 45*(3), 299–309.
Ducharme, S. H. (1993). Beyond the management of sexual problems: Creating a therapeutic environment for addressing sexuality issues. In C. J. Durgin, N. D. Schmidt, & L. J. Fryer (Eds.), *Staff development and clinical intervention in brain injury rehabilitation* (pp. 211–228). Gaithersburg: Aspen.
Ducharme, J. M., Spencer, T., Davidson, A., & Rushford, N. (2002). Errorless compliance training: Building a cooperative relationship between parents with brain injury and their oppositional children. *American Journal of Orthopsychiatry, 72*(4), 585–595.
Elbaum, J. (2010). Acquired brain injury and the family: Challenges and interventions. In J. Elbaum, & D. M. Benson (Eds.), *Acquired brain injury: An integrative neuro rehabilitation approach* (pp. 275–285). New York: Springer.
Engström, A., & Söderberg, S. (2011). Transition as experienced by close relatives of people with traumatic brain. *Journal of Neuroscience Nursing, 43*(5), 253–260.
Eriksson, G., Tham, K., & Fugl-Meyer, A. R. (2005). Couples' happiness and its relationship to functioning in everyday life after brain injury. *Scandinavian Journal of Occupational Therapy, 12*(1), 40–48.
Fengler, A. P., & Goodrich, N. (1979). Wives of elderly disabled men: The hidden patients. *The Gerontologist, 19*(2), 175–183.
Florian, V., & Katz, S. (1991). The other victims of traumatic brain injury: Consequences for family members. *Neuropsychology, 5*(4), 267–279.
Gan, C., Campbell, K. A., Gemeinhardt, M., & McFadden, G. T. (2006). Predictors of family system functioning after brain injury. *Brain Injury, 20*(6), 587–600.
Gan, C., Gargaro, J., Brandys, C., Gerber, G., & Boschen, K. (2010). Family caregivers' support needs after brain injury: A synthesis of perspectives from caregivers, programs, and researchers. *NeuroRehabilitation, 27*(1), 5–18.
Gill, C. J., Sander, A. M., Robins, N., Mazzei, D. K., & Struchen, M. A. (2011). Exploring experiences of intimacy from the viewpoint of individuals with traumatic brain injury and their partners. *Journal of Head Trauma Rehabilitation, 26*(1), 56–68.
Gill, D. J., & Wells, D. L. (2000). Forever different: Experiences of living with a sibling who has a traumatic brain injury. *Rehabilitation Nursing, 25*(2), 48–53.
Goldstein, K. (1952). The effect of brain damage on the personality. *Psychiatry, 15*(3), 245–260.
Gow, N. (2010). *Ten big toes and a prince's nose*. New York: Sterling Publishing.
Guerriere, D., & McKeever, P. (1997). Mothering children who survive brain injuries: Playing the hand you're dealt. *Journal of the Society of Pediatric Nurses, 2*(3), 105–115.
Hall, K. M., Karzmark, P., Stevens, M., Englander, J., O'Hare, P., & Wright, J. (1994). Family stressors in traumatic brain injury: A two-year follow-up. *Archives of Physical Medicine and Rehabilitation, 75*(8), 876–884.
Hallé, M. C., Duhamel, F., & Le Dorze, G. (2011). The daughter-mother relationship in the presence of aphasia: How daughters view changes over the first year poststroke. *Qualitative Health Research, 21*(4), 549–562.
Hammond, F. M., Davis, C. S., Whiteside, O. Y., Philbrick, P., & Hirsch, M. A. (2011). Marital adjustment and stability following traumatic brain injury: A pilot qualitative analysis of spouses perspectives. *Journal of Head Trauma Rehabilitation, 26*(1), 69–78.
Hawley, C. A., Ward, A. B., Magnay, A. R., & Long, J. (2003). Parental stress and burden following traumatic brain injury amongst children and adolescents. *Brain Injury, 17*(1), 1–23.
Howe, J. (1998). *There's a monster under my bed*. New York: Aladdin paperbacks.

Hynde, C., Kelly, T., & Steinberg, B. (1994). *I'll stand by you* [Recorded by The Pretenders]. *On last of the independents* [CD]. US: Sire.

Johnson, S. M. (2005). *Emotionally focused couple therapy with trauma survivors: Strengthening attachment bonds*. New York: Guilford Press.

Johnson, S. M., Makinen, J. A., & Millikin, J. W. (2001). Attachment injuries in couple relationships: A new perspective on impasses in couple therapy. *Journal of Marital and Family Therapy, 27*(2), 145–155.

Kao, H. F., & Stuifbergen, A. K. (2004). Love and load—the lived experience of the mother-child relationship among young adult traumatic brain-injured survivors. *Journal of Neuroscience Nursing, 36*(2), 73–81.

Karpf, M. K., & Shatz, I. M. (2005). The divorce is over—what about the kids? *American Journal of Family Law, 19*(1), 7–11.

Kay, T., & Cavallo, M. M. (1994). The family system: Impact, assessment, and intervention. In J. M. Siver, S. C. Yudofsky, & R. E. Hales (Eds.), *Neuropsychiatry of traumatic brain injury* (pp. 533–567). Washington, D. C.: American Psychiatric Press.

Kieffer-Kristensen, R., & Teasdale, T. W. (2011). Parental stress and marital relationships among patients with brain injury and their spouses. *NeuroRehabilitation, 28*(4), 321–330.

Kieffer-Kristensen, R., Teasdale, T. W., & Bilenberg, N. (2011). Post-traumatic stress symptoms and psychological functioning in children of parents with acquired brain injury. *Brain Injury, 25*(7–8), 752–760.

Kieffer-Kristensen, R., Siersma, V. D., & Teasdale, T. W. (2013). Family matters: Parental-acquired brain injury and child functioning. *NeuroRehabilitation, 32*(1), 59–68.

Klonoff, P. S. (2010). *Psychotherapy after brain injury: Principles and techniques*. New York: Guilford Press.

Klonoff, P. S. (2011). A therapist experiential model of treatment for brain injury. *Bulletin of the Menninger Clinic, 75*(1), 21–45.

Klonoff, P. S., & Koberstein, E. J. (2010). Family life. In P. S. Klonoff (Ed.), *Psychotherapy after brain injury: Principles and techniques* (pp. 150–170). New York: Guilford Press.

Klonoff, P. S., & Myles, S. M. (2010). Sense of self and identity. In P. S. Klonoff (Ed.), *Psychotherapy after brain injury: Principles and techniques* (pp. 75–99). New York: Guilford Press.

Klonoff, P. S., Lage, G. A., & Chiapello, D. A. (1993). Varieties of the catastrophic reaction to brain injury: A self psychology perspective. *Bulletin of the Menninger Clinic, 57*(2), 227–241.

Klonoff, P. S., Koberstein, E. J., Talley, M. C., & Dawson, L. K. (2008). A family experiential model of recovery after brain injury. *Bulletin of the Menninger Clinic, 72*(2), 109–129.

Kohut, H. (1987). The admiring selfobject and the idealized selfobject. In M. Elson (Ed.), *The Kohut seminars: On self psychology and psychotherapy with adolescents and young adults* (pp. 77–94). New York: W. W. Norton

Kolakowsky-Hayner, S. A., Miner, K. D., & Kreutzer, J. S. (2001). Long-term life quality and family needs after traumatic brain injury. *Journal of Head Trauma Rehabilitation, 16*(4), 374–385.

Kreutzer, J. S., Gervasio, A. H., & Camplair, P. S. (1994). Primary caregivers' psychological status and family functioning after traumatic brain injury. *Brain Injury, 8*(3), 197–210.

Kreutzer, J. S., Marwitz, J. H., Hsu, N., Williams, K., & Riddick, A. (2007). Marital stability after brain injury: An investigation and analysis. *NeuroRehabilitation, 22*(1), 53–59.

Kreutzer, J. S., Stejskal, T. M., Ketchum, J. M., Marwitz, J. H., Taylor, L. A., & Menzel, J. C. (2009). A preliminary investigation of the brain injury family intervention: Impact on family members. *Brain Injury, 23*(6), 535–547.

Krysan, M., Moore, K. A., & Zill, N. (1990). *Research on successful families* (Contract # HHS-100-89-0041). Prepared for Office of the Assistant Secretary for Planning and Evaluation U.S. Department of Health and Human Services. Washington, D. C.: U. S. Department of Health and Human Services.

Lansky, M. R. (1990). Escalation of trauma in the family of the patient with organic brain disease. *Family Systems Medicine, 8*(3), 231–240.

Laroi, F. (2003). The family systems approach to treating families of persons with brain injury: A potential collaboration between family therapist and brain injury professional. *Brain Injury, 17*(2), 175–187.

Larson, J., Franzén-Dahlin, A., Billiing, E., von Arbin, M., Murray, V., & Wredling, R. (2008). The impact of gender regarding psychological well-being and general life situation among spouses of stroke patients during the first year after the patients' stroke event: A longitudinal study. *International Journal of Nursing Studies, 45*(2), 257–265.

Layman, D. E., Dijkers, M. P. J. M., & Ashman, T. A. (2005). Exploring the impact of traumatic brain injury on the older couple: "Yes, but how much of it is age, I can't tell you...". *Brain Injury, 19*(11), 909–923.

Lefebvre, H., Pelchat, D., Swaine, B., Gelinas, I., & Levert, M. J. (2005). The experiences of individuals with a traumatic brain injury, families, physicians and health professionals regarding care provided throughout the continuum. *Brain Injury, 19*(8), 585–597.

Lezak, M. D. (1988). Brain damage is a family affair. *Journal of Clinical and Experimental Neuropsychology, 10*(1), 111–123.

Maitz, E. A., & Sachs, P. R. (1995). Treating families of individuals with traumatic brain injury from a family systems perspective. *Journal of Head Trauma Rehabilitation, 10*(2), 1–11.

McLaughlin, A. M., & Carey, J. L. (1993). The adversarial alliance: Developing therapeutic relationships between families and the team in brain injury rehabilitation. *Brain Injury, 7*(1), 45–51.

Medlar, T. (1998). The sexuality education program of the Massachusetts Statewide Head Injury Program. *Sexuality & Disability, 16*(1), 11–19.

Minnes, P., Woodford, L., Carlson, P., Johnston, J., & McColl, M. A. (2010). The needs of aging parents caring for an adult with acquired brain injury. *Canadian Journal of Aging, 29*(2), 185–192.

Minuchin, S. (1974). *Families & family therapy*. Cambridge: Harvard University Press.

Munsch, R. (2013). *Love you forever*. Buffalo: Firefly Books.

Nicoll, W. G. (2011). Resilience-focused brief family therapy: An Adlerian approach. *Journal of Individual Psychology, 67*(3), 206–221.

Niemeier, J. P., & Karol, R. L. (2011a). *Therapists' guide to overcoming grief and loss after brain injury*. New York: Oxford University Press.

Niemeier, J. P., & Karol, R. L. (2011b). *Overcoming grief and loss after brain injury*. New York: Oxford University Press.

Norup, A., Siert, L., & Mortensen, E. L. (2010). Emotional distress and quality of life in relatives of patients with severe brain injury: The first month after injury. *Brain Injury, 24*(2), 81–88.

Orsillo, S. M., McCaffrey, R. J., & Fisher, J. M. (1993). Siblings of head-injured individuals: A population at risk. *Journal of Head Trauma Rehabilitation, 8*(1), 102–115.

Pedro-Carroll, J. (2010). *Putting children first: Proven parenting strategies for helping children thrive through divorce*. New York: Penguin Group.

Perlesz, A., Kinsella, G., & Crowe, S. (2000). Psychological distress and family satisfaction following traumatic brain injury: Injured individuals and their primary, secondary, and tertiary carers. *Journal of Head Trauma Rehabilitation, 15*(3), 909–929.

Pessar, L. F., Coad, M. L., Linn, R. T., & Willer, B. S. (1993). The effects of parental traumatic brain injury on the behaviour of parents and children. *Brain Injury, 7*(3), 231–240.

Ponsford, J. (2013). Working with families. In J. Ponsford, S. Sloan, & P. Snow (Eds.), *Traumatic brain injury: Rehabilitation for everyday adaptive living* (2nd ed., pp. 263–290). New York: Psychology Press.

Prowe, G. (2010). *Successfully surviving a brain injury a family guidebook: From the emergency room to selecting a rehabilitation facility*. Gainesville: Brain Injury Success Books.

Reynolds, L. R. (2011). *Parenting through divorce: Helping your children thrive during and after the split*. New York: Skyhorse Publishing.

Romano, M. D. (1974). Family response to traumatic head injury. *Scandinavian Journal of Rehabilitation Medicine, 6*(1), 1–4.

Roos, S. (2002). *Chronic sorrow: A living loss*. New York: Brunner-Routledge.

Sachs, P. R. (1991). *Treating families of brain injury survivors*. New York: Springer.

Shaw, L. R., & McMahon, B. T. (1990). Family-staff conflict in the rehabilitation setting: Causes, consequences, and implications. *Brain Injury, 4*(1), 87–93.

Sherwin, E. D., & O'Shanick, G. J. (2000). The trauma of paediatric and adolescent brain injury: Issues and implications for rehabilitation specialists. *Brain Injury, 14*(3), 267–284.

Simpson, G., & Long, E. (2004). An evaluation of sex education and information resources and their provision to adults with traumatic brain injury. *Journal of Head Trauma Rehabilitation, 19*(5), 413–428.

Singer, G. H. S., & Nixon, C. (1993). "You can't imagine unless you've been there yourself": A report on the concerns of parents of children with acquired brain injury. In *Home/School support for families and children with traumatic brain injury*. Final Report (Report No. EC 304 319). (ED387969).

Skippon, R. (2013). Supporting families and parenting after parental brain injury. In G. Newby, R. Coetzer, A. Daisley, & S. Weatherhead (Eds.), *Practical neuropsychological rehabilitation in acquired brain injury: A guide for working clinicians* (pp. 295–320). London: Karnac Books.

Smith, R. L., & Stevens-Smith, P. (1992). A critique of healthy family functioning. In R. L. Smith & P. Stevens-Smith (Eds.), *Family counseling and therapy: Major issues and topics* (pp. 3–13). Ann Arbor: ERIC Counseling and Personnel Services Clearinghouse.

Springer, J. A., Farmer, J. E., & Bouman, D. E. (1997). Common misconceptions about traumatic brain injury among family members of rehabilitation patients. *Journal of Head Trauma Rehabilitation, 12*(3), 41–50.

Threats, T. (2010). The ICF framework and third party disability: Application to the spouses of persons with aphasia. *Topics in Stroke Rehabilitation, 17*(6), 451–457.

T-TAP. (2012). Addressing parental concerns fact sheet. http://www.worksupport.com/research/research/printView.cfm/501. Accessed 6 Jan 2013.

Tyerman, A., & Booth, J. (2001). Family interventions after traumatic brain injury: A service example. *NeuroRehabilitation, 16*(1), 59–66.

Urbach, J. R., & Culbert, J. P. (1991). Head-injured parents and their children. Psychosocial consequences of a traumatic syndrome. *Psychosomatics, 32*(1), 24–33.

Urbach, J. R., Sonenklar, N. A., & Culbert, J. P. (1994). Risk factors and assessment in children of brain-injured parents. *Journal of Neuropsychiatry and Clinical Neurosciences, 6*(3), 289–295.

Verhaeghe, S., Defloor, T., & Grypdonck, M. (2005). Stress and coping among families of patients with traumatic brain injury: A review of the literature. *Journal of Clinical Nursing, 14*(8), 1004–1012.

Visser-Meily, A., Post, M., Meijer, A. M., Maas, C., Ketelaar, M., & Lindeman, E. (2005a). Children's adjustment to a parent's stroke: Determinants of health status and psychological problems, and the role of support from the rehabilitation team. *Journal of Rehabilitation Medicine, 37*(4), 236–241.

Visser-Meily, A., Post, M., Meijer, A. M., van de Port, I., Maas, C., & Lindeman, E. (2005b). When a parent has a stroke: Clinical course and prediction of mood, behavior problems, and health status of their young children. *Stroke: A Journal of Cerebral Circulation, 36*(11), 2436–2440.

Vollmer, I. (2008). Parenting through separation and divorce. *Transition, 38*(3), 11–14.

Webster, G., & Daisley, A. (2007). Including children in family-focused acquired brain injury rehabilitation: A national survey of rehabilitation staff practice. *Clinical Rehabilitation, 21*(12), 1097–1108.

Webster, G., Daisley, A., & King, N. (1999). Relationship and family breakdown following acquired brain injury: The role of the rehabilitation team. *Brain Injury, 13*(8), 593–603.

Wedcliffe, T., & Ross, E. (2001). The psychological effects of traumatic brain injury on the quality of life of a group of spouses/partners. *South African Journal of Communication Disorders, 48*, 77–99.

Winnicott, D. W. (1994). The building up of trust. In C. Winnicott, C. Bollas, M. Davis, & R. Shepherd (Eds.), *Talking to parents* (pp. 121–134). Cambridge: Perseus Publishing.
Wolf, E. S. (1988). *Treating the self: Elements of clinical self psychology*. New York: Guilford Press.
Wongvatunyu, S., & Porter, E. J. (2005). Mothers' experience of helping young adults with traumatic brain injury. *Journal of Nursing Scholarship, 37*(1), 48–56.
Wongvatunyu, S., & Porter, E. J. (2008a). Changes in family life perceived by mothers of young adult TBI survivors. *Journal of Family Nursing, 14*(3), 314–332.
Wongvatunyu, S., & Porter, E. J. (2008b). Helping young adult children with traumatic brain injury: The life-world of mothers. *Qualitative Health Research, 18*(8), 1062–1074.
Yeates, G. (2009). Working with families in neuropsychological rehabilitation. In B. A. Wilson, F. Gracey, J. J. Evans, & A. Bateman (Eds.), *Neuropsychological rehabilitation: Theory, models, therapy and outcome* (pp. 138–156). New York: Cambridge University Press.
Yeates, G. (2013). Towards the neuropsychological foundations of couples therapy following acquired brain injury (ABI): A review of empirical evidence and relevant concepts. *Neuro-Disability & Psychotherapy, 1*(1), 108–150.
Yeates, G., & Daisley, A. (2013). Working with relationships in standard neuro-rehabilitation practice. In G. Newby, R. Coetzer, A. Daisley, & S. Weatherhead (Eds.), *Practical neuropsychological rehabilitation in acquired brain injury: A guide for working clinicians* (pp. 271–294). London: Karnac Books Ltd.
Zarski, J. J., DePompei, R., & Zook, A. II (1988). Traumatic head injury: Dimensions of family responsivity. *Journal of Head Trauma Rehabilitation, 3*(4), 31–41.
Zasler, N. D., & Martelli, M. F. (2011). Sexual dysfunction. In J. M. Silver, T. W. McAllister, & S. C. Yudofsky (Eds.), *Textbook of traumatic brain injury* (2nd ed., pp. 397–412). Washington, D. C.: American Psychiatric Publishing.
Zeigler, E. A. (1999). Psychosocial issues for spouses of brain injury survivors. *Journal of Neuroscience Nursing, 31*(2), 106–109.
Zinner, E. S., Ball, J. D., Stutts, M. L., & Philput, C. (1997). Grief reactions of mothers of adolescents and young adults with traumatic brain injury. *Archives of Clinical Neuropsychology, 12*(5), 435–447.

Chapter 4
Family Psychotherapy After Moderate to Severe Traumatic Brain Injury

4.1 Scenario: Early Questions about the Traumatic Brain Injury

Moderate to severe traumatic brain injuries have widespread and marked effects on the patient and, consequently, the family. Understandably, family members are usually uneducated and highly perplexed about the effects of moderate to severe brain injuries. As depicted in phase 1 of the Family Experiential Model (FEM) of Recovery (see Chap. 1, Sect. 1.5 and Fig. 1.3), notification about a significant brain injury in their loved one creates a myriad of emotional disturbances in the family, characterized by shock, disbelief, horror, and terror (Coetzer 2006; Klonoff et al. 2008). Depression, anxiety, and impaired quality of life have also been reported in relatives within 1 month of a severe traumatic brain injury in a loved one (Norup et al. 2010). At this initial stage, most family members have little to no knowledge about brain anatomy or function and do not understand the alterations in their loved one. They may ask questions such as: *What has happened to my loved one? What is a moderate to severe traumatic brain injury? What causes the damage to the brain? What is the course of recovery like and how long will it take?*

4.1.1 Therapeutic Intervention: Neuropathology of Moderate to Severe Traumatic Brain Injuries

In order to demystify the complexity of a traumatic brain injury, the psychotherapist can provide informative psychoeducation (Coetzer 2006; Klonoff and Koberstein 2010). This can begin very early after the injury, while the patient is still in the hospital (Norup et al. 2011) and/or later in the recovery process, whenever the relatives are ready for the information (see Chap. 2, Sect. 2.4.1.2). This starts with a user-friendly overview of the neuropathology of moderate to severe traumatic brain injuries, acquainting the primary caregiver and overall support network (e.g., tiers 1–3) with the typical physiological consequences of traumatic brain injuries on brain function, including the anticipated course of recovery.

P. S. Klonoff, *Psychotherapy for Families after Brain Injury*,
DOI 10.1007/978-1-4899-8083-0_4, © Springer Science+Business Media New York 2014

Traumatic brain injury is damage to brain tissue or alteration in brain function resulting from an external mechanical force (Menon et al. 2010; Roebuck-Spencer and Sherer 2008). Factors in altered brain function relate to a loss of or a decreased level of consciousness; loss of memory of events immediately before or after the injury; neurological deficits (e.g., weakness, loss of balance, vision changes, etc.); and alteration in mental state at the time of the injury (e.g., confusion, disorientation, slowed thinking, etc.; Menon et al. 2010). Risk factors include ages 15–24, children under the age of 5, and older adults (> 64 years); males; alcohol consumption; and prior brain injury (see Roebuck-Spencer and Sherer 2008, for a review). Moderate to severe traumatic brain injuries are typically defined by the Glasgow Coma Scale (GCS) score, duration of loss of consciousness (LOC), and posttraumatic amnesia (PTA, i.e., period of confusion; see Orman et al. 2011, for a review; see Roebuck-Spencer and Sherer 2008, for a review). The GCS measures eye opening, motor response, and verbal response. The score is usually obtained at the scene of the accident or in the Emergency Room. Scores range from 3 to 15; moderate brain injuries are categorized as scores of 9 to 12; severe injuries include scores from 3 to 8 (see Orman et al. 2011, for a review). Moderate traumatic brain injury is considered as LOC for more than 30 min and less than 24 h, with a PTA of more than 1 day, but less than 7 days. Severe traumatic brain injury is categorized as LOC for greater than 24 h and PTA for greater than 7 days (see Orman et al. 2011, for a review). Reviewing this information with the family gives them a framework by which to understand the initial severity of the injury.

Lesions to the brain result from either objects striking the head or the contact between the brain and the skull. This can produce focal or discrete injuries, including skull fractures, contusions, and hematomas (Carter et al. 2009; Roebuck-Spencer and Sherer 2008). There are also acceleration/deceleration injuries resulting from unrestricted movement of the head (Gennarelli and Graham 2005). These produce diffuse or widespread damage to the brain, also known as *shear injuries* or *diffuse axonal injuries* (DAIs; Cassidy 2009; see Roebuck-Spencer and Sherer 2008, for a review). DAIs result in unconsciousness whereby the brain goes "off-line" and cannot acquire new information due to disruption in the normal transmission of nerve impulses (Cassidy 2009; Swiercinsky et al. 1999). Other mechanisms of injury include penetrating or open head injuries, when an object (e.g., sharp instrument or missile) passes through the protective covering of the skull and into brain tissue (Lucas and Addeo 2006; Ponsford 2004; Smith 2011). At this juncture, the psychotherapist should review the actual mechanism of the (loved one's) injury for the relatives. For example, a brain injury caused by an auto accident would signify both focal and diffuse injuries, as opposed to an assault which is often a more focal type of injury.

Handouts can be effective in describing the effects of the brain injury in more detail. Figure 4.1 provides an overview of neuroanatomy, including the components of the central nervous system; definition of neurons and synapses; divisions and lobes of the brain; and other principal brain structures (Ashley 2010; Carter et al. 2009; Filley 2008; Goldberg 2010; Lezak et al. 2004; Schmahmann and Caplan 2006; Silver et al. 2011; Vaishnavi et al. 2011; Zasler and Martelli 2011). Figure 4.2

1) Neuroanatomy = study of the parts of the brain and their functions

2) Why study neuroanatomy?
   a) to help understand how the brain works
   b) to learn how the brain injury affects your loved one's ability to function
   c) so you and your loved one become "your own best expert" about brain injury

3) The central nervous system is divided into 3 major parts:
   a) brain
   b) brainstem
   c) spinal cord (not included in our study of neuroanatomy)

4) Neuron: basic working cell of the brain.
   a) Communication within and between neurons occurs chemically and electrically
   b) Synapse: space between neurons where neurotransmitters (chemicals) allow between-cell communication

5) Divisions of thc brain:
   a) Cerebrum: Main part of the brain, where the surface is called the cortex
   b) Hemispheres: Half of the brain, there are the two sides, left and right

Left hemisphere:
Language skills
(speaking, reading, etc.)
Math concepts
Linear processing
Verbal memory
Processes detailed information
Logical and analytical thinking
Familiar information

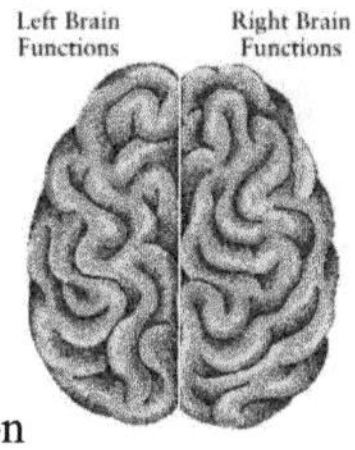

Right hemisphere:
Visuospatial processing
(mechanical skills)
Designs and pictures
Nonverbal (visuospatial) memory
Holistic/global perceptions ("big picture")
Creativity and intuition
Novel information

   c) Lobes: subdivision of a hemisphere, determined by functional and anatomical distinction. Each hemisphere has 4 lobes:
      a) frontal
      b) temporal
      c) parietal
      d) occipital

6) Other structures of the brain:
   a) Cerebellum: located at the base of the brain and behind the brainstem. It is important for motor function (smooth movements), balance, and coordination. Cerebellar damage also produces dizziness and jerky eye movements. Research suggests the cerebellum also plays a role in learning, procedural memory, cognitive processing, and emotional control.
   b) Brainstem: located between the cerebrum and spinal cord, comprised of the midbrain, pons, and medulla. The brainstem is a primitive part of the brain important for motor function, consciousness, arousal, and basic attention. It also regulates basic vegetative functions, such as breathing, heartbeat, and temperature.
   c) Corpus callosum: a band of fibers that connects the left and right hemispheres and allows them to share information.
   d) Hippocampus: a structure located deep in the temporal lobes, which is important for consolidating new learning. After a period of time, the information is either lost or transferred into long-term storage.

Fig. 4.1 Overview of neuroanatomy

e) Amygdala: a structure located next to the hippocampus, which is important for remembering emotional information/events. It is also important for attention and certain emotions (e.g., fear and aggressiveness).

f) Thalamus: located below the cortex deep within the brain. The thalamus is a major relay station for incoming sensory information. It is also important for learning, memory, and emotions.

g) Hypothalamus: located below the thalamus, it regulates important drives (e.g., appetite, sexual arousal, and thirst). Also involved in regulating body temperature and the sleep-wake cycle. Controls rage and fear reactions. Involved in memory processing.

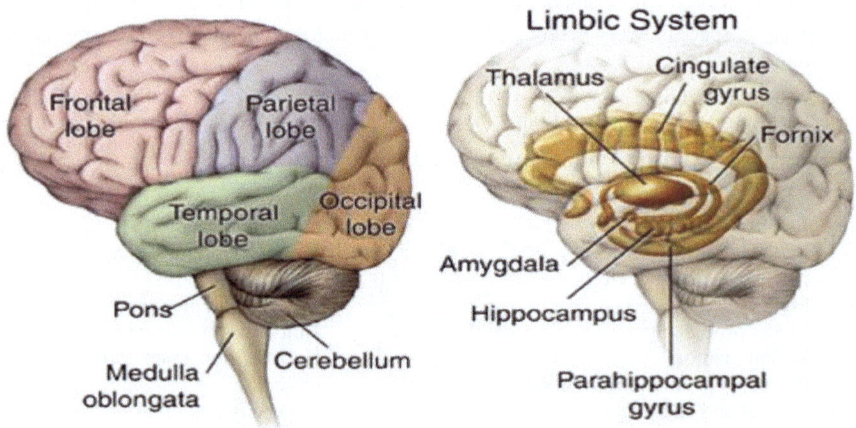

Fig. 4.1 (continued)

provides more detailed definitions about the effect of moderate to severe traumatic brain injuries on brain function and recovery, as well as some general definitions of some of the types of pathological changes to brain tissue (Lezak et al. 2004; Roebuck-Spencer and Sherer 2008; Snyder et al. 2006; Sturm et al. 1998; Swiercinsky et al. 1999). Common terminology should be reviewed from specific types of damage to the brain (e.g., contusion, hematoma, etc.). In addition, some of the secondary effects of the injury should be discussed, including increased intracranial pressure and seizure risk (Masel and DeWitt 2010; Roebuck-Spencer and Sherer 2008; Sturm et al. 1998). "User-friendly" resource materials about the physiological effects of brain injury for the clinician to consult and review with family members include *Traumatic Head Injury: Cause, Consequence, and Challenge* by Swiercinsky et al. (1999), *Head Injury: Information and Answers to Commonly Asked Questions: A Family's Guide to Coping* by Sturm et al. (1998), and the website http://www.dvbic.org.

The therapist should review these handouts with the family members, emphasizing the material that is most applicable to their loved one. As stated above, this psychoeducation should only be introduced when the primary caregiver and support network are prepared psychologically for the possible emotional distress that may ensue, as a review of the pathological effects of brain injury makes the damage "real"

1) The substance of the brain is soft and jelly-like. It is closely encased by the bones of the skull. It is also covered by several membranes (meninges) and cushioned by cerebral-spinal fluid (CSF), which surrounds the brain.

2) A blow to the head will cause loss of consciousness only if it is strong enough to affect the brainstem.

3) The lobes most likely to be bruised in a traumatic brain injury are the frontal and temporal lobes. This is because of the bony ridges on the inside of the skull near these lobes and because of the shape of the skull.

4) When cells in the central nervous system die, they are not replaced by new cells.

   If brain cells do not grow back, how does recovery take place?

   a) c ells that were damaged, but not destroyed, may recover.
   b) some cells might be trained to take over the function of the cells that were lost.

5) Soon after the injury, the brain begins to swell (a process called edema). The swelling makes it difficult for even the uninjured parts of the brain to function. This is why, in the hospital, the patient usually experiences temporary impairments, which begin to disappear as the swelling goes down.

6) The rate of *neurological* recovery after moderate to severe TBI is fastest during the first 6-12 months after a traumatic brain injury. The rate then slows over time, but can continue for a number of years following an injury. *Functional recovery* and improvement are not time limited.

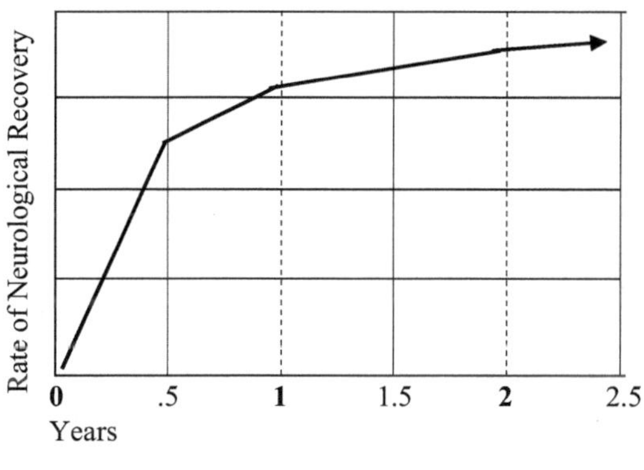

7) Focal vs. diffuse injury

   a) focal = damage is focused in a specific location (e.g. contusion, hemorrhage)
   b) diffuse = damage is spread throughout the brain (e.g. shearing)

Terminology for Moderate to Severe Traumatic Brain Injuries

1) Traumatic brain injury (TBI): injury to the brain caused by an accident

   a) coma = extended loss of consciousness (usually more than 24 hours)

Fig. 4.2 Effects of moderate to severe traumatic brain injuries

b) ICP (increased intracranial pressure)	= a common problem related to brain swelling (edema) or other complications which impedes normal blood flow to the injured brain. Medications and surgical procedures are used to control ICP
c) retrograde amnesia	= inability to remember events for a time period prior to the injury
d) PTA (posttraumatic amnesia)	= period of time after an injury in which new memories cannot be established and the patient is disoriented to person, place, and time
e) skull fracture	= when the skull fractures and fragments due to a powerful blow
f) contusion	= bruise, caused by brain tissue hitting against the inside of the skull
g) shearing/diffuse axonal injury	= the stretching and tearing of nerve fibers caused by the twisting of the brain inside the skull
h) contrecoup	= injury on the side opposite to the blow, which happens when the brain collides with the other side of the skull
i) hemorrhage	= bleeding into the brain, formed as a result of the trauma
j) hematoma	= collection of blood in the brain, formed by a hemorrhage
k) laceration	= brain tissue is cut or torn apart by an object (e.g. bullet) or bone fragment from a skull fracture that penetrates the brain tissue
l) seizure	= an episode of random and uncontrolled electrical firing in the brain They are more common after penetrating brain injuries. Seizure types are either generalized or partial. They result in confusion, hallucinations, strong emotions, muscle contractions, jerky movements, and sometimes, loss of consciousness.

Fig. 4.2 (continued)

and sometimes, overwhelming. At this juncture, it is often advisable to consult the actual medical records of the loved one, so as to personalize the discussion. The presentation of the material should be customized to maintain a positive working alliance. This translates to the therapist juxtaposing the devastating news with the need to be authentic. Figure 4.2 also depicts the rate of neurological recovery; although physiological recovery can improve for an extended time frame, it is most rapid during the first 6–12 months (Lezak et al. 2004; Ponsford 2004). However, it is important to emphasize the difference between the patient's physical versus functional recovery in order to offset the family's dismay. Functional recovery, i.e., implementation of compensations for the loved one's betterment, is self-determined. Time lines are fluid, and they depend more on the patient's motivation to implement and evolve his or her compensatory tools (Klonoff 2010).

4.2 Scenario: Overview of Skill Changes

Because the brain is the "master computer" controlling all abilities and functions, the individual's capabilities will be affected variably, depending on how and where the brain was damaged. In essence, moderate to severe traumatic brain injuries potentially impact all aspects of the patient's life, including his or her physical, cognitive, language, communication, emotional, and interpersonal domains. This in turn affects the patient's functional status, including the requirement for supervision in the home and the ability to resume driving, school, and/or work. This results in increased dependency on family members and dramatic lifestyle changes for all parties. Family members may notice a variety of thinking changes and may ask questions such as: *What has happened to my loved one's abilities? Why is he or she not able to think, act, move, or talk the same way?*

4.2.1 Neuroanatomy of Abilities

The psychoeducation process proceeds with more detailed information about the four lobes of the brain. Figure 4.3 provides a summary of some of the major functions of each of the lobes and possible resultant deficits after moderate to severe traumatic brain injury (Carter et al. 2009; Filley 2008; Goldberg 2010; Lucas and Addeo 2006; Malloy et al. 2006). The psychotherapist will explain the relevant challenges based on the pattern of test findings and neuroanatomical correlates. The frontal and temporal lobes are most susceptible to damage after a moderate to severe traumatic brain injury, because of the bony ridges of the skull atop which these lobes sit (Lucas and Addeo 2006; Sohlberg and Mateer 2001). The role of imaging reports summarizing computed tomography (CT) scans and magnetic resonance imaging (MRI) findings should be reviewed with the relatives, as these are useful vehicles to demonstrate the location and extent of their loved one's brain damage to specific internal structures (Cassidy 2009; Lezak et al. 2004).

A review of neuropsychological test findings is the next logical step in educating the family about their loved one's cognitive, sensory, and motor difficulties after a moderate to severe traumatic brain injury. This often occurs while the patient is in the hospital or soon after his or her discharge. Figure 4.4 is a graphical representation using a bell curve diagram, in which the primary postinjury limitations can be presented in a palatable format. The neuropsychologist will need to label the graph according to the individual's preinjury level of ability and then identify areas of preserved versus affected performance. The author prefers to limit the findings to global entities, as summarized in Table 4.1. Nonjargon terms make the data clearer, such as attention and concentration; speed of thinking; motor functions; vision; verbal skills; mechanical skills; memory; and reasoning. In general, the sequelae of neuropsychological deficits after moderate to severe traumatic brain injury are speed of thinking, attention and concentration, memory, and executive functions (Lezak et al. 2004; McCullagh and Feinstein 2011; Ponsford 2004; Vakil 2005).

It is also advantageous to discuss the role of effort and motivation towards the testing process. There can be several reasons for suboptimal effort, including mood disorders (e.g., depression, anxiety), fatigue, medication side effects, or an intentional decision to underperform (Franzen and Iverson 2006; Lezak et al. 2004; see Lezak et al. 2012, for a review; Lucas and Addeo 2006). Explaining the role of

A) Divisions of the cerebral cortex

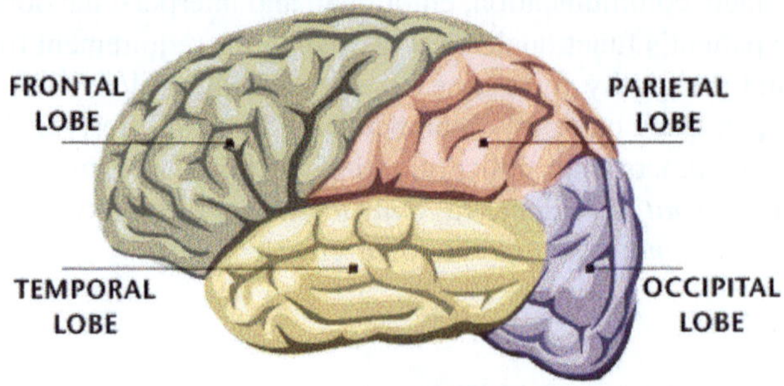

Frontal Lobes	
Responsible for:	**Injury results in:**
"Executive" functions	See Figure 4.6
Personality	• unawareness of injury effects • reduced emotional control • flattened affect • apathy and decreased spontaneity • labile mood or mood swings (fluctuations between laughing and crying) • childlike behavior • socially inappropriate behavior • depression (left hemisphere) • mania or psychosis (right hemisphere)
Voluntary movement (on opposite sides of the body)	• motor deficits (e.g., weakness, fine motor, motor programming, voluntary gaze, and visual search)
Voluntary speech and language	• deficits in speech production, word finding, and expressive language (aphasia)
Smell and taste	• loss of sense of smell and taste

Temporal Lobes	
Responsible for:	**Injury results in:**
Memory Verbal memory (left hemisphere) Nonverbal (visual) memory (right hemisphere)	• difficulty learning new information • forgetting recently learned material
Hearing and auditory processing	• auditory processing impairments
Language comprehension (left hemisphere)	• difficulty understanding language (aphasia)
Vision	• visual processing (due to damaged visual fibers passing through the temporal lobes)
Selective attention for verbal and visual input	• disturbance of selective attention of auditory and visual input
Categorize information	• impaired organization and categorization of verbal material
Personality and emotions	• misperception • suspiciousness • episodes of hyperirritability and aggressiveness

Parietal Lobes	
Responsible for:	**Injury results in:**
Mechanical and construction skills (right hemisphere)	• mechanical deficits
Visual attention (right hemisphere)	• reduced attention to one side of space (visual neglect)
Visuospatial processing (right hemisphere)	• visuospatial processing difficulties • difficulty making things (construction)

Fig. 4.3 Functions and deficits associated with the brain lobes

Right/left orientation (left hemisphere)	• impaired sense of direction • difficulty discriminating left from right
Language and reading comprehension (left hemisphere)	• reading, writing, and spelling deficits • word-finding deficits (anomia)
Math (left hemisphere)	• mathematical deficits
Sensation (on opposite sides of the body)	• impaired sensation (touch, vibration, and pain)
Body positioning and movement	• poor body awareness

Occipital Lobes	
Responsible for:	**Injury results in:**
Vision and visual processing	• visual field cut (hemianopsia) • blind spots • visual distortions • visual processing difficulties

Fig. 4.3 (continued)

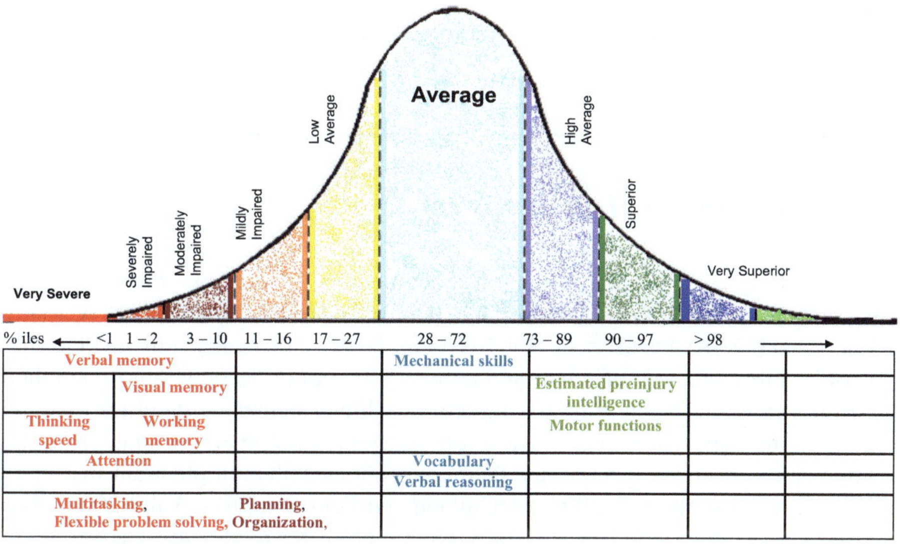

Verbal memory			Mechanical skills			
	Visual memory			Estimated preinjury intelligence		
Thinking speed	Working memory			Motor functions		
Attention			Vocabulary			
			Verbal reasoning			
Multitasking, Planning, Flexible problem solving, Organization,						

Fig. 4.4 Bell curve and associated percentile ranges

these factors as impediments to the accuracy of test results helps to expand the family members' depth of understanding and positively involves them in the dialogue process about their loved one's demeanor and mindset.

4.3 Scenario: Memory Challenges

Early on, it is common for family members to observe a change in their loved one's capacity to remember things happening around him or her. On the one hand, they are relieved that the patient remembers things about the past, yet they are perturbed and frightened when he or she cannot keep track of basic daily events or conversations. The family may ask questions such as: *Why can't my loved one learn and/or remember things I tell him or her? Why does he or she get confused so easily?*

Table 4.1 Neuropsychological domains

Effort and motivation
Estimate of preinjury intelligence
Attention and concentration
Speed of thinking
Motor functions
Verbal skills
Expression
Comprehension
Mechanical skills/visual skills
Memory
Working memory
Verbal memory
Visual memory
Reasoning
Verbal
Designs, diagrams, and pictures
Organization and planning
Flexible problem solving
Mood and personality

4.3.1 Overview of Memory Systems

Table 4.2 describes general information about memory. *Memory* has been defined as the ability to encode (take in), consolidate (store), and retrieve information (Cassidy 2009; Glisky 2004; Lezak et al. 2004; Wilson 2009). Practically, this involves the person's ability to learn information that he or she sees or hears; retain it; and then recall it, often after some time has lapsed. Disabling memory difficulties of some type after moderate to severe brain injury are a cardinal phenomenon, given the complexity of memory systems and their connections with multiple brain structures (Glisky 2004; Lezak et al. 2004; McCullagh and Feinstein 2011; Vakil 2005). The recovery of memory abilities is usually incomplete after moderate to severe brain injuries; instead, there is an emphasis on the "reduction of deficits" (see Wilson 2009, for a review). In general, the size of the cognitive problems corresponds to the severity of the traumatic brain injury (Dikmen et al. 1995; Lezak et al. 2004; Schretlen and Shapiro 2003); therefore, patients with moderate to severe traumatic brain injuries typically experience medium to large memory deficits.

The ability to learn and retain information is also linked to other aptitudes. These include perception or the integration of sensory impressions into meaningful data (Lezak et al. 2004). Additionally, the capacity to understand what is said; concentrate and focus one's cognitive energies; think quickly enough to follow information being imparted; demonstrate the intent and effort to remember; and be organized and flexible in one's approach to learning, all contribute to the process of learning and memory (Carter et al. 2009; McCullagh and Feinstein 2011, Stuss and Levine 2002).

A review of the neuropsychological test findings will be the first introduction to the nature and severity of memory problems. Given the complexity of memory as an entity (see Vakil 2005, for a review), the family will benefit from a review of

Table 4.2 General information about memory

Memory is defined as the ability to:
- Encode (take in)
- Consolidate (store)
- Retrieve information

Memory is a complex process requiring many cognitive functions, including:
- Perception
- Comprehension
- Attention and focus
- Speed of thinking
- Intention to remember/effort
- Flexible thinking
- Organization

Stages of memory:
- Registration: process by which large amounts of information are stored for less than 1 second, until transferred or lost
- Short-term or Working Memory: a "mental scratchpad" with temporary storage and manipulation of information (held for brief periods) involving neurochemical or electrical changes
- Long term: storing and consolidating information on a more permanent basis, requiring structural changes in the neurons
  - Old learning: historical information which occurred well before the injury
  - New learning: information which is learned after the brain injury

Other classifications of memory:
- Incidental: remembering without trying
- Procedural: remembering how to do something (e.g., ride a bicycle, drive a car)
- Declarative: remembering information about events, facts, or shared knowledge
- Retrospective: remembering the past
- Prospective: remembering to do something in the future

the relative areas of memory deficit for the loved one, vis-à-vis his or her ability to learn and retain novel verbal material and designs, implement procedures or steps for completing projects, or complete prospective assignments for the future.

Table 4.2 also reviews the stages of memory, which include the capability to register information for fleeting time periods; *working memory* or short-term storage and manipulation of information (Carter et al. 2009; see Glisky 2004, for a review); and long-term storage and consolidation of information. *Old learning* refers to information which was attained well before the brain injury (Squire 1987). This information is generally retained after moderate to severe traumatic brain injury, unless it occurred in close proximity to the accident and becomes affected by retrograde amnesia (Squire 1987). After moderate to severe traumatic brain injury, it is typical to be unable to efficiently and effectively learn and retain new information occurring after the injury (McCullagh and Feinstein 2011).

Other types of memory difficulties include *incidental* recall, which constitutes the individual's capacity to recall casual information that is occurring throughout the day (e.g., instructions or feedback given in passing). New learning and incidental memory problems interfere with the patient's ability to handle day-to-day responsibilities at home and in the community. These also cause stress for the tier 1 caregiver and close family members who often find themselves in the role of reminding their loved one of information or doing activities for him or her that he or she forgets to do. *Procedural* recall pertains to the individual's ability to recall steps for completing tasks, skills, or routines (e.g., changing the oil in a car; Wilson 2009). Therefore, patients who were "handy" at home and capable of fixing things leave an upsetting void for their family, who now must either add these duties to their own schedule or find others to fulfill these jobs. *Declarative* memory relates to the individual's ability to remember events, knowledge, or facts. Disruptions in this type of memory affect the loved one's capacity to participate in family discussions, resulting in the family feeling losses over shared experiences. *Retrospective* memory is a recollection of past experiences; *prospective* memory pertains to the patient's ability to remember to do something in the future (e.g., pack his or her lunch for the next day, or order medications from the pharmacy; Wilson 2009). Problems with this type of memory can place considerable pressure on the primary caregiver(s) to closely oversee their loved one to be sure he or she is "on top of his or her game." The family often feels that they are "picking up the pieces" when assignments or responsibilities fall through the cracks.

Table 4.3 summarizes frequent examples of memory difficulties after brain injury. Common perturbations for family members include loved ones perpetually forgetting daily chores and responsibilities, asking the same questions and/or repeating stories or events incessantly, as well as *confabulating* (i.e., filling in gaps in knowledge with incorrect guesses that they believe to be accurate). Other vexing manifestations include trouble adapting to changes in routine and attaining new proficiencies in the home and community (e.g., using a new coffee pot or getting lost in a store), as well as forgetting to use the very compensations which would improve his or her functionality (e.g., datebooks, electronic devices, or checklists). This latter setback compounds the family member's disillusionment and can engender feelings of futility with the rehabilitation process.

4.3.2 "Helpful Hints" and Tools for Families to Cope with Memory Challenges in their Loved Ones

A primary resource for memory problems in the loved one is neurorehabilitation. This encompasses: exercises to restore lost abilities; modification and organization of the environment to reduce taxing the memory system; activities to help the loved one learn more efficiently; and education about appropriate compensations (Klonoff 2010; Wilson 2009). A delightful and instructive resource for siblings of the loved one with memory problems is *Elvin: The Elephant Who Forgets* by Dr. Snyder (2005). Table 4.3 also summarizes "helpful hints" and techniques for the family to assist their loved one. These are divided into: techniques to improve efficiency; compensations for new learning; and study strategies (in case the family is assisting their loved one in academic pursuits). Efficiency strategies include cuing their loved one to

Table 4.3 Common memory problems after moderate to severe traumatic brain injury and "helpful hints" and tools

Common Memory Problems after Brain Injury:

Difficulty recalling information or remembering the steps of how to do things (e.g., computer password, using a washing machine)

Forgetting something recently seen or done (e.g., already bought milk)

Forgetting where something was placed (e.g., watch or keys)

Repeating things already said to people, without realizing it (e.g., stories, jokes)

Getting lost (e.g., forgetting where the car is parked)

Confabulation: "filling in the gaps" with logical guesses and/or information which are believed to be correct (but are incorrect) when memory fails

Difficulty learning new information (e.g., academic material) or new skills (e.g., work tasks, hobbies)

Forgetting a change in routine (e.g., taking a new medication)

Forgetting to use memory compensations (e.g., datebook, note taking)

Things That Can Negatively Affect Memory:

Fatigue and lack of sleep: the more tired a person is, the worse his/her learning and recall will be

Stress: being very anxious or stressed can interfere with learning and recall of information

Substances/medications: alcohol, street drugs, and certain medications (e.g., narcotic pain killers) can also interfere with learning and recall of information

"Helpful Hints" and Tools for Memory:

Improve Efficiency:

Encourage your loved one to pay attention

Reduce distractions

Simplify/streamline the information by eliminating what is irrelevant (i.e., focus on what is most important)

Make sure your loved one understands what you are saying or showing him/her

Organize the information with your loved one

Make sure your loved one is not anxious, depressed, tired, hungry, overly caffeinated, etc.

Compensations for new learning:

Learn about the loved one's external memory aids:

- Record important information in an accessible location (e.g., datebook, electronic devices, and procedure checklists)
- Make sure that your loved one's entries are detailed enough to be informative
- Help your loved one regularly check and review the entries
- Cue your loved one to use his/her datebook/electronic device to record details of upcoming events
- Be sensitive, clear, and concise when imparting information

Family members should use a comparable memory compensation system:

- Enhances the family's organization and reduces forgetfulness
- Provides positive role modeling for the loved one

Help your loved one develop routines (e.g., always take notes about important information) with specific times to do tasks

Help your loved one establish habits (e.g., always take medications at a certain time, keep keys in the same location)

Encourage your loved one to use prompts to remember to do tasks (e.g., set a timer)

Use a backup prompt (e.g., another alarm)

Help him/her obtain maps, written directions, and a global positioning system (GPS) for route finding

Table 4.3 (continued)

Study strategies:
Organize the material and minimize distractions
Implement learning techniques
Link new information to what he/she already knows
Encourage your loved one to rehearse/practice new information following the "little and often" rule
Reinforce "errorless learning"
Give him/her cues (e.g., first-letter prompts)
Acronyms: form an easily remembered word from the initial letters of a longer descriptive term e.g., SCUBA—self-contained underwater breathing apparatus
Mnemonics: broad term for helpful memory strategies (including acronyms), often in the form of easily remembered rhymes or sayings e.g.,"Thirty days hath September, April, June, and November; All the rest have thirty one Excepting February alone: Which hath but twenty-eight, in fine, Till leap year gives it twenty-nine"
Multimedia resources
Books
Elvin: The Elephant Who Forgets (Snyder 2005)

pay attention, reducing distractions in the environment, and simplifying information that is presented, so as not to overload or overwhelm the patient. Therapeutic instructions and feedback should be straightforward and succinct. Whenever possible, the caregiver should help his or her loved one be organized, as this is one of the best methods to compensate for memory difficulties.

There is good evidence that mood and general health considerations impact learning and memory (see Lezak et al. 2004, for a review). The psychotherapist will educate the family about their loved one's mood (e.g., degree of anxiety or depression) and health status, as his or her focus and retention will be enhanced if he or she is not anxious, depressed, fatigued, hungry, or overly caffeinated (Geisler and Polich 1992; Lamport et al. 2011; see Lezak et al. 2004, for a review; Nehlig 2010; Terry and Phifer 1986). Family members will be advised to discourage their loved one from using alcohol and street drugs (e.g., marijuana, ecstasy), as these substances will further impair his or her learning and recall skills (Allen et al. 2006; Battisti et al. 2010; Brown et al. 2010; see Dell Orto and Power 2000, for a review; Leitz et al. 2009; Pitel et al. 2007; Rodgers 2000).

With respect to new learning and memory compensations, external memory aids are considered to be the most efficient and effective techniques (see Sohlberg and Mateer 2001, for a review; Sohlberg and Turkstra 2011). These reduce caregiver burden by increasing the loved one's independence (Sohlberg and Turkstra 2011). Treating therapists can successfully assess what tools will be optimal, based on the unique factors and deficit pattern in the loved one (Sohlberg and Turkstra 2011). Then the family should be trained to support the compensation process. A case in point, to maximize their usefulness, the family should help the loved one record essential information in sufficient detail in an accessible location (e.g., datebooks, electronic devices, checklists) and cue him or her to refer to these as needed. This will include giving the loved one sufficient assistance in filling out his or her datebook with upcoming appointments and other "to do" items. The psychotherapist can provide the family written step-by-step procedures, flow charts, and diagrams to reduce the loved one's reliance on his or her impaired memory. This translates to less aggravation for all parties. The family should be encouraged to be sensitive in tone, clear, comprehensible, and concise when imparting information, so as not to overwhelm or unduly exasperate their loved one.

A detailed therapy protocol for developing and implementing a datebook system is contained elsewhere (Klonoff 2010). Stepwise recommendations for organizing the datebook and tracking assignments are provided, including a two-page system which allows for appointment schedules and prioritized daily task lists. Basically, the loved one needs a comprehensive system to track appointments, assignments, and a "to do" list. Working collaboratively with a neuropsychologist, occupational therapist, and speech–language pathologist will aid the family in supporting the use of the best system for their loved one.

Figure 4.5 contains a sample model of a two-page-per-day datebook for a patient, with a complementary one-page system for the primary caregiver (see the case study in Sect. 4.9). Given the multiple stressors and responsibilities on the caregiver's shoulders, it is strongly recommended that family members use their own datebook or electronic system. This provides an organized system for families and reduces the likelihood of overlooking key obligations. It is also reassuring and empowering to the loved one to witness the family modeling the tool that he or she is adjusting to.

A number of other "helpful hints" and compensations can be proffered by the psychotherapist. For example, to reduce patients' overreliance on family members, it is necessary to establish set routines. This lessens the pressures associated with new learning. A designated place and regular time should be set to review the patient's weekly responsibilities, whereby all parties dedicate their energies to clearly defining what tasks should be done on what day and at what time. This builds healthy routines and habits, which reinforce the learning process (Sohlberg and Mateer 2001). Frequently used articles (e.g., keys and datebooks) should be placed in the same location in the home, so as to reduce the likelihood of misplacing these items. Prompts, backup timers, and watch alarms also provide useful time-linked reminders for the loved one which do not impose on the family's energies. Families worry about their loved one's safety when he or she is directionally challenged. Practical tools include written directions, maps, or a global positioning system (GPS). This relieves trepidations on the part of the family and at the same time enhances their loved one's community independence and reintegration.

Table 4.3 also summarizes helpful study techniques which family members should be knowledgeable about so as to guide their loved one. When the patient is required to focus his or her attention to learn new information (including school coursework), it is beneficial for the family member to help their loved one organize the material; implement learning strategies (e.g., visualization, associations, mnemonics); as well as provide opportunities for him or her to study in a quiet setting. A building block approach of adding new material to mastered content is advisable. Successful studying is enhanced if the family can facilitate opportunities for their loved one to study the material a little at a time, with frequent reviews. Reinforcement of the technique of *errorless learning*, in which the loved one learns new material and skills by only

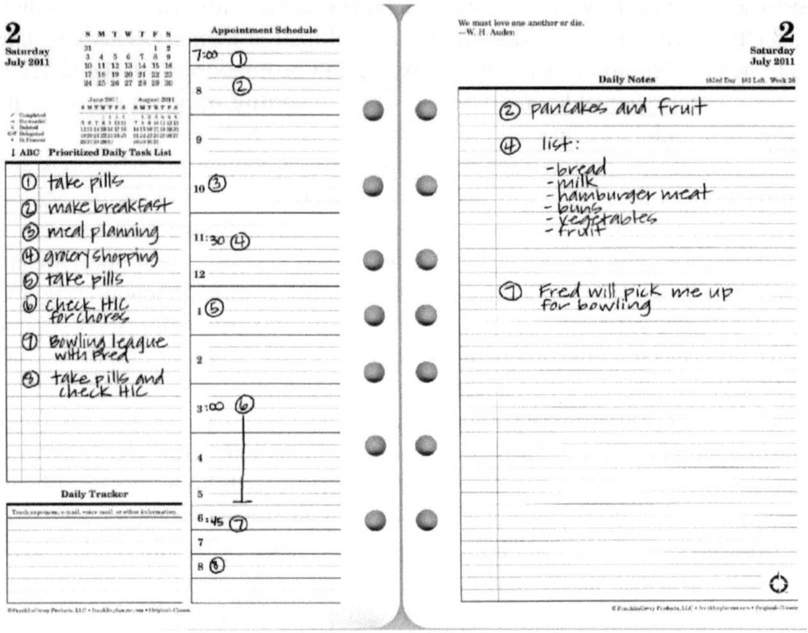

Wally's Datebook Pages

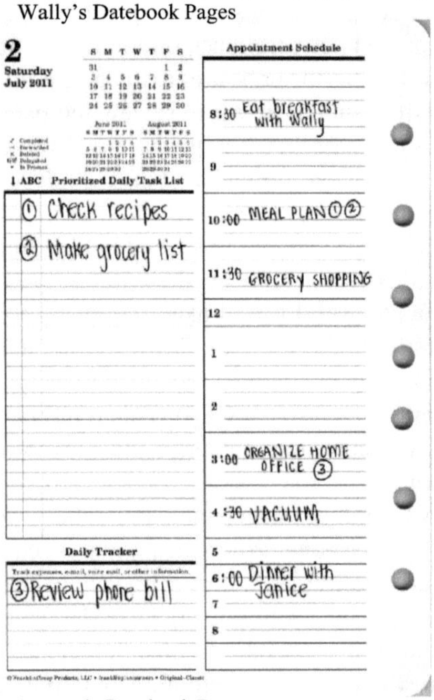

Annette's Datebook Page

Fig. 4.5 Wally and Annette's datebook pages

being exposed to correct information, will enhance the learning process (see Glisky 2004, for a review). Some relatives want to quiz their loved one for upcoming tests. In this case, the technique of providing cues (e.g., first-letter prompts), acronyms, or letter mnemonics will help enhance the learning process (Sohlberg and Mateer 2001; Sohlberg and Turkstra 2011).

4.4 Scenario: Executive Function Challenges

Although families cannot quite put their finger on what has changed, they notice gaps in their loved one's ability to think clearly, solve problems, and make good decisions. It seems as though the family is now explaining things much more and making choices on behalf of their loved one. They may ask the following questions:

4.4.1 How come he or she is so rigid and can't see the other side of things? Why does my loved one keep focusing on the same thing over and over? Why are things left to the last minute, with no pre-planning? How come he or she can't figure things out on his or her own without my input? How come he or she jumps into things without thinking? Why does my loved one make such poor choices?

Frontal lobe damage results in a variety of what are called executive function deficits. *Executive functions* can be considered as the skills a business executive engages in to perform his or her duties (Uomoto 2010). These represent the capacity for higher order thinking (McCullagh and Feinstein 2011; Stuss and Levine 2002; Turner and Levine 2004); as such they represent the dynamic "online" coordination of cognitive resources and are heavily involved in managing novel situations. Executive function subcomponents include: setting personal goals; weighing alternatives; selecting a course of action; sequencing intervening steps; and regulating behavior so as to attain goals (see Turner and Levine 2004, for a review). Figure 4.6 summarizes common executive function deficits, with their definitions. A rating scale is provided (0 = no problem; 5 = medium problem; 10 = large problem), as this is an enlightening method for the therapist to assess the family's (and patient's) perception of the magnitude of potential executive system difficulties. Relatives are often frazzled by their loved one's cognitive rigidity (Lezak 1986; Senelick and Dougherty 2001), which can manifest as a one-sided, "my way or the highway" mentality. A common example is the loved one's impatience and demand for transportation when and where he or she wants to go, without due consideration for the primary caregiver's other constraints. This inflexibility translates to an inability to put himself or herself in the family member's shoes or show empathy. To the family, the patient seems self-centered and insensitive.

Cognitive Executive Function Rating Scale for ________________________

Ratings: Choose the appropriate number for each executive function:

0	1	2	3	4	5	6	7	8	9	10
NO problem										BIG problem

Cognitive Executive Function Deficits		Family Rating	Patient Rating
Inflexibility	unable to take different perspective or "shift gears"		
Perseveration	"locking on" to a task or thought; "fixated;" unable to "break set"		
Planning and time management	thinking in advance; following a timeline		
Problem solving	finding solutions - "what and how do I do this?"		
Impulse control	thinking before speaking or acting		
Judgment	weighing alternatives and making good choices		
Initiation	getting things started		
Follow through	seeing tasks through to completion in a timely manner		
Complex attention and distractibility	difficulty paying attention in complex situations; cannot focus attention		
Sequencing	completing steps of a task in order		
Generating strategies	coming up with new ideas or techniques to solve problems		
Decision making	making good and realistic decisions		
Multitasking	doing multiple things well at once or "juggling balls"		
Organization	keeping things neat and orderly		
Setting priorities	completing tasks based on their relative importance		
Abstract reasoning	thinking on a general level or "outside the box"		
Concrete thinking	taking things literally and at face value		
Black-and-white thinking	all or nothing thinking; no gray zones		
Seeing the "big picture"	considering the many factors that go into a decision; seeing the grand scheme of things		

Fig. 4.6 A rating scale of cognitive executive function deficits, including definitions

The loved one may also perseverate on thoughts or activities, characterized by becoming fixated and "locked on." Sometimes, this is due to performing rituals for actual daily pursuits (e.g., preparing food or drinks, to the exclusion of other responsibilities) or playing computer games (e.g., solitaire). The person becomes so engrossed in the activity that he or she cannot "break set." Other times, it manifests as getting stuck on questions or topics (Coetzer 2006). Related to this, impaired planning, time management, and problem solving make the loved one "structure dependent" (Lezak 1988). This means the tier 1 caregiver is elevated to the position of a constant parental or supervisory role, orchestrating daily duties in which the loved one was self-sufficient before. Poor impulse control translates to judgment errors which then produce unsafe or socially unacceptable behavior (Lezak 1988). This is both embarrassing and harrowing for the family. Overall, these difficulties with rigidity, judgment, impulse control, lack of empathy, and reduced planning capacity erode the caregiver's mood and life satisfaction (Stuss and Levine 2002; Wells et al. 2005).

4.4.2 Why does my loved one talk about needing to get things done, but then doesn't have the "get up and go" to do them? How come he or she doesn't see projects through to completion, gets distracted, or gets all of the steps mixed up? How come he or she can't come up with new ways to do things when he or she hits roadblocks?

Figure 4.6 identifies common executive function problems with initiation, follow-through, complex attention, sequencing, and strategy generation. Families can become annoyed, thinking that their loved one is "lazy" or unmotivated to accomplish things. Sometimes, it feels that the patient is intentionally ignoring them or shirking his or her responsibilities. In actuality, their loved one may be having significant difficulties with initiation, that is, the capacity to get tasks started. This is a direct result of frontal lobe damage, rather than willful disobedience, idleness, or procrastination.

Distractibility causes the loved one to be unable to sustain his or her focus for extended periods of time, particularly for challenging undertakings (Stuss and Levine 2002). The patient may become confused in the process of doing the activity, as he or she loses track of the proper sequence. Examples of this are putting a bookcase together using directions or completing all aspects of the laundry in order (i.e., sorting, washing, drying, folding, and putting clothes away). The inability to complete tasks may also be coupled with decreased follow-through, especially if he or she has to employ strategizing to solve novel problems or complete them within a designated time frame.

4.4.3 Why can't my loved one make simple decisions? How come my loved one can only focus on one thing at a time and cannot "juggle multiple balls," like he or she did before the accident? Why is my loved one so disorganized and doesn't seem to be able to set the right priorities? What happened to thinking in shades of gray? How come my loved one thinks on such a simple level and can't see the "big picture?"

Additional executive function skills are also contained in Fig. 4.6. These include decision making, multitasking, organization, prioritization, abstract reasoning, and seeing the "big picture" (Lezak et al. 2012). Struggles in these areas translate to thinking on a more concrete or basic level and having difficulty appreciating the complexities of a situation, instead focusing on fragmented details. Black-and-white or all-or-nothing thinking precludes the gray zones. This can translate into impaired decision making, without acting in his or her own best interest. More complicated activities of daily living (e.g., bill paying and budgeting) can be negatively affected, as the patient easily misplaces valuable information and/or has difficulty prioritizing what bills need to be paid when. These skills are also mandatory in advanced academic settings (e.g., university) and most professional work settings. The patient is often viewed by family members and others as scattered, discombobulated, and untrustworthy, only because he or she cannot efficiently track and complete assignments and responsibilities.

4.4.4 "Helpful Hints" and Tools for Families to Cope with Executive Function Challenges in their Loved Ones

Table 4.4 summarizes therapeutic "helpful hints" and tools for family members to reduce their distress and discord because of executive function deficits in their loved ones. Undoubtedly, the best way for families to cope with their loved one's executive function difficulties is to collaborate closely with treating therapists and to embrace recommended practical and personalized compensations for the loved one. Usually, this involves simplifying responsibilities and dividing them into "bite-sized pieces." Imposing an external, organized structure and routine for the patient to follow also reduces caregiver burden. One such tool is the Home Independence Checklist (HIC), also described in detail elsewhere (Klonoff 2010). Basically, the HIC is a list of specific chores codeveloped between the loved one, primary caregiver, and relevant therapist (e.g., occupational therapist), which provides an external routine for home duties with designated days and times (see Klonoff 2010, for a review).

In addition to promoting self-sufficiency in the patient, the HIC is a valuable compensation for executive function limitations in complex attention, planning, decision making, organization, sequencing, initiation, follow-through, time management,

Table 4.4 "Helpful hints" and tools for family members to cope with executive function challenges in their loved ones

Collaborate closely with treating therapists to establish personalized compensations for the loved one
Develop external organizational tools which simplify responsibilities into "bite-sized pieces" (e.g., the Home Independence Checklist (HIC) and datebook)
Datebook and HIC strategies:
Keep tools in a prominent and consistent location
Link daily endeavors to specific times
Highlight and number appointments in the datebook
Immediately mark off completed assignments ("do it–mark it")
Do not "pre-check" or "back check"
Use the datebook for preplanning and prioritization
Have your loved one complete tasks consecutively rather than concurrently
Make sure the loved one does not overextend himself/herself
Organize and simplify the home's personal space—examples:
Use pillboxes
Label cupboards
Create folders for a filing system
Checklist for bill paying
Meal plans
Grocery lists
Become familiar with the loved one's time management techniques
Remember that family functions as "auxiliary frontal lobes"
Employ mottos: "action–consequence" and "if this, then that"
Use diagrams and charts as handy visual tools
Construct pros and cons lists and cost–benefit analyses
Work with the therapist to help the loved one see nuances and complexities
Develop realistic expectations of the loved one's capabilities
Participate on the loved one's "advisory board" to keep him/her safe
Have regular (at least weekly) "milieu meetings"

perseveration, setting priorities, and seeing the "big picture" (Klonoff 2010). An overall daily, weekly, and monthly schedule of obligations gives the loved one the "big picture" of the totality of home responsibilities. Assigned duties keep the patient focused on the task at hand, reducing a tendency to succumb to external distractions (e.g., television, computer games, etc.). The HIC identifies what needs to be done in what time frame, which provides another practical external structure to promote initiation and follow-through. By dividing items according to the day of the week, this tool facilitates the planning and prioritization of household requirements. The tendency to perseverate, or get locked onto a specific task, is reduced when the loved one recognizes that a number of responsibilities need to be completed each day. This encourages better time management skills. Structuring the list of chores enhances the loved one's decision-making, organization, and sequencing skills. For instance, weekly meals can be planned on Sunday; shopping can be completed on Monday; and cooking is then scheduled for Wednesday.

Figure 4.7 provides complementary sample HICs. I recommend one for the patient and another for the tier 1 caregiver (see the case study in Sect. 4.9). These should

	Mon	Tues	Wed	Thurs	Fri	Sat	Sun
7:00 A.M.	Make breakfast		Make breakfast		Make breakfast	Make breakfast	
7:30 A.M.	Pack lunch and pills	Pack lunch and pills	Pack lunch and pills	Pack lunch and pills	Pack lunch and pills		Fill pillbox
10:00 A.M.					Do laundry Clean bathroom	Meal planning Grocery shopping	Clean bedroom
3:00 P.M.	Check mailbox	Check mailbox	Check mailbox	Check mailbox	Check mailbox	Check mailbox	Bike riding
4:30 P.M.	Do homework	Do homework	Cook dinner	Do homework	Cook dinner	Swiffer and dust	Cook dinner
6:30 P.M.	Feed Laila dinner	Feed Laila dinner	Feed Laila dinner	Feed Laila dinner	Feed Laila dinner	Feed Laila dinner	Feed Laila dinner
6:45 P.M.	Load dishwasher Take out trash	Load dishwasher		Take out trash	Load dishwasher	Bowling league	Milieu meeting and check datebook
7:30 P.M.			Do homework				Do homework
8:30 P.M.	Check datebook	Check datebook	Check datebook	Check datebook	Check datebook	Check datebook	

Wally's Weekly HIC Schedule

	Mon	Tues	Wed	Thurs	Fri	Sat	Sun
7:00 A.M.		Make breakfast		Make breakfast			Make breakfast
10:00 A.M.						Meal planning Grocery shopping	Check Wally's pillbox
3:00 P.M.						Organize home office	Yard work
4:30 P.M.	Cook dinner	Cook dinner		Cook dinner		Vacuum	Go to drugstore/ errands
6:30 P.M.							Load dishwasher
6:45 P.M.	Do laundry		Load dishwasher	Do ironing	Load dishwasher		Milieu meeting and check datebook
7:30 P.M.	Pay bills	Clean bedroom					

Mom's Weekly HIC Schedule

Fig. 4.7 Wally and Mom's weekly Home Independence Checklist (HIC) schedules

be jointly developed with the treating occupational therapist or other relevant staff (e.g., neuropsychologist). This dual checklist reflects the mutuality of jobs to one another in the home environment. This is advantageous for both parties, as each can see their chores and feel a sense of collaboration and teamwork within the home environment. Similar to the datebook, this tool reduces caregiver stress by transferring some time-consuming responsibilities to the loved one in a manner that optimizes his or her independence and success. Conversely, the patient recognizes the commitment and contributions of the caregiver, based on his or her wide-ranging checklist of duties.

As referenced above, learning a regimented datebook system during neurorehabilitation is also an excellent way to ameliorate the loved one's difficulties with planning, time management, setting priorities, initiation, and follow-through. Adopting the technique of linking daily endeavors to specific times on the datebook page provides a beneficial structure, so the loved one is more likely to initiate and follow through with activities in a timely fashion. Highlighting and numbering appointments and tasks add clarity and structure, thereby increasing the probability that the loved one notices the entries and feels compelled to complete the task at the assigned time (Klonoff 2010). As an example, the family can cue the loved one to make an entry at 8:00 a.m. to take his or her medication and label this highlighted assignment as # 1, so he or she understands to do this first thing in the morning. Encouraging the loved one to mark off assignments not only empowers the loved one to maximize his or her independence but, importantly, enables the family a quick and nonintrusive way to track that all responsibilities are being fulfilled.

The psychotherapist will promote that the caregiver reinforce that the loved one keep the compensatory tools in a prominent and consistent location in the home (Klonoff 2010). He or she should adopt the "do it–mark it" protocol and not "pre-check" or "back-check" the completion of HIC or memory assignments, as he or she may later forget that the assignment has not in fact been completed (Klonoff 2010).

Additional datebook items which facilitate executive function skills are a medication card listing names and doses of medications; an address and phone number section listing key contacts for easy access; and business card holders for health-care providers (Klonoff 2010). These items provide an organized and accessible system, ultimately empowering the loved one to be more in control of his or her health and everyday commitments.

Datebooks are also wonderful tools to engender preplanning and prioritization, as these contain at least a few months of dated pages in which the loved one can anticipate, plan, and execute major pursuits which have assigned time lines and subgoals. For example, in planning a vacation, the psychotherapist can teach the caregiver and loved one how to enter dates of the trip, preparatory steps (e.g., when to book the flight, pack, pick up necessary medication prescriptions before leaving, and drop off pets at the pet resort), and follow up jobs (e.g., when to unpack, pick up pets, and return to work, etc.).

A handy strategy for reducing multitasking hassles is as follows. Whenever possible, have the loved one complete tasks consecutively versus concurrently. This means seeing each job to completion before starting the next one. For instance, when preparing a meal, the patient may need to fix one dish at a time. Obviously, some undertakings lend themselves better to this approach; however, the more severe the multitasking problems, the less likely the loved one is able to effectively split his or her attention and energies.

Other "helpful hints" include monitoring that the patient does not overextend himself or herself by "biting off more than he or she can chew." To the extent the loved one becomes overwhelmed and overburdened by chores and commitments, the burden of responsibility is hurled onto the primary caregiver and other tier supports. This involves organizing the loved one's physical space, including environmental modifications (Sohlberg and Mateer 2001). Options include using pillboxes for medications; labeling cupboards for easy access; setting up file cabinets with predetermined labeled folders; devising a stepwise checklist for bill paying; and creating meal plans and grocery lists to facilitate shopping and cooking (Klonoff 2010; Sohlberg and Mateer 2001).

Rehabilitation can teach time management techniques to assist the patient in being punctual and thoughtful about the family's schedule and demands. One technique is to have the caregiver (and loved one) estimate the proposed versus actual time for task completion. This provides firsthand experience with the challenges of completing daily responsibilities and helps all parties become realistic about the importance of preplanning, problem solving, initiation, organization, and follow-through.

The tier 1 caregiver and other tier supports may need to function as the "auxiliary frontal lobes" for the loved one who needs outside parameters to contain the tendency to "jump the gun" and/or make poor choices with potentially dire consequences. Psychotherapy will demonstrate how to guide the loved one to think methodically through various scenarios, with a paramount emphasis on safety. The motto "action–consequence" or "if this, then that" helps to configure this exercise. This cuing approach teaches the loved one stepwise problem solving and helps him or her better identify the key precursors to certain deleterious (or beneficial) actions.

Diagrams and charts are also handy visual tools to help with the loved one's restrictions in reasoning, problem solving, seeing the "big picture," generating strategies, and decision making. For instance, the therapist can guide the caregiver and loved one to construct a chart that identifies possible options to solve a "real-life" dilemma (e.g., whether or not the loved one should move out of the family's home). Together, both parties can develop a list of pros and cons or conduct a cost–benefit analysis (Klonoff 2010). This provides an external structure, but still enables input from the family and a chance for the loved one to take ownership of his or her choices. By walking through worrisome examples that impinge on family life, the therapist can demonstrate how to consider nuances and complexities, rather than resort to all-or-nothing and/or concrete thinking.

Ideally, a balance must be achieved with the realistic expectations of the patient in the context of the needs and desires of the family. To this end, if the family expects the patient to pay all of the bills, complete shopping and cooking on a daily basis, as well as keep up with his or her therapy homework and exercises, all parties are set up for failure. Therefore, dialogue with the treating therapists, with everyone "on the same page" is crucial to harmony and psychological well-being in the whole family, including the loved one. Of note, depending on the nature and severity of the brain injury, the tier support system will need to function indefinitely on the loved one's "advisory board" (Klonoff 2010), so as to keep him or her safe. This is especially essential for situations requiring higher order reasoning and analytical skills, such as financial management or complex quandaries in interpersonal relationships.

Lastly, regular *milieu meetings* should be scheduled. These are forums in which the patient and involved family members or housemates meet to coordinate personal and shared responsibilities (see Klonoff 2010, for a review). Figure 4.8 provides a sample "milieu meeting" agenda (see the case study in Sect. 4.9). Sample topics include mutually required phone calls; specific household tasks; meal planning; social events; finances; school or work events; and topics for upcoming psychotherapy sessions. These "milieu meetings" afford an invaluable opportunity for group planning and healthy two-way dialogue about the patient's and primary caregiver's preferences (see Klonoff 2010, for a review).

4.5 Scenario: Lack of Awareness, Denial, and Disavowal

It is baffling and disconcerting when family members notice ineptitudes that their loved one is not cognizant of. Families may ask questions such as: *How come he or she doesn't see the problems like I do? How come he or she thinks he or she can do everything just like before the traumatic brain injury?*

4.5.1 Overview of Awareness, Denial, and Disavowal

A hallmark of traumatic brain injury is organic unawareness (Flashman et al. 2011; Prigatano 1991). A working definition of *self-awareness* is the understanding and acknowledgment of postinjury neurological strengths and difficulties, as well as appreciating how these affect day-to-day functioning (Klonoff 2010). Typically, a neuropsychologist or therapist will ascertain the degree of organic unawareness through the interview process, clinical observations, and/or questionnaires (Flashman et al. 2011; Klonoff 2010). Comparison of the perceptions of the relatives versus the loved one regarding various postinjury skills is another informative approach, as normally the relatives will report a greater frequency and severity of problem domains. Table 4.5 includes a simple rating scale of awareness difficulties for the family and patient.

Deficits in awareness are associated with damage to the frontal lobes, as well as DAI (Flashman et al. 2011; Prigatano 2005a; Stuss 1991; Stuss and Levine 2002). The unawareness phenomenon can also extend from very early periods after the injury to many months or years, depending on the severity of the injury and the presence or dearth of rehabilitation (see Flashman et al. 2011, for a review; Klonoff 2010). The loved one's unawareness often varies according to the domain of disability;

"Milieu Meeting" Agenda

1. **What phone calls need to be made this week?**

Wally:	Mom:
a. my rehab doctor	a. the pharmacy
b. my school advisor	b. the insurance company

____
Document in our datebooks WHEN calls are to be made

2. **What specific household tasks need to be done?**

Wally:	Mom:
a. clean my desk	a. organize my study
b. bathe Laila	b. pull weeds

____
Document in our datebooks WHEN tasks are to be done

3. **Meal planning**:

Wally:	Mom:
a. shop with mom on Sat. a.m.	a. finalize shopping list with Wally Sat.
b. cook dinner on Sun., Wed., Fri.	b. cook dinner on Mon. Tues. Thurs.

____
Document in our datebooks when meals are to be prepared

____
Add missing ingredients to the shopping list

4. **Social events planned for the week**:

Wally:	Mom:
a. bowling league with Fred on Sat.	a. go to dinner with Janice on Sat.

____
Document in our datebooks when these events will take place

5. **Finances:**

Wally:	Mom:
a. discuss allowance for doing chores	a. review the phone bill with Wally

____
Document these discussions in our datebooks

Fig. 4.8 Sample "milieu meeting" agenda for Wally and Annette

6. **School/Work:**

Wally:	Mom:
a. review my quiz schedule this week	a. review my evening work meetings

____
Document in our datebooks when these events will take place

7. **Topics for next psychotherapy appointment:**

Wally:	Mom:
a. when can I take my driving eval?	a. Wally's behavior at the store

____
Document these topics in our datebooks

Wally and Mom: Transfer appointments from "Month at a Glance" onto daily pages

Fig. 4.8 (continued)

physical deficiencies are more obvious to the individual as compared to emotional, thinking, and interpersonal problems (Flashman et al. 2011; Hart et al. 2004; Trahan et al. 2006). Once the educational process about the brain injury begins, common emotions expressed by the patient range from indifference to surprise and bewilderment to agitation and argumentativeness (Flashman et al. 2011; Klonoff 2010; O'Callaghan et al. 2006). The emergence of negative emotions symbolizes the transition from "ignorance is bliss" to the stark realization of debilitating limitations or "catastrophic reactions" (CRs), as well as increased depression and anxiety (Godfrey et al. 1993; Goldstein 1952; Klonoff 2010; Niemeier and Karol 2011a; see Sect. 4.6 for more information about CRs). Research has demonstrated that remediating organic unawareness is critical for the patient's adherence to rehabilitation; long-term adjustment (including independent living and work); and the family's psychological well-being (see Flashman et al. 2011, for a review; see Klonoff and Koberstein 2010, for a review; Prigatano and Fordyce 1986; Sander et al. 2003; Trahan et al. 2006).

Different from unawareness are the phenomena of disavowal and denial. These are psychological reactions produced by the inability of the loved one to cope with the painful realities of injury-related shortcomings. *Disavowal* is the intermittent acknowledgment of problems, while *denial* is "the persistent psychological disbelief in his or her disability, even in the face of objective evidence to the contrary" (Klonoff 2010, p. 103). The loved one may display defensiveness, avoidance, minimization of deficits, and excuses as manifestations of denial of his or her limitations (Kortte et al. 2003; O'Callaghan et al. 2006; Prigatano and Klonoff 1998). Often, unawareness, disavowal, and denial coexist (Flashman et al. 2011; Klonoff 2010; Prigatano and Klonoff 1998), making it difficult for the relatives to ascertain exactly why their loved one seems impervious to the nature and seriousness of his or her challenges.

Table 4.5 Ratings and "helpful hints" for families to cope with unawareness in their loved ones

Unawareness Rating

0	1	2	3	4	5	6	7	8	9	10	Family	Patient
NO problem										BIG problem		

- Realize that unawareness is a direct result of the traumatic brain injury
- Your loved one may not recognize the specific deficits, especially nonphysical ones, and likely will not translate (i.e., generalize) his/her difficulties to daily activities and responsibilities
- Neurorehabilitation, including psychotherapy, are critical to help reduce unawareness
- Let the treatment team take the lead in the educational process to avoid "killing the messenger"
- Realize that improving awareness is a gradual process, with "peaks and valleys"
- Advocate for your loved one to receive both individual and group-oriented therapies
- Your loved one will likely need "real life" activities in the community to gain awareness
- Be aware of "dignity of risk" and "planned failures"
- Seek emotional support for the relatives through their own therapy regarding consequences of unawareness
- Gain knowledge about the difference between unawareness, disavowal, and denial through therapeutic input
- Encourage your loved one about the "wait and see" attitude and the mantra "patience, trust, and collaboration"
- Try to provide praise and positive feedback, as your loved one may not recognize subtle improvements

4.5.2 *"Helpful Hints" for Families to Cope with Awareness, Denial, and Disavowal Problems in their Loved Ones*

Table 4.5 summarizes therapeutic "helpful hints" for the family to better understand and cope with their loved one's unawareness. Just the realization that the failure to acknowledge the effects of the brain injury is caused by the brain damage itself is worthwhile for the family and will also facilitate a more tolerant approach to their loved one. A practical analogy is that the brain acts as the computer "mainframe," and damage results in the computer's inability to recognize its own malfunctioning. Furthermore, because of the unawareness, the loved one will typically underestimate the impact of his or her injury. This is known as the incapacity for generalization or the inability to appreciate the functional implications for community pastimes (e.g., driving, work, school, and home life; Flashman et al. 2011; Klonoff 2010).

Within the context of neurorehabilitation, the family should rely on the treating therapists to take the lead in addressing organic awareness. Usually this means that the team will review and educate the patient about injury-related restrictions. The role of the family is to participate in the learning process and then to support the loved one during his or her emotional turmoil. This will avoid the loved one's predilection to "kill the messenger" (i.e., blame the family for the "bad news" and vent his or her hurt and anger towards them; Klonoff 2010). Understanding the prevalence of organic unawareness through psychotherapy will help the family make sense of their loved one's difficult behaviors, including resistance to therapeutic interventions, as well as poor insight, judgment, and decision making about his or her current capabilities (Lezak et al. 2004). Also, organic unawareness difficulties fall on a continuum, ranging from profound to relatively mild (Klonoff 2010). The process of psychoeducation and therapy can greatly ameliorate unawareness; however, the family should be enlightened that the process is slow, with "peaks and valleys." Often, the loved one will progress from relative unawareness to burgeoning awareness, and then to a fuller appreciation (Klonoff 2010). As such, the family can then reassure their loved one that increasing awareness is a gradual process.

When possible, the tier supports should seek out and encourage the loved one to participate in individual and group neurorehabilitation therapies that will facilitate self-reflection and improved awareness (Klonoff 2010; Prigatano 2005b). Examples of group therapies are cognitive retraining, a psychoeducation group, and group psychotherapy. In cognitive retraining, a therapist administers exercises and elicits dialogue about the patient's specific strengths, challenges, and his or her potential impact in the community. The psychoeducational group teaches neuroanatomy and the recovery process. Group psychotherapy incorporates didactics and collective sharing about the definition and manifestations of organic unawareness (Klonoff 2010). Video recording exercises are beneficial and concrete mechanisms to help the patient better appreciate his or her strengths and limitations (Cassidy 2009; see Flashman et al. 2011, for a review; Klonoff 2010).

Allowing the loved one to try "real-life" endeavors, which will help him or her better appreciate the consequences of the traumatic brain injury, is crucial to improving self-awareness (Cassidy 2009; Godfrey et al. 1993; Klonoff 2010; Turner et al. 2009). Sometimes, this means affording the loved one the "dignity of risk" of pursuits that appear beyond his or her capabilities in order for the loved one to gain firsthand knowledge of his or her strengths and challenges (Klonoff 2010). A "planned failure" allows the loved one the latitude (i.e., choice and responsibilities) of making his or her own choices in a protected manner, with the expectation that this venture will be unsuccessful (Klonoff 2010). Often, this entails the therapist and family retreating to the sidelines, yet remaining accessible when circumstances go awry. Of note, "planned failures" should definitely be orchestrated carefully by the treatment team and not undertaken solely by the family, so as to avoid dire or dangerous consequences and to best address the inevitable angst that this "therapeutic reality check" will precipitate (Klonoff 2010).

The family will require substantial emotional support as well as assistance in better appreciating the relative contributions of unawareness, disavowal, and denial. Hence, relatives should seek the expertise of a neuropsychologist or psychotherapist to help discern the relative contribution of these complex organic and psychological factors. Supportive psychotherapy is instrumental in helping the family cope with these entities (Flashman et al. 2011; Klonoff 2010). Once the family understands that the psychological reactions of denial and disavowal also represent the patient's natural reaction to overly dismaying information, the family can react more compassionately and apportion feedback based on their loved one's readiness to have dialogue about the negative implications of his or her injury.

Another constructive approach is for the tier 1 and 2 supports to encourage the loved one to follow the therapeutic recommendations of taking a "wait-and-see" attitude about the long-term effects of the brain injury, as well as embrace the mantra "patience, trust, and collaboration" with the rehabilitation team, in order to maximize his or her gains (see Chap. 2, Sect. 2.4.1.1; Klonoff 2010). In the face of sorrowful circumstances, it is typical for individuals to need praise and positive reminders. Being so close to the injury, the loved one may also have difficulty appreciating subtle improvements and gains; this is exacerbated by memory failures. Thus, the support network should regularly emphasize the positive aspects of the recovery and rehabilitation process for their loved one, as oftentimes the loved one may ignore or minimize these, secondary to his or her unawareness.

4.6 Scenario: Mood, Behavioral, and Communication Challenges

In addition to thinking and memory changes, families are perplexed by changes in their loved one's mood, behavior, and communication skills. It seems that the personality and interaction style of their loved one are altered. Families may ask questions such as: *How come my loved one does not show emotion? Why does my loved one get so upset when he or she is trying to do things? Why does my loved one seem so down and grouchy? How come I feel like I am walking on eggshells around him or her?*

4.6.1 Overview of Mood and Behavioral Challenges

As depicted in Fig. 4.9, moderate to severe traumatic brain injury often impacts the patient's affect and mood (Cassidy 2009; Jorge and Robinson 2011; Lucas and Addeo 2006). Many of these behavioral and mood changes are associated with frontal lobe damage (Alderman 2004). Emotional and behavioral changes are also reactive, that is, they occur in reaction to the loved one's realization of injury-related limitations (Alderman 2004; Klonoff 2010; Prigatano 1986). Again, a ten-point scale can be

Communication, Mood, and Behavioral Rating Scale for ___________________

Ratings: Choose the appropriate number for each challenge:

0 1 2 3 4 5 6 7 8 9 10
NO problem BIG problem

	Communication, Mood, and Behavioral Challenges	Family Rating	Patient Rating
Disinhibition	lack of filter or inability to inhibit or control inappropriate behaviors or responses		
Blunt	overly direct comments which appear insensitive or hurtful		
Poor self-monitoring	not watching what you do or say; reduced self-analysis of behavior		
Poor read of social cues	not picking up on subtle cues, including nonverbal communication and behavior which is within the bounds of social norms and expectations		
Inappropriateness	comments which are offensive or too personal		
Poor nonverbal communication	decreased ability to convey information without using words (e.g., reduced eye contact, poor body language)		
Self-centered	appearing selfish and concerned with personal needs to the exclusion of others'		
Childlike behavior	acting less mature than your age		
Hyperverbality	talking too much		
Tangentiality	switching topics randomly		
Poor thought formulation	difficulty thinking in advance what to say so it is communicated clearly and concisely		
Flat affect	decreased range of facial expression; lack of animation		
Apathy	diminished motivation affecting initiative, goal-directed behavior, and emotional reactions		
Catastrophic reactions (CRs)	the behavioral state that occurs when a patient struggles and fails to perform tasks which were completed easily preinjury		
Depression	deep sadness, joyless, feelings of hopelessness, and helplessness		
Snarky	irritable, grouchy, sarcastic		

Fig. 4.9 A rating scale of communication, mood, and behavioral challenges, including definitions

utilized so that the therapist can obtain perceptions from the family (and patient) regarding the relative seriousness of these problems. Commonly, especially in the acute phases postinjury, the patient shows flattened affect or a limited range of facial expressions. Disorders of diminished motivation are relatively common, including apathy and abulia (i.e., profound apathy, lack of movements and speech, and reduced interest and social engagement; Lezak 1988; Marin and Wilkosz 2011; Waldron-Perrine et al. 2008). The loved one may have difficulty "getting in touch" with emotions and feeling more "blah" about his or her condition. As the patient recovers, more of his or her preinjury personality emerges. In fact, sometimes, the brain injury causes an exaggeration in the loved one's preexisting personality and behaviors (Alderman 2004; Prigatano 1999). This has been referred to as the "volume turned up" on preinjury problems (Prigatano 1999) and is likened to a loudness knob on a stereo or sound system (Klonoff 2010).

A telltale sign of increased awareness in the patient is the emergence of CRs, whereby the patient becomes acutely aware of postinjury incapacities, relative to his or her preinjury skills (Goldstein 1952). Depression also commonly emerges after moderate to severe traumatic brain injury (Cassidy 2009; see Lezak et al. 2004, for a review; Turner et al. 2009). This is related to the anatomical, neurochemical, neurohormonal, and physiological changes in the brain, in conjunction with environmental stressors, including cascading "CRs" (Cassidy 2009; Jean-Bay 2000; Jorge and Robinson 2011; see Klonoff 2010, for a review; Rosenthal et al. 1998; Senelick and Dougherty 2001). Changes in his or her sense of self and the grief and loss process triggered by shattered plans and aspirations also catalyze depression (see Klonoff 2010, for a review). The patients' frustration tolerance is often diminished after moderate to severe traumatic brain injury. They can easily become "snarky" or irritable, and usually they take their frustrations out on their relatives, with whom they feel safe. Changes in mood and behavior can become overwhelming and exasperating to the caregiver and overall support network (Hassan et al. 2011; Martin et al. 2001), who are only acting in the best interest of their loved one. A negative feedback loop is created, whereby the primary caregiver(s) feel helpless, depressed, and hopeless. In fact, research shows that there is a reciprocal relationship between behavioral and mood changes in the loved one and the family's emotional distress (Schonberger et al. 2010).

4.6.2 "Helpful Hints" and Tools for Families to Cope with Mood and Behavioral Challenges in their Loved Ones

Table 4.6 summarizes the signs and symptoms of CRs and depression, as well as therapeutic "helpful hints" and tools for the family to cope with their loved one's mood and behavioral difficulties after moderate to severe traumatic brain injury. Critical to understanding the loved one's postinjury emotionality is recognizing CRs, which are manifested differently, depending on the makeup of each patient. The patient's neuropsychologist should take the lead in explaining the concept of CRs and unique expressions in the loved one, based on his or her familiarity with the patient. In general, once the patient experiences the stark realization of his or her failings, he or she may erupt into some combination of anger, frustration, impatience, sadness, tearfulness, anxiety, fear, embarrassment, guilt, helplessness, hopelessness, defensiveness, and especially feeling overwhelmed (Klonoff 2010). Overpowering

Table 4.6 Symptoms, "helpful hints," and tools for coping with catastrophic reactions (CRs) and depression in loved ones

Common forms of CRs	
Overwhelmed	Snarky
Frustrated/impatient	Blaming
Anger/rage	Defensive
Sad	Tearful
Depressed	Anxious
Guilt	Fear/panic
Embarrassed	Withdrawn
Avoidance	Shut down
Minimizing	Concealment
Helplessness	Devastated
Hopeless	
"Helpful Hints" and Tools	
Understand your loved one's form(s) of the CR and try to react with empathy	
Encourage and collaborate with your loved one to:	
Discuss CRs in individual psychotherapy sessions	
Learn the precipitants of CRs	
Tweak circumstances to avoid reoccurrence	
Stop the activity, take a break, and regroup	
Participate in compensation training sessions at home to improve functionality	
Be organized and incorporate a comforting structure, routine, and accountability	
Modify the environment	
Simplify work/school activities so they are manageable	
Set "bite-sized" goals that are attainable	
Consider helpful medications (e.g., antidepressants, mood stabilizers)	
Communicate to family members when he/she feels overwhelmed	
Engage with people who are empathic and flexible	
Exercise, get proper rest, and incorporate good nutrition	
Engage in enjoyable hobbies and relaxing activities (e.g., yoga, soft music)	
Improve awareness, acceptance, and realism	
Signs of Depression	
Insomnia or excessive sleep	Self-deprecation
Low energy	Apathy
Psychomotor agitation or slowing	Lack of motivation, joy, or pleasure
Reduced libido	Hopelessness
Appetite change/Weight loss	Helplessness
Cognitive changes (impacting concentration, memory, and decision making)	Worthlessness
Social withdrawal	Guilt
Crying	Suicidal thoughts
Low self-esteem	
Other associated signs and manifestations	
Frustration	Fear
Brooding	Anxiety
Despair	Avoidance
Disillusionment	Grief
Emptiness	Shame
Hostility	Self-hatred
Snarkiness	Rage
Gloominess	Psychosomatic pain
Pessimism	Sorrow

Table 4.6 (continued)

"Helpful hints" and tools
Pursue education from your loved one's therapists and physicians, especially warning signs and symptoms, so as to respond with compassion
Remember that depression and grief are a predictable phase of the recovery and psychological healing process, related to improved awareness
Immediately seek out and implement intensive psychotherapy for your loved one and expect possible avoidance or resistance
Seek treatment with a psychiatrist for your loved one's mood and adjustment concerns, especially given the potentially dangerous upshots of severe depression (e.g., risk of self-harm, substance abuse)
Model and show "buy in" regarding the benefits of psychological and psychiatric interventions
Be open to psychotropic medications (e.g., antidepressants, mood stabilizers) for your loved one
Supervise your loved one's medications:
Verify he/she is taking them routinely
Make sure there are no missed doses or other compliance concerns
If necessary, observe the loved one taking his/her medications
Check his/her pillbox
Make sure medications are not accumulated or hoarded
Assist as needed with reordering and picking up medications
Remove any access to firearms
Seek education from professionals about the symptoms of substance use and abuse and their impact on mood (e.g., information resources, support for random urinalyses)
If necessary, facilitate substance abuse treatment for your loved one
Seek education about precursors and warning signs of suicide
Obtain information about community interventions and resources in the case of psychiatric emergencies:
Call 911
Take him/her to a hospital Emergency Room or behavioral health clinic
Obtain a list of contacts from health professionals
Assist and encourage your loved one to resume his or her preinjury lifestyle and overall community reintegration, meaningful activities, and quality of life
Multimedia Resources
Website
www.biausa.org/_literature_43189/depression_and_ brain_injury

ineptitudes can be devastating. "Snarky" behavior is another sign of CRs, as the loved one can become irritable, grouchy, or sarcastic when confronted or when trying to accept his or her limitations (Klonoff 2010). Other more subtle, but equally salient indicators are avoiding upsetting tasks, withdrawing and shutting down, minimizing or discounting ineptitudes, and concealing or hiding failures. Often, patients describe CRs as "hitting the wall" or "meltdowns" (see Klonoff 2010, for a review).

Table 4.6 also describes "helpful hints" for the family to cope with CRs in their loved one. This begins with caregiver and family education from the treating therapists about CRs. The relatives are then better equipped to avoid precipitating or escalating CRs in their loved one (Klonoff et al. 1993). This includes reacting empathically and managing tendencies towards impatience and ire when they observe bursts of emotionality in the loved one. Within the therapeutic setting, it is useful to review pre-session examples of CRs in the home and community so as to glean the precipitants. Circumstances can then be tweaked for the future to avoid the reemergence of the CR. If necessary, the loved one can be encouraged to stop the activity or take a break and regroup (e.g., studying for a difficult test). The therapist may need to counsel the family member to disengage from a situation and give the loved one a "time-out" so that strong emotions (e.g., anger) can dissipate (Coetzer 2006).

Another technique to reduce the incidence of CRs is collaborative compensation training sessions within the home with the patient, caregiver, and relevant therapists (e.g., occupational and physical therapists and/or speech–language pathologists). These set the tone for meaningful improvement in functionality and help generalize clinic-based ideas. This can include adaptive equipment, checklists, and other memory tools. Activities should be organized with a comforting structure, routine, and built-in accountability so as to anchor the loved one, especially during busier times (e.g., the holiday season).

Modifying the environment also reduces CRs (Klonoff 2010; Klonoff et al. 1993). This includes learning through the rehabilitation process how to help the loved one simplify work or school assignments so they are manageable, as well as set "bite-sized" goals. Certain medications can help to reduce the frequency of CRs (e.g., antidepressants and mood stabilizers), and the loved one should be encouraged to discuss this with his or her psychotherapist and psychiatrist.

Through the psychotherapeutic process, the loved one should be encouraged to notify family members when he or she feels overwhelmed. He or she can also engage with other tier supports that are empathic and flexible. Other strategies include working with the therapists to elevate the loved one's physical and emotional resources with exercise, proper rest, and good nutrition. Promoting the loved one to participate in enjoyable hobbies and relaxing interests (e.g., yoga, soft music) has a calming effect and provides a life balance. Therapy will teach mutually improved awareness, acceptance, and realism in the family (as well as the patient) and set the stage for adaptation, whereby there is the optimal fit for the loved one in the home and community. This ensures success and happiness (Klonoff 2010).

Table 4.6 also summarizes signs of depression in the loved one and "helpful hints" and tools for the family. It is also vital for family members to pursue education so as to recognize the signs and symptoms of depression and its prevalence after moderate to severe traumatic brain injury (Niemeier and Karol 2011b). A helpful user-friendly resource is *Coping with Depression after Traumatic Brain Injury* by Brown (2004) at www.biausa.org/_literature_43189/depression_and_brain_injury. Psychoeducation by a neuropsychologist, psychiatrist, and/or rehabilitation physician is strongly recommended. Depression symptoms can be divided into vegetative signs (e.g., sleep, appetite, and libido changes); psychological symptoms (e.g., low self-esteem and loss of joy or pleasure); behaviors (e.g., social withdrawal, crying, relationship difficulties); and cognitive components (e.g., self-criticism, hopelessness, and decreased concentration; Jean-Bay 2000; Cassidy 2009; Niemeier and Karol 2011b; Ponsford 2013). Relatives should be informed of the many other interconnected symptoms and manifestations of depression, including sorrow, brooding, gloominess, despair, disillusionment, emptiness, pessimism, frustration, snarkiness, hostility, fear, anxiety, avoidance, grief, shame, self-hatred, rage, and psychosomatic pain (American Psychiatric Association 2000; Cassidy 2009; see Klonoff 2010, for a review; Jean-Bay 2000; Ponsford 2013; Senelick and Dougherty 2001). Once the family and support network understand the many facets of depression as being part of the grief and loss process, they are much more likely to respond with compassion towards their loved one. The family should derive some solace that depression and grief are a predictable phase of the recovery and psychological healing process, as they reflect the loved one's improved awareness of the magnitude of his or her life changes (Klonoff 2010; Senelick and Dougherty 2001).

Crucial in helping a loved one cope with CRs, grief, and depression is to immediately seek out and implement intensive psychotherapy (Cassidy 2009; Klonoff 2010; Niemeier and Karol 2011b). The caregiver should recognize that often the patient will express resistance to this, in part because of the impact of his or her distress on drive and motivation, but also because he or she may be fearful or embarrassed about the need to seek professional help, related to cultural or environmental factors. Therefore, the family may need to take the lead as an advocate in this regard. This will require positive modeling on the part of the family, in that they must verbalize and "buy into" the idea of psychiatric and psychological interventions. It is also invaluable to work with a psychiatrist regarding the loved one's mood and adjustment concerns, especially given the potentially dangerous upshots of severe depression (e.g., risk of self-harm, substance abuse, etc.; Cassidy 2009; Horner et al. 2005; Klonoff and Lage 1995; Niemeier and Karol 2011b; Ponsford 2013; Simpson and Tate 2007).

Oftentimes, psychotropic medications can have phenomenal benefits for CRs, depression, and suicidal risk. Hence, family members should be responsive to a close liaison with a psychiatrist to identify remedying medications. Effective antidepressants include selective serotonin reuptake inhibitors (SSRIs; e.g., sertraline, paroxetine, fluoxetine, citalopram, and escitalopram), as well as selective serotonin and norepinephrine reuptake inhibitors (SSNRIs; e.g., venlafaxine, mirtazapine, and duloxetine; Arciniegas and Silver 2011; Cassidy 2009; Klonoff and Lage 1995; Senelick and Dougherty 2001; Waldron-Perrine et al. 2008). Trazodone is also a helpful antidepressant which assists with postinjury sleep disruptions (Arciniegas and Silver 2011; P. Bollam, personal communication, n.d.). Some antiepileptic drugs are also prescribed to help with aggression and mood swings, including carbamazepine, oxcarbazepine, valproate, and lamotrigine (Arciniegas and Silver 2011; Cassidy 2009).

The therapist will coach family members to be vigilant about supervising their loved one's medications, including verifying that he or she is taking the medications routinely, with no missed doses or other compliance issues. This includes either administering/observing the loved one take the medication(s) or checking the pillbox. Medications should never be accumulated or hoarded by the loved one, especially when there is concern about self-harm (Klonoff 2010). Often, relatives need to coordinate the reordering and pickup of prescriptions, especially for more acutely injured loved ones with significant memory and executive function deficits. Lastly, no weapons or firearms should be accessible in the home when the loved one has severe depression, or any thoughts of self-harm, especially when there are judgment and impulse control challenges (Klonoff and Lage 1995).

With respect to substance abuse, the family should be educated in psychotherapy regarding possible warning signs linked to specific drug and alcohol use (see American Council for Drug Education, n.d.; Aspen Education Group, n.d.). This is crucial, as substance abuse will interfere with recovery and successful community reintegration (Klonoff 2010; see Ricker 2010, for a review). Many of the symptoms associated with drug and alcohol use are similar to those of brain injury; therefore, there can be a synergistic effect between substance use and brain injury, including the worsening of psychiatric symptoms (Miller and Werner 2011). The signs of alcohol intoxication are alcohol odor, nausea, vomiting, stupor, slurred speech, poor balance and coordination, irritability, aggression, mood swings, as well as reduced judgment, impulse control, concentration, and memory (Allen et al. 2006; Goforth et al. 2010; Miller and Werner 2011). Marijuana use is associated with increased appetite, bloodshot eyes, relaxation, sleepiness, changes in mood states (i.e., euphoria, anxiety, paranoia), laughter and talkativeness, decreased motivation, and impaired judgment, problem solving, attention, and memory (Allen et al. 2006; Goforth et al. 2010). Stimulant use (e.g., cocaine) is characterized by hyperactivity, restlessness, jumpiness, euphoria, irritability, anxiety, depression, paranoia, poor attention span, excessive talking alternating with sleepiness, pupil dilation, decreased appetite, and weight loss (Allen et al. 2006; Goforth et al. 2010). Sometimes, the patient becomes addicted to opioids or narcotic pain medications. These medications produce decreased alertness, drowsiness, sedation, lethargy, nausea, apathy, euphoria, inability to concentrate, pupil constriction, and drug-seeking behavior (Allen et al. 2006; Goforth et al. 2010; National Institute on Drug Abuse, n.d.).

The therapist will instruct relatives to be attuned to exaggerated responsiveness to deleterious repercussions from drugs and alcohol after significant brain injury (Cassidy 2009). Educational materials, emotional support, and collaboration with treating physicians to schedule regular random urinalyses will bolster the family's knowledge and comfort level (Klonoff 2010; Miller 1993; Sparadeo 1993). If problems persist, most likely, the loved one will need a specialized substance abuse counselor (Klonoff 2010; Ricker 2010).

The therapist will educate tier supports about the higher risk of suicide in traumatic brain injury survivors (Bahraini et al. 2013). With respect to concerns about suicidality in the loved one, the family should be alerted in their therapy to precursors and warning signs, including intense and abrupt life changes (e.g., failed relationships, faltering careers, failing grades, unemployment, etc.); unnerving health complications (e.g., uncontrolled seizures); a shattered sense of identity; loss of freedoms and independence (e.g., supervision by family members, not driving, etc.); chronic and deep depression with feelings of worthlessness, joylessness, helplessness, and hopelessness; cognitive rigidity and a "no-way-out" mentality; and social isolation and withdrawal (see Klonoff 2010, for a review; Klonoff and Lage 1995; see Simpson and Tate 2007, for a review). Suicide becomes the ultimate expression of "narcissistic rage" when the loved one feels permanently deprived of his sense of integrity, choices, and future (Klonoff and Lage 1995). Another serious risk is pre- and postinjury suicidal thoughts or attempts (see Klonoff and Lage 1995, for a review).

Given that family members are on the frontlines of coping with intense emotions in their loved ones, they should be notified by the treating physicians and neuropsychologist about community interventions when they are concerned about the safety of their loved one. This includes calling 911, taking him or her to a hospital Emergency Room or a behavioral health clinic, and other community agencies and resources (Kuipers and Lancaster 2000). The family should inquire about a written list of contacts from the treating neuropsychologist, psychiatrist, and/or physician, so as to have immediate access, in case of emergencies (Simpson and Tate 2007).

Recent research indicates that depressive symptomatology is ameliorated by the patient's progress in resuming his or her preinjury lifestyle and overall community reintegration, including a sense of belonging (Jean-Bay 2000; Ownsworth et al. 2011). Thus, to the extent that family members can encourage their loved one, or even assist in attaining meaningful activities and quality of life, depressive symptomatology can be diminished.

4.6.3 How come my loved one seems so immature and blurts out things without thinking? How come my loved one doesn't watch what he or she is saying and says things that are hurtful or embarrass me in public? Why is my loved one so much more talkative now and why can't he or she stay on topic? How come he or she takes so long to think of what to say?

Figure 4.9 contains some other common communication and behavioral changes, many of which are correlated with frontal lobe damage. Quite upsetting to the relatives and support network are changes in the loved one's pragmatics, or functional social communications, which affect interpersonal relationships (see Klonoff 2010, for a review; Sohlberg and Mateer 2001). This is particularly the case when patients, without realizing the impact, are inappropriate or disinhibited; they may blurt out blunt, rude, or hurtful comments to those who are dedicated to helping them.

Related to the frontal lobe injury, patients often do not notice or self-monitor their comments, nor do they pick up on social cues that they are offending others (Klonoff 2010). To complicate matters, they become aggravated when family members point out social ineptitudes, rather than taking ownership for their communication style (Klonoff 2010). This can escalate into the relatives "walking on eggshells" whenever they need to communicate with their loved one.

Patients may also lose the capacity to appreciate the nuances of language and interactions, such as missing abstract or humorous content. Nonverbal communication skills can also be affected. The patient may show reduced eye contact and not notice negative body language or gestures towards his or her audience. This can make it difficult for the family to discern the intent of their loved one's interactions, including not realizing the patient is teasing or joking. This also has major ramifications for interpersonal and intimate relationships, as the patient does not grasp the subtleties of communication.

Behaviorally, the patient may appear much more egocentric, precluding the consideration of the needs and feelings of others (Lezak 1988; Senelick and Dougherty 2001). In addition, the patient's behavior often seems more childlike and less sophisticated to outsiders (Klonoff 2010; Lezak 1988). Friends and tier 3 supports may react with disdain and then withdraw from the patient (Lezak et al. 2004). The caregiver and extended family feel alienated from preinjury social circles and their own social isolation fosters loneliness and misery.

Other communication challenges relate to the loved one's inability to monitor the amount and quality of his or her contributions to conversations. Often, there is a lack of appreciation of the listener's needs and feelings and the patient will talk excessively (i.e., hyperverbality) and/or wander aimlessly from topic to topic (i.e., tangentiality). At other times, the patient is struggling to formulate his or her thoughts and then express them coherently and cohesively (Hartley and Jensen 1991; Le et al. 2011; Stuss and Levine 2002). This translates to long pauses between interactions and a dearth of flow and content (Coelho et al. 2002), which can try the patience of the already harried relatives.

4.6.4 "Helpful Hints" and Tools for Families to Cope with Communication Challenges in their Loved Ones

Table 4.7 summarizes therapeutic "helpful hints" and tools for the primary caregiver and other tier supports to cope with their loved one's communication challenges after moderate to severe traumatic brain injury. Paramount in the process is the family's collaboration with neurorehabilitation therapists, especially speech–language pathologists and neuropsychologists. In addition, it takes specialized training to diagnose and treat communication difficulties and the family will be at a disadvantage navigating this territory unassisted. As described in Chap. 2, Sect. 2.4.1.3, family members can bear the brunt of the patient's wrath, when they are giving solo "therapeutic advice" about these sensitive issues.

One jocular and "real-life" technique that the therapist can employ to ease the patient and family into the delicate discussion of communication skills are vignettes from television programs or movies. For example, in the movie, *Liar, Liar* (Bostick et al. 1997), Fletcher's uncontrollable verbalizations in the courtroom provide a humorous, but worthwhile example of the deleterious role of disinhibited comments. Likewise, Joe Friday, from *Dragnet* (Meshekoff et al. 1951–1959) is an excellent example of flat affect.

One useful tool that the speech–language pathologists can develop on behalf of the patient is a communication pragmatics log (see Klonoff 2010, for a review). This is comprised of a list of appropriate and inappropriate target behaviors, with an accompanying yes/no checklist which allows therapists and the support network to provide feedback. Overall, the log reinforces healthy social interactions, as well as encourages self-monitoring and self-correction of communication challenges within the treatment setting and community. Examples of acceptable behaviors include "think

Table 4.7 "Helpful hints" and tools for families to cope with communication challenges in their loved ones

Collaborate with speech-language pathologists and neuropsychologists
Remind the loved one of illustrative television or movie vignettes presented during therapy
Work with therapists to develop a communication pragmatics log
Gauge the loved one's receptivity to and context for feedback
Prioritize a few key skills at a time (e.g., "pick battles")
Provide feedback in a timely fashion
Develop a cuing system (e.g., "time-out signal")
Compliment good communication skills
Involve the loved one in group activities to practice communication skills (e.g., family functions, sports events, and group therapies)
Educate the support network about the loved one's pragmatic communication difficulties
Remind the loved one of communication challenges and compensations (per the therapists) prior to attending social functions
Review and practice appropriate conversational topics before going to social events (e.g., current events, movies, family milestones) using role-playing techniques
Review inappropriate language and topic areas that are setting specific (e.g., cursing, flirtatious behavior)
Model proper etiquette in social interactions
*Do not personalize blunt, insensitive, or embarrassing comments

before I speak" and "remember to be a good listener." Samples of problematic behaviors to be avoided include "don't invade people's personal space" and "don't curse." Relatives play an integral adjunct role in monitoring communication pragmatic behaviors listed on the log when out in public. Troubling instances can be shared with the treating therapists, who, if necessary, can be the "bad guy" in therapeutically confronting problem areas with the patient (see Chap. 2, Sect. 2.4.1.3).

The therapist can help the family learn to be considerate of the readiness of their loved one to accept suggestions. This means taking the mood and energy level of the patient into account, as well as the setting and context. Providing input when the patient is frustrated, overwhelmed, or tired will be much less palatable. Discussing sensitive topics should also be done in a private setting, so as not to needlessly embarrass the loved one. The inner feeling of trepidation in the caregiver is a sign that the patient may not be amenable to recommendations at that time. The discussion should be deferred to include therapists, or at least postponed.

It is easiest to focus on selected, "high-priority" behaviors that have the most impact on the loved one's social relationships. This is part of "picking battles" with the loved one, so as not to burn out the family and/or patient with constant pointers (see Chap. 2, Sect. 2.4.2.3). Assuming the loved one is agreeable, providing specific examples of what was said in a timely fashion will help the loved one better appreciate the family's concerns. Otherwise, he or she may not remember the circumstances or may underestimate the significance of the problem. If the loved one is receptive, the therapist can propose a subtle hand signal that close relatives can employ as a cuing device, when needed. Examples include a "time-out" signal to indicate the patient is off topic or overly talkative. On the other hand, when the patient demonstrates proper pragmatics, it is important for the family to be complimentary, so that he or she can build on these achievements. Again, close communication with the patient's treating therapists on an ongoing basis will facilitate the dialogue process between the relatives and the loved one.

Families can make a strong contribution to their loved one's progress in communication pragmatics by involving him or her in social gatherings (e.g., family functions, sports events, etc.). When feasible, the psychotherapist and relatives should also advocate for group therapy experiences for the loved one (e.g., communication pragmatics group), so that he or she can gain the necessary social competencies to further his or her recovery (Klonoff 2010). The therapists, together with the patient and primary caregiver, should educate the extended support group regarding the loved one's challenges with communication. This proactive approach reduces the likelihood of social stigmatism and ostracism.

As part of the therapeutic dialogue, the therapist can also instruct the support network regarding how best to prepare the loved one for upcoming social events and review a predetermined list of challenges and compensations. Furthermore, the caregiver can initiate role-play exercises for possible scenarios which could arise at an event, including reviewing and practicing fitting conversational topics. This is especially apt when patients struggle to generate topics for a meaningful exchange. Discussing recent current events, movies, or family milestones provides a positive structure and impetus for the loved one to initiate dialogue with others. For patients with tendencies towards disinhibited and socially inappropriate behaviors, it behooves the family to review the therapist's recommendations for proper etiquette, including casual reminders to avoid cursing and/or excessively flirtatious behavior. A great teaching tool for the loved one is to model the family displaying positive social behaviors.

Of utmost importance for the tier supports is to develop the psychological armor necessary not to personalize blunt or insensitive comments by their loved ones. Similarly, if the patient makes embarrassing comments or displays offensive behavior, the tier 1 caregiver(s) should remind himself or herself that this reflects the nature and severity of the brain injury, so as not to unduly berate himself or herself or criticize his or her loved one.

4.7 Scenario: Physical Challenges

Families are often yearning for improved physical abilities in their loved ones. They may ask questions such as: *Why is my loved one's balance so poor? Why is he or she so tired? Why is his or her endurance so low?*

4.7.1 Overview of Physical Challenges

There are a number of possible physical sequelae after moderate to severe traumatic brain injury. A detailed discussion of this area is beyond the scope of this book.

However, the functional relevance of problems with balance, fatigue, and reduced stamina are addressed. Given the breadth of changes, some of these are further discussed in the following chapters, including visual deficits (e.g., Chap. 6, Sect. 6.5).

Table 4.8 lists some common physical challenges after moderate to severe traumatic brain injury. As with Figs. 4.6 and 4.9, a ten-point rating scale is a beneficial technique for the therapist to obtain the family's (and patient's) self-perception of the severity of the problems with balance, fatigue, and endurance. It is strongly recommended that relatives consult with their loved one's rehabilitation physician, neurologist, and physical therapist regarding the nature and underlying causes of physical challenges.

Balance problems can be caused by difficulty controlling body position, decreased ability to process and synthesize sensory information, as well as vision and motor deficits (see Campbell and Parry 2005, for a review; Richter 2005). Damage to the cerebellum, somatosensory, or vestibular systems can cause balance deficits (Richter 2005). Fatigue and unspecific tiredness are common after moderate to severe traumatic brain injury, and can be related to sleep–wake disturbances caused by hypersomnia, excessive daytime sleepiness, and insomnia (Kempf et al. 2010). Sleep problems are caused by physiological, chemical, or hormonal changes in the brain, emotional factors, or medication side effects (Belmont et al. 2006; Parcell et al. 2008; Vaishnavi et al. 2011). Areas in the brain which regulate sleep include the hypothalamus, reticular activating system, brainstem (e.g., pons), pituitary, and the pineal gland (Belmont et al. 2006; Parcell et al. 2008). Reduced stamina is commonly caused by deconditioning, especially when patients have been bedridden or physically inactive for extended periods of time postinjury (Mossberg et al. 2010).

4.7.2 "Helpful Hints" and Tools for Families to Cope with Physical Challenges in their Loved Ones

Table 4.8 also summarizes therapeutic "helpful hints" and tools for relatives to cope with their loved ones' physical challenges. After a brain injury, balance difficulties may be subtle and emerge only in more demanding or even daunting situations (e.g., home and community settings with physical obstructions, uneven terrain, and/or multiple distractions; Richter 2005). Relatives may underestimate the seriousness of balance deficits and unknowingly put their loved one in physical danger. For that reason, family members should always adhere to physical restrictions and protocols suggested by treating physicians and physical therapists. This includes assistive devices (e.g., walker, gait belt, shower chair, etc.). Sometimes, based on the caregiver's and patient's enthusiasm and doggedness to resume a normal physical lifestyle, they may inadvertently undercut the recommendations and not follow through consistently in the home environment. This not only puts the loved one's safety in jeopardy but can also undermine the physical therapist's plan of care and lead to bad habits in ambulation, which are then very difficult to remediate. Since balance difficulties are often exacerbated by uneven terrain, relatives should always check with their loved

Table 4.8 Ratings, "helpful hints," and tools for families to cope with physical challenges in their loved ones

Balance Rating

0	1	2	3	4	5	6	7	8	9	10	Family	Patient
NO problem										BIG problem	☐	☐

Do not underestimate balance difficulties which are exacerbated in demanding home and community settings

Be careful not to inadvertently put your loved one in dangerous situations

Always adhere to physical restrictions and protocols recommended by the treating physician and physical therapist

Do not undercut therapeutic recommendations by altering physical protocols outside of the clinic

Check with your loved one's physician and physical therapist before advancing exercise programs or community sports

Fatigue Rating

0	1	2	3	4	5	6	7	8	9	10	Family	Patient
NO problem										BIG problem	☐	☐

Reduced Endurance

0	1	2	3	4	5	6	7	8	9	10	Family	Patient
NO problem										BIG problem	☐	☐

Consult your loved one's physician about sleep and fatigue problems

Normalize these problems for your loved one

Recognize that fatigue increases due to structural, biological, pain, cognitive, mood, and medication factors

Use proper sleep hygiene techniques (see below)

Consult with your physicians about possible beneficial medications and interventions to improve alertness as well as decrease pain and insomnia

Reinforce the use of a sleep log

Encourage a proper diet and regular exercise

Collaborate with your loved one's physical therapist about effective conditioning programs to

Table 4.8 (continued)

build endurance
Attend gym visits with the therapist and support the use of a heart rate monitor
Remember "more is better" may not apply in this scenario – do not over exercise your loved one
Help your loved one manage information overload: o reduce complex thinking demands o build in rest breaks o practice skills to make them automatic o use compensations (checklists) o complete cognitively demanding tasks in the mornings o gradually increase work hours
Encourage your loved one to regulate his or her lifestyle, including reducing stressors and addressing mood problems
Sleep Hygiene
Wake up and go to bed at about the same time every day (7 days per week)
Avoid going to bed too early
Do not try to "catch up" on sleep
Naps should be short (<1 hour) and occur in the early afternoon
Spend time outside every day to regulate your internal clock
Engage in physical and mental activities during the day (but not too close to bedtime)
Use your bed for sleeping only; do not study, read, listen to music or watch TV in bed
Reduce environmental disruptions, for example, too much light or noise
Avoid stimulating activities (e.g., exercise, video games) before bedtime
Avoid stimulants, caffeinated beverages, power drinks, nicotine, and alcohol
Do not use sleeping pills or sleep aids unless recommended by your doctor
Make 30–60 minutes before bedtime quiet and for "winding down"
Consider trying warm milk, a warm bath, quiet music, or relaxation exercises to facilitate sleep

one's physicians and physical therapist before increasing the physical complexity of an exercise program or community pastimes. This would include sports such as cycling, hiking, or rock climbing. The rule of thumb is not to risk the loved one sustaining another serious traumatic brain injury or other system injury.

Sleep problems, fatigue, and excessive daytime sleepiness should of course be evaluated and treated by a physician. The experience of excessive fatigue should be normalized for the family (and patient), as this is a very common postinjury occurrence (Cassidy 2009; Hicks et al. 2008; Ouellet and Morin 2006; Prowe 2010; Vaishnavi et al. 2011). Structural, biological, cognitive, pain, mood (anxiety and depression), and medication factors are all pertinent considerations for poor sleep quality after traumatic brain injury (Ouellet and Morin 2006; Parcell et al. 2008; Shekleton et al. 2010; Vaishnavi et al. 2011). Disrupted sleep patterns and insomnia also increase daytime fatigue (Ouellet and Morin 2006; Parcell et al. 2008). Proper sleep hygiene techniques are vital to the patient's proper sleep cycle and optimum daytime wakefulness (Arciniegas and Silver 2011; Walker and Kunz 2011). Table 4.8 also lists proper sleep hygiene techniques (Arciniegas and Silver 2011; Channing Bete 2012; Vaishnavi et al. 2011; Walker and Kunz 2011). Treatment of pain (taking into account the effect of pain medications on alertness) is also recommended to facilitate nighttime sleep (Vaishnavi et al. 2011).

Some medications are used to improve daytime alertness (e.g., the psychostimulants bromocriptine and amantadine), and they should be discussed with your loved one's rehabilitation physician or neurologist (Arciniegas and Silver 2011; Cassidy 2009; Ricker 2010; Senelick and Dougherty 2001; Vaishnavi et al. 2011; Waldron-Perrine et al. 2008). Other medications combat insomnia, including antihistamines (e.g., diphenhydramine), melatonin, ramelteon, and sometimes, sedative/hypnotic medications (Waldron-Perrine et al. 2008).

The psychotherapist can assist the patient and family in developing healthy habits. This can include introducing a sleep log notating sleep duration and quality (Vaishnavi et al. 2011). Proper diet and regular exercise are essential antidotes for reducing sleepiness and building stamina (Vaishnavi et al. 2011). Consultation with a dietician can be instructive to ascertain calorie-dense foods which facilitate energy improvements and overall good health and recovery. Choices include sufficient protein, fruits, and vegetables, as well as vitamin E-rich foods (Borek 2010; Gomez-Pinilla and Sharma 2010; see Joseph et al. 2009, for a review; Rajpal and Johnston 2009; Ryan 2007; Watson and Preedy 2010). Building cardiovascular fitness is instrumental to offset diminished endurance (Mossberg et al. 2010). The family member should be aware of what conditioning programs are most applicable for his or her loved one, making sure that he or she is not overdoing it. Wearing a heart rate monitor is an excellent strategy to maintain heart rate in the proper range. When feasible, it is best for the caregiver to attend gym visits with the loved one and physical therapist, so as to be cognizant of the best exercise regimen to ensure cardiovascular fitness and safe exercise practices. The adage "more is better" is not applicable in these situations and the caregiver should be careful not to advance programs before the patient is physically and cognitively ready.

As patients become more physically and cognitively active, their fatigue can increase, in part related to the mental effort it takes to complete challenging activities (Belmont et al. 2006; Ouellet and Morin 2006; Senelick and Dougherty 2001; Ziino and Ponsford 2006). Psychoeducation can provide "helpful hints" to reduce mental (and therefore physical) fatigue. These include: managing information overload by decreasing daily demands on the loved one for task completion involving complex attention, working memory, multitasking, and time pressures (Ponsford 2011). Rest breaks also help the loved one prolong mental stamina (Ouellet and Morin 2006; Ponsford 2011; Swiercinsky et al. 1999). The more tasks become automatic, the less cognitively demanding they become. Therefore, lots of practice for the loved one, as well as use of compensations that organize the information (e.g., checklists), will keep mental and physical energy levels primed (Ponsford 2011). Given that depression and anxiety affect sleep and increase fatigue levels (Ouellet and Morin 2006; Shekleton et al. 2010), helping the loved one manage his or her stressors will also combat tiredness and low energy. Research also suggests that more cognitively demanding undertakings should be completed in the mornings to maximize mastery, with a gradual increase in hours (Ouellet and Morin 2006). Overall, the family should encourage their loved one to regulate his or her lifestyle, taking into account the limitations (Ponsford 2011).

4.8 Scenario: Family Members' Angst and Disillusionment

Despite psychoeducation and input from professionals, oftentimes family members still feel completely overtaxed and devastated about the changes in their loved one, as well as the disruption to the family's lifestyle and cohesiveness. This can extend to several years postinjury, especially when the loved one suffers from cognitive disorders, anxiety, and social isolation (Ponsford and Schonberger 2010). They may say something like: *You've given me all of this information, but I can't deal with this.... I want my loved one back the way he or she was and my life also...*

4.8.1 Overview of Family Members' Angst and Disillusionment

Family members experience elevated emotional distress after traumatic brain injury, including anxiety and depression (Ennis et al. 2013; Kreutzer et al. 1994; Ponsford et al. 2003; Riley 2007; see also Chap. 2, Sect. 2.3). The loved one's reduced community reintegration compounds the family's distress (Marsh et al. 1998; Winstanley et al. 2006). As depicted in the FEM, the burden of "24/7" responsibilities, as well as uncertainty about the future, can cause the primary caregiver and relatives to plummet into hopelessness, bitterness, and resentment due to their schedule and life upheaval, financial setbacks, segregation, as well as physical, mental, and emotional exhaustion (Klonoff and Koberstein 2010; Klonoff et al. 2008).

4.8.2 *"Helpful Hints" and Tools for Families to Cope with their Angst and Disillusionment*

The psychotherapist will become an astute observer of the family system interactions. For instance, sometimes, pervasive depression in the primary caregiver and loved one "feed off of each other," creating a downward recurring cycle of gloom and despair. Table 4.6 contains symptoms of depression for the loved one (see Sect. 4.6.2); these are directly applicable to the caregiver and other tier supports enveloped in the totality of the loved one's needs. For easy reference, these are recapitulated in Table 4.9, along with common symptoms of anxiety. A ten-point rating scale or categories (no problem; small, medium, or large problem) can be utilized. As part of therapy, the caregiver and other relevant family members can complete these ratings periodically, so as to identify salient sentiments and trends. Anxious responses include excessive worry, fearfulness, edginess, irritability, concentration lapses, sleep problems, and other physiological changes (e.g., muscle tension, dizziness, rapid heartbeat, shortness of breath, nausea, faintness, chest pain, sweating, and shaking; American Psychiatric Association 2000). When depression and/or anxiety become entrenched in the caregiver, he or she is unable to galvanize the necessary resources to cope with hardships.

Table 4.10 summarizes an overview of some of the therapeutic "helpful hints" and tools for the primary caregiver and support network to begin to cope with their dismay about the alterations in their loved one as well as their own overall existence. (Other facets of this will be addressed in other chapters, including Chaps. 3, 6, 7, 8, 9, 10, and 11.) The therapist may suggest that the caregiver track his or her mood, including daily ratings (0 = no problem; 10 = severe problem) to increase self-awareness. This can also be done using a smartphone or computer application. Some relatives (including younger family members) respond better to a "feelings vocabulary chart" (Bloomquist 1996), which depicts multiple moods from which to choose. This alerts the family to a wealth of emotional responses (e.g., disappointed, disbelieving, disgusted, exasperated, jealous, miserable, nervous, regretful, shocked, suspicious, and undecided), which they may otherwise be ill attuned to. Journaling is also a powerful vehicle for self-reflection and when entries are shared with the psychotherapist, specific dilemmas can be more easily targeted. Sometimes, psychotropic medications are necessary and are indicated if mood disturbances become chronic and interfere with functionality and/or goal setting and attainment on an ongoing basis (e.g., SSRIs and mood stabilizers; P. Bollam, personal communication, n.d.). Normalization of the family's emotional distress and feelings of loss should be a primary goal of psychotherapy (Johnson and McCown 1997). A review of the FEM, especially within the context of a therapeutic relationship, is an excellent mechanism for the support network to self-evaluate their mood and coping strategies (Klonoff and Koberstein 2010). This is especially efficacious when the family is in the "yellow" or worse, approaching the "red zone," characterized by problematic coping and poor adjustment. As illustrated in Table 4.10, recognition of the relatives' unique forms of CRs by proxy (see also Chap. 2, Sect. 2.4.2.1 and Chap. 9, Sect. 9.4) will keep them vigilant

Table 4.9 Family members' depression and anxiety rating scale.
Have the family member provide ratings of his or her symptoms of depression and anxiety. Use the following scale: No problem; Small problem; Medium problem; Large problem

Domain:	No problem	Small	Medium	Large
Signs of Depression:				
Insomnia				
Excessive sleep				
Low energy				
Psychomotor agitation or slowing				
Reduced libido				
Appetite change				
Weight loss				
Concentration difficulties				
Memory difficulties				
Decision making difficulties				
Social withdrawal				
Crying				
Low self-esteem				
Self-deprecation				
Apathy				
Lack of motivation				
Lack of joy or pleasure				
Hopelessness				
Helplessness				
Worthlessness				
Guilt				
Suicidal thoughts				
Associated Signs:				
Frustration				
Brooding				
Despair				
Disillusionment				
Emptiness				
Hostility				
Fear				
Anxiety				
Avoidance				
Grief				
Shame				
Self-hatred				
Snarkiness				
Rage				
Psychosomatic pain				
Sorrow				
Gloominess				
Pessimism				

Table 4.9 (continued)

Signs of Anxiety:				
Excessive worry				
Fearfulness				
Edginess				
Irritability				
Concentration lapses				
Sleep problems				
Muscle tension				
Dizziness				
Rapid heartbeat				
Shortness of breath				
Nausea				
Faintness				
Chest pain				
Sweating				
Shaking				

about their propensity to become upset or mournful and then resort to unhealthy coping techniques, including overprotectiveness, anger, or blaming of others. Once the family is comfortable with navigating through the FEM model, they can use it as a self-reflection tool and as a technique to guide them back towards adaptive coping.

Through cognitive–behavioral therapy, conceptualizing the recovery and rehabilitation process for the loved one, as well as themselves, is best done using the model of a "marathon" versus a "sprint" (S. Myles, personal communication, n.d.). In fact, traumatic brain injury has been depicted as a "disease process" which is permeating and usually lifelong, rather than a short-lived "event" (Leith et al. 2004; Masel and DeWitt 2010). This provides the family with a realistic time frame and removes undue pressures for "instant results." As mentioned in Sect. 2.2.1.2, the adages "things take time" (T.T.T.; Hein 2003) and "one day at a time" facilitate acceptance and are sustaining thoughts during periods of turmoil and disillusionment. Setting short-term, incremental goals by the family (and loved one) anchors the family unit and nourishes a hopeful stance.

A source of consternation in family members is the reemergence of problematic personality attributes in the loved one that preceded the traumatic brain injury. These can include rule-breaking behavior, acting out, or poor motivation and integrity. These difficulties, in combination with the general aftermath of the brain injury, often inundate the family's coping mechanisms. The psychotherapist will require a detailed understanding of preexisting family psychodynamics in the context of the family system to trace the roots, manifestations, and degree of entrenchment of these behaviors. Only then can the therapist undertake to address their reemergence and provide meaningful therapeutic recommendations. In addition, psychoeducation by the psychotherapist regarding the relative contributions of preinjury characterological versus postinjury organic and reactive personality and mood changes, is vital to helping the family provide the necessary support and guidance to their loved one.

Remaining informed and proactive in the rehabilitation process will empower the primary caregiver and the overall support network (i.e., tiers 1–3). Treating therapists should encourage information sharing, input, and direct participation by the

Table 4.10 "Helpful hints" and tools for families to cope with their own emotional challenges

Become educated about the signs of depression and anxiety
Track your mood using a mood log, a feelings vocabulary chart, or journaling
If needed, be open to pharmacological treatment for depression and anxiety
Recognize that emotional distress and feelings of loss are normal and expected
Use the Family Experiential Model (FEM) of Recovery as a mechanism to self-evaluate mood and reinforce healthy coping strategies
Know your forms and reasons for catastrophic reactions (CRs) by proxy
Examples:
Frustration and angst because of the loved one's dependency on the caregiver
Sadness and disillusionment because of altered career plans
Hypervigilance because the loved one shows poor executive functions and communication pragmatics in the community
Despair because of the slow rate of progress and chronicity of some challenges
Conceptualize traumatic brain injury as a lifelong disease process, not a short-lived event
View the recovery and rehabilitation process as a marathon, not a sprint
Rely on stabilizing mantras such as "things take time" (T.T.T.) and "one day at a time"
Set short incremental goals so as to foster hope
Work with your psychotherapist to better understand the role of organic brain injury versus preinjury personality problems which are interfering with the recovery and rehabilitation process
Remain informed, proactive, and collaborative in the neurorehabilitation process, including the family's pre- and postinjury psychological health
Cope actively with family system issues, including outside stressors:
Focus on self-care
Actively incorporate regular respite
Delegate responsibilities
Cultivate resiliency
Participate in ongoing family education and support with professionals, incorporating group therapy and educational tools
Multimedia resources
Models
Family Experiential Model (FEM) of Recovery (Klonoff and Koberstein 2010; Klonoff et al. 2008)
Books
Your Brain at Work (The Conference Board, Inc. & The Dana Alliance for Brain Initiatives 2008)

support network (Coetzer 2006; Klonoff and Koberstein 2010; Nabors et al. 2002; Niemeier and Karol 2011b; Shaw et al. 1997) to counteract their pervasive feelings of helplessness attributed to the uncontrollable nature of the traumatic brain injury. Collaborating harmoniously with the treatment team invigorates the rehabilitation process and facilitates a positive momentum for all parties. Often, the primary caregiver(s) is bombarded by multiple stressors above and beyond the seemingly endless duties stemming from the care of the loved one after the traumatic brain injury. The psychotherapist should consult the interactive models of psychotherapy and family psychological health (see Chap. 1, Fig. 1.1 and Chap. 3, Fig. 3.1) and acquaint himself or herself with the caregiver's and overall family's unique history, culture, psychodynamics, environment, personality variables, values, and aspirations. Actively coping with family system issues in therapy, including dysfunctional elements, is critical for the emotional and physical longevity in the caregiver. This includes self-care, encompassing respite and delegation of responsibilities. Cultivating resiliency in the face of the inevitable downturns and disappointments is a central goal of family therapy (Perlesz et al. 1999). This can be accomplished by teaching the family adaptive problem-solving techniques which identify and prioritize issues; self-regulation of emotional reactions; as well as ways to brainstorm about and evaluate solutions (Rivera et al. 2008). Regular and ongoing family education and support by professionals, also in group formats, are highly advisable (Klonoff 2010; Ponsford and Schonberger 2010). Written resources on "cognitive fitness" that incorporate a holistic and healthy lifestyle are handy educational tools, including *Your Brain At Work* (The Conference Board, Inc. & The Dana Alliance For Brain Initiatives 2008). Family therapy groups are further addressed in Chaps. 9 and 11.

4.9 Case Study

Wally was age 18 when he suffered a traumatic brain injury as a result of a single car rollover motor vehicle accident, in which he was an unrestrained passenger. His initial GCS score was 7 and his period of unconsciousness was 72 h, with a period of PTA of 20 days. A CT scan demonstrated hemorrhages in the left and right frontal lobes as well as the left temporal lobe. An MRI scan of the brain indicated DAIs involving the frontal lobes and corpus callosum. Early complications included edema and raised intracranial pressure. Overall, Wally suffered a severe traumatic brain injury, with both focal and diffuse damage.

While receiving therapies on an inpatient neurorehabilitation unit, Wally underwent a neuropsychological screening examination. At that time, he was quite confused and was still considered to be in a period of PTA. After 4 weeks of multidisciplinary therapies, Wally showed good progress and was discharged home to the care of his mother, Annette (i.e., his tier 1 caregiver).

Wally and his mother were fortunate that they lived in a large metropolitan center which had a holistic neurorehabilitation treatment center available. His mother was proactive about seeking additional therapies, and even though Wally was ambivalent about continuing treatment, he hesitantly agreed to enroll in therapies within 10 days of his hospital discharge. Wally was assigned to a neuropsychologist, Dr. Egal, who would provide psychotherapy as well as family support and education. As a first step to building a working alliance, information regarding the goals, philosophy, and expectations of the neurorehabilitation process were provided to Wally and his mother during the initial consultation with Dr. Egal (see Chap. 2, Fig. 2.3). Paperwork was also provided to Wally's mother so that she would understand the nature and limits of her therapeutic relationship with Dr. Egal (see Chap. 2, Fig. 2.1).

Dr. Egal conducted a thorough interview, including Wally's demographic, background social and medical history, injury-related data, and overall psychological status (see Klonoff 2010, for a review). Dr. Egal was careful to monitor the mood and reactions of Wally's mother, based on interactions during the early sessions (see Chap. 2, Table 2.1). Wally's mom was sometimes tearful and anxious, and it was Dr.

Egal's impression that she was struggling not to become overwhelmed. Nonetheless, she was very caring and inquisitive. She volunteered that her son received exemplary care in the hospital and Dr. Egal opined (to himself) that this would help to catalyze a positive working alliance in this new setting.

Dr. Egal met separately with Wally's mother within the first 2 days of his program admission. He obtained relevant social history using a structured interview (see Chap. 2, Table 2.2). Annette was born outside of Des Moines, IA. Her parents had emigrated from the Netherlands before she was born. They were farmers with close ties to the extended family, strong values, and an exemplary work ethic. Annette described a happy childhood, cavorting with her many cousins around the farmlands. She was the first in her family to attend college, completing a degree in library science. Annette married her high school sweetheart, but later divorced from him when Wally was 3 years old. Wally and his father had not had any contact since that time.

Prior to Wally's injury, he and Annette were living together, along with Annette's close cousin who had recently moved to the area from Oklahoma. Annette was a full-time librarian and also took care of most of the household jobs. She prided herself in her parenting skills, inculcating the same values of hard work and responsibility in Wally. For instance, she stated that Wally was quite involved in the home prior to the accident, including doing multiple chores and taking care of his pet Labrador Retriever, Laila. Annette was pleased to admit that she had minimal pre-accident stressors and stated that she and Wally had a very good relationship. Prior to the accident, she was doing well financially and had a wide support network of friends and work colleagues. Other than her divorce, she denied other major life stressors. She drank modest amounts of alcohol, but did not smoke or use drugs. She had pursued counseling after her divorce, which she found to be very helpful. She was also very involved in her nondenominational church, which had always provided solace and inspiration. Dr. Egal's overall conceptualization was that Annette had many favorable personality attributes and a healthy family system, which would serve her well, including compassion, congeniality, cohesiveness, resiliency, good family boundaries, and adaptability. He felt intuitively that a positive working alliance could be forged, based on mutual trust and partnership and a holistic view of the family's needs (see also Chap. 1, Fig. 1.1 and Sect. 1.4.3; Chap. 2, Sect. 2.4.1; and Chap. 3, Sect. 3.1.1 and Fig. 3.1).

The next session was used to gain more injury-related information from Annette's perspective. She began to sob when she reminisced that a police officer telephoned the home in the middle of the night after Wally's accident. As described in phase 1 of the FEM, she recalled being filled with intense emotions, including shock, disbelief, horror, and panic. She described how she rushed to the hospital, where she kept a constant bedside vigil. She commented that she found attending the hospital chapel very comforting.

Annette stated that she was now taking a leave of absence from work, as her top priority was Wally's recovery and rehabilitation. Fortunately, for her, she had accumulated a good deal of paid time off. A number of her fellow librarians also donated their vacation time. Other than eliciting adjunct support and help from her cousin, Linda (i.e., her tier 2 support), Annette was in social seclusion. She stated she could not even think about hobbies or leisure, with so much going on with Wally. Basically, she could not fathom enjoying life until the same was true for her son. Annette admitted to insomnia; she had also lost 10 pounds since Wally's accident. She confided in Dr. Egal that she was sad and scared. She stated her biggest concerns were how Wally would progress and whether or not he would make a full recovery. As his devoted mother, she felt the supreme duty to re-raise him (see Chap. 3, Sect. 3.3.2).

Nonetheless, Dr. Egal was impressed with Annette's good early level of awareness, acceptance, and realism (see Chap. 2, Table 2.3). She completed the Deficit Rating Scale for Wally (see Chap. 2, Table 2.4) and endorsed not only physical (i.e., balance and fatigue) problems but also impaired attention and concentration, memory, and speed of thinking. Annette also noticed that Wally was more easily frustrated and was now exhibiting mood swings. He sometimes reacted with "snarky" retorts to her as well as Linda. Annette spontaneously stated that she did not feel that Wally was ready to return to school. She also shared that the accident had definitely altered both of their lives and she welcomed professional support and guidance. When Dr. Egal cautiously inquired about her willingness to help Wally use compensations (e.g., a datebook), she was eager to engage the learning process. Although she wept, she expressed appreciation to Dr. Egal when he gently imparted that the rehabilitation and recovery process would likely be slow and arduous. Annette clearly was a pragmatist. She was optimistic, yet she realized that Wally and herself would need to make adjustments and proceed in a stepwise manner back into the home and community. Her beliefs and behavior depicted the "green adaptive coping" zone on the FEM (see Chap. 1, Fig. 1.3). Dr. Egal and Annette agreed to meet weekly to discuss Wally's progress and challenges, as well as to continue the process of receiving psychoeducation and emotional support.

Meanwhile, Wally had undergone additional neuropsychological testing. Dr. Egal reviewed the test findings in graphical form (see Fig. 4.4) with Wally and Annette during their third session. Wally had worked diligently during the evaluation; however, he demonstrated moderately impaired memory performance, characterized by difficulty learning and retaining verbal information, including confabulatory responses. Moderate deficits in attention and concentration were also observed. In addition, Wally showed severely slowed speed of information processing and moderate to severe problems with reasoning and flexible thinking.

Over the course of the following several weeks, Annette embarked upon an intensive training program to better understand Wally's impairments. As a librarian, she was hungry for knowledge, and she took notes during sessions, as well as obtained supplementary reading resources. First, Annette noticed that Wally was having difficulty with declarative, procedural, and prospective memory. He would forget leisure activities he had participated in with his friends within a day or two, and he was having difficulty completing household assignments (e.g., the laundry sequence). He was forgetting to feed Laila in the evenings. Wally's mom was feeling overburdened, as she felt she was busy "picking up the pieces" every day, based on Wally's forgetfulness. Based on conjoint sessions with Wally and his mother together with Dr. Egal, the specific memory challenges were explored in more detail. Then Dr. Egal coordinated with Wally's speech–language pathologist and occupational therapist to devise effective tools for the home. "Helpful hints" which were instituted included a HIC and datebook protocol so that Wally would keep track more independently of home responsibilities. Annette also helped Wally develop routines so as to complete items every day at the same time; this helped immensely, especially with pet care. Wally's smartphone had an alarm, which he used to cue himself to take his medications in the morning and evening. Annette tried to reduce distractions in the home whenever possible. Their roommate, Linda, was also sensitive to the need for routine and structure, and she helped to reinforce a healthy diet and sleep schedule for Wally. As a support network, Annette and Linda typified healthy engagement, receptiveness, patience, flexibility, collaboration, and realism with the therapeutic process (see also Chap. 3, Sect. 3.1.3 and Fig. 3.1). Together, they were providing mutual support for each other as tier 1 and 2 supports.

Wally's mother also noticed higher order thinking difficulties. He was more impulsive and was making poor judgments. For instance, he decided to try to drive the family car, prior to being released by a physician to do so. Wally had enrolled in an online class as part of his therapy. He struggled with setting a study schedule and then would not initiate or follow through in a timely fashion. His notes were also very disorganized. He began to fail class assignments. Annette also noticed that he was not seeing the "big picture" and seemed unaware of the extent and nature of his limitations, as Wally kept perseverating on adding college coursework and decreasing treatment time, despite the obstacles he was facing in his one class. Behaviorally, he was starting to experience CRs, particularly when he received failing grades. He also became avoidant about doing assignments. He was easily irritated and reacted defensively to his mother's feedback. Annette felt embroiled in the "no-win" situation as a thankless "pseudotherapist" (see Chap. 2, Sect. 2.4.1.3).

Thankfully, due to Annette's trust, patience, and collaborative approach, she liaisoned closely with Dr. Egal and the rest of the treatment team. He reminded her that as Wally's mother and dedicated tier 1 caregiver, he was bound to "hurt the one he loves" (see Chap. 2, Sect. 2.4.2.2). This scapegoat behavior emerged from Wally's ambivalence about his reliance or her, yet resentment over his dependency (see Chap. 3, Sect. 3.3.2). Dr. Egal cautioned her to disengage when Wally was fuming, so as not to escalate the situation. He recommended that Annette let the rehabilitation therapists be the "bad guys" and take the lead in constructive feedback. The therapists fine-tuned the HIC and datebook system to better accommodate the need for a study plan. This included apportioning certain assignments to particular times of the day and counterbalancing his social and home management activities. Annette was guided to coordinate her home chore checklist with Wally's, which helped to streamline the shared responsibilities (see Fig. 4.7). His speech–language pathologist and occupational therapist also helped him structure his day to complete all of his tasks consecutively, thereby reducing the incidence of CRs associated with complex attention and multitasking. Dr. Egal recommended that Annette and Wally partake in a "milieu meeting" on Sunday evenings to synchronize their datebooks, schedules, and review plans for the week (see Fig. 4.5 for sample datebook entries and Fig. 4.8 for a "milieu meeting" agenda).

The therapists and Annette helped Wally better appreciate the importance of a stepwise approach to school, using the "real-life" data about his poor grade. Dr. Egal emphasized the importance of "not biting off more than he could chew," so as to reduce the likelihood that he would succumb to a depressive state. They mapped a chart of how and when to add courses, as well as take a driving examination, based on the successful building blocks of good academic performance and improved scores in cognitive retraining and on a simulated driving program. Annette was taught useful study techniques by the speech–language pathologist to assist Wally, including organizing his study space and the utility of acronyms and mnemonics.

Dr. Egal also facilitated Wally's inclusion in a psychoeducational group which focused on neuroanatomy, so as to learn more about the results of his injury and counteract the deleterious effects of unawareness. Fortunately, Dr. Egal and the therapists took the lead in addressing these complex and upsetting issues. That way, the extent of snarky behavior was reduced, as well as the tendency to "kill the messenger" in the home environment. To Annette and Linda's credit, they excelled at maintaining an understanding and empathic stance, even when Wally was overwhelmed and saddened. They realized this was an inherent part of the recovery and awareness training process and remained vigilant about Wally's mood. They also screened social pursuits with his friends, to be sure he did not imbibe alcohol or use any street drugs.

After about 4 months of neurorehabilitation, Wally added a community college class in communications, which he attended on campus. He was making an excellent physical recovery, with only slight high-level balance challenges. He was also becoming more involved in recreation and had rejoined a bowling league. This was a fun activity that also increased his coordination and endurance. Annette overheard Wally with his friends and noticed that he was hyperverbal and much more disinhibited, blunt, and seemingly selfish, including demanding that his friends provide rides for him at a moment's notice. He was also socially inappropriate around young women and Annette observed him coming on "much too strong" towards one of the cashiers at the local grocery store.

This behavior was particularly worrisome to Annette and she found herself experiencing CRs by proxy, becoming tense and melancholic. The 24/7 responsibilities and her hypervigilance about Wally's social skills in the community were creating physical, mental, and emotional exhaustion. She was succumbing to "chronic sorrow" and "loss spirals" over Wally's missteps (see Chap. 3, Sect. 3.3.2). She confessed to feelings of hollowness, wariness, and rumination. Annette used her weekly psychotherapy sessions to process these sentiments with Dr. Egal. Thankfully, through "companioning" and empathic responsiveness, he created a secure "holding environment" where she could safely emote. He also recommended she use the "stop think" method and structure time-limited "worry periods." Dr. Egal also normalized her angst using the FEM model, which was very reassuring to Annette. Together, Dr. Egal and Annette reviewed "warning signs" of anxiety and depression. She found that a daily mood log honed her introspection skills. He reframed the recovery and rehabilitation process as a "marathon," delicately reminding her of the seriousness of Wally's accident. Dr. Egal also reviewed all of Wally's gains, as a way to adopt a

Table 4.11 Wally's communication pragmatics log

Appropriate	Inappropriate
1) Be concise and give others a chance to converse	1) Do not talk excessively and dominate the conversation
2) Be polite, kind, and thoughtful about others' feelings	2) Watch disinhibited comments; do not be blunt, insulting, or hurtful; no foul language
3) Consider other people's needs and time constraints	3) Do not be selfish or demanding
4) Get to know young women gradually and be sensitive to their privacy	4) Do not come on "too strong"

Did Wally demonstrate appropriate communication pragmatics?

Date:_________

Time	Comments	Initials
8:00-noon	Y/N	
noon-4:00 p.m.	Y/N	
4:00-8:00 p.m.	Y/N	
8:00-10:00 p.m.	Y/N	

more constructive stance of "one day at a time." With the guidance of Dr. Egal, she concluded she still had the emotional reserves to cope overall with her daily strains.

Dr. Egal assured Annette of the importance of an informed and proactive role in this phase of Wally's rehabilitation. The speech–language pathologist introduced Wally and Annette to a communication pragmatics log (see Table 4.11) and a "time-out" technique that his mother (and trusted friends) could employ when needed. Only the germane behavioral concerns were included in the log, as an example of "picking battles." A meeting was also instituted by Dr. Egal and the speech–language pathologist to review these communication strategies with Wally and his broader support network (e.g., Linda and a few close friends). Wally was beginning to realize that he was alienating others, so he agreed to try the new tools. In addition, Annette, Linda, and Wally's friends were given written "helpful hints" about how to remind Wally of his challenges before attending social events, including practicing more appropriate topics and monitoring his blunt comments and foul language.

Dr. Egal helped enroll Wally in weekly group psychotherapy and communication pragmatics groups. These venues afforded the much-needed therapeutic input and practice. Annette, Linda, and Wally's friends were also encouraged to rely on their instincts of "walking on eggshells" as a gauge of how and when to give input. When Wally erupted into insulting and snarky behavior, they were reminded not to take his behavior personally, but rather to react calmly and recognize that this was a manifestation of his emotional distress and CRs.

To counteract any further emotional deterioration, Dr. Egal regularly reviewed the importance of respite and self-care for Annette through community involvements (i.e., tier 3 supports). She was invited to join a newly formed support group for family members. She was also held "accountable" to schedule and participate in enjoyable pastimes without Wally. Dr. Egal helped her recognize her capacity as a "good-enough parent," reminding her that the inevitable flaws propelled Wally to the next level of self-reliance as well as tolerance for aggravations and imperfections in himself and others (see also Chap. 3, Sect. 3.3.2). Annette was now contemplating returning to work, even on a part-time basis, given how much she enjoyed and valued her job. Despite the predictable "peaks and valleys," the neurorehabilitation process and family therapy were proceeding exceedingly well. She was reframing the initial hopeless catastrophe as a manageable family hurdle and could envision a more hopeful future for herself and Wally.

References

Alderman, N. (2004). Disorders of behavior. In J. Ponsford (Ed.), *Cognitive and behavioral rehabilitation: From neurobiology to clinical practice* (pp. 269–298). New York: Guilford Press.

Allen, D. N., Frantom, L. V., Forrest, T. J., & Strauss, G. P. (2006). Neuropsychology of substance use disorders. In P. J. Snyder, P. D. Nussbaum, & D. L. Robins (Eds.), *Clinical neuropsychology: A pocket handbook for assessment* (2nd ed., pp. 649–673). Washington, D. C.: American Psychological Association.

American Council for Drug Education. (n. d.). Signs and symptoms of substance abuse. In Phoenix House: Signs and symptoms of substance abuse. http://www.phoenixhouse.org/prevention/signs-and-symptoms-of-substance-abuse/. Accessed 3 June 2013.

American Psychiatric Association. (2000). *Diagnostic and statistical manual of mental disorders* (4th ed., text revision). Washington, D. C: American Psychiatric Association.

Arciniegas, D. B., & Silver, J. M. (2011). Psychopharmacology. In J. M. Silver, T. W. McAllister, & S. C. Yudofsky (Eds.), *Textbook of traumatic brain injury* (2nd ed., pp. 553–569). Washington, D. C.: American Psychiatric Publishing.

Ashley, M. J. (2010). Neuroanatomic review of cognitive function: Anatomy and plasticity. In M. J. Ashley (Ed.)., *Traumatic brain injury: Rehabilitation, treatment, and case management* (3rd ed., pp. 513–548). New York: CRC Press.

Aspen Education Group. (n. d.). Signs of alcohol or drug use. www.aspeneducation.com/factsheetsubstance.html. Accessed 4 June 2011.

Bahraini, N. H., Simpson, G. K., Brenner, L. A., Hoffberg, A. S., & Schneider, A. L. (2013). Suicidal ideation and behaviours after traumatic brain injury: A systematic review. *Brain Impairment*, (First View), 1–21. doi:10.1017/BrImp.2013.11.

Battisti, R. A., Roodenrys, S., Johnstone, S. J., Respondek, C., Hermens, D. F., & Solowij, N. (2010). Chronic use of cannabis and poor neural efficiency in verbal memory ability. *Psychopharmacology, 209*(4), 319–330.

Belmont, A., Agar, N., Hugeron, C., Gallais, B., & Azouvi, P. (2006). Fatigue and traumatic brain injury. *Annales de Readaptation et de Medecine Physique, 49*(6), 370–374.

Bloomquist, M. L. (1996). *Skills training for children with behavior disorders: A parent and therapist guidebook*. New York: Guildford Press.

Borek, C. (2010). Garlic and aging: Current Knowledge and future considerations. In R. R. Watson & V. R. Preedy (Eds.), *Bioactive foods in promoting health: Fruits and vegetables* (pp. 223–234). Burlington: Academic Press.

Bostick, M., Brubaker, J. D., Grazer, B. (Producers), & Shadyac, T. (Director) (1997). *Liar liar* [Motion picture]. United States: Universal Studios.

Brown, J., McKone, E., & Ward, J. (2010). Deficits of long-term memory in ecstasy users are related to cognitive complexity of the task. *Psychopharmacology, 209*(1), 51–67.

Brown, M. (2004). *Coping with depression after traumatic brain injury* [Booklet]. US: Brain Injury Association of America.

Campbell, M., & Parry, A. (2005). Balance disorder and traumatic brain injury: Preliminary findings of a multi-factorial observational study. *Brain Injury, 19*(13), 1095–1104.

Carter, R., Aldridge, S., Page, M., & Parker, S. (2009). *The human brain book: An illustrated guide to its structure, function, and disorders*. New York: DK Publishing.

Cassidy, J. W. (2009). *Mindstorms: The complete guide for families living with traumatic brain injury*. Philadelphia: Da Capo Press.

Channing Bete Company, Inc. (2012). *Understanding sleep disorders* [Booklet]. South Deerfield: Channing Bete Company.

Coelho, C. A., Youse, K. M., & Le, K. N. (2002). Conversational discourse in closed-head-injured and non-brain-injured adults. *Aphasiology, 16*(4–6), 659–672.

Coetzer, R. (2006). *Traumatic brain injury rehabilitation: A psychotherapeutic approach to loss and grief.* New York: Nova Science.

Dell Orto, A. E., & Power, P. W. (2000). *Brain injury and the family: A life and living perspective* (2nd ed.). Boca Raton: CRC Press.

Dikmen, S. S., Machamer, J. E., Winn, H. R., & Temkin, N. R. (1995). Neuropsychological outcome at 1-year post head injury. *Neuropsychology, 9*(1), 80–90.

Ennis, N., Rosenbloom, B. N., Canzian, S., & Topolovec-Vranic, J. (2013). Depression and anxiety in parent versus spouse caregivers of adult patients with traumatic brain injury: A systematic review. *Neuropsychological Rehabilitation: An International Journal, 23*(1), 1–18.

Filley, C. M. (2008). Neuroanatomy for the neuropsychologist. In J. E. Morgan & J. H. Ricker (Eds.), *Textbook of clinical neuropsychology* (pp. 61–82). New York: Taylor & Francis Group.

Flashman, L. A., Amador, X., & McAllister, T. W. (2011). Awareness of Deficits. In J. M. Silver, T. W. McAllister, & S. C. Yudofsky (Eds.), *Textbook of traumatic brain injury* (2nd ed., pp. 307–323). Washington, D. C.: American Psychiatric Publishing.

Franzen, M. D., & Iverson, G. L. (2006). Detecting negative response bias and diagnosing malingering: The dissimulation exam. In P. J. Snyder, P. D. Nussbaum, & D. L. Robins (Eds.), *Clinical neuropsychology: A pocket handbook for assessment* (2nd ed., pp. 102–119). Washington, D. C.: American Psychological Association.

Geisler, M. W., & Polich, J. (1992). P300, food consumption, and memory performance. *Psychophysiology, 29*(1), 76–85.

Gennarelli, T. A., & Graham, D. I. (2005). Neuropathology. In J. M. Silver, T. W. McAllister, & S. C. Yudofsky (Eds.), *Textbook of traumatic brain injury* (pp. 27–50). Washington, D. C.: American Psychiatric Publishing.

Glisky, E. L. (2004). Disorders of memory. In J. Ponsford (Ed.), *Cognitive and behavioral rehabilitation: From neurobiology to clinical practice* (pp. 100–128). New York: Guilford Press.

Godfrey, H. P. D., Partridge, F. M., Knight, R. G., & Bishara, S. (1993). Course of insight disorder and emotional dysfunction following closed head injury: A controlled cross-sectional follow-up study. *Journal of Clinical and Experimental Neuropsychology, 15*(4), 503–515.

Goforth, H. W., Murtaugh, R., & Fernandez, F. (2010). Neurologic aspects of drug abuse. *Neurologic Clinics, 28*(1), 199–215.

Goldberg, S. (2010). *Clinical Neuroanatomy made ridiculously simple: Interactive edition* (3rd ed.). Miami: MedMaster.

Goldstein, K. (1952). The effect of brain damage on the personality. *Psychiatry, 15*(3), 245–260.

Gomez-Pinilla, F., & Sharma, S. (2010). The therapeutic potential of diet and exercise on brain repair. In M. J. Ashley (Ed.), *Traumatic brain injury: Rehabilitation, treatment, and case management* (3rd ed., pp. 485–498). New York: CRC Press.

Hart, T., Sherer, M., Whyte, J., Polansky, M., & Novack, T. A. (2004). Awareness of behavioral, cognitive, and physical deficits in acute traumatic brain injury. *Archives of Physical Medicine and Rehabilitation, 85,* 1450–1456.

Hartley, L. L., & Jensen, P. J. (1991). Narrative and procedural discourse after closed head injury. *Brain Injury, 5*(3), 267–285.

Hassan, S. T., Khaw, W. F., Rosna, A. R., & Husna, J. (2011). Traumatic brain injury: Caregivers' problems and needs. *Journal of Nepal Medical Association, 51*(181), 53–55.

Hein, P. (2003). T. T. T. In *PoemHunter.com*, poems by Piet Hein. http://www.poemhunter.com/poem/t-t-t/. Accessed 3 July 2011.

Hicks, E., Senior, H. E., Purdy, S., Barker-Collo, S., & Larkins, B. (2008). Interventions for fatigue management after traumatic brain injury (Protocol). *Cochrane Library,* (4).

Horner, M. D., Ferguson, P. L., Selassie, A. W., Labbate, L. A., Kniele, K., & Corrigan, J. D. (2005). Patterns of alcohol use 1 year after traumatic brain injury: A population-based, epidemiological study. *Journal of the International Neuropsychological Society, 11*(3), 322–330.

Jean-Bay, E. (2000). The biobehavioral correlates of post-traumatic brain injury depression. *Journal of Neuroscience Nursing, 32*(3), 169–176.

Johnson, J., & McCown, W. (1997). *Family therapy of neurobehavioral disorders: Integrating neuropsychology and family therapy*. New York: Haworth Press.

Jorge, R. E., & Robinson, R. G. (2011). Mood disorders. In J. M. Silver, T. W. McAllister, & S. C. Yudofsky (Eds.), *Textbook of traumatic brain injury* (2nd ed., pp. 173–187). Washington, D. C.: American Psychiatric Publishing.

Joseph, J. A., Shukitt-Hale, B., & Willis, L. M. (2009). Grape juice, berries, and walnuts affect brain aging and behavior. *Journal of Nutrition, 139*(9), 1813S–1817S.

Kempf, J., Werth, E., Kaiser, P. R., Bassetti, C. L., & Baumann, C. R. (2010). Sleep-wake disturbances 3 years after traumatic brain injury. *Journal of Neurology, Neurosurgery, & Psychiatry, 81*(12), 1402–1405.

Klonoff, P. S. (2010). *Psychotherapy after brain injury: Principles and techniques*. New York: Guilford Press.

Klonoff, P. S., & Koberstein, E. J. (2010). Family life. In P. S. Klonoff (Ed.), *Psychotherapy after brain injury: Principles and techniques* (pp. 150–170). New York: Guilford Press.

Klonoff, P. S., & Lage, G. A. (1995). Suicide in patients with traumatic brain injury: Risk and prevention. *Journal of Head Trauma Rehabilitation, 10*(6), 16–24.

Klonoff, P. S., Lage, G. A., & Chiapello, D. A. (1993). Varieties of the catastrophic reaction to brain injury: A self psychology perspective. *Bulletin of the Menninger Clinic, 57*(2), 227–241.

Klonoff, P. S., Koberstein, E. J., Talley, M. C., & Dawson, L. K. (2008). A family experiential model of recovery after brain injury. *Bulletin of the Menninger Clinic, 72*(2), 109–129.

Kortte, K. B., Wegener, S. T., & Chwalisz, K. (2003). Anosognosia and denial: Their relationship to coping and depression in acquired brain injury. *Rehabilitation Psychology, 48*(3), 131–136.

Kreutzer, J. S., Gervasio, A. H., & Camplair, P. S. (1994). Primary caregivers' psychological status and family functioning after traumatic brain injury. *Brain Injury, 8*(3), 197–210.

Kuipers, P., & Lancaster, A. (2000). Developing a suicide prevention strategy based on the perspectives of people with brain injuries. *The Journal of Head Trauma Rehabilitation, 15*(6), 1275–1284.

Lamport, D. J., Hoyle, E., Lawton, C. L., Mansfield, M. W., & Dye, L. (2011). Evidence for a second meal cognitive effect: Glycaemic responses to high and low glycaemic index evening meals are associated with cognition the following morning. *Nutritional Neuroscience, 14*(2), 66–71.

Le, K., Mozeiko, J., & Coelho, C. (2011). Discourse analyses: Characterizing cognitive-communication disorders following TBI. *ASHA Leader, 16*(2), 18–21.

Leith, K. H., Phillips, L., & Sample, P. L. (2004). Exploring the service needs and experiences of persons with TBI and their families: The South Carolina experience. *Brain Injury, 18*(12), 1191–1208.

Leitz, J. R., Morgan, C. J. A., Bisby, J. A., Rendell, P. G., & Curran, H. V. (2009). Global impairment of prospective memory following acute alcohol. *Psychopharmacology, 205*(3), 379–387.

Lezak, M. D. (1986). Psychological implications of traumatic brain damage for the patient's family. *Rehabilitation Psychology, 31*(4), 241–250.

Lezak, M. D. (1988). Brain damage is a family affair. *Journal of Clinical and Experimental Neuropsychology, 10*(1), 111–123.

Lezak, M. D., Howieson, D. B., Loring, D. W., Hannay, H. J., & Fischer, J. S. (2004). *Neuropsychological assessment* (4th ed.). New York: Oxford University Press.

Lezak, M. D., Howieson, D. B., Bigler, E. D., & Tranel, D. (2012). *Neuropsychological assessment* (5th ed.). New York: Oxford University Press.

Lucas, J. A., & Addeo, R. (2006). Traumatic brain injury and postconcussion syndrome. In P. J. Snyder, P. D. Nussbaum, & D. L. Robins (Eds.), *Clinical neuropsychology: A pocket handbook for assessment* (2nd ed., pp. 351–380). Washington, D. C.: American Psychological Association.

Malloy, P. F., Cohen, R. A., Jenkins, M. A., & Paul, R. H. (2006). Frontal lobe function and dysfunction. In P. J. Snyder, P. D. Nussbaum, & D. L. Robins (Eds.), *Clinical neuropsychology: A pocket handbook for assessment* (2nd ed., pp. 607–625). Washington, D. C.: American Psychological Association.

Marin, R. S., & Wilkosz, P. A. (2011). Disorders of diminished motivation. In J. M. Silver, T. W. McAllister, & S. C. Yudofsky (Eds.), *Textbook of traumatic brain injury* (2nd ed., pp. 295–305). Washington, D. C.: American Psychiatric Publishing.

Marsh, N. V., Kersel, D. A., Havill, J. H., & Sleigh, J. W. (1998). Caregiver burden at 6 months following severe traumatic brain injury. *Brain Injury, 12*(3), 225–238.

Martin, C., Viguier, D., Deloche, G., & Dellatolas, G. (2001). Subjective experience after traumatic brain injury. *Brain Injury, 15*(11), 947–959.

Masel, B. E., & DeWitt, D. S. (2010). Traumatic brain injury: A disease process, not an event. *Journal of Neurotrauma, 27,* 1529–1540.

McCullagh, S., & Feinstein, A. (2011). Cognitive changes. In J. M. Silver, T. W. McAllister, & S. C. Yudofsky (Eds.), *Textbook of traumatic brain injury* (2nd ed., pp. 279–294). Washington, D. C.: American Psychiatric Publishing.

Menon, D. K., Schwab, K., Wright, D. W., Mass, A. I., & The Demographics and Clinical Assessment Working Group of the International and Interagency Initiative toward Common Data Elements for Research on Traumatic Brain Injury and Psychological Health. (2010). Position statement: Definition of traumatic brain injury. *Archives of Physical Medicine and Rehabilitation, 91*(11), 1637–1640.

Meshekoff, M., Meyer, S. D., Webb, J., Strock, H. L., & Canfield, H. (Producers). (1951–1959). *Dragnet* [Television series]. Los Angeles: National Broadcasting Company.

Miller, L. (1993). *Psychotherapy of the brain-injured patient: Reclaiming the shattered self.* New York: W. W. Norton.

Miller, N. S., & Werner, T. (2011). Alcohol and drug disorders. In J. M. Silver, T. W. McAllister, & S. C. Yudofsky (Eds.), *Textbook of traumatic brain injury* (2nd ed., pp. 461–474). Washington, D. C.: American Psychiatric Publishing.

Mossberg, K. A., Amonette, W. E., & Masel, B. E. (2010). Endurance training and cardiorespiratory conditioning after traumatic brain injury. *Journal of Head Trauma Rehabilitation, 25*(3), 173–183.

Nabors, N., Seacat, J., & Rosenthal, M. (2002). Predictors of caregiver burden following traumatic brain injury. *Brain Injury, 16*(12), 1039–1050.

National Institute on Drug Abuse. (n. d.). *NIDA infofacts: Prescription and over-the-counter medications.* www.drugabuse.gov/Infofacts/PainMed.html. Acessed 4 June 2011.

Nehlig, A. (2010). Is caffeine a cognitive enhancer? *Journal of Alzheimer's Disease, 20*(1 suppl), 85–94.

Niemeier, J. P., & Karol, R. L. (2011a). *Therapists' guide to overcoming grief and loss after brain injury*. New York: Oxford University Press.

Niemeier, J. P., & Karol, R. L. (2011b). *Overcoming grief and loss after brain injury*. New York: Oxford University Press.

Norup, A., Siert, L., & Mortensen, E. L. (2010). Emotional distress and quality of life in relatives of patients with severe brain injury: The first month after injury. *Brain Injury, 24*(2), 81–88.

Norup, A., Kristensen, K. S., Siert, L., Poulsen, I., & Mortensen, E. L. (2011). Neuropsychological support to relatives of patients with severe traumatic brain injury in the sub-acute phase. *Neuropsychological Rehabilitation, 21*(3), 306–321.

O'Callaghan, C., Powell, T., & Oyebode, J. (2006). An exploration of the experience of gaining awareness of deficit in people who have suffered a traumatic brain injury. *Neuropsychological Rehabilitation, 16*(5), 579–593.

Orman, J. A. L., Kraus, J. F., Zaloshnja, E., & Miller, T. (2011). Epidemiology. In J. M. Silver, T. W. McAllister, & S. C. Yudofsky (Eds.), *Textbook of traumatic brain injury* (2nd ed., pp. 3–22). Washington, D. C.: American Psychiatric Publishing.

Ouellet, M. C., & Morin, C. M. (2006). Fatigue following traumatic brain injury: Frequency, characteristics, and associated factors. *Rehabilitation Psychology, 51*(2), 140–149.

Ownsworth, T., Fleming, J., Haines, T., Cornwell, P., Kendall, M., Nalder, E., & Gordon, C. (2011). Development of depressive symptoms during early community reintegration after traumatic brain injury. *Journal of the International Neuropsychological Society, 17*, 112–119.

Parcell, D. L., Ponsford, J. L., Redman, J. R., & Rajaratnam, S. M. (2008). Poor sleep quality and changes in objectively recorded sleep after traumatic brain injury: A preliminary study. *Archives of Physical Medicine and Rehabilitation, 89*(5), 843–850.

Perlesz, A., Kinsella, G., & Crowe, S. (1999). Impact of traumatic brain injury on the family: A critical review. *Rehabilitation Psychology, 44*(1), 6–35.

Pitel, A. L., Witkowski, T., Vabret, F., Guilery-Girard, B., Desgranges, B., Eustache, F., & Beaunieux, H. (2007). Effect of episodic and working memory impairments on semantic and cognitive procedural learning at alcohol treatment entry. *Alcoholism, Clinical and Experimental Research, 31*(2), 238–248.

Ponsford, J. (2004). Rehabilitation following traumatic brain injury and cerebrovascular accident. In J. Ponsford (Ed.), *Cognitive and behavioral rehabilitation: From neurobiology to clinical practice* (pp. 299–342). New York: Guilford Press.

Ponsford, J. (2011, June). *Fatigue and sleep disturbance related to TBI* [PowerPoint slides]. Paper presented at the 3rd Federal Interagency Conference on Traumatic Brain Injury, Wash. D. C.

Ponsford, J. (2013). Dealing with the impact of TBI on psychological adjustment and relationships. In J. Ponsford, S. Sloan, & P. Snow (Eds.), *Traumatic brain injury: Rehabilitation for everyday adaptive living* (2nd ed., pp. 226–262). New York: Psychology Press.

Ponsford, J., & Schonberger, M. (2010). Family functioning and emotional state two and five years after traumatic brain injury. *Journal of the International Neuropsychological Society, 16*(2), 306–317.

Ponsford, J., Olver, J., Ponsford, M., & Nelms, R. (2003). Long-term adjustment of families following traumatic brain injury where comprehensive rehabilitation has been provided. *Brain Injury, 17*(6), 453–468.

Prigatano, G. P. (1986). Personality and psychosocial consequences of brain injury. In G. P. Prigatano, D. J. Fordyce, H. K. Zeiner, J. R. Roueche, M. Pepping, & B. C. Wood (Eds.), *Neuropsychological rehabilitation after brain injury* (pp. 29–50). Baltimore: Johns Hopkins University Press.

Prigatano, G. P. (1991). Disturbance of self-awareness of deficit after traumatic brain injury. In G. P. Prigatano & D. L. Schacter (Eds.), *Awareness of deficit after brain injury: Clinical and theoretical issues* (pp. 111–126). New York: Oxford University Press.

Prigatano, G. P. (1999). *Principles of neuropsychological rehabilitation*. New York: Oxford University Press.

Prigatano, G. P. (2005a). Disturbances of self-awareness and rehabilitation of patients with traumatic brain injury: A 20-year perspective. *Journal of Head Trauma Rehabilitation, 20*(1), 19–29.

Prigatano, G. P. (2005b). Impaired self-awareness after moderately severe to severe traumatic brain injury. *Acta Neurochirurgica, 93,* 39–42.

Prigatano, G. P., & Fordyce, D. J. (1986). The neuropsychological rehabilitation program at Presbyterian Hospital, Oklahoma City. In G. P. Prigatano, D. J. Fordyce, H. K. Zeiner, J. R. Roueche, M. Pepping, & B. C. Wood (Eds.), *Neuropsychological rehabilitation after brain injury* (pp. 96–118). Baltimore: Johns Hopkins University Press.

Prigatano, G. P., & Klonoff, P. S. (1998). A clinician's rating scale for evaluating impaired self-awareness and denial of disability after brain injury. *The Clinical Neuropsychologist, 12*(1), 56–67.

Prowe, G. (2010). *Successfully surviving a brain injury a family guidebook: From the emergency room to selecting a rehabilitation facility*. Gainesville: Brain Injury Success Books.

Rajpal, V., & Johnston, J. F. (2009). Nutrition management of traumatic brain injury patients. *Support Line, 31*(1), 10–19.

Richter, E. F. III. (2005). Balance problems and dizziness. In J. M. Silver, T. W. McAllister, & S. C. Yudofsky (Eds.), *Textbook of traumatic brain injury* (2nd ed., pp. 393–404). Washington, D. C.: American Psychiatric Publishing.

Ricker, J. H. (2010). Traumatic brain injury in adults. In R. G. Frank, M. Rosenthal, & B. Caplan (Eds.), *Handbook of rehabilitation psychology* (2nd ed., pp. 43–62). Washington, D. C.: American Psychological Association.

Riley, G. A. (2007). Stress and depression in family carers following traumatic brain injury: The influence of beliefs about difficult behaviours. *Clinical Rehabilitation, 21*(1), 82–88.

Rivera, P. A., Elliott, T. R., Berry, J. W., & Grant, J. S. (2008). Problem-solving training for family caregivers of persons with traumatic brain injuries: A randomized controlled trail. *Archives of Physical Medicine and Rehabilitation, 89*(5), 931–941.

Rodgers, J. (2000). Cognitive performance amongst recreational users of "ecstasy.". *Psychopharmacology, 151*(1), 19–24.

Roebuck-Spencer, T., & Sherer, M. (2008). Moderate and severe traumatic brain injury. In J. E. Morgan & J. H. Ricker (Eds.), *Textbook of clinical neuropsychology* (pp. 411–429). New York: Taylor & Francis Group.

Rosenthal, M., Christensen, B. K., & Ross, T. P. (1998). Depression following traumatic brain injury. *Archives of Physical Medicine and Rehabilitation, 79,* 90–103.

Ryan, M. (2007). *Sports nutrition for endurance athletes* (2nd ed.). Boulder: Velo Press.

Sander, A. M., Sherer, M., Malcc, J. F., High, W. M. Jr., Thompson, R. N., Moessner, A. M., & Josey, J. (2003). Preinjury emotional and family functioning in caregivers of persons with traumatic brain injury. *Archives of Physical Medicine and Rehabilitation, 84,* 197–203.

Schmahmann, J. D., & Caplan, D. (2006). Cognition, emotion and the cerebellum. *Brain: A Journal of Neurology, 129*(Pt 2), 290–292.

Schonberger, M., Ponsford, J., Olver, J., & Ponsford, M. (2010). A longitudinal study of family functioning after TBI and relatives' emotional status. *Neuropsychological Rehabilitation, 20*(6), 813–829.

Schretlen, D. J., & Shapiro, A. M. (2003). A quantitative review of the effects of traumatic brain injury on cognitive functioning. *International Review of Psychiatry, 15*(4), 341–349.

Senelick, R., & Dougherty, K. (2001). *Living with brain injury: A guide for families* (2nd ed.). Birmingham: HealthSouth Press.

Shaw, L. R., Chan, F., & Lam, C. S. (1997). Development and application of the family involvement questionnaire in brain injury rehabilitation. *Brain Injury, 11*(3), 219–231.

Shekleton, J. A., Parcell, D. L., Redman, J. R., Phipps-Nelson, J., Ponsford, J. L., & Rajaratnam, S. M. (2010). Sleep disturbance and melatonin levels following traumatic brain injury. *Neurology, 74*(21), 1732–1738.

Silver, J. M., Yudofsky, S. C., & Anderson, K. E. (2011). Aggressive disorders. In J. M. Silver, T. W. McAllister, & S. C. Yudofsky (Eds.), *Textbook of traumatic brain injury* (2nd ed., pp. 225–238). Washington, D. C.: American Psychiatric Publishing.

Simpson, G., & Tate, R. (2007). Suicidality in people surviving a traumatic brain injury: Prevalence, risk factors and implications for clinical management. *Brain Injury, 21*(13–14), 1335–1351.

Smith, C. (2011). Neuropathology. In J. M. Silver, T. W. McAllister, & S. C. Yudofsky (Eds.), *Textbook of traumatic brain injury* (2nd ed., pp. 23–36). Washington, D. C.: American Psychiatric Publishing.

Snyder, H. (2005). *Elvin the elephant who forgets*. Wake Forest: Lash & Associates Publishing/Training.

Snyder, P. J., Nussbaum, P. D., & Robins, D. L. (Eds.). (2006). *Clinical neuropsychology: A pocket handbook for assessment* (2nd ed.). Washington, D. C.: American Psychological Association.

Sohlberg, M. M., & Mateer, C. A. (2001). *Cognitive rehabilitation: An integrative neuropsychological approach*. New York: Guilford Press.

Sohlberg, M. M., & Turkstra, L. S. (2011). *Optimizing cognitive rehabilitation: Effective instructional methods*. New York: Guilford Press.

Sparadeo, F. R. (1993). Substance use: A critical training issue for staff in brain injury rehabilitation. In C. J. Durgin, N. D. Schmidt, & L. J. Fryer (Eds.), *Staff development and clinical intervention in brain injury rehabilitation* (pp. 189–205). Gaithersburg: Aspen Publishers.

Squire, L. R. (1987). *Memory and brain*. New York: Oxford University Press.

Sturm, C. D., Forget, T. R. Jr., & Sturm, J. L. (1998). *Head injury: Information and answers to commonly asked questions*. St. Louis: Quality Medical Publishing.

Stuss, D. T. (1991). Disturbance of self-awareness after frontal system damage. In G. P. Prigatano & D. L. Schacter (Eds.), *Awareness of deficit after brain injury: Clinical and theoretical issues* (pp. 63–83). New York: Oxford University Press.

Stuss, D. T., & Levine, B. (2002). Adult clinical neuropsychology: Lessons from studies of the frontal lobes. *Annual Review of Psychology, 53*, 401–433.

Swiercinsky, D. P., Price, T. L., & Leaf, L. E. (1999). *Traumatic head injury: Cause, consequence, and challenge* (revised ed.). Kansas City: Brain Injury Association of Kansas & Greater Kansas City.

Terry, W. S., & Phifer, B. (1986). Caffeine and memory performance on the AVLT. *Journal of Clinical Psychology, 42*(6), 860–863.

The Conference Board, Inc., & The Dana Alliance for Brain Initiatives. (2008). *Your brain at work* [Booklet]. USA: The Conference Board, Inc., & The Dana Alliance for Brain Initiatives.

Trahan, E., Pepin, M., & Hopps, S. (2006). Impaired awareness of deficits and treatment adherence among people with traumatic brain injury or spinal cord injury. *Journal of Head Trauma Rehabilitation, 21*(3), 226–235.

Turner, B., Fleming, J., Cornwell, P., Haines, T., & Ownsworth, T. (2009). Profiling early outcomes during the transition from hospital to home after brain injury. *Brain Injury, 23*(1), 51–60.

Turner, G. R., & Levine, B. (2004). Disorders of executive functioning and self-awareness. In J. Ponsford (Ed.), *Cognitive and behavioral rehabilitation: From neurobiology to clinical practice* (pp. 224–268). New York: Guilford Press.

Uomoto, J. M. (2010). The contribution of the neuropsychological evaluation to traumatic brain injury rehabilitation. In M. J. Ashley (Ed.), *Traumatic brain injury: Rehabilitation, treatment, and case management* (3rd ed., pp. 843–882). New York: CRC Press.

Vakil, E. (2005). The effect of moderate to severe traumatic brain injury (TBI) on different aspects of memory: A selective review. *Journal of Clinical and Experimental Neuropsychology, 27*(8), 977–1021.

Vaishnavi, S., Makley, M., & Rao, V. (2011). Sleep disturbance and fatigue. In J. M. Silver, T. W. McAllister, & S. C. Yudofsky (Eds.), *Textbook of traumatic brain injury* (2nd ed., pp. 325–342). Washington, D. C.: American Psychiatric Publishing.

Waldron-Perrine, B., Hanks, R. A., & Perrine, S. A. (2008). Pharmacotherapy for postacute traumatic brain injury: A literature review for guidance in psychological practice. *Rehabilitation Psychology, 53*(4), 426–444.

Walker, W. C., & Kunz, R. D. (2011). Postconcussion syndrome: Symptom management. In F. S. Zollman (Ed.), *Manual of traumatic brain injury management* (pp. 119–124). New York: Demos Medical Publishing.

Watson, R. R., & Preedy, V. R. (Eds.). (2010). *Bioactive foods in promoting health: Fruits and vegetables*. Burlington: Academic Press.

Wells, R., Dywan, J., & Dumas, J. (2005). Life satisfaction and distress in family caregivers as related to specific behavioural changes after traumatic brain injury. *Brain Injury, 19*(13), 1105–1115.

Wilson, B. A. (2009). *Memory rehabilitation: Integrating theory and practice*. New York: Guilford Press.

Winstanley, J., Simpson, G., Tate, R., & Myles, B. (2006). Early indicators and contributors to psychological distress in relatives during rehabilitation following severe traumatic brain injury: Findings from the brain injury outcomes study. *Journal of Head Trauma Rehabilitation, 21*(6), 453–466.

Zasler, N. D., & Martelli, M. F. (2011). Sexual dysfunction. In J. M. Silver, T. W. McAllister, & S. C. Yudofsky (Eds.), *Textbook of traumatic brain injury* (2nd ed., pp. 397–412). Washington, D. C.: American Psychiatric Publishing.

Ziino, C., & Ponsford, J. (2006). Selective attention deficits and subjective fatigue following traumatic brain injury. *Neuropsychology, 20*(3), 383–390.

Chapter 5
Family Psychotherapy for Concussions and the Postconcussive Syndrome

5.1 Scenario: Early Questions about Concussions (or Mild Traumatic Brain Injuries)

Concussions, also known as mild traumatic brain injuries and postconcussion syndrome, have both unique and some overlapping symptoms. With the increased interest in sports-related concussions, this topic is especially timely. Family members can be puzzled and confused about what symptoms apply to which entities. They are also unsure regarding how to best aid a loved one with these diagnoses.

Families may be notified that a loved one has sustained a concussion or mild traumatic brain injury and be understandably worried about his or her well-being. They may ask questions such as: *What is a concussion? What problems might he or she have? How long will it take to get better?*

5.1.1 Therapeutic Intervention: The Definition and Symptoms of a Concussion and Mild Traumatic Brain Injury

Mild traumatic brain injuries are the most common neurological disorder across the spectrum of traumatic brain injuries (Ruff 2011; Shukla and Devi 2010; see Snell et al. 2009, for a review). The estimate is that approximately 80–85% of traumatic brain injuries fall into this category (Lewine 2011; Ruff et al. 2009). Historically, there was a paucity of psychoeducation for the support network, given the often subtle consequences of the injury (Johnson and McCown 1997) and the fact their loved one may or may not come to the attention of medical personnel. Of note, the terms concussion and mild traumatic brain injury are mostly used interchangeably in the literature and by health-care professionals (Iverson and Lange 2011a; Lucas and Addeo 2006; McAllister 2011; Ruff et al. 2009). Education about the symptoms and recovery course after a concussion is advantageous so that the relatives comprehend the ripple effect of mild sequelae on the family system and at the same time support the loved one and help him or her take the necessary precautions to maximize recovery (Cavallo and Kay 2005; Johnson and McCown 1997; see Rohling et al. 2012, for a review).

P. S. Klonoff, *Psychotherapy for Families after Brain Injury*,

DOI 10.1007/978-1-4899-8083-0_5,

A *concussion* is defined as an immediate disturbance in neurological functioning resulting from rapid acceleration and deceleration due to external physical forces (Echemendia et al. 2011; see Lezak et al. 2004, for a review; see Ruff et al. 2009, for a review). The injury produces biochemical and neurometabolic changes in the brain (Echemendia et al. 2011). A mild concussion has no loss of consciousness and can be characterized by signs such as "seeing stars" and/or a short period of confusion and disorientation. A classic concussion involves a reversible coma which dissipates within the first 20–30 min after the event (Lezak et al. 2004). Mild traumatic brain injuries are defined as a Glasgow Coma Scale score of 13–15; a coma of 30 min or less; and a period of posttraumatic amnesia that does not exceed 24 h (Iverson and Lange 2011a; McAllister 2011; Mittenberg and Roberts 2008; Ruff et al. 2009; Shukla and Devi 2010). Seizures, intracranial lesions not requiring surgery, as well as focal and transient neurological symptoms affecting vision, hearing, language, sensation/perception, or motor skills may also be present (Iverson and Lange 2011a; see Ruff et al. 2009, for a review).

Worth mentioning is that mild traumatic brain injury can occur without loss of consciousness. However, there is altered or disturbed consciousness (e.g., incomplete memory of the event, as well as feeling dazed, confused, or disoriented; McAllister 2011; Menon et al. 2010; Ruff et al. 2009). Mild traumatic brain injury has also been categorized according to those individuals without any abnormal neuroimaging findings (e.g., a computed tomography (CT) or magnetic resonance imaging (MRI) scan) and those with abnormal findings (e.g., hemorrhage, hematoma, contusion, or depressed skull fracture), referred to as complicated mild traumatic brain injuries (Iverson and Lange 2011a; Lewine 2011; McAllister 2011). These latter patients usually have more significant injury effects (e.g., vertigo and decreased hearing; see Crandall 2011, for a review; de Guise et al. 2010; see Iverson and Lange 2011a, for a review; McCrea 2008; Shukla and Devi 2010).

Families will find out that there is considerable variability and even disagreements between health-care professionals about the expected course of mild traumatic brain injury (Bigler et al. 2013; see Klonoff and Lamb 1998, for a review; Prigatano and Gale 2011; Rohling et al. 2012; Ruff 2011). This author likes the paradigm proposed by Dikmen and colleagues (Dikmen et al. 1995). They found a "dose–response" relationship between the severity of the injury and level of cognitive impairment. Based on this model, a mild injury would produce mild cognitive challenges. In addition, a good deal of the current literature suggests that the loved one's thinking deficits should resolve completely within approximately 3 months after a mild insult (see Crandall 2011, for a review; see McAllister 2011, for a review; McCrea 2008; see Mittenberg and Roberts 2008, for a review; Rohling et al. 2011, 2012). The concussion should be considered transient, with a full recovery to be expected (Iverson and Lange 2011b; Rohling et al. 2012).

Table 5.1 summarizes typical symptoms of concussion or mild traumatic brain injury, both early on and after a delay of several days to weeks (Dikmen et al. 2001; Henrie and Elovic 2011; Johnson et al. 2011; Lucas and Addeo 2006; McAllister 2011; Mild Traumatic Brain Injury Committee of the Head Injury Interdisciplinary Special Interest Group of the American Congress of Rehabilitation Medicine 1993; Nilsson et al. 2011; O'Jile et al. 2006; Prigatano and Gale 2011; Ruff et al. 2009; Shukla and Devi 2010; Zafonte 2011; www.dvbic.org).

Table 5.1 Common symptoms of a concussion/mild traumatic brain injury

Early physical symptoms:
Headaches
Vomiting
Dizziness
Nausea
Drowsiness
Blurred vision
Confusion
Disorientation
Lethargy
Later symptoms:
Physical:
Headache
Dizziness
Sleep problems
Fatigue
Low energy
Vision and hearing problems
Ringing in the ears
Balance difficulties
Sensitivity to sounds and lights
Cognitive:
Memory difficulties
Reduced concentration and attentional difficulties
Slower thinking and reaction time
Difficulty finding words
"Fogginess"
Emotional:
Irritability
Anxiety
Depression
Mood swings

5.1.2 "Helpful Hints" and Tools for Families to Assist their Loved One after a Concussion or Mild Traumatic Brain Injury

The primary caregiver (tier 1) and other involved family members (tier 2; see Chap. 1, Sect. 1.3 and Figs. 1.1 and 1.2) can be instrumental in advocating for and helping the loved one obtain education about concussions or mild traumatic brain injuries. This is valuable, as early patient education has been found to relate to a better outcome (Iverson and Lange 2011b; McAllister 2011; Snell et al. 2009). It also reduces strain on the family system (Johnson and McCown 1997). Beneficial resources include http://www.cdc.gov/TraumaticBrainInjury/statistics.html; http://www.aans.org/Patient%20Information/Conditions%20and%20Treatments/Concussion.aspx; and http://www.cdc.gov/concussion/pdf/facts_about_concussion_tbi-a.pdf.

Once relatives have a general understanding of the definition and signs associated with concussion or mild traumatic brain injury, they should be given other "helpful hints" and tools to assist their loved one in the recovery process and reintegration into prior activities and responsibilities. Table 5.2 summarizes these "helpful hints" and tools for the family.

Given that sometimes patients with a mild concussion do not lose consciousness, it may be difficult to know if a loved one needs medical attention. However, the rule of thumb should be to have the patient see a medical professional at an Emergency Room or by a primary-care physician (PCP) if there is any suspicion of a concussion or mild traumatic brain injury (Bruns 2011). If the loved one is seen at an Emergency Room, typically discharge recommendations will be provided (Bruns 2011). These often include checking in on the loved one every 4 h over the ensuing 24 h to monitor his or her well-being. Family members should expect other medical advice to include: avoid alcohol; rest and avoid strenuous activities for several days; and do not drive for at least 24 h and until feeling capable (e.g., able to concentrate). The loved one should avoid taking narcotics, sedatives, muscle relaxants, and nonsteroidal anti-inflammatory drugs (Bruns 2011). Acetaminophen is often preferred to alleviate headaches and antiemetics can reduce nausea (Bruns 2011).

The family should be counseled as to when to access immediate medical care (Bruns 2011). Serious consideration should be given to neurological deterioration, including the emergence of: fainting, drowsiness, lethargy, or a failure to wake up; a change in behavior (e.g., acting strange); a constant severe headache or a worsening of a headache; vomiting more than twice; increased confusion (e.g., cannot remember new events or recognize familiar people); passing out, a blackout, or seizure; clumsiness or the inability to move parts of the body; blurred vision or slurred speech; or continual bleeding or fluid from the ear or nose (Bruns 2011; Putukian 2011). The support network should expect that physicians will request a CT and MRI scan if there is a posttraumatic alteration in consciousness or perturbation of neurological sequelae (Lewine 2011; McCrea 2008).

Educational materials for family members and the loved one help to reduce worry and overreactions. These include common symptoms, the likely time course of recovery, reassurance regarding the positive prognosis for complete recovery, and suggested coping strategies (Iverson and Lange 2011b; Johnson and McCown 1997; Shukla and Devi 2010). Neuropsychological testing is often effective in delineating specific postevent consequences in concussed patients (Echemendia et al. 2011; Iverson and Lange 2011a). At times, relatives will need to advocate on behalf of their loved one to undergo an assessment, especially in smaller communities where a neuropsychologist may not be readily accessible. The skill domains which are typically evaluated include attention and concentration, speed of thinking, motor speed, memory, reading speed and comprehension, general language skills, and executive functions (e.g., problem solving, planning, organization, impulse control, etc.; Tsaousides et al. 2011; see also Chap. 4, Sect. 4.2.1, Table 4.1, and Fig. 4.4). Mood and the level of emotional distress should also be evaluated so as to provide a well-rounded assessment (Klonoff and Dawson 2004; Tsaousides et al. 2011).

Table 5.2 "Helpful hints" and tools for families to assist their loved ones after a concussion or mild traumatic brain injury

- Be prepared to advocate for care for your loved one (and yourself)
- Your loved one will need to be seen at an Emergency Room or by a primary-care physician if there is suspicion of a concussion or mild traumatic brain injury
- Follow-up recommendations for the loved one include:
  - Check in every 4 h for 24 h to monitor his/her well-being
  - Avoid alcohol
  - Rest and avoid strenuous activities for several days
  - Do not drive for at least 24 h and until feeling able to concentrate
  - Per physicians, do not take narcotics, sedatives, muscle relaxants, or nonsteroidal anti-inflammatory drugs
  - Per physicians, take acetaminophen for headaches and antiemetics for nausea
- Seek immediate medical care if you observe neurological deterioration, including symptoms of:
  - Fainting
  - Drowsiness
  - Lethargy
  - Inability to wake up
  - Change in behavior (acting strange)
  - Constant severe headache or worsening of a headache
  - Vomiting more than twice
  - Increased confusion
  - Passing out or blackout
  - Seizure
  - Clumsiness
  - Inability to move body parts
  - Blurred vision
  - Slurred speech
  - Continual bleeding or fluid from the ear or nose
- Be prepared that typically a physician will request a CT scan and/or MRI if symptoms worsen
- Try to access educational materials for you and your loved one
- Advocate for neuropsychological testing that takes a broad-based approach, with collateral input from the family
- The best approach is an individualized medical and treatment approach with gradual resumption of typical activities (e.g., driving, work, school)
- The neuropsychologist may prescribe helpful treatment entities and compensations:
  - Datebook
  - Electronic devices
  - Note taking
  - Filing system
  - Post-it notes
  - Telephone message pad
  - Alarms
  - Specific accommodations for school and work
  - Short-term holistic treatment
- Watch for dysfunctional interactions and reactions to the loved one
- Recognize there may be temporary disruptions to the family system
- Work with a family therapist to guide and mediate trouble patches as they arise
- Remember to engage in regular self-care, including spiritual beliefs and existential pursuits
- Pursue a "continuum of care" model

Multimedia resources

Websites

http://www.cdc.gov/TraumaticBrainInjury/statistics.html

http://www.aans.org/Patient%20Information/Conditions%20and%20Treatments/Concussion.aspx

http://www.cdc.gov/concussiopn/pdf/facts about concussion tbi-a.pdf

A thorough neuropsychological assessment will also require a broad-based orientation that takes into account the loved one's demographics; family, educational, and occupational histories; psychosocial history; and other medical history (Klonoff and Dawson 2004; Klonoff and Lamb 1998; see also Chap. 2, Sect. 2.1). The support network (and the loved one) should identify a neuropsychologist who follows the clinical protocol of acquiring detailed medical (e.g., neurological, neuroradiographic, and psychiatric records), work and school data, as well as conducts a detailed interview as part of the evaluation of mild traumatic brain injury (Klonoff and Lamb 1998). Collateral input from family members is key to helping the neuropsychologist ascertain the loved one's level of daily functioning. This includes his or her capacity to be independent and productive at home with chores and responsibilities, as well as drive or work (Klonoff and Dawson 2004). Therefore, a knowledgeable relative is encouraged to attend the appointments so as to provide often crucial input about pre- and postinjury topics (see Chap. 2, Sect. 2.1; Klonoff and Lamb 1998).

Most professionals will propose a gradual resumption of typical activities, including work, school, and driving (Bruns 2011; Iverson and Lange 2011b). A neuropsychologist who has performed an evaluation can often provide treatment planning, including helpful stepwise suggestions for resumption of daily duties (e.g., work and/or school) and possibly cognitive rehabilitation by a neuropsychologist, speech-language pathologist, or occupational therapist, including compensation training (Torrence et al. 2011; Tsaousides et al. 2011). Beneficial tools and strategies include a datebook, electronic devices, and note taking/filing to assist with memory and organization; post-it notes for quick reminders; a telephone message pad for phone calls; and alarms as cues for medications (Wilson 2009). Specific accommodations may be needed for successful community reintegration, such as rest breaks at school or work or extended time allowances for tests (Tsaousides et al. 2011). The family should be aware that an individualized and balanced medical/treatment style is optimal, which validates the loved one's health concerns, without unduly fostering illness behavior (McAllister 2011).

In cases of bigger deficits, short-term therapy using a team approach incorporating a speech-language pathologist, occupational therapist, and neuropsychologist may be necessary to address cognitive, language, and functional challenges. A case in point, a short-term holistic framework with group therapies has proved favorable for patients after mild brain injury (Nilsson et al. 2011). This model provided 16 weekly sessions with homework and follow-up. The objectives were to: increase the process of change through an emphasis on support and psychoeducation (for the loved one and family members); enhance awareness, acceptance, and adaptation; and apply compensations to home and work activities (Nilsson et al. 2011).

Some families display dysfunctional interactions and reactions to a loved one with a mild traumatic brain injury (see Chap. 1, Sect. 1.4.3 and Chap. 3, Sect. 3.1.1). For example, periodically, relatives dismiss the input from health professionals and discount the impact of the injury. This may be in stark contrast to the loved one, who is experiencing markedly altered values, goals, relationships, and a sense of mortality (Johnson and McCown 1997). To him or her, the injury may be mild but is not trivial. Sometimes, through misinformation and misattribution, the family becomes insensitive and resorts to viewing the loved one as "weak" or "faking" (Johnson and McCown 1997). Conversely, therapists should be mindful of families (and a loved one) who are overestimating and/or overreacting to limitations caused by other possible stressors, including family dysfunction (Johnson and McCown 1997; see Sect. 5.2 on postconcussion syndrome). Unhealthy dependency or interpersonal hostility can fragment the support network (Johnson and McCown 1997). The psychotherapist and/or family therapist should be cognizant of the impact of these deleterious family dynamics on the loved one, family system, and ultimately the treating professionals, lest the latter succumb to negative countertransference reactions and/or compassion fatigue (see Klonoff 2011, for a review). The therapist guides and mediates on behalf of the family unit (including the loved one). Together, they find a "middle ground" for accurate appraisals of one another's perceptions and needs, so as to facilitate everyone's overall adjustment.

As has been detailed elsewhere, the primary caregiver is encouraged to engage in regular self-care for the necessary emotional, physical, and mental resources to provide input and advocate for the loved one (Channing Bete Company, Inc. 2010). Spiritual beliefs and existential pursuits are often constructive guideposts during the healing process (Johnson and McCown 1997). Overall, relatives should be aware that a "continuum of care model" can be efficacious in meeting the multiplicity of needs for the loved one after a mild traumatic brain injury (Rose 2005). The support network may need to help coordinate care in this regard, including the involvement of physical–medical management; case management; specialist consultations (e.g., with a neurologist or rehabilitation physician); psychoeducation; a baseline and follow-up neuropsychological assessment; stress management and counseling; as well as worksite reintegration and follow-up (Rose 2005).

5.1.3 Sports Concussions

A subtype of concussions results from sports injuries. The family may ask questions such as: *Did my loved one sustain a concussion during the game? How will that affect his or her brain? When can he or she go back to playing?*

5.1.3.1 Therapeutic Intervention: The Effects of Sports-Related Concussions—Single and Multiple Impacts

Sports concussion has become a growing public concern and has been coined a "silent epidemic of youth" (Moser et al. 2011). It has five features: caused by direct impacts to the head, face, neck, or elsewhere with an impulsive force transmitted toward the head; rapid onset of temporary neurological impairment that resolves spontaneously; symptoms reflecting a functional disturbance; graded clinical syndromes that may not involve loss of consciousness; and usually has normal structural neuroimaging studies (Covassin and Elbin 2011). Depending upon the sport, the player is at risk of sustaining one or multiple concussions; additional concussions complicate the recovery process (Lezak et al. 2004; McCrea 2008). Predominant concussion culprits are the contact sports of football, soccer, ice hockey, and especially boxing (Barr et al. 2008; Covassin and Elbin 2011; Harvey et al. 2011; Lezak et al. 2004; Lucas and Addeo 2006). Other sources of concussion are skiing, horseback riding, wrestling, baseball, basketball, lacrosse, rugby, skateboarding, bicycling, martial arts, cheerleading, and all-terrain vehicle crashes (Covassin and Elbin 2011; Macciocchi 2006; Toshkezi et al. 2011; Zafonte 2011). Research indicates that most individuals recover from a single sports concussion within 7–10 days (see Barr et al. 2008, for a review; Echemendia et al. 2011).

There is evidence that sustaining one concussion increases the likelihood of subsequent concussions (Henry and de Beaumont 2011). A "dose-related" continuum is observed, whereby the degree of cognitive deficits will correspond to the number and severity of concussions (Lezak et al. 2004). Boxers and football players are at particular risk of cumulative damage and can develop chronic traumatic encephalopathy (CTE). CTE reflects focal and diffuse damage, as well as atrophy of multiple brain structures (see Doolan et al. 2011, for a review; Harvey et al. 2011; Toshkezi et al. 2011). CTE has dementia-like symptoms, including motor difficulties (e.g., poor balance, clumsiness, incoordination, and tremors) as well as challenges with dizziness, vision, disorientation, confusion, attention, memory, speech, slower thinking, and reasoning (d'Hemecourt 2011; Harvey et al. 2011; see Lezak et al. 2004, for a review; McCrory 2011a; Toshkezi et al. 2011). Troubles with emotions and judgment also abound (Toshkezi et al. 2011). Rapid succession of injuries have also been referred to as "second impact syndrome," whereby a second concussion is sustained before the physiological reactions to a prior injury have resolved (see Barr et al. 2008, for a review; Harvey et al. 2011; see Henry and de Beaumont 2011, for a review; see Lezak et al. 2004, for a review; McCrea 2008; see Zafonte 2011, for a review). Complications may emanate from rapid brain swelling and cerebral hemorrhage, which can produce devastating consequences (Harvey et al. 2011; see Zafonte 2011, for a review).

5.1.3.2 "Helpful Hints" and Tools for Helping a Loved One After a Sports Concussion

Many of the principles in Sect. 5.1.2 delineating recovery from a concussion or mild traumatic brain injury apply to sports injuries. This section will include additional considerations (see Table 5.3). There is much more interest and attention being paid to the effects of sports concussion on the player as well as the need for public education (Weber and Edwards 2012). The support network should be reminded that their loved one may ignore or trivialize symptoms so as to continue playing the sport. This stance emerges for a myriad of reasons, including a misunderstanding regarding the seriousness of the situation, the desire to emulate older athletes, wanting to seem "tough," and not wanting to let down his or her teammates (Putukian 2011; Toshkezi et al. 2011). Similarly, sometimes parents pressure coaches and medical

Table 5.3 "Helpful hints" and tools for families to assist their loved ones after a sports concussion

Pursue education about sports concussions so as to guide your loved one
Watch for a tendency in your loved one to ignore or trivialize concussion symptoms so as to keep playing
Do not pressure your loved one or medical professionals about premature return to play
Focus on the long-term health and safety of your loved one
Utilize learning modules to educate the family and your loved one, including symptoms
Be aware of legislations that specify policies
Advocate for a comprehensive "sideline" assessment by medical or coaching staff
Take your loved one to the Emergency Room for a status assessment
Request hospital-based information on sports concussion
Try to find a sports neuropsychologist
Advocate for a baseline and/or follow-up neuropsychological evaluation to help with decisions related to sports and school reintegration
Remember that physical rest is integral to recovery
Sometimes, short-term cognitive remediation is beneficial
Watch for possible mood changes related to the concussion and non-play status
Seek mental health services, a support group, and psychotropic medications for psychiatric sequelae, as needed
Utilize therapists and liaison with the school to provide medical input and request the necessary accommodations
Limit overstimulating hobbies at home
Encourage proper sleep hygiene and abstinence from alcohol
If necessary, contact a physician about sleep problems and headaches
Seek out information about "return-to-play" guidelines
Be open to medical professionals' input so that your loved one does not return to play prematurely
Your loved one's needs, recovery, and return to play will be individualized, also based on the specifics of his/her injury and his/her age
Your loved one should not return to play until:
He or she is completely asymptomatic at rest and during exertion
Any psychiatric sequelae have dissipated
All other rule-out symptoms have been addressed
Advocate for injury prevention:
Encourage helmet wear
Remember helmets do not make the loved one "invincible" to injury
Watch for feelings of "false security" with helmet use leading to riskier behavior
Be aware of general prevention suggestions:
Have your loved one undergo a preseason physical examination
Be sure the trainer is qualified and has written emergency procedures
Advocate for safe facilities and equipment
Advocate for access to a physician during practices and games
Check if the coach has training in risks of injury
Advocate for strict enforcement of game rules by officials
Discourage violence or aggression during play
Familiarize yourself with specific prevention recommendations that are sport specific

professionals to release their loved one to play before he or she is ready (Doolan et al. 2011). Fortunately, the athletic culture (with the help of the medical profession) has moved from a position of "tough it out" to "sit it out" (Young 2011). Overall, the emphasis should be on the current and long-term safety and health of the athlete (Doolan et al. 2011).

Family education about sports concussion is critical so as to grasp the phenomenon and guide the loved one in the best direction (d'Hemecourt 2011). Currently in Arizona, all athletes are required to undergo concussion education and complete an e-learning module developed by Javier Cardenas, M.D., the Arizona Interscholastic Association, the Arizona Cardinals, Arizona State University, and Barrow Neurological Institute (Brainbook) (http://www.stjosephs-phx.org/Who_We_Are/Press_Center/218754) in order to participate in school sports (PRNewswire 2011). If possible, parents should also try to study this material (Cardenas, in Witkowski 2011). Relatives (and the loved one) should be aware that there is now state and federal government as well as collegiate and professional legislation encompassing concussion management policies (see Doolan et al. 2011, for a review). These include: education of athletes, parents, coaches, and school/organization officials regarding the management of sports' concussions; removal of youths from play who have sustained a concussion; and review of requirements for return-to-play clearance, based on a written release by an appropriate health-care professional (Echemendia et al. 2011).

Sports concussion symptoms are very similar to those of other concussions (see Sect. 5.1.2 and Table 5.1). However, family members should be aware that a sports injury more often causes confusion and amnesia than loss of consciousness (Kegel and Lovell 2011). Typical signs are disorientation and/or appearing stunned, dazed, or glassy eyed while on the sidelines (Kegel and Lovell 2011). The first line of attack for sports-related concussion is on-site or "sideline" assessment by emergency medical personnel, the athletic trainer, or team physician (Putukian 2011; Zafonte 2011). They will ascertain if the athlete is showing alterations in mental status, such as confusion, posttraumatic amnesia, headaches, dizziness, or problems with concentration and balance (Barr et al. 2008; Guskiewicz 2011).

Sideline assessment tools include the Concussion Symptom Inventory; the Balance Error Scoring System (to assess dizziness and balance); and the Standardized Assessment of Concussion (SAC; Barr and McCrea 2011; McCrea et al. 2000). The SAC provides a brief evaluation of key cognitive areas, including attention and concentration, memory, and rapid novel problem solving. It can be administered by an athletic trainer (see Harvey et al. 2011; McCrea et al. 2000). If possible, a team approach with a multidimensional assessment is ideal. This is comprised of: clinical observations; a symptom checklist; balance assessment; diagnostic structural brain imaging (e.g., a CT scan or MRI); a physical/neurological exam; and screening of thinking abilities (e.g., orientation to person, place, and time; concentration; and memory) at the time of the injury and at follow-up (Barr 2006; Barr and McCrea 2011; Barr et al. 2008; Doolan et al. 2011; Guskiewicz 2011; Putukian 2011).

When the loved one is seen in the Emergency Room, the physician will determine his or her medical condition and be sure that the loved one is ready for hospital discharge (see Jagoda 2010, for a review). Physicians will often base this on negative CT scan findings and a Glasgow Coma Scale score of 15 (see Jagoda 2010, for a review). The family should also be proactive about requesting hospital-based informational material on sports concussions (Jagoda 2010).

Relatives should also be aware of the value of neuropsychological testing after a sports concussion to evaluate the athlete's cognitive and psychological status (Barr and McCrea 2011; Barr et al. 2008; Doolan et al. 2011; Echemendia et al. 2011; Johnson et al. 2011; Zafonte 2011). A sport neuropsychologist is an excellent resource in this regard (Carr and Shunk 2011). This is especially useful when determining when an athlete is safe to return to competition (Barr et al. 2008; Doolan et al. 2011; Echemendia 2006a). Currently, baseline testing is available for some professional athletes. This defines the player's cognitive skill set prior to sustaining a concussion and also contains demographic, medical, and developmental information (Barr et al. 2008; Lucas and Addeo 2006). Others are urging baseline evaluations for all school athletes, which includes a review of typical symptoms, a neurologic examination, a cognitive evaluation, and balance testing (Putukian 2011). Otherwise, the loved one should undergo an evaluation after the concussion, in order to document possible thinking changes.

There are paper and pencil, computer, or Web-based versions of the assessments (Pardini et al. 2011). These assess orientation, memory, concentration, processing speed, reaction time, problem solving, etc. (Barr et al. 2008; see Echemendia 2006b, for a review; see Harvey et al. 2011, for a review; Lucas and Addeo 2006; Pardini et al. 2011). Some experts recommend baseline and follow-up evaluations which incorporate effort testing (see Schatz 2011, for a review). The loved one's neurologist or family doctor will be the most suitable resource from which to learn about neuropsychological testing.

Physical rest is integral to recovery. Family members should know that often physicians will promote physical rest, removal from activities that would risk another head injury, as well as abstinence from strenuous activities and resistance training, including running, weight lifting, etc. (Meehan 2011). The return to physical activity should be graded (Meehan 2011).

As stated in Sect. 5.1.2, short-term cognitive remediation with a speech-language pathologist, neuropsychologist, or occupational therapist to address cognitive sequelae may also enhance the recovery course after sports concussion. This can include paper and pencil and computer-based tasks that address attention and concentration, new learning, speed of information processing, etc. These can be done as part of therapy and supplemented as homework (see Chap. 8, Sect. 8.2.2, and Table 8.5 for a list of activities).

In addition to physical and cognitive changes, the family should be sensitive to possible mood issues in their loved one, including depression and anxiety (Doolan et al. 2011; see McCrory 2011b, for a review). Some athletes report reduced "vigor" after a concussion (Mainwaring 2011). Mood deterioration can also emanate from the restrictions placed on physical and cognitive activities during the recuperation phase (Meehan 2011). Family support during this transition is indispensable. Involvement with a sports psychologist/neuropsychologist or a support group may be worthwhile psychotherapeutic resources for the athlete (see Doolan et al. 2011, for a review). If needed, the services of other mental health professionals (e.g., a psychiatrist) for the loved one should be utilized (Meehan 2011). This individual should incorporate the contextual reality of the loved one and his or her family system and be sensitive to their phenomenological stance (see Chap. 1, Sect. 1.3; Klonoff 2010). Sertraline has also been found to be effective in treating depression and may also have cognitive benefits (see Meehan 2011, for a review).

The support network should also be vigilant about the loved one's capability to handle schoolwork after a concussion and can solicit the assistance of a neuropsychologist or speech-language pathologist in this regard (d'Hemecourt 2011; Echemendia et al. 2011). The therapists and family can facilitate the dissemination of specific medical instructions to the school. As stated above, school accommodations may be required during the recovery process (d'Hemecourt 2011; Doolan et al. 2011; Meehan 2011) and include a gradual academic return, with reduced assignments and tests (Doolan et al. 2011; d'Hemecourt 2011). Some professionals counsel against stimuli which require concentration, including video games, text messaging, and computers (Doolan et al. 2011; Meehan 2011; Putukian 2011; see Zafonte 2011, for a review). Alcohol intake should be avoided and proper sleep hygiene is recommended (Putukian 2011; see Zafonte 2011, for a review). That includes removing the distractions of text messaging, computers, televisions, video games, etc. from the bedroom and resting in a quiet dark room (Meehan 2011). At times, sleep medications are needed, including melatonin or trazodone (Meehan 2011). If the loved one is suffering from headaches, he or she should seek medical assistance regarding helpful medications (see Zafonte 2011, for a review).

As a concerned family member, care should be taken that the loved one does not return to play prematurely, as this can increase the risk of additional injuries or complications (Barr et al. 2008; Echemendia 2006a). This applies also to collegiate and professional sports, where the pressures can be intensified to return to active play (Pardini et al. 2011). There are "return-to-play" guidelines through the 2008 Zurich statement, the American Academy of Neurology, Cantu (see Barr et al. 2008, for a review; see Echemendia 2006a, for a review; see Harvey et al. 2011, for a review), and others (see Echemendia 2006a, for a review; Kegel and Lovell 2011). These specify if and when a player should return to the sport after one or more concussions. This decision-making process is both complicated and fluid (Echemendia 2006a). A multidisciplinary methodology is preferred, which is individualized to each athlete (Doolan et al. 2011; Echemendia 2006a; Harvey et al. 2011). For instance, younger athletes may require more time to recover because of their developing brains (Doolan et al. 2011). Family members can advocate that medical professionals include the loved one in the decision-making process (Doolan et al. 2011), so as to maximize his or her "buy in."

There is widespread agreement that the player should not return to the sport until he or she is completely asymptomatic, both at rest and during exertion (d'Hemecourt 2011; Doolan et al. 2011; Echemendia 2006a; Putukian 2011). This also includes monitoring psychiatric sequelae (e.g., depression, irritability, and restlessness; Harvey et al. 2011). When ready, a gradual progression to resuming play should be followed (d'Hemecourt 2011). Although controversial, researchers have suggested discontinuation from a sport when there are three or more concussions (e.g., the "three-strike rule"), prolonged symptoms, diminished athletic or academic performance, and/or CT or MRI abnormalities (see Henry and de Beaumont 2011, for a review; Kegel and Lovell 2011; Sedney et al. 2011). A "brain hygiene model" depicting many of the above principles is a handy reference for relatives (Moser et al. 2011).

Prevention of injury is vital to reducing concussive injuries. To the extent that relatives influence their loved one about safe sports practices, they should strongly encourage him or her to wear a helmet. This also applies to cyclists, skiers, snow boarders, and equestrians (see McCrory 2011b, for a review). However, the family and the loved one should remember that helmets do not make the player "invincible" (Phykitt in Young 2011). Hence, the support network should be wary of "false security" leading to riskier behavior (Harvey et al. 2011). There are also some general prevention ideas for athletes. These include: a preparticipation physical examination; a qualified trainer for all teams; written emergency procedures; safe facilities and equipment; access to a physician on the field during practice and play or access to immediate services when emergencies dictate so; coaches' training to include risks of injury; strict enforcement of game rules by officials; and discouragement of violence or aggression during play (Jayarao et al. 2011). Some authors have developed sport-specific prevention guidelines, which are helpful for the relatives of athletes to be aware of (see Jayarao et al. 2011, for a review).

5.2 Postconcussion Syndrome

Some individuals (e.g., approximately 10–20%) who sustain a concussion or mild traumatic brain injury evolve into what has been described as a postconcussion syndrome (Lucas and Addeo 2006; Wang and Zollman 2011). Family members may ask questions such as: *Why does my loved one still have so many difficulties since his or her concussion? A doctor diagnosed my loved one with a postconcussion syndrome—what is that? It's been months since my loved one's concussion and he or she is not working—how come?*

5.2.1 Therapeutic Intervention: The Effects of Postconcussion Syndrome

The entity of postconcussion syndrome is under fairly hot debate, with some researchers and clinicians staunchly supporting its existence and others not (see Garden et al. 2010, for a review; Iverson 2006; Klonoff and Dawson 2004; Klonoff and Lamb 1998; see McAllister 2011, for a review; see McAllister and Arciniegas 2002, for a review; see Rohling et al. 2012, for a review; see Ruff 2011, for a review). Some researchers and clinicians view postconcussion syndrome as a "biopsychosocial model," with cognitive, emotional, medical, psychosocial, and motivational factors (see Powell and McCrea 2011, for a review). Some consider the symptoms of postconcussion syndrome as nonspecific and also prevalent in healthy individuals

Table 5.4 Common symptoms of a postconcussion syndrome

Headaches
Dizziness
Balance difficulties
Sleep problems (e.g., insomnia)
Fatigue
Nausea
Memory difficulties
Concentration difficulties
Personality change
Irritability
Anxiety
Mood fluctuations
Depression
Apathy
Low tolerance for stress, emotion, or alcohol
Sensitivity to noise or light
*Symptoms must be present for 3 months
*Symptoms must interfere with social functioning

without a brain injury, as well as many other types of illnesses (Cicerone and Kalmar 1995; Dikmen et al. 2010; Donnell et al. 2012; see Garden et al. 2010, for a review; Larrabee et al. 2013; Lucas and Addeo 2006; see McCrea 2008, for a review; see Meares et al. 2011, for a review; see Rohling et al. 2012, for a review; see Ruff 2011, for a review; Wang and Zollman 2011). Others caution that postconcussion syndrome may be a misdiagnosis for anxiety, depression, posttraumatic stress disorder, or somatoform disorder (Donnell et al. 2012; Iverson 2006; see Rohling et al. 2012, for a review).

Table 5.4 lists a compilation of postconcussion symptoms, based on the literature (Cicerone and Kalmar 1995; Garden et al. 2010; see McAllister 2011, for a review; see Wang and Zollman 2011, for a review). There is a history of traumatic brain injury causing a significant concussion. Memory and concentration are affected and the loved one may also complain of headaches, dizziness, fatigue, insomnia, balance difficulties, nausea, and sensitivity to noise or light. Personality changes may include irritability, depression, anxiety, mood fluctuations, apathy, or low tolerance for stress, emotion, or alcohol (see McAllister 2011, for a review; see Wang and Zollman 2011, for a review). Some conceptualizations include a preoccupation with their symptoms, fear of permanent brain damage, and/or adoption of a sick role (see Wang and Zollman 2011, for a review). Postconcussion syndrome aftereffects by definition must persist for 3 months and must be of sufficient severity to interfere with social functioning. Some authors have described a postconcussion syndrome lasting for up to 2 years with symptoms of high anxiety, depression, feeling overwhelmed, indecisiveness, poor organizational skills, as well as a self-perception of reduced practical capabilities and impaired interpersonal relationships (Rees and Bellon 2007).

Table 5.5 "Helpful hints" and tools for families to assist their loved ones with a diagnosis of postconcussion syndrome

Liaison with medical professionals, including neurologists, psychologists, and psychiatrists, as early intervention and education are key
Collect informational resources, including from the Emergency Room
Medical professionals will evaluate multiple pre- and postinjury factors in trying to understand your loved one's symptom presentation
Family input is integral to a thorough and accurate diagnostic formulation
Neuropsychological testing is a helpful assessment tool, also including relevant background information
Be savvy about the possible role of symptom exaggeration (including from litigation) in hampering the loved one's recovery process
The treatment approach will be to promote recovery by lessening symptoms and encouraging a stepwise return to productive community activities
Treatment for physical symptoms (e.g., dizziness and balance problems) may be warranted
Psychoeducation, psychological counseling, cognitive therapies, and psychiatric interventions are useful to restructure self-perceptions toward abilities and potentials and to foster the use of compensations for mainstreaming into society
Proper sleep hygiene is essential
Meditation, relaxation training, white noise, and biofeedback techniques improve sleep, headaches, and pain
Selective use of pharmacological agents are helpful, including antidepressants, mood stabilizers, and medications to regulate sleep and alertness
Family members should advocate for the best care using a multidisciplinary approach which is individualized to the loved one's needs

5.2.2 "Helpful Hints" and Tools for Assisting a Loved One with a Postconcussion Syndrome

Table 5.5 summarizes "helpful hints" and tools for the family to assist the loved one with a postconcussion syndrome. The diagnosis and interventions for postconcussion syndrome may vary, based on the nature and variety of symptoms experienced by the loved one (McAllister and Arciniegas 2002). As with the other entities discussed in this chapter, a close liaison with a neurologist is important to better understand this syndrome. Other relevant resources are neuropsychologists, rehabilitation psychologists, health psychologists, and psychiatrists (Powell and McCrea 2011). Early intervention and education is integral to preventing the emergence of a postconcussion syndrome, including disseminated information from the Emergency Room (McAllister and Arciniegas 2002; McCrea 2008; Powell and McCrea 2011). The family can be proactive in accessing these services for their loved one and themselves.

The family member should expect that medical professionals will be striving to determine what other diagnoses may explain the loved one's symptoms, as often these will vary (Rohling et al. 2012; Zasler 2011). The possibilities include: the role of self-expectations; attribution of symptoms to a traumatic brain injury versus other causes; general stress; chronic pain; neck injuries; other current or premorbid medical conditions (e.g., hypertension, diabetes, sleep disorders); developmental disorders (e.g., attention deficit disorder); lower cognitive reserves; preexisting and/or postaccident depression and anxiety; posttraumatic stress disorder; medication side effects; substance abuse; and/or financial compensation (Belanger et al. 2013; Dikmen et al. 2010; Evered et al. 2003; Gunstad and Suhr 2001; Iverson 2006; Klonoff and Lamb 1998; Lucas and Addeo 2006; McCrea 2008; Meares et al. 2011; Mooney et al. 2005; see Rohling et al. 2012, for a review; Vanderploeg et al. 2003; Wang and Zollman 2011). On occasion, the loved one maintains a biased view of the "good old days" compared with his or her postaccident status (Gunstad and Suhr 2001; Lange et al. 2010).

Other considerations include normal aging, prior head injuries, and learning disabilities (Dikmen et al. 2001; Lucas and Addeo 2006). In addition, a preaccident history of psychological traumatization (e.g., childhood physical or sexual abuse) may also relate to postconcussion symptoms (Mooney et al. 2005). Other contributory factors include preinjury personality traits or a style that is perfectionistic, dramatic, dependent, insecure, avoidant, or negativistic, and is focused on physical problems (Evered et al. 2003; Garden et al. 2010). Current psychosocial stressors (e.g., marital problems) may intensify or represent the underlying etiology. In this case, the family's insights about the loved one's history prior to the injury are weighty in the professional's diagnostic formulation, which in turn guide the treatment methodology (McAllister and Arciniegas 2002).

As stated previously, neuropsychological testing is a beneficial diagnostic tool for delineating the thinking, behavioral, and mood changes associated with postconcussion syndrome (Klonoff and Dawson 2004; Wang and Zollman 2011). Again, the neuropsychologist should obtain applicable collateral input to glean the full symptom picture (see Sect. 5.1.2). The family member should be sure to accompany the loved one to his or her appointments and provide thorough feedback, so as to help the neuropsychologist make a judicious diagnosis. This will include records and information pertaining to the actual concussion and a detailed description of the onset and progression of symptoms (Wang and Zollman 2011). The relative's ability to integrate and describe the loved one's current status in the context of possible preexisting mood concerns is central, especially in the realms of depression, anxiety, or other emotional stressors. Pre- and postaccident substance abuse/dependence should also be discussed as part of the medical workup (Powell and McCrea 2011). In addition, some medications can affect mood and cognition (e.g., opioids; Meares et al. 2006).

Sometimes, the loved one may be exaggerating his or her symptoms for a variety of reasons; this has been linked to the onset of postconcussion symptoms (McCrea 2008; Mooney et al. 2005; see Wang and Zollman 2011, for a review). These include some form of financial reward (e.g., from a lawsuit) or additional care and attention from the primary caregiver. Obviously, this assertion by a medical specialist can engender offense and defensiveness in the loved one (as well as the family). This becomes a test of the psychological health of the family and the solidity of the working alliance. In essence, tier 1 and 2 supports will need "buy in" that in order for the loved one to receive the correct treatment, his or her doctors and therapists will need to arrive at the appropriate formulation of underlying reasons for a postconcussion syndrome, including symptom magnification and financial reward (Iverson 2006). It is recommended that the support network also be informed about the potential role of litigation in causing an exaggeration of symptoms (Mittenberg and Roberts 2008). If necessary, a family member should intervene with the loved one's attorney to be sure that all parties have the same priorities with respect to the resumption of normal duties and pastimes.

If the loved one's treating professionals arrive at a diagnosis of postconcussion syndrome, their treatment approach will be to promote recovery (Walker and Kunz 2011). Walker and Kunz (2011) have proposed a number of interventions. These involve guidance, education, and support, also including how to manage troubling symptoms. To help abate worries about the loved one's health, the therapist will likely employ reassurance and motivational techniques. This includes clarification that symptoms are part of the recovery process, so as to lessen fears about permanent brain damage. Therapeutic exercises to address dizziness, disequilibrium, and vestibular disorders may be needed. Educational interventions and psychological counseling to address mood changes and to assist with goal setting are recommended, especially when anxiety and depression are pronounced (McAllister and Arciniegas 2002; McCrea 2008; Powell and McCrea 2011; Walker and Kunz 2011). One method is referred to as "cognitive restructuring," in which the psychotherapist helps the loved one dismantle distorted self-perceptions and instead substitute accurate self-appraisals about his or her injury, abilities, and potentials (see Powell and McCrea 2011, for a review). In some instances, limited cognitive rehabilitation may be indicated, especially if the emphasis is on compensation training for memory challenges (see Walker and Kunz 2011, for a review).

Other suggestions by Walker and Kunz (2011) include incorporation of normalizing exercise and recreational activities, as well as resumption of occupational, academic, and social responsibilities. This should be done gradually, to reduce distress and facilitate mastery. The importance of mainstreaming into the community and being productive is crucial. As with other neurological syndromes, good sleep hygiene is essential for improved daytime functioning (McAllister and Arciniegas 2002; Powell and McCrea 2011; Walker and Kunz 2011). Meditation, relaxation training, and white noise devices can also improve sleep (Walker and Kunz 2011). Behavioral health specialists can also introduce progressive muscle relaxation or biofeedback to reduce headaches and neck pain (Powell and McCrea 2011).

Using pharmacological agents can also be a positive treatment adjunct to reduce symptoms of a postconcussion syndrome (Walker and Kunz 2011). These include antidepressants for depression and anxiety (e.g., selective serotonin reuptake inhibitors); antiepileptic mood stabilizers to help with irritability and anger (e.g., valproic acid and carbamazepine); and some activating antidepressants as well as stimulant medications to help with fatigue (e.g., fluoxetine, modafinil, methylphenidate, and amantadine; see Walker and Kunz 2011, for a review). Of course, all of these treatments must be carefully coordinated with treating physicians and therapists, with a holistic orientation being optimum (Ruff 2011). The family can help by coordinating the finest care for their loved one.

5.3 Case Study of a Concussion

Michelle was age 28 when she was involved in a car accident in which her car was broadsided. Fortunately for her, she was driving a larger vehicle and the air bag deployed. Witnesses at the scene noticed she "passed out" for about 3 min. When the paramedics arrived on the scene shortly thereafter, they noted she was somewhat confused and disoriented to the date. She also had limited recollection of events earlier in the day. Michelle was taken by ambulance to a local hospital and was diagnosed with a concussion. Thankfully, her CT and MRI scans were normal. However, she had a severe headache, nausea, and dizziness. Justifiably panicked, her husband, Martin, promptly raced to the Emergency Room to be with her. By that time, her confusion and disorientation had mostly dissipated. She was anxious to return home, as she had a 3-year-old daughter, Camille, waiting for her. After approximately 3 h, the Emergency Room physician provided her with ibuprofen for her headache and ondansetron for her nausea. He also provided them with written material on warning signs of neurological deterioration and instructed her husband to keep a close watch over her, which he eagerly agreed to do.

The next day at Martin's insistence, Michelle went to see her PCP with him in tow. Michelle described continued headaches and slight dizziness. She noticed her ability to pay attention was compromised and she felt "in a fog." Although she was thankful that she was not more seriously injured, she was also emotionally shaken and tearful. Michelle worked as a third-grade teacher and her PCP felt it was too early to return to the classroom, given the cognitive and physical demands of her job. With some convincing by Martin, Michelle reluctantly agreed to take a few days off, although she was keen to get back to her students as soon as possible.

Michelle recuperated at home for the next 10 days. Martin took 2 days off work to monitor her. She rested and avoided her typical hearty workouts of hiking and jogging. They agreed she should abstain from driving for the first few days and then only drive short distances without Camille in the car. She and Martin were vigilant about following her physicians' advice regarding not drinking alcohol or taking narcotic pain medications, even though she was achy. Based on information from the Emergency Room and the PCP, Martin was sensitive to any signs of neurological deterioration, and, thankfully, none emerged.

At the suggestion of her PCP, Michelle went to a neuropsychologist to be sure she was clearing enough cognitively to teach and return to her regular lifestyle. Martin gladly accompanied her, as he remained concerned about her condition. They were impressed with the neuropsychologist, Dr. Warren, as he took time to conduct a detailed interview about her current symptoms as well as obtain relevant background history (see Chap. 1, Sect. 1.3, and Fig. 1.1; and Chap. 2, Sect. 2.2, and Table 2.2). Michelle and Martin were born in Phoenix, AZ. Both of them belonged to the Church of Jesus Christ of Latter Day Saints (LDS). Martin (and Michelle) had strong family ties and prioritized their religious affiliation. Both considered themselves well adjusted and happily married. Neither one of them had prior significant illnesses or psychological problems. However, when asked about prior "critical events" in the marriage, Dr. Warren noticed their coping capacity, resiliency, and relationship constancy when describing a miscarriage at 15 weeks of gestation (see Chap. 3, Sect. 3.2.2).

Upon inquiry from Dr. Warren, Martin added germane observations regarding his wife's mild cognitive changes that he had observed at home. These included, during family home evenings, trouble focusing on teachings, songs, and togetherness as well as increased distractibility and forgetfulness about little things (e.g., where she put Camille's toys). Dr. Warren immediately recognized that Martin was clearly devoted to his wife's predicament (see Chap. 2, Sect. 2.2, and Table 2.1). Further exploration revealed that Martin was especially concerned about the longer-term prognosis, specifically whether or not Michelle would have permanent sequelae which would preclude her returning to work and motherhood. Dr. Warren surmised that Martin had some gaps in his awareness about the effects of Michelle's mild traumatic brain injury, insofar as the farther reaching aftereffects (see Chap. 2, Sect. 2.2.1.1, and Table 2.3). Also, reading between the lines, using a combination of psychoanalytic and family schema approaches, Dr. Warren hypothesized that Michelle's vocation as a teacher was particularly meaningful to Michelle, given her recent miscarriage. Dr. Warren provided some reassurance that the neuropsychological testing would be instrumental in delineating her strengths and challenges. Employing a psychoeducational approach, he also provisionally explained the typical course of recovery, namely that Michelle should show gradual improvement with a resolution of symptoms over the next several weeks.

Noteworthy was that preaccident, Michelle had just started instructing third grade, after teaching kindergarten for 5 years. She had found the transition somewhat daunting related to the new coursework and testing protocols for this age group. Dr. Warren shared that Michelle's neuropsychological profile 10 days postconcussion indicated subtle difficulties in complex attention, speed of thinking, new learning, and multitasking. Functionally, she still noticed some mild sensitivity to noise. Emotionally, she was feeling much better, although she reported occasional anxiety about her symptoms and interruption in her daily routine.

In keeping with Michelle's faith, she was community minded and felt the urge to get back to the classroom as soon as possible. Nonetheless, her neuropsychologist, Dr. Warren, cautioned her to take a gradual process, which Martin reinforced, as he remained worried about Michelle's health. Together, all three of them fashioned a return-to-work plan, whereby Michelle started working three mornings per week. She gradually ramped up her hours over the next 2 weeks, until she was teaching full time. Dr. Warren suggested several pertinent compensations to help her with focus, memory, and multitasking. These included assistive technology, whereby she put more information into her tablet in the form of a "to do" list to compensate for memory lapses. She also did more lesson preparation in advance and used a whiteboard in the classroom for assignments and instructions for the children (and herself). Dr. Warren also recommended some computer tasks in her areas of challenge that she completed at home.

It was very evident to Dr. Warren that Michelle and Martin had a sturdy and healthy marriage; historically, their "mentalizing" capacities enabled close attunement (see

Chap. 3, Sect. 3.2.2). As her tier 1 support, Martin was trustworthy, compassionate, agreeable, and flexible, which was fortifying to Michelle during her recovery. He developed a positive working alliance with Dr. Warren and was a pleasure to work with, as he was trusting and agreeable by nature (see also Chap. 3, Fig. 3.1). Dr. Warren was mindful to provide suggestions in "bite-sized pieces" using a collaborative approach (see Chap. 2, Sect. 2.4.1). For instance, Dr. Warren gently recommended that Martin take over more of the household chores and fulfill Camille's nighttime bathing ritual so that Michelle could get her rest.

Dr. Warren also encouraged Martin to act upon his good boundaries and "recharge his battery." Initially, Martin was reticent to do this, feeling guilty that he could "enjoy life" when Michelle was recuperating (see Chap. 2, Sect. 2.3.5). Dr. Warren stressed that Martin needed the necessary respite in order to attend to his multiple responsibilities. Conjoint sessions with Michelle helped, as she was considerate about Martin's need to take care of himself, in order to mitigate caregiver burden (see Chap. 2, Sect. 2.3.7). This included being observant of his own health and psychological needs and grabbing small respite breaks when he could. Dr. Warren also promoted that Martin continue his own exercise regime, even when Michelle could not. Martin reached out to tier 2 supports (e.g., his parents and in-laws) as well as tier 3 supports from the LDS church, all of whom gladly volunteered to spend time with Camille, to reduce the burden of responsibility at home. Dr. Warren was appropriately inquisitive about other sources of emotional sustenance. Martin sensed Dr. Warren's genuine interest, and brought his favorite inspirational scripture into a session to share with him.

Nonetheless, Dr. Warren noticed that Martin was exhibiting some "yellow warning" zone behaviors, based on the Family Experiential Model (FEM) of Recovery (see Chap. 1, Sect. 1.5; Klonoff and Koberstein 2010; Klonoff et al. 2008). He was anxious and overprotective about Michelle's health, which he now felt was fragile. He took a firm stance about "prohibiting" her extracurricular activities, including hiking and jogging, despite medical clearance from her PCP for a modified routine. Martin was petrified that she would fall and hurt herself. Dr. Warren explained the concepts of "shifting sands" (see Chap. 2, Sect. 2.4.2.3) and "dignity of risk" (see Chap. 4, Sect. 4.5.2; Klonoff and Koberstein 2010) and gradually guided Martin toward a more tolerant and less fearful perspective. Martin was also reticent to engage in sexual relations with Michelle, identifying himself more as a "caregiver" than "partner/lover." Dr. Warren gingerly and adroitly explored the obstacles to their sexual intimacy and through conjoint sessions, Martin and Michelle discovered the practical (i.e., time constraints), psychological (i.e., Martin's new identity as a "caregiver" versus "spouse" and Michelle's fretfulness), and physical (i.e., Michelle's headaches and mild dizziness) barriers. With Dr. Warren's guidance, they forged a game plan to rekindle their romance, including date nights and stepwise increases in intimacy (see Chap. 3, Sect. 3.2.2).

As time went on, Dr. Warren explored the couple's existential perspective about the recovery process (see Chap. 1, Sect. 1.2.10). Michelle and Martin often conversed about how fortunate they felt that the accident was not more serious. They discovered the "silver lining" of the incident, as they took each other and Camille much less for granted and pledged to cherish their time and activities together (see Chap. 2, Sect. 2.4.2.4). Martin (and Michelle) were clearly in phase 6 (soon to be phase 7) "green coping" zone of the FEM and the Patient Experiential Model (PEM) of Recovery (Klonoff 2010). Given the knowledge that Michelle gained through her own concussion, she wanted to educate her LDS Relief Society meeting and the physical education teachers and coaches at the school about sports concussions from basketball and soccer. Dr. Warren helped her with the research to obtain pamphlets and website material, including ImPact testing (http://impacttest.com/). Michelle shared these resources with the churchwomen as well as the physical education teachers and coaches; they were all very appreciative. Hearing what happened to another mother, colleague, and friend was a "wake-up call," and they were more mindful about the risks of injury to their children and students.

References

Barr, W. B. (2006). Assessing mild traumatic brain injury on the sideline. In R. J. Echemendia (Ed.), *Sports neuropsychology: Assessment and management of traumatic brain injury* (pp. 87–111). New York: Guilford Press.

Barr, W. B., & McCrea, M. (2011). Diagnosis and assessment of concussion. In F. M. Webbe (Ed.), *The handbook of sport neuropsychology* (pp. 91–111). New York: Springer.

Barr, W. B., McCrea, M., & Randolph, C. (2008). Neuropsychology of sports-related injuries. In J. E. Morgan & J. H. Ricker (Eds.), *Textbook of clinical neuropsychology* (pp. 660–678). New York: Taylor & Francis Group.

Belanger, H. G., Barwick, F. H., Kip, K. E., Kretzmer, T., & Vanderploeg, R. D. (2013). Post-concussive symptom complaints and potentially malleable positive predictors. *The Clinical Neuropsychologists, 27*(3), 343–355.

Bigler, E. D., Farrer, T. J., Pertab, J. L., James, K., Petrie, J. A., & Hedges, D. W. (2013). Reaffirmed limitations of meta-analytic methods in the study of mild traumatic brain injury: A response to Rohling et al. *The Clinical Neuropsychologist, 27*(2), 176–214.

Bruns, J. J. (2011). Mild traumatic brain injury: Initial medical evaluation and management. In F. S. Zollman (Ed.), *Manual of traumatic brain injury management* (pp. 51–57). New York: Demos Medical Publishing.

Carr, C. M., & Shunk, A. W. (2011). Qualifications and training of the sport neuropsychologist. In F. M. Webbe (Ed.), *The handbook of sport neuropsychology* (pp. 17–34). New York: Springer.

Cavallo, M. M., & Kay, T. (2005). The family system. In J. M. Silver, T. W. McAllister, & S. C. Yudofsky (Eds.), *Textbook of traumatic brain injury* (pp. 533–558). Washington, D. C.: American Psychiatric Publishing.

Channing Bete Company, Inc. (2010). *Service member and family handbook: Recovering from traumatic brain injury* [Booklet]. South Deerfield: Channing Bete Company.

Cicerone, K. D., & Kalmar, K. (1995). Persistent postconcussion syndrome: The structure of subjective complaints after mild traumatic brain injury. *Journal of Head Trauma Rehabilitation, 10*(3), 1–17.

Covassin, T., & Elbin, R. J. (2011). History and epidemiology of concussion in sport. In F. M. Webbe (Ed.), *The handbook of sport neuropsychology* (pp. 53–74). New York: Springer.

Crandall, M. (2011). Epidemiology of traumatic brain injury. In F. S. Zollman (Ed.), *Manual of traumatic brain injury management* (pp. 25–29). New York: Demos Medical Publishing.

de Guise, E., Lepage, J. F., Tinawi, S., LeBlanc, J., Dagher, J., Lamoureux, J., & Feyz, M. (2010). Comprehensive clinical picture of patients with complicated vs. uncomplicated mild traumatic brain injury. *The Clinical Neuropsychologist, 24*(7), 1113–1130.

d'Hemecourt, P. (2011). Subacute symptoms of sports-related concussion: Outpatient management and return to play. *Clinics in Sports Medicine, 30*(1), 63–72.

Dikmen, S. S., Machamer, J. E., Winn, H. R., & Temkin, N. R. (1995). Neuropsychological outcome at 1-year post head injury. *Neuropsychology, 9*(1), 80–90.

Dikmen, S., Machamer, J., & Temkin, N. (2001). Mild head injury: Facts and artifacts. *Journal of Clinical & Experimental Neuropsychology, 23*(6), 729–738.

Dikmen, S., Machamer, J., Fann, J. R., & Temkin, N. R. (2010). Rates of symptom reporting following traumatic brain injury. *Journal of the International Neuropsychological Society, 16*(3), 401–411.

Donnell, A. J., Kim, M. S., Silva, M. A., & Vanderploeg, R. D. (2012). Incidence of postconcussion symptoms in psychiatric diagnostic groups, mild traumatic brain injury, and comorbid conditions. *The Clinical Neuropsychologist, 26*(7), 1092–1101.

Doolan, A. W., Day, D. D., Maerlender, A. C., Goforth, M., & Brolinson, P. G. (2011). A review of return to play issues and sports-related concussion. *Annals of Biomedical Engineering*. doi:10.1007/s10439-011-0413-3. (in press).

Echemendia, R. J. (2006a). Return to play. In R. J. Echemendia (Ed.), *Sports neuropsychology: Assessment and management of traumatic brain injury* (pp. 112–128). New York: Guilford Press.

Echemendia, R. J. (Ed.). (2006b). *Sports neuropsychology: Assessment and management of traumatic brain injury*. New York: Guilford Press.

Echemendia, R. J., Iverson, G. L., McCrea, M., Broshek, D. K., Gioia, G. A., Sautter, S. W., Macciocchi, S. N., & Barr, W. B. (2011). Role of neuropsychologists in the evaluation and management of sport-related concussion: An inter-organization position statement. *Clinical Neuropsychologist, 25*(8), 1289–1294.

Evered, L., Ruff, R., Baldo, J., & Isomura, A. (2003). Emotional risk factors and postconcussional disorder. *Assessment, 10*(4), 420–427.

Garden, N., Sullivan, K. A., & Lange, R. T. (2010). The relationship between personality characteristics and postconcussion symptoms in a nonclinical sample. *Neuropsychology, 24*(2), 168–175.

Gunstad, J., & Suhr, J. A. (2001). "Expectation as etiology" versus "the good old days": Postconcussion syndrome symptom reporting in athletes, headache sufferers, and depressed individuals. *Journal of the International Neuropsychological Society, 7*(3), 323–333.

Guskiewicz, K. M. (2011). Balance assessment in the management of sport-related concussion. *Clinics in Sports Medicine, 30*(1), 89–102.

Harvey, D. J., Freeman, J., Broshek, D. K., & Barth, J. T. (2011). Sports injuries. In J. M. Silver, T. W. McAllister, & S. C. Yudofsky (Eds.), *Textbook of traumatic brain injury* (2nd ed., pp. 427–438). Washington, D. C.: American Psychiatric Publishing.

Henrie, M., & Elovic, E. P. (2011). Somatic manifestations of mild traumatic brain injury. In F. S. Zollman (Ed.), *Manual of traumatic brain injury management* (pp. 91–99). New York: Demos Medical Publishing.

Henry, L. C., & de Beaumont, L. (2011). Effects of repeated concussive and subconcussive impacts in sport. In F. M. Webbe (Ed.), *The handbook of sport neuropsychology* (pp. 155–171). New York: Springer.

Iverson, G. L. (2006). Misdiagnosis of the persistent postconcussion syndrome in patients with depression. *Archives of Clinical Neuropsychology, 21*, 303–310.

Iverson, G. L., & Lange, R. T. (2011a). Concussion versus mild traumatic brain injury: Is there a difference? In F. S. Zollman (Ed.), *Manual of traumatic brain injury management* (pp. 43–40). New York: Demos Medical Publishing.

Iverson, G. L., & Lange, R. T. (2011b). The natural history of mild traumatic brain injury. In F. S. Zollman (Ed.), *Manual of traumatic brain injury management* (pp. 65–71). New York: Demos Medical Publishing.

Jagoda, A. S. (2010). Mild traumatic brain injury: Key decisions in acute management. *Psychiatric Clinics of North America, 33*(4), 797–806.

Jayarao, M., Chin, L. S., & Cantu, R. C. (2011). Prevention of sports-related concussion and brain injury. In F. S. Zollman (Ed.), *Manual of traumatic brain injury management* (pp. 30–34). New York: Demos Medical Publishing.

Johnson, E. W., Kegel, N. E., & Collins, M. W. (2011). Neuropsychological assessment of sport-related concussion. *Clinics in Sports Medicine, 30*(1), 73–88.

Johnson, J., & McCown, W. (1997). *Family therapy of neurobehavioral disorders: Integrating neuropsychology and family therapy*. New York: Haworth Press.

Kegel, N. E., & Lovell, M. R. (2011). Sports-related concussion: Identification and return-to-play decision-making. In F. S. Zollman (Ed.), *Manual of traumatic brain injury management* (pp. 58–64). New York: Demos Medical Publishing.

Klonoff, P. S. (2010). *Psychotherapy after brain injury: Principles and techniques*. New York: Guilford Press.

Klonoff, P. S. (2011). A therapist experiential model of treatment for brain injury. *Bulletin of the Menninger Clinic, 75*(1), 21–45.

Klonoff, P. S., & Dawson, L. K. (2004). Commentary-neuropsychological evaluation of patients with traumatic brain injury: Polarization versus holistic integration. *Archives of Clinical Neuropsychology, 19*, 1095–1101.

Klonoff, P. S., & Koberstein, E. J. (2010). Family life. In P. S. Klonoff (Ed.), *Psychotherapy after brain injury: Principles and techniques* (pp. 150–170). New York: Guilford Press.

Klonoff, P. S., & Lamb, D. G. (1998). Mild head injury, significant impairment on neuropsychological test scores, and psychiatric disability. *The Clinical Neuropsychologist, 12*(1), 31–42.

Klonoff, P. S., Koberstein, E. J., Talley, M. C., & Dawson, L. K. (2008). A family experiential model of recovery after brain injury. *Bulletin of the Menninger Clinic, 72*(2), 109–129.

Lange, R. T., Iverson, G. L., & Rose, A. (2010). Post-concussion symptom reporting and the "good-old-days" bias following mild traumatic brain injury. *Archives of Clinical Neuropsychology, 25*, 442–450.

Larrabee, G. J., Binder, L. M., Rohling, M. L., & Ploetz, D. M. (2013). Meta-analytic methods and the importance of non-tbi factors related to outcome in mild traumatic brain injury: Response to Bigler et al. (2013). *The Clinical Neuropsychologist, 27*(2), 215–237.

Lewine, J. D. (2011). Brain imaging in mild traumatic brain injury. In F. S. Zollman (Ed.), *Manual of traumatic brain injury management* (pp. 82–90). New York: Demos Medical Publishing.

Lezak, M. D., Howieson, D. B., Loring, D. W., Hannay, H. J., & Fischer, J. S. (2004). *Neuropsychological assessment* (4th ed.). New York: Oxford University Press.

Lucas, J. A., & Addeo, R. (2006). Traumatic brain injury and postconcussion syndrome. In P. J. Snyder, P. D. Nussbaum, & D. L. Robins (Eds.), *Clinical neuropsychology: A pocket handbook for assessment* (2nd ed., pp. 351–380). Washington, D. C.: American Psychological Association.

Macciocchi, S. N. (2006). Epidemiology of cerebral concussion. In R. J. Echemendia (Ed.), *Sports neuropsychology: Assessment and management of traumatic brain injury* (pp. 71–86). New York: Guilford Press.

Mainwaring, L. (2011). Short-term and extended emotional correlates of concussion. In F. M. Webbe (Ed.), *The handbook of sport neuropsychology* (pp. 251–273). New York: Springer.

McAllister, T. W. (2011). Mild brain injury. In J. M. Silver, T. W. McAllister, & S. C. Yudofsky (Eds.), *Textbook of traumatic brain injury* (2nd ed., pp. 239–264). Washington, D. C.: American Psychiatric Publishing.

McAllister, T. W., & Arciniegas, D. (2002). Evaluation and treatment of postconcussive symptoms. *Neurorehabilitation, 17*(4), 265–283.

McCrea, M. (2008). *Mild traumatic brain injury and postconcussion syndrome: The new evidence base for diagnosis and treatment*. New York: Oxford University Press.

McCrea, M., Kelly, J. P., & Randolph, C. (2000). *Standardized Assessment of Concussion (SAC): Manual for Administration, Scoring, and Interpretation* (3rd ed.). Waukesha: CNS Inc.

McCrory, P. (2011a). Sports concussion and the risk of chronic neurological impairment. *Clinical Journal of Sports Medicine, 21*(1), 6–12.

McCrory, P. (2011b). Future advances and areas of future focus in the treatment of sport-related concussion. *Clinics in Sports Medicine, 30*(1), 201–208.

Meares, S., Shores, E. A., Batchelor, J., Baguley, I. J., Chapman, J., Gurka, J., & Marosszeky, J. E. (2006). The relationship of psychological and cognitive factors and opioids in the development of the postconcussion syndrome in general trauma patients with mild traumatic brain injury. *Journal of the International Neuropsychological Society, 12,* 792–801.

Meares, S., Shores, E. A., Taylor, A. J., Batchelor, J., Bryant, R. A., Baguley, I. J., et al. (2011). The prospective course of postconcussion syndrome: The role of mild traumatic brain injury. *Neuropsychology, 25*(4), 454–465.

Meehan, W. P. III. (2011). Medical therapies for concussion. *Clinics in Sports Medicine, 30*(1), 115–124.

Menon, D. K., Schwab, K., Wright, D. W., Mass, A. I., & The Demographics and Clinical Assessment Working Group of the International and Interagency Initiative toward Common Data Elements for Research on Traumatic Brain Injury and Psychological Health. (2010). Position statement: Definition of traumatic brain injury. *Archives of Physical Medicine and Rehabilitation, 91*(11), 1637–1640.

Mild Traumatic Brain Injury Committee of the Head Injury Interdisciplinary Special Interest Group of the American Congress of Rehabilitation Medicine. (1993). Definition of mild traumatic brain injury. *Journal of Head Trauma Rehabilitation, 8*(3), 86–87.

Mittenberg, W., & Roberts, D. M. (2008). Mild traumatic brain injury and postconcussion syndrome. In J. E. Morgan & J. H. Ricker (Eds.), *Textbook of clinical neuropsychology* (pp. 430–436). New York: Taylor & Francis Group.

Mooney, G., Speed, J., & Sheppard, S. (2005). Factors related to recovery after mild traumatic brain injury. *Brain Injury, 19*(12), 975–987.

Moser, R. S., Fryer, A. C., & Berardinelli, S. (2011). Youth sport concussion: A heads up on the growing public health concern. In F. M. Webbe (Ed.), *The handbook of sport neuropsychology* (pp. 187–207). New York: Springer.

Nilsson, C., Bartfai, A., & Löfgren, M. (2011). Holistic group rehabilitation-a short cut to adaptation to the new life after mild acquired brain injury. *Disability and Rehabilitation, 33*(12), 969–978.

O'Jile, J. R., Ryan, L. M., Betz, B., Parks-Levy, J., Hilsabeck, R. C., Rhudy, J. L., & Gouvier, W. D. (2006). Information processing following mild head injury. *Archives of Clinical Neuropsychology, 21,* 293–296.

Pardini, J. E., Johnson, E. W., & Lovell, M. R. (2011). Concussion management programs in college and professional sport. In F. M. Webbe (Ed.), *The handbook of sport neuropsychology* (pp. 209–233). New York: Springer.

Powell, M. R., & McCrea, M. (2011). Factors suggesting a need for referral to mental health providers in postconcussive disorder. In F. S. Zollman (Ed.), *Manual of traumatic brain injury management* (pp. 140–144). New York: Demos Medical Publishing.

Prigatano, G. P., & Gale, S. D. (2011). The current status of postconcussion syndrome. *Current Opinion in Psychiatry, 24*(3), 243–250.

PRNewswire. (2011, Aug 16). Required concussion exam; Arizona's big idea. http://www.sportsconcussions.org/ibaseline/concussion-exam-arizonas-big-idea. Accessed 24 Nov 2011.

Putukian, M. (2011). The acute symptoms of sport-related concussion: Diagnosis and on-field management. *Clinics in Sports Medicine, 30*(1), 49–61.

Rees, R. J., & Bellon, M. L. (2007). Post concussion syndrome ebb and flow: Longitudinal effects and management. *NeuroRehabilitation, 22*(3), 229–242.

Rohling, M. L., Binder, L. M., Demakis, G. J., Larrabee, G. J., Ploetz, D. M., & Langhinrichsen-Rohling, J. (2011). A meta-analysis of neuropsychological outcome after mild traumatic brain injury: Re-analyses and reconsiderations of Binder et al. (1997), Frencham et al. (2005), and Pertab et al. (2009). *The Clinical Neuropsychologist, 25*(4), 608–623.

Rohling, M. L., Larrabee, G. J., & Millis, S. R. (2012). The "miserable minority" following mild traumatic brain injury: Who are they and do meta-analyses hide them? *The Clinical Neuropsychologist, 26*(2), 197–213.

Rose, J. M. (2005). Continuum of care model for managing mild traumatic brain injury in a workers' compensation context: A description of the model and its development. *Brain Injury, 19*(1), 29–39.

Ruff, R. M. (2011). Mild traumatic brain injury and neural recovery: Rethinking the debate. *NeuroRehabilitation, 28*(3), 167–180.

Ruff, R. M., Iverson, G. L., Barth, J. T., Bush, S. S., Broshek, D. K., & The NAN Policy and Planning Committee. (2009). Recommendations for diagnosing a mild traumatic brain injury: A National Academy of Neuropsychology education paper. *Archives of Clinical Neuropsychology, 24,* 3–10.

Schatz, P. (2011). Computerized neuropsychological assessment in sport. In F. M. Webbe (Ed.), *The handbook of sport neuropsychology* (pp. 173–186). New York: Springer.

Sedney, C. L., Orphanos, J., & Bailes, J. E. (2011). When to consider retiring an athlete after sports-related concussion. *Clinics in Sports Medicine, 30,* 189–200.

Shukla, D., & Devi, B. L. (2010). Mild traumatic brain injuries in adults. *Journal of Neurosciences in Rural Practice, 1*(2), 82–88.

Snell, D. L., Surgenor, L. J., Hay-Smith, E. J. C., & Siegert, R. J. (2009). A systematic review of psychological treatments for mild traumatic brain injury: An update on the evidence. *Journal of Clinical & Experimental Neuropsychology, 31*(1), 20–38.

Torrence, C. B., DeCristofaro, C., & Elliott, L. (2011). Empowering the primary care provider to optimally manage mild traumatic brain injury. *Journal of the American Academy of Nurse Practitioners, 23*(12), 638–647.

Toshkezi, G., Chin, L. S., & Cantu, R. C. (2011). Cumulative effects of repeated mild traumatic brain injury. In F. S. Zollman (Ed.), *Manual of traumatic brain injury management* (pp. 72–76). New York: Demos Medical Publishing.

Tsaousides, T., Dams-O'Connor, K., & Gordon, W. A. (2011). Cognition in mild traumatic brain injury: Neuropsychological assessment. In F. S. Zollman (Ed.), *Manual of traumatic brain injury management* (pp. 100–106). New York: Demos Medical Publishing.

Vanderploeg, R. D., Curtiss, G., Duchnick, J. J., & Luis, C. A. (2003). Demographic, medical, and psychiatric factors in work and marital status after mild head injury. *Journal of Head Trauma Rehabilitation, 18*(2), 148–163.

Walker, W. C., & Kunz, R. D. (2011). Postconcussion syndrome: Symptom management. In F. S. Zollman (Ed.), *Manual of traumatic brain injury management* (pp. 119–124). New York: Demos Medical Publishing.

Wang, E., & Zollman, F. S. (2011). Postconcussion syndrome: Diagnostic characteristics and clinical manifestations. In F. S. Zollman (Ed.), *Manual of traumatic brain injury management* (pp. 113–118). New York: Demos Medical Publishing.

Weber, M., & Edwards, M. G. (2012). Sport concussion knowledge in the UK general public. *Archives of Clinical Neuropsychology, 27*(3), 355–361.

Wilson, B. A. (2009). *Memory rehabilitation: Integrating theory and practice*. New York: Guilford Press.

Witkowski, G. (2011, Aug 18). Arizona first state telling athletes to pass concussion education exam. Peoria Times. http://www.peoriatimes.com/sports/headlines/article_84a4de38-c9cd-11e0-abda-001cc4c002e0.html?mode=story. Accessed 24 Nov 2011.

Young, R. (Reporter/Host). (2011, Oct 28). Teen's fatal brain injury in football game raises questions (Radio series episode). In WBUR Boston and PRI (Producer), *Here & Now*. Boston: National Public Radio.

Zafonte, R. (2011). Diagnosis and management of sports-related concussion: A 15-year-old athlete with a concussion. *JAMA: The Journal of the American Medical Association, 306*(1), 79–86.

Zasler, N. D. (2011). Confounding factors in postconcussive disorders. In F. S. Zollman (Ed.), *Manual of traumatic brain injury management* (pp. 125–131). New York: Demos Medical Publishing.

Chapter 6
Family Psychotherapy after Stroke and Anoxic Brain Injury

6.1 Scenario: Early Questions about Stroke and Anoxic Brain Injuries

Stroke (or cerebrovascular accident; CVA) represents the most common serious neurological problem in the world and is the leading cause of disability in the USA (see Festa et al. 2008, for a review). Depending on the nature and location of the stroke, there is a multiplicity of consequences (Festa et al. 2008). However, strokes tend to have lateralized or one-sided effects to the right or left side of the brain (Lezak et al. 2012). Similarly, hypoxic/anoxic brain injuries caused by oxygen deprivation negatively impact the loved one's functionality (Caine and Watson 2000). The ramifications for the caregiver and family are diverse and they are thrust into "on-the-job training" (Palmer and Palmer 2011).

As depicted in phase 1 of the Family Experiential Model (FEM) of Recovery (see Chap. 1, Sect. 1.5 and Fig. 1.3), there is a bombardment of confusing information couched in medical jargon (Klonoff and Koberstein 2010; Klonoff et al. 2008; Stein 2004). The initial emotional aftermath includes feeling shocked, terrified, panicky, and helpless (Klonoff et al. 2008; Senelick 2010). As with other neurological entities, stroke and hypoxic/anoxic injuries drain the relatives, manifested as depression, anxiety, frustration, feelings of grief and loss, alienation, role alterations, health decline, social isolation, and other psychosocial issues (see Bakas 2009, for a review; Cao et al. 2010; Palmer and Palmer 2011). At the outset, family members usually have minimal direct experience with the loved one's medical condition and can be quite overwhelmed about the limitations. They may ask questions such as: *What is a stroke? What is anoxia? What happens now? Will he or she recover? What do I do next?*

6.1.1 Therapeutic Intervention: Neuropathology of Stroke and Anoxic Brain Injuries

Stroke education and support is vital for the tier 1 caregiver and tier supports, especially, as most stroke survivors are discharged home from the hospital (see Bakas

P. S. Klonoff, *Psychotherapy for Families after Brain Injury*,
DOI 10.1007/978-1-4899-8083-0_6, © Springer Science+Business Media New York 2014

2009, for a review). This should start immediately after the event, in order to adequately prepare the support network for the complexities of this process. Generally, a multidisciplinary team of health-care professionals is preferred, including the physiatrist, neurologist, nurse, social worker, psychotherapist/neuropsychologist, and rehabilitation therapists (e.g., physical, occupational, and recreational therapists and a speech–language pathologist; Benson and Pavol 2010; Duarte and Fishman 2010; Klonoff 2010; see Langhorne et al. 2011, for a review; Niemeier and Karol 2011a). The psychoeducation process should be tailored to the sensibilities of the relatives (and loved one), taking into account their culture, family dynamics, psychological readiness, and medical factors, including prognosis (see also Chap. 1, Sect. 1.3 and Fig. 1.1, and Chap. 2, Sect. 2.4.1.2). The children's books, *My Grandpa Had a Stroke* by Butler (2007) and *Now One Foot, Now the Other* by dePaola (2006) provide some age-appropriate, yet informative explanations about stroke for youngsters that should reduce perplexity and fearfulness.

Stroke has been defined as permanent local or global damage to the brain due to a blocked blood vessel or bleeding (Markus et al. 2010; Stein 2004; Williams 2010). A stroke can last 24 h or longer, or lead to death (Markus et al. 2010). There are sometimes, warning signs of strokes, including *transient ischemic attacks* (TIAs; Senelick 2010; Stein 2004). These occur in approximately 15 % of stroke victims (Senelick 2010). TIAs represent a temporary interruption in the blood supply to part of the brain from a blockage (Senelick 2010; Stein 2004). Risk factors for TIAs are hypertension and atherosclerosis (i.e., thickened arterial walls with plaque-like lesions; Lezak et al. 2012; Weinstein and Swenson 2006). Symptoms usually develop rapidly and often disappear within 15 min, or maximally 24 h (Caplan 2010; Senelick 2010; Stein 2004). Signs of a TIA include sudden numbness or weakness of the face, arm, or leg usually on one side of the body; confusion; trouble speaking or understanding others; difficulty walking; dizziness; loss of balance or coordination; vision problems; and severe headache, nausea, or vomiting (Senelick 2010). Patients with TIAs are at high risk of eventually having a stroke and so it is imperative to seek medical attention (Lezak et al. 2012; Senelick 2010; Stein 2004).

In order to grasp the effects of stroke on the loved one, it is helpful to review some basic neuroanatomy. Figure 6.1 illustrates a simplified version of the brain blood supply system. The circulation system is divided into the anterior territory, supplied by the carotid arteries (Markus et al. 2010). They feed the anterior and middle cerebral arteries as well as the posterior communicating artery (Markus et al. 2010). The anterior cerebral artery supplies parts of the frontal and parietal lobes (Weinstein and Swenson 2006). The middle cerebral artery is the largest branch of the internal carotid artery and it divides into several other branches which feed the lateral (outside) surface of the brain, including the frontal, parietal, and temporal lobes (Markus et al. 2010; Weinstein and Swenson 2006). The posterior circulation includes the vertebral artery which combines to form the basilar artery (Markus et al. 2010). The basilar artery feeds the posterior cerebral arteries which supply the temporal and occipital lobes (Markus et al. 2010). Strokes can also occur in the brainstem and cerebellar regions (Markus et al. 2010).

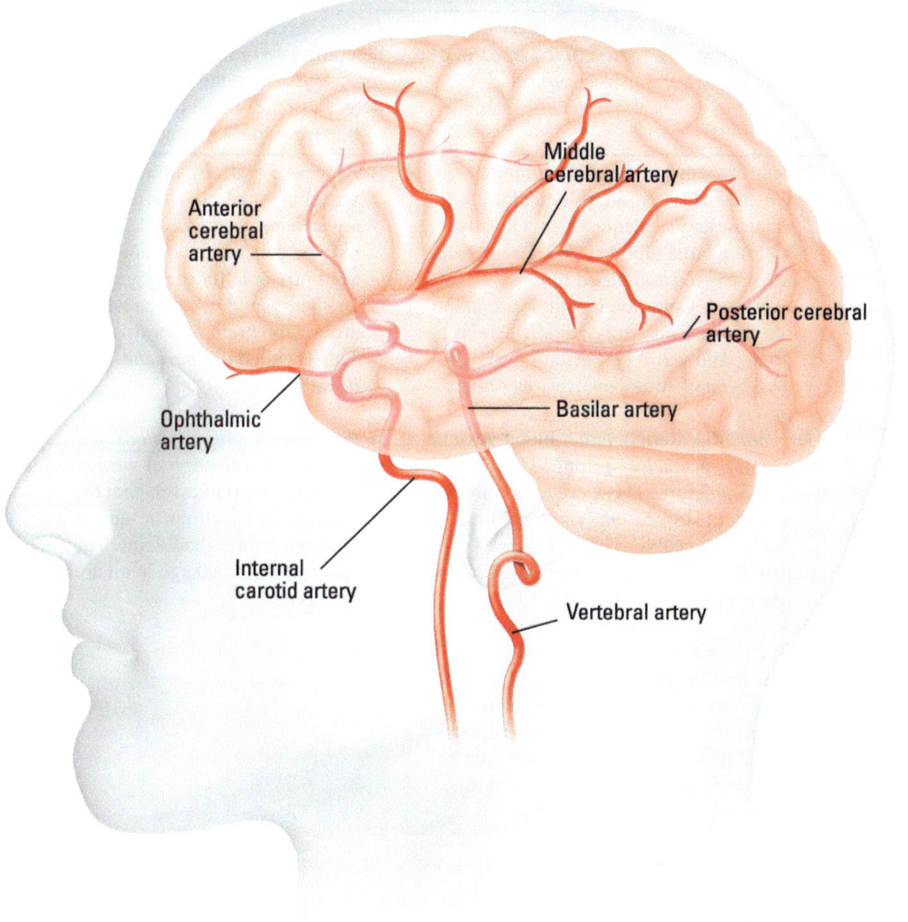

Fig. 6.1 Brain blood supply system. (©2013 National Stroke Association. Content provided with permission from the National Stroke Association. Visit www.stroke.org for stroke education resources)

Table 6.1 describes the various types of strokes and their mechanisms and can be provided as a handout to the family (Cullum et al. 2008; Dimancescu 2010; Festa et al. 2008; Lezak et al. 2012; Palmer and Palmer 2011; Senelick 2010; Stein 2004; Weinstein and Swenson 2006). *Ischemic* strokes occur from a reduction of blood flow to the brain due to obstruction of blood vessels (e.g., by thrombotic, lacunar, or embolic strokes) or by global decreased perfusion (Festa et al. 2008; Palmer and Palmer 2011; Uchino et al. 2011). Ischemic strokes occur from large vessel atherothrombosis, embolisms, and small vessel disease (Caplan 2010; Festa et al. 2008). Arteriosclerosis or "hardening of the arteries" is a common cause of ischemic stroke (Dimancescu 2010).

Table 6.1 Types of strokes and their mechanisms

	Ischemic: a stroke caused by interruption of blood flow to a region of the brain due to occlusion (i.e., obstruction) or decreased perfusion. Forms of ischemic stroke are:	*Hemorrhagic*: a stroke caused by massive bleeding into brain tissue. Causes include hypertension, congenital cerebral artery defects, toxins, or blood disorders. Forms of hemorrhagic stroke are:
a.	*Thrombotic*: this is the most common type of stroke. A fatty blood clot (i.e., atherosclerotic plaque) forms locally within a large blood vessel. The vessels are narrowed and blood flow is restricted. Common locations are in the internal carotid artery, middle cerebral artery, and vertebral basilar arteries. This type of stroke evolves over hours or days	*Aneurysm*: a malformation of the blood vessel in which there is a ballooning of a weakened arterial wall. Aneurysms may be genetic and can be asymptomatic for many years. When an aneurysm bursts, it causes bleeding around the brain rather than inside it. This is called a *subarachnoid hemorrhage*
b.	*Lacunar*: disease in smaller blood vessels usually caused by prolonged high blood pressure. These are also known as "silent strokes" as symptoms may not be noticeable. These strokes usually affect small areas of the brain and can be cumulative over time	*Arteriovenous malformations*: a congenital collection of weakened and abnormal blood vessels that form irregular connections or tangles between arteries and veins. They are susceptible to leakage in all areas of the brain
c.	*Embolic*: a clot which forms elsewhere (e.g., carotid artery, aorta, or heart) gets into the bloodstream and travels to the brain. When it reaches a narrow blood vessel, it can get stuck and block blood flow. Embolic substances can be a piece of thrombus, air, fat, plaque particles, bacteria, tissue, or tumor cells. Most embolic strokes occur in the middle cerebral artery	
d.	*Global decreased perfusion:* decreased blood flow to the brain which is generalized and diffuse. Causes include cardiac problems and hypotension. The "watershed" borderzone areas (i.e., the boundaries between major blood vessel distributions) are most often affected	

When the brain does not get sufficient oxygen and nutrients carried in the blood, the brain cells die (Stein 2004). The area of damaged or dead tissue is called an *infarct* (Lezak et al. 2012). Ischemic strokes often emanate from the middle cerebral artery (see Lezak et al. 2012, for a review). This type of stroke may not be painful, and so the loved one may postpone accessing medical treatment (Stein 2004). Acute treatment for ischemic strokes include a "clot buster" tissue plasminogen activator (t-PA), which must be given within the first 3.0–4.5 h of the stroke (Uchino et al. 2011; Williams 2010).

Hemorrhagic strokes result from massive bleeding inside the head (Palmer and Palmer 2011; Weinstein and Swenson 2006). They account for 10 % of strokes, but create the highest mortality (Senelick 2010). Bleeding within the brain tissue is called an *intracerebral* or *intraparenchymal* hemorrhage (Dimancescu 2010; Palmer and Palmer 2011). Etiologies include hypertension, congenital cerebral artery deficits, toxins, and blood disorders (Senelick 2010; Weinstein and Swenson 2006). Often, the onset is abrupt and prognosis is poor if loss of consciousness exceeds 2 days (Weinstein and Swenson 2006).

Table 6.1 also contains subtypes of hemorrhagic strokes, including *aneurysms* and *arteriovenous malformations* (AVMs). An *aneurysm* is a swelling or outpouching arising from weakness in the elastic membrane of a larger brain artery (Cullum et al. 2008; Stein 2004; Weinstein and Swenson 2006; Williams 2010). One common type is called "berry" or saccular aneurysms, which develop at branch points of vessels (see Cullum et al. 2008, for a review; Markus et al. 2010). Aneurysms can be genetic and are often asymptomatic for a number of years (Cullum et al. 2008; Stein 2004; Williams 2010). As the vessel wall stretches, it becomes increasingly thin and fragile. It is then susceptible to rupturing, similar to a balloon filling with air (Cullum et al. 2008). Factors which increase the risk of rupture include a family history, high blood pressure, smoking, and cocaine use (Williams 2010).

When the aneurysm bursts, it causes a *subarachnoid hemorrhage,* or bleeding around the brain into the third space of the meninges (Dimancescu 2010; Palmer and Palmer 2011; Stein 2004). The classic sign of a subarachnoid hemorrhage is a severe headache (i.e., "the worst headache possible"; Cullum et al. 2008; Markus et al. 2010; Uchino et al. 2011). Other symptoms are: nausea and vomiting; stiff neck; loss of or altered consciousness; confusion; motor problems; or visual disturbances (Cullum et al. 2008; Lezak et al. 2012; Markus et al. 2010). Physicians have a grading system which rates the severity of the subarachnoid hemorrhage, with higher grades representing a more severe presentation and outcome (Cullum et al. 2008; Markus et al. 2010). Treatments are to "clip," place wire coils, or use special glues to clot or seal off the aneurysm (Cullum et al. 2008; Stein 2004; Uchino et al. 2011).

Possible complications of subarachnoid hemorrhages are hydrocephalus (i.e., impaired reabsorption or obstruction of the flow of cerebrospinal fluid), seizures (see Chap. 8), and vasospasms (i.e., spasmodic constriction of the blood vessels; Lezak et al. 2012; Markus et al. 2010; Uchino et al. 2011). Vasospasms can interrupt the blood supply to an area of the brain (Stein 2004). They can cause neurological aftereffects, including aphasia (i.e., language problems), hemiplegia (i.e., paralysis of half of the body), and increased confusion (Cullum et al. 2008).

Another form of intracranial hemorrhage emerges from an AVM (Weinstein and Swenson 2006). An AVM is a congenital collection of weakened and abnormal blood vessels that form an irregular connection between arteries and veins (Cullum et al. 2008; Markus et al. 2010; Stein 2004; Weinstein and Swenson 2006; Williams 2010). Although AVMs are quite uncommon, they can occur in all regions of the brain and are susceptible to leakage (Cullum et al. 2008; Lezak et al. 2012; Weinstein and Swenson 2006). Chronic headaches or seizures may precede the rupture (Cullum et al. 2008). AVMs can be observed using a computerized tomography (CT) or magnetic resonance imaging (MRI) scan or angiogram (Markus et al. 2010). Treatment of AVMs includes observation, surgical excision, radiosurgery, or embolization (Markus et al. 2010; Stein 2004; Williams 2010). Once they bleed, they can cause damage to brain tissue (Stein 2004).

There are numerous risk factors for stroke, including older age; gender (male); ethnicity (e.g., African Americans, Hispanics, Far Eastern Asian, and South Asian); family history of stroke; hypertension (high blood pressure); cardiovascular disease; structural cardiac abnormalities; diabetes; hyperlipidemia; carotid stenosis; TIAs; obesity; physical inactivity; oral contraceptives; cigarette smoking; drug use (e.g., cocaine, heroin); and alcohol abuse (see Caplan 2010, for a review; Festa et al. 2008; see Lezak et al. 2012, for a review; Markus et al. 2010; Palmer and Palmer 2011; Rosenberg et al. 2010; Senelick 2010; Stein 2004; Williams 2010). The caregiver should be knowledgeable about these risk factors so as to promote a healthy way of life, including proper diet and exercise (Festa et al. 2008; Senelick 2010).

Stroke prevention is important and should utilize a family-centered approach (Lawrence et al. 2010). Food suggestions for stroke prevention include: at least five daily portions of fruits and vegetables; six servings daily of grains; limited salt, saturated fats, cholesterol, fried foods, sweets, and sugary beverages; twice-weekly servings of oily fish (e.g., tuna or salmon); and increased intake of soy, fresh tomato, walnuts, almonds, and green, Korean ginseng, or jasmine tea (Markus et al. 2010; Williams 2010). The therapist will remind the caregiver to be vigilant regarding the loved one's medication compliance in order to minimize the possibility of a recurrent stroke. This is especially salient if he or she has major cognitive or language limitations which interfere with adherence (Festa et al. 2008; Palmer and Palmer 2011). Being a positive role model for the loved one is ideal and also preserves his or her own energies (Lawrence et al. 2010; Palmer and Palmer 2011). Encouraging regular exercise (at least 30 min five or more times per week); managing stress levels; monitoring blood pressure; and attending all physician visits (including a yearly physical) are also preventative measures (Markus et al. 2010; Senelick 2010).

An ischemic event results in decreased oxygen delivery to brain tissue (Hopkins and Bigler 2008). *Anoxia* is defined as complete oxygen deprivation to the brain (Caine and Watson 2000; Lezak et al. 2012), while *hypoxia* is reduced oxygenation of the blood (see Hopkins and Bigler 2008, for a review; Howard et al. 2011; Lezak et al. 2012). Greater oxygen deprivation creates more severe brain damage and consequences (Family Caregiver Alliance 2004). Causes of hypoxia/anoxia include cardiac arrest; cardiac disease or surgery; carbon monoxide poisoning; attempted hanging; and near drowning (Hopkins and Bigler 2008). For the purposes of this chapter, the discussion focuses on the effects of cardiac arrest. Locations susceptible to hypoxia/anoxia include the hippocampus, cerebellum, thalamus, basal ganglia, and cerebral cortex (Caine and Watson 2000; see Hopkins and Bigler 2008, for a review; see Lezak et al. 2012, for a review; see Lim et al. 2004, for a review). Unlike stroke, anoxia affects both sides of the brain and affects the oxygen-dependent sites (Lezak et al. 2012). For three-dimensional views of brain anatomy, see http://www.brainline.org/multimedia/interactive_brain/the_human_brain.html or http://www.finr.net/educational-resources/finr-educational-materials/3d-brain/.

6.2 Scenario: Overview of Skill Changes

Stroke and anoxia affect neurological skills based on the extent and nature of the brain damage (Garcia-Molina et al. 2006; Howard et al. 2011; see Lezak et al. 2012, for a review). Potential domains are physical, cognitive, language, communication, emotional, and interpersonal (Caine and Watson 2000; see Lezak et al. 2012, for a review). This in turn affects independence in the home and community and the capability to resume driving, school, and/or work. Concomitantly and understandably, the tier 1 caregiver and other tier supports incur added or new obligations. They may notice a variety of thinking changes and may ask questions such as: *How will this stroke affect my loved one? What does it mean to have an anoxic injury? Why are his or her speech, movement, and vision so different?*

6.2.1 Neuroanatomy of Abilities

The psychotherapist is a strong resource for providing psychoeducation about the expected deficits related to various injuries. Figure 6.2 depicts the relative locations in the brain of a number of abilities. Table 6.2 depicts some of the blood supplies/neuroanatomical substrates for various functions and a summary of likely impairments caused by various types of strokes and anoxic injuries (Fox et al. 2006; Verfaellie and Heilman 2006; Weinstein and Swenson 2006). CT and MRI scans are informative tools to clarify damage locations (Stein 2004). A conventional angiogram as well as magnetic resonance and computerized tomographic angiographies are employed to provide pictures of the brain's blood vessels (Senelick 2010; Stein 2004). Neurological, neuropsychological, speech and language, occupational, and physical therapy evaluations will delineate potential strengths and challenges. As stated in Chap. 4, Fig. 4.4, the bell curve is a utilitarian mechanism to delineate the cognitive changes, as it can be used to identify a range of strengths and difficulties, specifying their relative severity. Preinjury levels should be used as the reference point, so that a sophisticated assessment of the current condition is provided. Representative subsets include deficits in: sensation and motor skills on the contralateral (opposite) side of the body; language (i.e., aphasia), attention, vision, and visuoperceptual abilities; memory; and executive functions (Weinstein and Swenson 2006). In interpreting test findings, the role of behavioral and other physical factors should be considered, including fatigue, effort, and mood. It is advisable to obtain input from the caregiver regarding his or her perception of the loved one's functioning when drawing therapeutic conclusions and making recommendations.

Of note, families and the loved one will be gratified to know that the recovery process after strokes and anoxia (and other forms of acquired brain injuries) is mediated by multiple factors, including spontaneous neurological recovery, training, adaptation, pharmacotherapeutic agents, and neuroplasticity. *Neuroplasticity* is the potential capacity of the central nervous system to modify its structural and functional organization through neuronal regeneration or collateral sprouting and the emergence of previously latent brain pathways (Rosenberg et al. 2010).

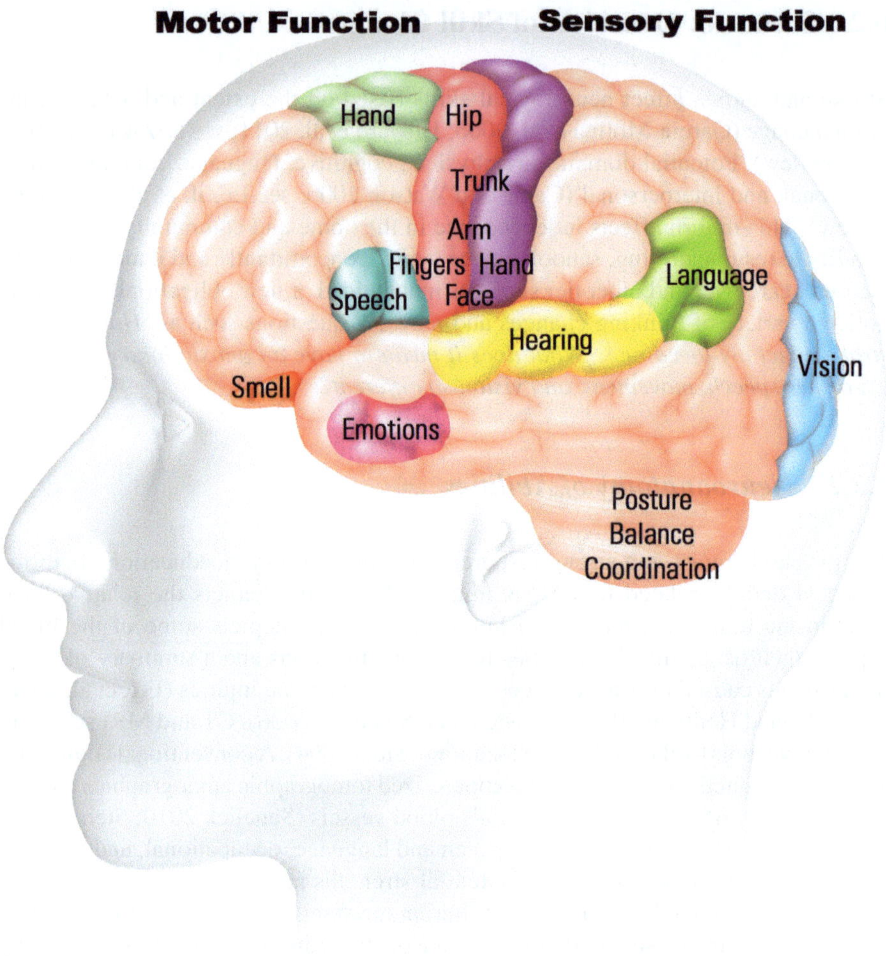

Fig. 6.2 Brain locations for abilities. (©2013 National Stroke Association. Content provided with permission from the National Stroke Association. Visit www.stroke.org for stroke education resources)

6.3 Scenario: Aphasia

A common consequence of left hemisphere stroke is aphasia (Senelick 2010). *Aphasia* is a communication disorder affecting speaking, comprehension of spoken or written language, repetition, naming, reading, and writing (Sinanović 2010; Stewart and Riedel 2011). Everyday activities are cumbersome or impossible, including conversing, using technology, or watching television (see Gillespie et al. 2010, for a review). Compounding the distress is the natural tendency of the relatives to shield the loved one from the burden of care, for fear of upsetting him or her (Gillespie et al. 2010). Overall, aphasia in a loved one creates upheaval; the caregiver desires

Table 6.2 Functions and deficits related to blood supply and neuroanatomical substrates after stroke and anoxia

Blood supply/neuroanatomical substrate	Responsible for	Injury results in
Middle cerebral artery/dominant frontal lobe	Expressive language	Broca's aphasia
Middle cerebral artery/dominant temporal lobe	Receptive language	Wernicke's aphasia
Middle cerebral artery/dominant frontal and temporal lobes	Expressive and receptive language	Global aphasia
Right middle cerebral artery/posterior cerebral artery/parietal and occipital lobes, brainstem, thalamus	Visual perception	Homonymous hemianopia and other visual deficits
Middle cerebral artery/anterior cerebral artery	Motor functioning	Paralysis of the opposite (contralateral) face, arm, and leg
Hippocampus, temporal and frontal lobes, thalamus	Memory	Memory loss and an amnestic syndrome

to protect the loved one, advance his or her social reintegration, and support communication (see Gillespie et al. 2010, for a review). Yet, they are stymied by the incapacities and may ask questions such as: *Why can't my loved one speak? Why can't he or she understand what I say? How come he or she can't read or write anymore?*

6.3.1 Overview of Aphasia

Table 6.3 describes general information about aphasia. Aphasia is most often associated with left hemisphere damage and occurs in roughly one-third of stroke victims (Festa et al. 2008; see Sinanović 2010, for a review). There are a number of types of aphasia and the family is advised to work closely with their medical professionals, including a speech–language pathologist, to comprehend the unique deficits (and retained strengths) in their loved one. This section reviews three types of aphasia: *Broca's, Wernicke's, and Global aphasia.*

Broca's, nonfluent, motor, or expressive aphasia is regularly related to a middle cerebral artery stroke affecting the left frontal lobe (Markus et al. 2010; Stein 2004; Stewart and Riedel 2011). It is characterized by poor speech production (Festa et al. 2008). Early on, the loved one may be mute (Stewart and Riedel 2011). The loved one may know what he or she wants to say, but cannot find the words (Stein 2004). The flow of speech is impaired. It is often halting and hesitant, with short and simple utterances and abnormal sentence structure (Caplan 2010; Cherney and Small 2009; Festa et al. 2008; Stewart and Riedel 2011). This is known as *telegraphic speech*, in which small connector words are missing (Festa et al. 2008; Stein 2004). Verbalizations may also have problematic rhythm and pitch (Stewart and Riedel

Table 6.3 Types of aphasia

Broca's aphasia	Wernicke's aphasia	Global aphasia
Often associated with a left middle cerebral artery stroke affecting the frontal lobes	Often associated with a left middle cerebral artery stroke affecting the temporal lobe and aspects of the parietal and occipital lobes	Often there is occlusion to the trunk of the middle cerebral artery
Limited speech output	Lots of speech output, but with word errors (e.g., made up words)	Speech may be limited to automatic words and phrases
Characterized by deficits in: Speech production Speech flow—hesitant and halting with short and simple utterances Sentence structure ("telegraphic speech") Speech rhythm and pitch Repeating words Written and oral grammar Auditory comprehension Naming Reading and writing	Characterized by deficits in: Word repetition Awareness of errors Auditory comprehension Naming Reading and writing	Characterized by deficits in: All aspects of language Word repetition Voluntary speech sounds Auditory comprehension Reading and writing

2011). Word repetition may be more effortful and there is often impairment in oral and written grammar (Festa et al. 2008; see Stewart and Riedel 2011, for a review). Other challenges include auditory comprehension, reading, and writing (see Stewart and Riedel 2011, for a review). Caregiver strain may be exacerbated when the loved one cannot express himself or herself (see Stewart and Riedel 2011, for a review).

Wernicke's, receptive, or sensory aphasia is often associated with a left middle cerebral artery stroke affecting the temporal lobe and aspects of the parietal and occipital lobes (Festa et al. 2008). It is characterized by speech that is fluent, but with word errors, as well as impaired auditory comprehension, repetition, naming, reading, and writing (Cherney and Small 2009; Festa et al. 2008). Language output contains real words, word substitutions (*paraphasias*), and *neologisms* (i.e., made-up words; Cherney and Small 2009; Kramer et al. 2010; Stewart and Riedel 2011). The speech output can sound vague and meaningless (*jargon* with multiple paraphasias), but the loved one may not be aware of this (Cherney and Small 2009; Festa et al. 2008; Kramer et al. 2010; Stewart and Riedel 2011). Personality characteristics linked to Wernicke's aphasia include anger and paranoia (Festa et al. 2008).

Global, mixed, or total aphasia typically emerges after a massive stroke affecting both sites associated with Broca's and Wernicke's aphasia (Festa et al. 2008). Often, there is occlusion to the trunk of the middle cerebral artery (Festa et al. 2008; Stewart and Riedel 2011). It is a syndrome of complete language disruption, whereby both language output and auditory comprehension are significantly affected (Festa et al. 2008; Markus et al. 2010; Stewart and Riedel 2011). Therefore, the loved one may rely on facial expressions, intonations, and contextual cues to understand others (Stewart and Riedel 2011). He or she will not be able to voluntarily produce speech sounds, and output is limited to *automaticisms* (i.e., automatic words or phrases; Stein 2004; Stewart and Riedel 2011). Word repetition, reading, and writing can also be restricted (Stewart and Riedel 2011). As the global aphasia dissipates, the loved one may evolve into more of a Broca's aphasia (Festa et al. 2008).

Another common type of speech problem is *anomia,* in which the loved one may struggle to find words and name specific objects (Senelick 2010; Stein 2004). Families will notice a pattern of "talking around" a missing word by using a phrase to describe it. This is called *circumlocution* (Stein 2004). Of note, sometimes, the loved one will display other communication disorders in conjunction with aphasia (Cherney and Small 2009). Speech *apraxia* is the incapacity to coordinate movements to pronounce words caused by deficits in the programming and sequencing of the articulators (e.g., jaw, lips, tongue, cheeks; see Kramer et al. 2010, for a review; Stein 2004). It often coexists with Broca's aphasia (Stein 2004). *Dysphagia* is the disruption of swallowing due to impairments in sensation, muscle strength, and coordination (see Kramer et al. 2010, for a review). *Dysarthria* is irregular speech production because of weakness or incoordination of the lips, tongue, and throat muscles related to areas of the brain responsible for articulation, including the cerebellum (Markus et al. 2010; Palmer and Palmer 2011; see Stewart and Riedel 2011, for a review). Dysarthric output may sound slurred or unintelligible (Kramer et al. 2010; Palmer and Palmer 2011).

Aphasia is not usually associated with anoxia, although there are sometimes language impairments, including auditory comprehension, verbal expression, spontaneous output, naming, and dysarthria (see Caine and Watson 2000, for a review; FitzGerald et al. 2010; Garcia-Molina et al. 2006; Peskine et al. 2010).

6.3.2 "Helpful Hints" and Tools for Families to Cope with Aphasia in their Loved One

A detailed discussion of treatment interventions for apraxia, dysarthria, and dysphagia is beyond the scope of this book. Close liaison with the speech–language pathologist and other adjunct rehabilitation specialists is a must for the tier 1 caregiver and other tier supports in order to grasp these phenomena and incorporate safe and effective exercises and compensations in the home for the loved one. The chapter, "Rehabilitation of Speech, Language, and Swallowing Disorders" by Kramer et al. (2010) is an excellent resource.

Table 6.4 summarizes "helpful hints" and tools for families to cope with aphasia in their loved one. The psychotherapist will educate the relatives that the prognosis for aphasia is based on several factors, including the site and size of the stroke (see Cherney and Small 2009, for a review). Critical to maximizing the recovery of the loved one's language problems is speech therapy, including an emphasis on practical communication (Brown et al. 2011; Cherney and Small 2009; Stewart and Riedel 2011). The speech–language pathologist will inform the support network (and loved one) that aphasia can manifest as complex combinations of language strengths and difficulties (Stewart and Riedel 2011). Because of this, it is easy for others to overestimate the loved one's comprehension (see Stewart and Riedel 2011).

Table 6.4 "Helpful Hints" and tools for family members to cope with aphasia in their loved ones

The prognosis for aphasia is partially based on the site and size of the stroke
Seek speech and language therapy to maximize the loved one's recovery from aphasia. The family should:
Engage in two-way dialogue with the speech-language pathologist about the loved one's lifestyle
Participate in goal setting
Obtain education about stroke and aphasia
Solicit communication training on personalized strategies that can be applied at home
Inquire about therapeutic speech groups
The family should seek occupational therapy so as to:
Understand how aphasia affects completion of daily activities
Participate in home visits to learn adaptations, such as for medications and recipes
Become acquainted with a Home Independence Checklist and "milieu meeting" form
Recognize that attending therapy with the loved one enhances the well-being of the family unit
General suggestions
Be patient with the loved one's language deficits and allow time for responses
Slow down the rate of speech so the loved one can better comprehend
Keep input shorter and simpler
Use concrete yes/no choices
Communicate in a quiet nondistracting environment
Encourage conversations and socialization
Watch the tendency to speak for the loved one and/or correct speech errors
Work with the speech-language pathologist to understand and assist with reading and writing skills
Broca's aphasia
Don't overestimate the loved one's level of understanding
Encourage other forms of communication (e.g., gestures, drawing, writing)
Provide missing words (if the loved one is comfortable)
Watch the loved one's body language and facial expression to gain cues
Simplify grammar
Suggest singing to assist with language production
Repeat back what you understood the loved one to be saying
Ask the loved one for clarification if verbalizations are unclear
Wernicke's aphasia
Signal the loved one so as to stop the flow of speech
Cue him or her to change topics
Use pictures to impart information
Realize the loved one will "talk around" a missing word (e.g., circumlocution)
Keep communication short and simple and make it relevant to him or her
Face the loved one and speak clearly at a normal loudness
Use common words and simple sentences
Global aphasia
Use visual cues, pictures, gestures, facial expressions, and body language
Employ a communication board with pictures of common objects and family members
Emphasize important words and keep communication simple
Try to include the loved one in social conversations and singing activities
Encourage automatic speech activities (e.g., counting and praying)
Other considerations
Provide the optimum amount of supervision, protectiveness, as well as practical and emotional support
Promote community independence and autonomy as appropriate
Use compensations to ensure the loved one's safety in the home and community:
Cell phone with programmed numbers
A written explanation of key medical challenges

Table 6.4 (continued)

An emergency alert system in the home
Encourage the loved one to attend an aphasia support group
Reinvolve the loved one (and yourself) in community activities for socialization and quality of life
Address caregiver/family loneliness and anxiety through psychotherapy and other interventions (e.g., a social worker) to:
Improve acceptance, find new life priorities, and celebrate improvements
Seek social and meaningful activities
Find respite time
Encourage the loved one to participate in home responsibilities and roles
Work through legitimate fears and worries about the loved one's safety versus autonomy
Address financial stressors and other practical concerns
Participate in a caregiver support group
Employ coping skills, including a sense of humor, determination, resiliency, patience, spirituality, positivity, and hopefulness
Multimedia resources
Book
Aphasia Couple Therapy (ACT) Workbook (Boles 2010)

Two-way dialogue with the speech–language pathologist allows the relatives to share pertinent feedback about the loved one's and family's home, work, social, and leisure life so that interventions target relevant domains (Howe et al. 2012; Johansson et al. 2011). The speech–language pathologist will solicit contributions for treatment goal setting; provide education about stroke and aphasia (through oral, written, and helpline information); and institute communication training on personalized strategies to augment conversations that can also be applied at home (Howe et al. 2012; Johansson et al. 2011; Manders et al. 2011; Sherratt et al. 2011; Simmons-Mackie et al. 2010; Wilkinson and Wielaert 2012). For instance, a speech–language pathologist can use video feedback, language tasks, and role-playing to facilitate collaborative conversations between spouses, one of whom has aphasia (Wilkinson et al. 2011).

One good resource is the *Aphasia Couple Therapy (ACT) Workbook* by Boles (2010). It contains various templates, examples, exercises, role-play activities, and ways for the loved one and caregiver to boost the stroke survivor's functionality in the home and community. Examples include dining out (including making a choice, setting a reservation, deciding the mode of transportation, ordering food, and conversing during the meal); grocery shopping (incorporating a prefabricated list, navigating at the store, and paying for the groceries); and going to a movie (addressing which movie, when, and where as well as formatted discussion questions).

Useful therapeutic speech groups to address aphasia include an Aphasia Group or Current Events Group, whereby patients practice talking, listening, reading, writing, and abstract reasoning in a group format, to simulate community life. This prepares the loved one to talk on the phone, order at a restaurant, and speak with teachers, coworkers, and in other social settings (A. Blank and M. Rynn, personal communication, 10/11/12). Ultimately, speech and language therapy will optimize the loved one's goal attainment, meaningful relationships, and strivings for a positive way of existing (Brown et al. 2010).

Treatment with an occupational therapist is also very worthwhile, so that the family guides the loved one when completing daily activities in the context of his or her aphasia (Stewart and Riedel 2011). This includes home visits to teach adaptations (e.g., instructions for medication(s) or written recipes; Nätterlund 2010; Stewart and Riedel 2011). Figure 6.3 is an example of a Home Independence Checklist (HIC) that can be utilized to cue the aphasic loved one regarding simple home chores (see Chap. 4, Sect. 4.4.4 for more information). Picture icons or actual photos from the home environment replace written language to make it easier for the loved one to follow the checklist. Figure 6.4 is an example of a form that can be utilized for "milieu meetings" in the home when the loved one has a milder form of aphasia. This can be developed and practiced with the caregiver using the expertise of the speech–language pathologist and occupational therapist (for more information on "milieu meetings," see Chap. 4, Sect. 4.4.4; Klonoff 2010). Although attending therapy with the loved one is time consuming and can interrupt the caregiver and relatives' work schedule, research indicates that the well-being and lifestyle of the patient and support network are definitely enhanced (Johansson et al. 2011).

Table 6.4 also summarizes specific ideas for improving communication with various types of aphasias (Hill 2011; Stein 2004; see Stewart and Riedel 2011, for a review). Family members of a loved one should be patient and allow time for responses; slow down their rate of speech so the loved one can better comprehend; keep input shorter and simpler; use concrete yes/no choices; communicate in a quiet nondistracting environment; encourage conversations and socialization; and be mindful of not continuously speaking for the loved one or correcting speech errors (Gillespie et al. 2010; Green et al. 1997; Hill 2011; Stein 2004; Williams 2010). Singing can facilitate language production (Stein 2004). When the loved one suffers from global aphasia, using gestures, pointing, visual cues, and communication boards with familiar objects and people is helpful (Stein 2004).

The psychotherapist should alert the caregiver and support network regarding providing the requisite amount of supervision, protectiveness as well as practical and emotional support for the loved one, yet at the same time promoting his or her community independence and autonomy (Brown et al. 2011, 2012; Gillespie et al. 2010). The caregiver will usually need to make arrangements for 24-hour supervision for the loved one with severe aphasia (Stein 2004). However, when the loved one has some degree of retained verbal abilities, the psychotherapist can recommend certain compensations to the loved one and family to maximize safety. This includes carrying a cell phone with programmed germane phone numbers and contact information; a written explanation of chief medical considerations in case of emergency; and an emergency alert system in the home (Stein 2004). The psychotherapist and speech–language pathologist will likely recommend that the loved one attend a support group to practice communication skills and glean social support, including friendships (Brown et al. 2011, 2012; Stein 2004). To this end, the caregiver may need to advocate for this, including providing transportation. The loved one should be heartened to reinvolve himself or herself in community activities which promote socialization and quality of life, including travel, work (if viable), interest classes, and other leisure pursuits (Brown et al. 2011). This will facilitate mutual independence, stimulation, and normality (Brown et al. 2011).

Home Independence Checklist

Mon Tues Wed Thurs Fri Sat Sun

Morning Tasks:

1) Get your own breakfast 3-4 times a week

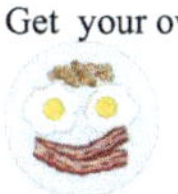

2) Check iPad each morning

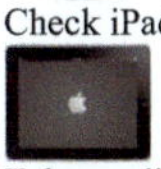

3) Take medication

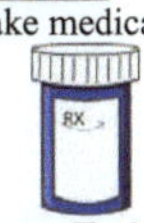

Afternoon Tasks:

4) Check iPad every afternoon

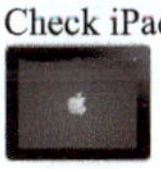

5) Practice using the computer 3 times a week

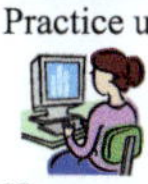

6) Home exercise/homework 3-4 times a week

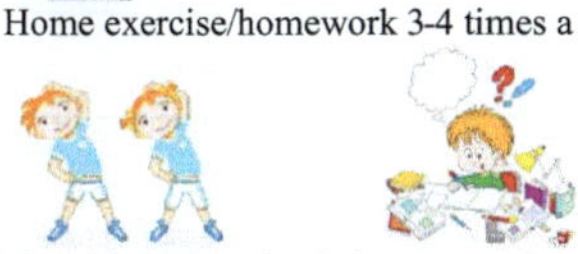

7) Help with the laundry 2 times a week

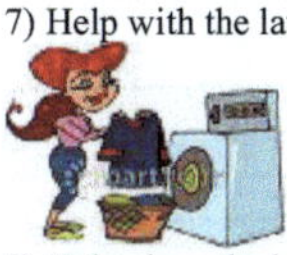

8) Help clean the bathroom 1 time a week

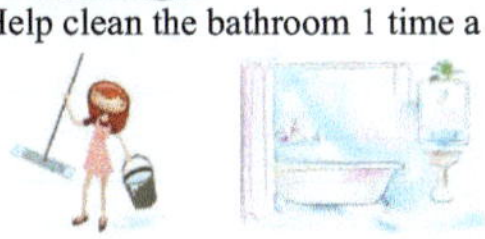

9) Vacuum house 1 time a week

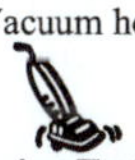

Evening Tasks:

10) Help with dinner 3 times a week

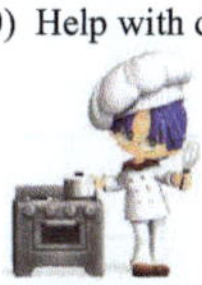

Weekend Tasks:

11) Perform leisure activity of your choice

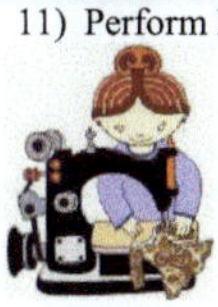

Fig. 6.3 Home Independence Checklist

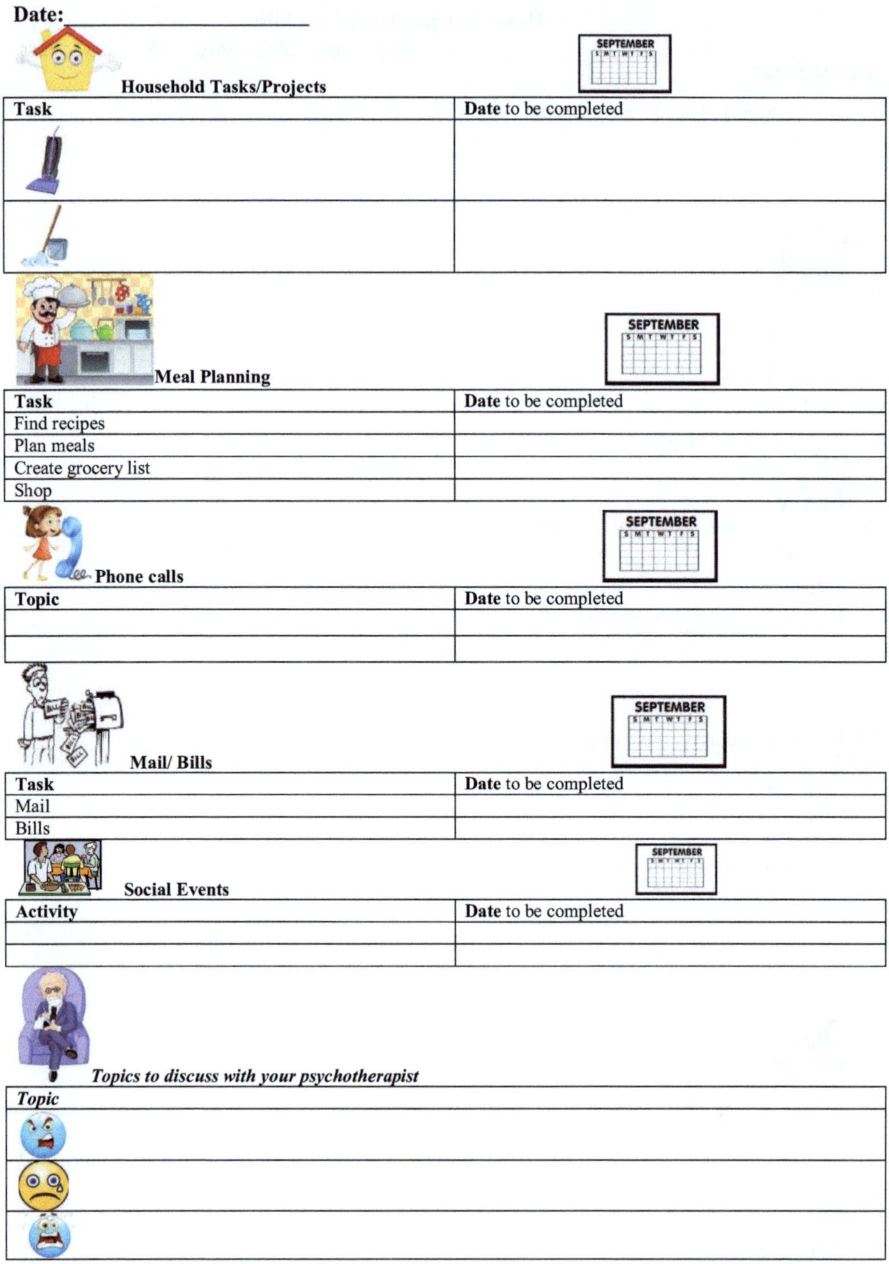

Date:____________________

Household Tasks/Projects

Task	**Date** to be completed

Meal Planning

Task	**Date** to be completed
Find recipes	
Plan meals	
Create grocery list	
Shop	

Phone calls

Topic	**Date** to be completed

Mail/ Bills

Task	**Date** to be completed
Mail	
Bills	

Social Events

Activity	**Date** to be completed

Topics to discuss with your psychotherapist

Topic

Fig. 6.4 "Milieu meeting" form

The caregiver and support network have specific needs post stroke and the psychotherapist should be attuned to loneliness and anxiety about their circumstances (Nätterlund 2010). Suggestions include psychotherapy for the family (improving acceptance, finding new life priorities, and celebrating improvements); involvement in their own social and meaningful activities; finding respite time for themselves to address their own priorities; encouraging the loved one to participate in home responsibilities and roles to the best of his or her ability; and working through legitimate fears and worries about the loved one's safety versus autonomy (Brown et al. 2011, 2012; Howe et al. 2012). Families may need therapeutic interventions (also from a social worker), for juggling financial stresses, role modifications, transportation demands, and caregiving of other family members (Howe et al. 2012). Participating in a caregiver support group provides an ambience of caring, belonging, sharing, and confidence (Howe et al. 2012; Nätterlund 2010; see also Chaps. 9 and 11). Worthy attributes that the therapist can cultivate include a sense of humor, determination, resiliency, patience, spirituality, positivity, and hopefulness (Brown et al. 2011, 2012; Howe et al. 2012).

Computer technology is being utilized to treat aphasia (Dietz et al. 2011; van de Sandt-Koenderman 2011). Table 6.5 summarizes more modern and innovative assistive technology devices (ATDs) and relevant websites containing adaptations and compensations for aphasia (Kuster 2012; Scherer 2012). These range considerably in terms of the language skills they address and the severity of the aphasia. This technology is advantageous, as it is age appropriate, part of the current social norm, and portable (Blank and Rynn 2012). It also can be used in the community, allowing for home programs and improved communication opportunities with the support network (Blank and Rynn 2012). Language and communication aids include smartphones, tablets, or computer applications; various types of Augmentative and Alternative Communication (AAC) devices; speech-to-text "writing"; text-to-speech "reading"; spelling aids as well as video and audio recorders (Blank and Rynn 2012; Scherer 2012).

AAC devices are favored when verbal expression is not functional and when there are impairments in gestures and written communication modes (Kramer et al. 2010). For example, Say-It! Sam and Proloquo2Go are suitable for patients with expressive aphasia, dysarthria, and spelling problems (A. Blank, personal communication, 10/15/12; M. Rynn, personal communication, 6/14/13). These systems provide recorded words and phrases based on symbols or text. Recordings on tablets can be ideal for speech and language exercise practice in the home environment. This includes expanding speech clarity and verbal expression (A. Blank, personal communication, 10/15/12). Table 6.5 also provides other beneficial devices and resources to increase communication, follow directions, and foster spelling, writing, and reading. These include Dragon Dictation for more intact speech, but compromised writing and spelling deficits; wordQ + speakQ for word prediction to assist with spelling; Evernote© for note taking; and audio books to allow access to literature in the context of reading impairments. Of course, it is vital for the family to consult with the loved one's speech–language pathologist in order to select the optimum tools based on the patient's unique challenges and needs.

Table 6.5 Assistive technology to address aphasia

Technology
Augmentative and Alternative Communication (AAC) devices (e.g., Say-it! Sam and Proloquo2go)
Tablets, smartphones, and computers with language apps
Technology to aid in writing and spelling problems (e.g., Dragon Dictation, wordQ+speakQ)
Audio books
Skype
Google+
FaceTime
Sources for new technologies and accessing information
Apps for AAC: www.appsforaac.net
Spectronics: www.spectronicsinoz.com
GeekSLP: www.geekslp.com
Therapyapp411.com: www.therapyapp411.com
Aphasia Tool Box: www.aphasiaapps.com
Tactus Therapy Solutions: www.tactustherapy.com
(e.g., Comprehension TherAppy, Conversation TherAppy, Naming TherAppy)
Speechie apps: www.speechieapps.com/?s=aphasia
EmpTech: www.emptech.info/index.php
AssistiveWare: www.assistiveware.com
(e.g., Pictello, Proloquo2Go)
Possum: www.possum.co.uk
Words+: www.words-plus.com/index.htm
Turning Point: www.turningpointtechnology.com/index.asp
Kurzweil Educational Systems: www.kurzweiledu.com/products.html
Parrot Software: www.parrotsoftware.com/default/default.aspx
Reading Made Easy.com: www.readingmadeez.com
wordQ+speakQ: www.goqsoftware.com
Speech function on computer: www.microsoft.com/enable/products/office2010
iPad text to speech function: www.apple.com/accessibility/macosx/literacylearning.html
Lingraphica: www.aphasia.com/products/apps
(e.g., Phonemes, Oral Motor, Consonant Blends)
Wiki Spaces: www.sccatn.wikispaces.com/file/view/Sorting_AAC_aaps_OCT302011.pdf
The National Aphasia Association
www.aphasia.org/naa_materials/technology_resource_information.html
ASHA.org: www.asha.org/Publications/leader/2012/120605/App-titude–Apps-to-Aid-Aphasia.htm
Other resources
Icons and pictures for cookbooks and shopping list (e.g., www.epicurious.com/services/mobile)
Facebook (for aphasia compensations)
You-tube (for demonstrations of compensations)
Consumer questions to ask: www.asha.org/public/speech/consumerqa
National Institute on Deafness and Other Communicative Disorders—directory of organizations www.nidcd.nih.gov/directory/keyword.asp?keyword14=14

6.4 Scenario: Cognitive and Behavioral Deficits

Relatives may become alarmed at thinking and behavioral changes in their loved one after a stroke or anoxic event. The tier 1 caregiver and tier supports may ask questions such as: *Why is he or she so distractible? Why is my loved one so forgetful? Why does he or she have so much trouble handling responsibilities like he or she used to? Why is his or her personality and behavior so different?*

6.4.1 Overview of Cognitive and Behavioral Deficits

Stroke and anoxia can affect the loved one's cognition, especially in the realms of attention, memory, and executive functions, with greater inabilities linked to the location, size, and severity of the brain injury as well as the extent of neurological complications (see Caine and Watson 2000, for a review; Cohen et al. 2006; Cullum et al. 2008; see Hopkins and Bigler 2008, for a review; Howard et al. 2011; Lim et al. 2004; Niemeier and Karol 2011a; O'Connor and Lafleche 2006; Peskine et al. 2010; Senelick 2010; Stein 2004).

Attention has been defined as a state of focused awareness on a subset of incoming information (Gerrig and Zimbardo 2002). It encompasses the capacity to remain focused on a stimulus or task and is required for new learning and effective cognition (Green et al. 1997). Attention is predicated on wakefulness and alertness (Stein 2004). There are several types of attention, which are summarized in Table 6.6. These include sustained (or vigilance), selective (or focused), alternating, and divided attention (Cohen et al. 2006; Fuchigami 2012; Green et al. 1997; Kearney et al. 2010; Lezak et al. 2012; Sohlberg and Mateer 2001). Table 6.6 also provides some "real-life" examples of these attention processes.

Stroke usually affects short-term memory; old learning is typically better preserved (Niemeier and Karol 2011a, b; Stein 2004). Memory deficits after anoxia are due to hippocampal and frontal lobe damage (see Caine and Watson 2000, for a review; FitzGerald et al. 2010; see Garcia-Molina et al. 2006, for a review; Peskine et al. 2010). Impairments can be profound and enduring, affecting both visual and verbal encoding, retention, and recall (FitzGerald et al. 2010; Garcia-Molina et al. 2006; Howard et al. 2011; Peskine et al. 2010). Memory loss can also extend to periods before the anoxic event (i.e., retrograde amnesia) as well as after (i.e., anterograde amnesia; see Caine and Watson 2000, for a review; Peskine et al. 2010). Confabulatory responses (i.e., "filling in the gaps" when recall is spotty or nonexistent) is also common (Peskine et al. 2010; see Chap. 4, Sect. 4.3 and Tables 4.2 and 4.3 for a more detailed discussion of memory).

Executive functions are the higher order thinking skills that are employed to manage complex daily responsibilities (see also Chap. 4, Sect. 4.4. and Fig. 4.6). They include abstract reasoning, flexible thinking, planning, problem solving, seeing the "big picture," organization, prioritization, initiating and following through with actions, sequencing, complex attention, multitasking, judgment, generating strategies, and decision making (see Caine and Watson 2000, for a review; Nunn et al. 2008). Executive function deficits after anoxia are often implicated in frontal lobe and basal ganglia damage (see Caine and Watson 2000, for a review; O'Connor and Lafleche 2006). Reduced insight into the nature and extent of the difficulties is also common with both anoxia and stroke (Howard et al. 2011; Stein 2004).

Anterior communicating artery aneurysms often present with a triad of symptoms: memory loss, confabulation, and personality changes as well as executive function deficits (see Cullum et al. 2008, for a review). Cerebral hemorrhages due to AVMs affect intellectual functions, memory, and attention (Cullum et al. 2008). Patients

Table 6.6 Types of attention processes

Attention: definition
The ability to remain focused on a stimulus or task; it is required for new learning and effective cognitive functioning
Types of attention and real world examples
Sustained or vigilance: The ability to maintain attention over time while doing one task in a quiet, distraction-free setting
Home: pay bills, watch television, read a book, talk on the phone, do a word search puzzle
Work: pay attention during a meeting or work shift
School: attend to the class discussion, read a book chapter, do mental math activities, focus during a test
Selective or focused or concentration: The ability to maintain attention while screening out background distractions
Home: pay bills with background music on; watch television while someone is talking on the phone
Work: focus on a work task with background noise (e.g., phones, people talking)
School: work on a classroom assignment while the teacher and other students are talking
Alternating: The capacity for mental flexibility which allows for shifting between tasks with different cognitive requirements
Home: prepare a meal and stop to help a child with homework; switch between paying bills and doing the laundry
Work: work on a project and handle interruptions (e.g., phone calls, co-workers questions)
School: read a chapter and take notes
Divided: The ability to simultaneously respond to two or more tasks or multiple elements within a task
Home: prepare a meal while visiting with a friend
Work: check email while talking on the telephone
School: answer questions on an open book exam while checking notes

with aneurysms and various types of strokes experience a series of behavioral sequelae, including apathy, irritability, anger, sadness, depression, anxiety, and mood lability (Aniskiewicz 2007; Caplan 2010; Cullum et al. 2008; Festa et al. 2008; see Waldron et al. 2012, for a review; see Wilson 2009, for a review). Behaviorally, after anoxia, the loved one may show impulsivity, emotional fluctuations (i.e., lability), irritability, flat affect, apathy, a lack of emotional expression as well as diminished initiative and drive (see Caine and Watson 2000, for a review; FitzGerald et al. 2010; Peskine et al. 2010). These can be quite severe and impede his or her functionality and autonomy (Peskine et al. 2010). Notably, there is an interaction between cognitive, emotional, and behavioral problems which can reverberate and exacerbate the loved one's limitations (Wilson 2009).

6.4.2 "Helpful Hints" and Tools to Assist the Loved One with Cognitive and Behavioral Challenges

Certainly, milieu-oriented therapy is preferable for addressing the loved one's cognitive, emotional, and behavioral obstacles after acquired brain injury, as this paradigm provides integrated care to improve awareness, acceptance, and realism (Klonoff 2010; Wilson 2009). The holistic approach employs a combination of specialists, including a physiatrist, nurse, neuropsychologist, speech–language pathologist, physical, occupational, and recreational therapists, social worker, and dietician (Klonoff 2010; Rosenberg et al. 2010). Integrated and intensive therapy maximizes the loved one's outcome (Klonoff et al. 2001) and is most efficacious in supporting the caregiver and relatives. This includes both individual and group-oriented therapies, including a memory group in which the loved one practices memory mnemonics and nifty compensations as well as group psychotherapy to provide integral education and emotional support to facilitate the loved one's adjustment to his or her "new normal" (Klonoff 2010; Wilson 2009). Family education and support regarding the loved one's predicament and treatment interventions underlie this model (Klonoff and Koberstein 2010).

Table 6.7 is comprised of "helpful hints" and tools for the family to assist the loved one with his or her cognitive and behavioral challenges, grouped according to each domain. Table 6.7 also lists a number of worthwhile cognition websites, including various compensatory devices. There are a number of techniques that the caregiver and family can employ to improve the loved one's attention. Examples that the psychotherapist and other therapists will suggest include: gently cue the loved one to use self-management systems (e.g., deliberately focus his or her attention); remind him or her to self-pace (e.g., do demanding undertakings when freshest; get proper rest; and set realistic expectations); build in breaks to lessen mental fatigue; if possible, allow him or her to finish one assignment before starting another; recognize the value of maintaining a "key ideas log" (i.e., whereby thoughts are jotted down to be attended to later); avoid creating overstimulating and distracting environments (e.g., use ear plugs; turn off the cell phone, radio, and television when concentrating on a conversation or job; fulfill responsibilities when children are away or asleep; shop during less busy times); and encourage him or her to utilize other environmental modifications to reduce the load on attention (e.g., filing and bill-paying systems, labeling cupboards, etc.; Green et al. 1997; Niemeier and Karol 2011a; Sohlberg and Mateer 2001; Stein 2004). Sometimes, the loved one's physician will prescribe a medication to improve attention and arousal, for instance, amantadine, dextroamphetamine, mondafinil, and methylphenidate (Stein 2004; Uchino et al. 2011).

There are a number of assistive products designed for adaptation to cognitive challenges, which are referred to as "cognitive support technology" (Scherer 2012) or "external memory aids" (Wilson and Kapur 2009). The psychotherapist and rehabilitation team will propose various compensations for memory and executive functions. Some of these are described in Chap. 4 (Sects. 4.3.2 and 4.4.4) and include datebooks, HICs, and "milieu meeting" agendas. Other procedures are available to reduce confusion and chaos in the loved one's daily routine. Examples of "low-tech" memory aids are checklists, calendars, diaries, notebooks, schedules, post-it notes, pillboxes, alarm clocks, watch alarms, oven timers, shopping lists, mail sorters, color-coded filing and labeling systems, and posted instructions on appliances (Niemeier and Karol 2011a; Scherer 2012; Sohlberg and Turkstra 2011; Stein 2004; Wilson and Kapur

Table 6.7 "Helpful Hints" and tools for the family to assist the loved one with cognitive and behavioral challenges

Attention

Work with the therapists to provide gentle reminders about self-management and self-pacing strategies:

- Deliberately focus his or her attention
- Do demanding tasks when freshest
- Get proper rest
- Set realistic expectations
- Build in breaks
- Finish one task before starting another
- Keep a "key ideas log"
- Avoid overstimulating and distracting environments
- Use environmental modifications to reduce the attention load
- Work with your loved one's physician about medication options

Memory and Executive Functions

Work with the therapists to learn about "cognitive support technology" and "external memory aids" and obtain assistance in choosing and implementing the best system

"Low tech" options:

Datebook	Home Independence Checklist
"Milieu meeting" agenda	Checklists
Calendars	Diaries
Notebooks	Schedules
Post-it notes	Pillboxes
Alarm clocks	Watch alarms
Oven timers	Shopping lists
Mail sorters	Color coded filing and labeling systems
Posted instructions	

"High tech" options:

Electronic reminder alarms	Location detection devices
Way-finding aids	Electronic storage devices
Smartphones	Tablets

Learn interventions such as "vanishing cues" and "backward chaining"

Give input into what systems work best for the loved one and family unit

Multimedia Resources

Books

- *Wilfrid Gordon McDonald Partridge* (Fox, 1989)
- *Assistive Technologies and Other Supports for People with Brain Impairment* (Scherer, 2012)

Cognitive Websites:

PEAT: www.brainaid.com
Picture Planner: www.cognitopia.com
Pocket Endeavor: www.ablelinktech.com/index.php?id=38
Community Integration Suite: www.ablelinktech.com/index.php?id=36
Visual Assistant: www.ablelinktech.com/index.php?id=35
The Listening Program: www.thelisteningprogram.com
Quizlet: http://quizlet.com
Voice Cue: www.enablemart.com/Catalog/Attainment-Company/Voice-Cue
Evernote: https://evernote.com
Awesome Note: http://bridworks.com/anote/eng
Notability: www.gingerlabs.com
Calvetica Calendar: www.mysterioustrousers.com/calvetica
WatchMinder 2: www.watchminder.com

Table 6.7 (continued)

Cadex Reminder Watch: www.bindependent.com/cgi-bin/shopper.cgi?preadd=action&key=gctl11
Other Watches: www.abilityhub.com/cognitive/index.htm
WayFinder: http://www.ablelinktech.com/index.php?id=33
ChatterBlocker: http://chatterblocker.com
Behavioral and Mood Changes
Obtain psychoeducation and emotional support from the psychotherapist
Learn about the symptoms of depression and "catastrophic reactions" in the loved one
Be open to the involvement of a psychiatrist
Develop personalized strategies (a "tool kit") of techniques to assist the loved one
Learn to differentiate psychological from neurological problems
Understand underlying reasons for "mean" behavior in the loved one, including dysfunctional family patterns, organicity, grief and loss reactions, "narcissistic rage," executive function deficits, and misery
Engage in marital or family therapy to address underlying dynamics
Do not personalize the loved one's outbursts
Develop insight, react empathically, and avoid "counter narcissistic rage" attacks
Be open to psychotropic medications (i.e., for aggression and agitation), behavioral modification techniques, and speech and language therapy to ameliorate anger outbursts in the loved one

2009). Sometimes, the more simplistic messages are the most powerful ones, such as "loose papers = lost papers" (A. Blank, personal communication, 11/2/12). The psychotherapist and other therapists will be judicious in choosing the best combination of devices, so as not to overload the loved one (Baldwin et al. 2011).

The therapist will introduce the loved one and tier 1 primary caregiver to the concept of *vanishing cues* (Sohlberg and Turkstra 2011; see Wilson 2009, for a review). This is an error minimization technique, whereby necessary prompts are given, and then gradually faded out (Wilson 2009). Because the goal is errorless learning, mistakes are avoided when the loved one is learning a new skill or information (Wilson 2009). As the learned behavior is gradually integrated and then mastered, the caregiver reduces his or her cuing and involvement. This empowers the loved one and frees the family from constant oversight.

Backward chaining is also a useful therapeutic technique, whereby the loved one is first prompted through the steps of a complete activity (Wilson 2009). Then he or she is guided through all of the steps of the chain, except for the final one, which he or she does independently (Wilson 2009). Then additional steps at the back end of the sequence are systematically omitted, with the expectation that the loved one will complete these by himself or herself (Wilson 2009).

The loved one with severe memory deficits will rely on the familiarity, knowledge basis, and fortitude of the caregiver and support network. Hence, the caregiver's contributions regarding the utility and embracement of various tools are critical to the rehabilitation process. Factors such as the loved one's mood, energy level, insight level, motivation, and history with memory systems, in combination with the relatives' preferences, are pertinent variables (Klonoff 2010; Wilson and Kapur 2009). The caregiver will usually find himself or herself in the role of the educator, coach, and cheerleader in helping the loved one master these new compensations outside of the treatment clinic. The children's book, *Wilfrid Gordon McDonald Partridge* by Fox (1989) is a whimsical illustration of these honorable functions.

In the age of technology, there are now other handy instruments with which the family should become familiarized. Therapists will introduce "high-tech devices," many of which require more sophisticated knowledge and are more complex (Sohlberg and Turkstra 2011). The support network will often need to be trained in the loved one's use of these in the home and community. Electronic reminder alarms (e.g., on phones, watches, and pillboxes), location detection devices to locate items, way-finding aids (e.g., stand-alone or built-in automobile satellite navigation devices), and electronic storage devices (e.g., cameras, computers, dictaphones) increase the loved one's capacities (Wilson and Kapur 2009). Other examples of multipurpose gadgets are smartphones and tablets (Scherer 2012; Sohlberg and Turkstra 2011). Various applications are available and updated regularly, including checklists, "to do lists," calendars, alarm reminder systems, recording programs, and note organizing systems. A valuable resource for specialized technologies for various cognitive limitations is *Assistive Technologies and Other Supports for People with Brain Impairment* by Scherer (2012).

With respect to behavioral and mood alterations in the loved one, the psychotherapist is a great resource to provide the emotional support and psychoeducation to the caregiver and relatives (as well as the loved one). This includes the propensity for poststroke/anoxia depression and catastrophic reactions (CRs; Sinanović 2010; Starkstein et al. 1993; Waldron et al. 2012). The psychotherapist will utilize diverse approaches to evaluate the loved one's psychological status, including clinical interviews and questionnaires (Klonoff 2010; Wilson 2009). Psychiatric assessment is an important adjunctive service to analyze the loved one's emotional status (Klonoff 2010). Once a clear-cut diagnostic formulation has been achieved, the psychotherapist and treatment team are equipped to provide the necessary interventions for the loved one, including psychoeducation and training for the family members.

Overall, several treatment methods are recommended for the loved one, including cognitive behavioral therapy, insight-oriented therapy, collaboration with a psychiatrist for psychotropic medications to address anxiety, depression, CRs as well as psychoeducation, skill training, and compensation implementation for difficulties with initiation and apathy (Klonoff 2010; see Waldron et al. 2012, for a review; Wilson 2009). Case in point, the caregiver and family's frustration level and resentment will wane if they realize that the loved one's neurological problems with initiation and follow through is not "laziness" (Elbaum 2010; Niemeier and Karol 2011b).

The psychoeducation and supportive psychotherapy process for the caregiver and family should mirror the services the loved one is receiving, so that all parties realize the nature and etiology of emotional and personality changes. This will translate into personalized strategies (e.g., a "tool kit") that the relatives can employ to maximize the loved one's productivity in the home and community. This includes ascertaining which behaviors are most likely organically based or caused directly by the brain injury (e.g., reduced awareness, apathy, flat affect, diminished impulse control, and emotional lability) compared with emotional reactions to the devastating circumstances (e.g., depressive and anxious reactions as well as CRs; Prigatano et al. 1986; see Chap. 4, Sects. 4.5 and 4.6 and Table 4.6 for a more detailed discussion of these topics).

The psychotherapist will need to address "mean" behavior in the loved one, often exhibited as verbal attacks, put-downs, agitation, or even rage towards the tier 1 caregiver and other tier supports. One therapist described a son's escalating attacks as "mine fields of emotions, employing psychological bullets, grenades, or bombs" (S. Myles, personal communication, 2/7/13), in order to capture the hurtful and destructive influence for the unaware loved one and to empathically relate with the targeted parents. First, the overall psychological health of the family system needs to be assessed, as historical and current "structural" dysfunctional factors may be impinging on family relations, including distrust, egocentrism, disagreeableness, poor boundaries, fragmentation, and fragileness. Problematic "therapeutic process components" include disconnection, resistance, impatience, rigidity, adversarialism, and unrealism about injury aftereffects (see Chap. 3, Sect. 3.1.1). Other possible explanations (besides CRs) should be delved into, including: organicity (i.e., lability from damage to the emotional regulation centers of the brain); grief and loss reactions and feelings of powerlessness around "controlling" caregivers; "narcissistic rage" caused by the loved one's shattered sense of self and core abilities; disinhibition (i.e., compromised filtering) and decreased perspective taking capacity due to frontal lobe damage, creating a rigid and defensive stance towards others; and the propensity to "hurt the one he or she loves," due to his or her bottomless misery embedded in a sense of comfort and security with the primary caregiver.

Using the therapeutic process, a mindful analysis of possible contributing factors (often occurring concomitantly) is essential in order for the family to understand the underlying dynamics and react empathically to the loved one's verbal assaults. When the outbursts reflect preexisting acrimony (perhaps with the volume turned up), marital or family systems therapy may be warranted to treat dysfunctional patterns. The psychotherapist will caution the primary caregiver and other tier supports not to personalize these attacks, as this is fundamental to avoiding counterattacks. If instead, the caregiver or support network acknowledges the loved one's understandable psychic pain, he or she feels validated and the situation naturally defuses. Organically based aggression and agitation can be ameliorated by antipsychotic medications (e.g., risperidone; Siegel et al. 2007; Waldron-Perrine et al. 2008). The psychotherapist will also help the caregiver and other relatives (including younger siblings) self-monitor their propensity for their own "narcissistic rage" attack on the loved one, which is precipitated by internal feelings of resentment, grief, or powerlessness. Disengaging from escalating scenarios is key to all parties maintaining emotional restraint. Sometimes, behavioral modification and limit setting techniques need to be incorporated to reduce the frequency of these confrontations. Adjunct therapy with the speech–language pathologist to address communication pragmatic "faux pas," in combination with rebuilding self-sufficiency through physical and occupational therapies, also diminishes the feelings of incompetence and dependency in the loved one.

6.5 Scenario: Vision and Motor Deficits

Family members may notice some inexplicable peculiarities in their loved one's visual and motor skills and be perplexed by the situation. The caregiver may ask questions such as: *Why can't he or she see things? Why is my loved one having difficulty dressing himself or herself? Why are drawings so distorted? How come he or she can't read or write properly? Why is one side of his or her body paralyzed?*

6.5.1 Overview of Vision and Motor Deficits

Vision is the primary sensory system and visual impairments interfere with day-to-day activities, including grooming, dressing, eating, locating objects, shopping, cooking, reading, writing, driving, mobility, and managing finances (Lindman 2011; Warren 2005). *Hemianopia* is loss of vision in the visual field opposite to the side of the stroke (Palmer and Palmer 2011). Loss of the entire right or left visual field in both eyes is called *homonymous hemianopia* (Caswell 2005; Stein 2004). The loved one may be unaware of his or her visual field loss (Markus et al. 2010). Manifestations include not seeing entities on one side, bumping into things (especially when going through doorways), and reading problems (Markus et al. 2010). Overall, a homonymous hemianopia can negatively impact the loved one's mobility, driving, and navigation, especially in dynamic and chaotic environments (Lindman 2011; Solomon and Goldstein 2009; Warren 2005).

Common visual sequelae, especially after right hemisphere stroke and sometimes anoxic injuries, include visuoperceptual, visuospatial, and constructional deficits (Caine and Watson 2000; Capruso et al. 2006; Festa et al. 2008; FitzGerald et al. 2010; Peskine et al. 2010). *Visuoperception* includes form and pattern discrimination, also including color and shape (Capruso et al. 2006). *Visuospatial* ability is the processing of the visual orientation or location of articles in space, including depth and motion (Capruso et al. 2006). Visuospatial skills contribute to motor coordination, balance, and directional sense when reading or writing (Lindman 2011; Scheiman 2011). *Constructional* skill is the capacity to draw or assemble things from their component subparts (Capruso et al. 2006).

Hemineglect, neglect, or inattention is a disorder of visuospatial awareness, whereby the loved one does not orient, recognize, or attend to stimuli on the side opposite to the stroke site (Festa et al. 2008; Heilman 2009; Markus et al. 2010; Verfaellie and Heilman 2006). This phenomenon is not related to vision loss per se, although the two can coexist (Capruso et al. 2006; Caswell 2005). Neglect is more frequent after right hemisphere stroke involving the parietal lobe and other brain structures, whereby the left side of space is not registered by the right brain (Capruso et al. 2006; Festa et al. 2008; Heilman 2009; Markus et al. 2010; Sinanović 2010; Stein 2004; Williams 2010). It is considered an attentional disturbance, also involving the reticular activating system in the brainstem and the thalamus (Capruso et al. 2006; Verfaellie and Heilman 2006). Early on, the loved one may not recognize his or her left arm or leg or be unaware of illness or disability; this is called *anosognosia* (Prigatano 2010; Verfaellie and Heilman 2006; Williams 2010).

Other examples of neglect include: failure to copy the left side of a design; shaving or putting makeup on only the right side of the face; eating food only on the right side of the plate; omission of keys on the left side of the computer keyboard; colliding with items on the left side; and not responding to a person standing on the left side (Festa et al. 2008; Klonoff et al. 1990; Senelick 2010; Stein 2004; Verfaellie and Heilman 2006; Williams 2010). Sometimes, the neglect phenomenon dissipates over time (Senelick 2010); however, its persistence can interfere with the loved one's independence (Heilman 2009).

Stroke often produces motor problems, specifically *hemiparesis* or *hemiplegia* (Senelick 2010). *Hemiplegia* is paralysis while *hemiparesis* is weakness of the side of the body opposite to the stroke (Palmer and Palmer 2011; Senelick 2010). Approximately 80–88% of patients have hemiparesis acutely (National Stroke Association 2006; see Rosenberg et al. 2010, for a review). When the stroke affects the middle cerebral artery, the most common pattern is greater weakness in the hand, followed by the arm and leg correspondingly (Stein 2004). Weakness after a stroke is usually connected to loss of the capability to control and coordinate movements (Stein 2004). Owing to these physical challenges, the loved one may not be able to walk; dress himself or herself; use the restroom independently; open the hand or move the fingers separately; grab things (e.g., hold a utensil); and/or tie his or her shoes (National Stroke Association 2006; Senelick 2010; Stein 2004).

Strokes can also produce *spasticity,* which is an imbalance of muscle tension and movement (Senelick 2010). It results in tightness and pain in the muscles and an increase in resistance when passively moving the limbs (Rosenberg et al. 2010; Senelick 2010). Paralysis and spasticity often coexist after stroke (Senelick 2010). Motor *apraxia* can occur after a left hemisphere stroke, which is the inability to perform skilled movements, either in isolation or in a sequence (Festa et al. 2008). For instance, the loved one may be unable to demonstrate how to wave goodbye or mail a letter (Festa et al. 2008). Lastly, disequilibrium, dizziness, vertigo, and impaired balance are common after a stroke, increasing the risk of falls (Megna 2010).

Movement disorders can also develop from anoxic brain injury (see FitzGerald et al. 2010, for a review; Howard et al. 2011; Peskine et al. 2010). These include *ataxia,* or motor incoordination as well as impaired balance and gait from damage to the cerebellum (Hopkins and Bigler 2008). Damage to the basal ganglia can result in *myoclonus* or "shock-like" involuntary muscle jerks; *dystonia*, which is prolonged muscle contraction causing pain, abnormal posture, twisting, or repetitive movements; and an *akinetic-rigid* syndrome, characterized by muscle rigidity, tremor, and postural instability (Tröster and Arnett 2006; Venkatesan and Frucht 2006).

6.5.2 "Helpful Hints" and Tools for Families to Assist the Loved One with Vision and Motor Challenges

First and foremost, when possible, the loved one should receive some combination of occupational, physical, and speech therapy to address neglect, hemiparesis/hemiplegia, other motor deficits, and hemianopia. For example, occupational therapists address the consequences of the loved one's specific deficiencies in the form of upper extremity function, self-care (e.g., bathing, toileting, grooming, feeding, hygiene, and medication management), instrumental activities of daily living (e.g., meal preparation, money management), visuoperceptual skills, cognitive capabilities, mobility, community reintegration (including driving and other modes of transportation), and prework aptitude (Kearney et al. 2010).

A detailed discussion of treatment for vision and motor incapacities is beyond the scope of this book. However, Table 6.8 summarizes some basic "helpful hints" and tools for the family to assist the loved one with these phenomena. Currently, there are a number of "low-tech" assistive technologies (e.g., pencil grips, Velcro^{TM}) as well as "high-tech" examples (e.g., portable and one-handed keyboards, talking calculators, etc.; Glenn and Hill 2010; Scherer 2012). Pertinent resources are "Stroke Rehabilitation" by Langhorne et al. (2011) and *Assistive Technologies and Other Supports for People with Brain Impairment* by Scherer (2012); the latter includes informative websites (e.g., www.abledata.com; www.frogpad.com; and www.agrabilityproject.org/assistivetech/tips/handtools.cfm).

The psychotherapist will propose to the tier 1 caregiver and tier supports that they be proactive about joining sessions with the physical and occupational therapists as well as a speech–language pathologist to become acquainted with various compensations. It is always ideal for the therapist to introduce and reinforce the correct use of strategies to combat stroke effects. The family should solicit the "buy in" of the loved one with respect to a willingness to accept tutelage about carryover into the home. In this regard, the psychotherapist can be an excellent "mediator" so that the caregiver does not become the untoward target of "kill the messenger" (Klonoff 2010). Other suggestions for the relatives are: follow the guidance of the rehabilitation team so as to create a structured, consistent, and secure environment once at home; focus on fundamental and concrete "survival" skills to further the loved one's independence (e.g., self-care and activities of daily living to start); and be patient with the process (Senelick 2010).

The aim of treatment is to maximize the loved one's functionality and, importantly, increase his or her safety in the environment (Heilman 2009). Some compensations for left neglect include: place items at home on the right side of the individual; invite visitors to sit on the right side of the loved one; remove objects that the loved one might bump into in narrow passageways at home; gently remind or assist the loved one to put a red line/Velcro^{TM} on the left side of pages; encourage the loved one to scan from left to right when in the community; and walk on the loved one's left side in busy environs (e.g., the mall) so that he or she does not run into obstacles (Heilman 2009; Stein 2004; Williams 2010).

Table 6.8 "Helpful Hints" and tools for the family to assist the loved one with vision and motor challenges

General considerations
Liaison with the loved one's physical and occupational therapists as well as a speech-language pathologist
Therapies should be individualized, task-oriented, and functionally-oriented
Learn about the loved one's strategies, compensations, as well as "low tech" and "high tech" assistive technologies
Encourage the loved one to "buy in" to the therapeutic interventions
Work with the psychotherapist so as not to become the untoward target of "kill the messenger"
Create a structured, consistent, and secure environment at home
Focus on fundamental and concrete "survival" skills to further the loved one's independence
Be patient with the process
Help the loved one maximize his or her functionality and safety

Left visual neglect
Place items at home on the right side of the loved one
Invite visitors to sit on the right side of the loved one
Remove objects that the loved one might bump into in narrow passageways
Gently remind or assist the loved one in putting a red line/Velcro™ on the left side of pages
Encourage the loved one to scan from left to right when in the community
Walk on the loved one's left side in busy environs
Realize the loved one may be unable to drive

Vision loss
Learn about compensatory training and restoration therapy
Advocate for your loved one to work with a neurorehabilitation optometrist and/or occupational therapist
Pursue interactive technology (the Neuro-Vision Rehabilitator™ and Vision Coach™)
Work with the occupational therapist in the home:
- Clear pathways
- Eliminate clutter
- Incorporate high-contrast, tactile labeling systems, talking clocks, and microwave ovens
- Remove area rugs
- Install safety programs
- Become familiar with assistive techniques and devices

Obtain input and clearance from a neuro-opthalmologist if pursuing driving or using machinery

Motor deficits
Keep regular appointments with the treating physicians (e.g., physiatrist)
Seek therapy for the loved one with a physical and occupational therapist to maximize the loved one's physical and functional independence
Become familiar with new treatment interventions, assistive technology devices, and home programs and obtain the necessary training to assist and cue the loved one
Engage in home visits:
- Create adequate lighting
- Ensure that external and household pathways are even and not slippery
- Place railings and grab bars in appropriate locations
- Accommodate raised or adjusted toilet seats
- Remove obstructing items
- Learn how to assist the loved one in transfers in the home and car
- Help tailor home therapies to the family's lifestyle by giving input to the therapists

Multimedia resources
Books/articles
"Stroke Rehabilitation" (Langhorne et al. 2011)
Assistive Technologies and Other Supports for People with Brain Impairment (Scherer 2012)

Table 6.8 (continued)

Stroke Recovery and Rehabilitation (Stein et al. 2009)
Living with Stroke: A Guide for Families (Senelick 2010)
Stroke Rehabilitation: A Function-Based Approach (Gillen 2011)
Websites
Assistive technologies
www.abledata.com
www.frogpad.com
www.agrabilityproject.org/assistivetech/tips/handtools.cfm
www.carsonoptical.com/customer
www.therapro.com
Driving information
www.ialvs.com/State-Driving-Laws
www.mdsupport.org/library/drivingrequirements.html
Visuoperceptual activities
Hoppers by Binary Arts
Set—https://www.setgame.com/set
Lonpos 101 pyramid—http://www.lonpos-europe.com/en.html
Jigsaw puzzles 50 to 100 pieces
I Spy jigsaw puzzles
Puzzlemania by Highlights—www.puzzlemania.com
Puzzles—(e.g., www.jigzone.com, www.ageofpuzzles.com, www.jigsaw2order.com)
Tangrams
Mighty Mind—www.mightymind.com
I Spy books by Scholastic
Spot the Differences by Sterling Publishing Co., Inc
Word-finds by TV Guide—www.kappapuzzles.com
Hidden Pictures by Highlights
Geoboards
Parquetry boards
Card sorting
Solitaire
Blink card game
Checkers, Chess, Backgammon, Dominoes
Paint by numbers
Fine motor activities
Operation board game
Perfection board game

Visual rehabilitative procedures for vision loss (including hemianopia) consist of compensatory training and restoration therapy (Esther Han 2010; Solomon and Goldstein 2009). Typically, this therapy is done by a neurorehabilitation optometrist and/or occupational therapist (Esther Han 2010; Lindman 2011). A neurorehabilitation optometrist is specialized in vision therapy exercises, including range of motion and fusion exercises (Esther Han 2010; Lindman 2011). He or she can also prescribe lenses (e.g., reading or prism glasses; Caswell 2005; Esther Han 2010; Lindman 2011). There is also new interactive technology available to occupational therapists and neurorehabilitation optometrists to address visual scanning and processing deficits, including the Neuro-Vision Rehabilitator™ and Vision Coach™. Other activities are summarized in Table 6.8 and include computer programs, puzzles, eye–hand coordination exercises, and scanning activities.

The occupational therapist may also educate the caregiver and support network on how to modify the home environment, secondary to the loved one's vision challenges; home visits are invaluable in this case (Kearney et al. 2010). Suggestions include: clear pathways for safe mobility; eliminate clutter; incorporate high-contrast, tactile labeling systems, talking clocks, and microwave ovens; remove area rugs that can cause fall hazards; and install safety programs (e.g., life line medical alert services; Copolillo and Ivanoff 2011; Kearney et al. 2010). There are a number of assistive techniques and devices for neurovisual deficits, including using slant boards, increasing contrast and light, decreasing patterns, or enlarging materials using eyewear, hand-held, stand, and computer magnifiers (Copolillo and Ivanoff 2011; Lindman 2011; www.carsonoptical.com/customer_Faq/Magnifiers/1; www.therapro.com). In the community, the loved onc can use way-finding devices so as to orient him or her and provide directions (Copolillo and Ivanoff 2011). Therapies should be individualized and task oriented with targeted outcomes, including independent living, transportation, etc. (Solomon and Goldstein 2009).

Neglect and visual field loss usually impede driving or use of machinery (Heilman 2009). The psychotherapist will urge the family (and loved one) to obtain clearance from key physicians, including a rehabilitation physician and/or neuro-opthalmologist. Typically, a neuro-opthalmologist will need to perform a visual field test in order to be sure the loved one has sufficient vision for driving (Markus et al. 2010). Minimum visual requirements vary by state, so the relatives will need to discuss this with the loved one's physician. (For more information on national and international driving stipulations, see Bron et al. 2010; www.ialvs.com/State-Driving-Laws; and www.mdsupport.org/library/drivingrequirements.html).

Table 6.8 also summarizes some "helpful hints" and tools for motor deficits, including hemiplegia and hemiparesis. The psychotherapist will push the caregiver to keep regular appointments with the loved one's doctors. Whenever feasible, the loved one should be followed by a physiatrist, who can manage his or her stroke symptoms and make rehabilitative recommendations (Senelick 2010). As stated previously, it behooves the loved one to obtain rehabilitation from occupational and physical therapists in order to address his or her motor problems and provide the rudiments of psychoeducation to the support network. The physical therapist can improve mobility (e.g., with a wheelchair, walker, cane, or independently), strength, posture, range of motion, coordination, balance, and endurance (National Stroke Association 2006; Senelick 2010). The occupational therapist addresses upper extremity functioning, including range of motion, muscle strength and tone, coordination, sensation as well as mobility in the home and community (Kearney et al. 2010).

There are a number of new protocols and ATDs to address hemiparesis, including leg braces, orthotics, special shoes, biofeedback, electrical stimulation, and constraint-induced therapy (National Stroke Association 2006; Senelick 2010; Stein 2004; www.abledata.com). In this latter treatment, the loved one's useable limb is immobilized in a sling, so that the affected arm is "forced" to work according to the "use it or lose it" principle (National Stroke Association 2006; Rosenberg et al.

2010; Stein 2004). The caregiver will need instruction on the various technologies and home programs, as often he or she needs to physically aid the loved one in putting on equipment as well as cue him or her to complete home stretching routines and exercises (Senelick 2010; Williams 2010). Injections of botulinum toxin (Botox), intrathecal baclofen, and certain medications (e.g., tizanidine, dantrolene, diazepam) can reduce spasticity (National Stroke Association 2006; Senelick 2010). Aquatic therapy can be very effective (Senelick 2010), although the caregiver will need education for interacting with the loved one in a home pool.

Occupational therapists address upper extremity weakness as well as gross and fine motor control and coordination, so as to expand the loved one's capacity to be independent in the home environment (Kearney et al. 2010; Senelick 2010). Specific responsibilities and strategies which the occupational therapist addresses are for self-care and activities of daily living (Kearney et al. 2010; Senelick 2010). Examples include slings, splints, and lapboards (to avoid medical complications); long-handled sponges; pistol-grip reachers; adaptive laces for tying shoes; Velcro™ (instead of buttons and zippers) for dressing; nonslip dycem to stabilize articles; adaptive eating utensils (e.g., a rocker knife for cutting food); jar openers; and special pan and pot holders (Scherer 2012; Senelick 2010). Caregiver education regarding the purpose and protocols for these specific devices is instrumental for the loved one. Notably, the occupational therapist's energies are directed towards teaching the loved one activities of daily living in the context of physical limitations and concurrently educating and supporting the caregiver to maximize self-sufficiency and both parties' well-being.

Home visits involving the caregiver, other family members, loved one, and occupational/physical therapists are also efficacious for introducing mechanisms to advance gross and fine motor skills as well as bolster the loved one's safety and functionality (Scherer 2012). Recommendations include: create adequate lighting; ensure that external and household pathways are even and not slippery; place railings and grab bars in appropriate locations; accommodate raised or adjusted toilet seats; and remove obstructing items (Scherer 2012). The physical and occupational therapists also instruct the family about community adaptations, for instance car transfers (Senelick 2010). The therapy approach should be tailored to the loved one's and relatives' daily needs (Stein 2004). Therefore, involvement of the tier supports is crucial, so that the emphasis of therapy is on the actual duties with which the loved one needs to develop proficiency. For more information on treatments for motor aftereffects post stroke as well as the role of therapeutic interventions, see the books, *Stroke Recovery and Rehabilitation* by Stein, Harvey, Macko, Winstein, and Zorowitz (2009), *Living with Stroke: A Guide for Families* by Senelick (2010), and *Stroke Rehabilitation: A Function-Based Approach* by Gillen (2011).

6.6 Scenario: Family Members' Angst and Disillusionment

Despite psychotherapy, understandably, the caregiver and support network suffer from emotional distress and lifestyle threats from a stroke or anoxic injury in a loved one. This occurs both acutely and into the chronic phases of recovery. The caregiver and family may say something like: *I'm still having so much trouble dealing with this, I just don't know how to go forward...*

6.6.1 Overview of Family Members' Angst and Disillusionment

Spouses and other family members with a loved one who has sustained a stroke or anoxic event are vulnerable to caregiver strain and reduced quality of life in the physical, psychological, economic, and social arenas (Bakas et al. 2004; Collins and Swartz 2011; Draper and Brocklehurst 2007; Larson et al. 2005; Smeets et al. 2012). This is due to the abruptness of the stroke onset, ill preparedness in the caregiver, an unwanted role, and shortened hospital stays (Bakas et al. 2004; Collins and Swartz 2011; Draper and Brocklehurst 2007; Niemeier and Karol 2011a). Caregivers are also often older (Rombough et al. 2007), given the demographics of stroke recipients.

The caregiver can feel lonely, overburdened, and in a thankless pickle (Elbaum 2010). Particular risk factors for caregiver distress include spousal relationships; more severe stroke/anoxic effects; and significant physical, self-care, speech, cognitive (e.g., confusion and forgetfulness), and mood/behavioral changes (e.g., depression, anxiety, and aggression) in the loved one (Bakas et al. 2004; Blonder et al. 2007; Clark et al. 2004; Coombs 2007; Draper and Brocklehurst 2007; Franzén-Dahlin et al. 2008; Haley et al. 2009; Perrin et al. 2008; Smeets et al. 2012). Tensions escalate if the loved one scapegoats the caregiver through disrespect, unreasonable behavior, or rage attacks (Elbaum 2010). Spouses can suffer from depression and anxiety concomitant to multiple losses, affecting leisure time, freedom to leave the loved one unattended, and the altered marital relationship, including loss of a partner (Coombs 2007; Smeets et al. 2012). Physical exhaustion, guilt over leaving the loved one, fear about life uncertainties and the health-related issues, unfamiliar and time-consuming roles and responsibilities, and home confinement augment the caregiver's pressures (Cao et al. 2010; Coombs 2007).

The tier 1 caregiver is the "linchpin" of the loved one's posthospital existence (Caplan 2010). As time elapses, practical (e.g., self-care including feeding, grooming, dressing, toileting, and bathing) and emotional dysfunction impinge even more on the caregiver, resulting in depression, tense social relations, reduced relationship harmony, and sometimes, burnout (see Collins and Swartz 2011, for a review; Coombs 2007; Perrin et al. 2008; Rigby et al. 2009; Visser-Meily et al. 2009). This includes loss of an interpersonal connection with the loved one (Perrin et al. 2008). In addition, working caregivers have "double duty" demands, as although they receive support from other relatives, their load often remains as high as nonworking family members (Ko et al. 2007). To complicate matters, their work life suffers, with missed hours and reduced productivity (Ko et al. 2007). Overall, there is profound grief about uncertainties and fractured hopes, translating into a loss of sense of self (Niemeier and Karol 2011a).

6.6.2 *"Helpful Hints" and Tools for Families to Cope with their Angst and Disillusionment*

Table 6.9 summarizes "helpful hints" and tools for families to cope with their angst and disillusionment when caring for a loved one with stroke or anoxic injury. Psychotherapy becomes an essential support and educational resource (Bakas et al. 2004; see Collins and Swartz 2011, for a review; Eldred and Sykes 2008; Klonoff and Koberstein 2010; Perrin et al. 2008). It is advisable to incorporate cultural sensitivity when planning treatment (Perrin et al. 2010). That being said, principles and interventions described earlier are applicable to caregivers and family members of stroke/anoxia victims (see Chap. 4, Sect. 4.8.2). These include the FEM as a self-reflection mechanism (Klonoff and Koberstein 2010), the realization that the recovery process is a "marathon" not a "sprint" (S. Myles, personal communication, n.d.) as well as other adages (e.g., "one day at a time").

The support network will encounter hurdles which alter over time (Cameron and Gignac 2008). They should expect a "roller coaster" of emotions vacillating between gratitude for progress, and feelings of fear, sadness, and discouragement when obstacles surface (Klonoff and Koberstein 2010; Niemeier and Karol 2011b). A primary therapeutic objective is to keep the caregiver and others in the "green zone" of coping, rather than plummeting and becoming trapped in the "yellow warning" or "red crisis" zones (see Chap. 1, Sect. 1.5). This will require interventions which are "timed right" based on the family's current requirements (Cameron and Gignac 2008; Klonoff 2010). Methodologies should be informational, emotional, instrumental (i.e., towards specific life modifications), and appraisal (i.e., providing validating and constructive feedback regarding the caregiver's efforts; Cameron and Gignac 2008). This includes books written from the vantage point of the loved one who sustained the stroke and/or the caregivers. Inspirational examples include: *The Diving Bell and the Butterfly* by Bauby (1998); *My Year Off: Recovering Life After a Stroke* by McCrum (1999); *My Stroke of Luck* by Douglas (2003); *Conquering Stroke: How I Fought My Way Back and How You Can Too* by Greene (2008); *Change in the Weather: Life After Stroke* by McEwen and Paisner (2008); *After the Stroke: My Journey Back to Life* by McEwen and Paisner (2009); *A Stroke of Insight: A Brain Scientist's Personal Journey* by Taylor (2009); and *One Hundred Names for Love: A Stroke, a Marriage, and the Language of Healing* by Ackerman (2011).

Table 6.9 "Helpful Hints" and tools for family members to cope with their angst and disillusionment

Find a psychotherapist who incorporates cultural sensitivity into his or her interventions
Techniques must be "timed right" and are informational, emotional, instrumental, and appraisal
Challenges change over time so expect a roller coaster of emotions
Work with the therapist to stay in the "green coping" zone of the FEM
Recognize your CRs by proxy
Work through feelings of grief, loss, guilt, and anger
Attempt to "make the best" of a harrowing experience
Attend to your own physical health:
Go to doctors' appointments
Exercise regularly
Maintain a nutritious diet
Engage in practical problem solving and preparedness by learning coping techniques
Seek psychoeducation from a team of neurorehabilitation therapists, including early on
Find ways to "recharge the batteries" and maximize well-being:
Reinforce the carry-over of the loved one's learned strategies and exercise programs to the home
Employ constructive feedback techniques
Create structured routines
Keep a busy and productive lifestyle for everyone, including socialization experiences and cognitive stimulation
Maintain a positive working alliance with the treatment team
Be mindful about the balance between overprotectiveness and inattention
Learn techniques to reduce emotional distress
Keep accord in the family system
Find time for humor and laughter
Show affection to one another
Remain hopeful
For spouses
Foster the loved one's expression of emotions
Focus on improving marital harmony and life satisfaction
Be open to different venues (e.g., individual counseling, marital therapy, family therapy)
Adjust to the new individual in the dyad
Understand and address changes in the sexual relationship
Employ active coping techniques, including self-management and mastery
Search for the "silver linings:"
Renewed commitment to the marriage
Accentuate the positive
All caregivers and tier supports can:
Reframe caregiving in a positive light
Find meaning in life
Use sources of inspiration, including faith, hope, and optimism
Utilize compassionate and competent tier 2 and 3 community supports
Pursue emotional contacts, including support groups
Multimedia resources
Model
Family Experiential Model (FEM) of Recovery (Klonoff and Koberstein 2010; Klonoff et al. 2008)
Questionnaire
Family's Sense of Self Following Brain Injury-Sentence Completion Task
Books
The Diving Bell and the Butterfly (Bauby 1998)
My Year Off: Recovering Life After a Stroke (McCrum 1999)
My Stroke of Luck (Douglas 2003)

Table 6.9 (continued)

Conquering Stroke: How I Fought My Way Back and How You Can Too (Greene 2008)
Change in the Weather: Life After Stroke (McEwen and Paisner 2008)
After the Stroke: My Journey Back to Life (McEwen and Paisner 2009)
A Stroke of Insight: A Brain Scientist's Personal Journey (Taylor 2009)
One Hundred Names for Love: A Stroke, a Marriage, and the Language of Healing (Ackerman 2011)
Cookbooks
Hungry Girl to the Max! The Ultimate Guilt-Free Cookbook (Lillien 2012)
Cooking for Beginners (Academy of Nutrition and Dietetics 2012)

Psychoeducation and therapy are central so that the caregiver recognizes CRs by proxy (see also Chap. 2, Sect. 2.4.2.1; and Chap. 9, Sect. 9.4 and Tables 9.7 and 9.8). These episodes occur when he or she witnesses the loved one's incapacities. Caregiver angst translates to problematic behaviors, including overprotectiveness, discouragement, external blaming, and/or irritability. As depicted in the FEM, family members traverse their own journey of grief and loss secondary to shattered dreams. Using this model and the listening perspective during both individual counseling and group therapy is integral to the family's adaptation process (see also Chap. 9, Sect. 9.5). The psychotherapist will utilize cognitive–behavioral therapy so that the caregiver can work through unnecessary feelings of guilt and anger. Tactics encompass avoiding: "awfulizing" the circumstances; harsh self-talk and self-judgments; second-guessing and "should ofs"; self-defeating behaviors; and unrealistic expectations (Klonoff and Koberstein 2010; Niemeier and Karol 2011a). Instead, the psychotherapist will guide the relatives to reframe their harrowing situation and "make the best" of it (Klonoff and Koberstein 2010). The Sense of Self Questionnaire becomes a beneficial medium to illuminate the way forward (see Chap. 2, Sect. 2.3.8 and Fig. 2.2 and Chap. 11, Sect. 11.6.1).

Given the older age of many stroke caregivers, it is imperative that they attend to their own physical health (Cao et al. 2010; Collins and Swartz 2011; Franzén-Dahlin et al. 2007). The psychotherapist will advocate that he or she attend regular doctors' appointments and immediately address any health concerns (Palmer and Palmer 2011). Also, regular exercise maintains the physical and emotional energies of tier 1 and 2 supports (Cao et al. 2010; Collins and Swartz 2011). The caregiver will need to coordinate with others to enable opportunities for all parties to exercise, even if this is for 10–15 min a few times per week. When housebound, home exercise equipment (e.g., stationary bicycle or treadmill) and DVDs are viable options. Interactive home games (e.g., a Wii™ system) allows for both social and physical outlets. A nutritious diet is also a prerequisite for the well-being of the loved one, caregiver, and involved relatives (Collins and Swartz 2011). First-rate meal preparation resources which are quick and healthy include *Hungry Girl to the Max! The Ultimate Guilt-Free Cookbook* by Lillien (2012) and *Cooking for Beginners* through the Academy of Nutrition and Dietetics (2012).

Research has shown that practical problem solving and overall preparedness reduces the caregiver's degree of depression after stroke (see Elbaum 2010, for a review; Perrin et al. 2008; Shanmugham et al. 2009). Teaching coping techniques should start during inpatient rehabilitation (Shanmugham et al. 2009). The ideal system is to include a team of neurorehabilitation therapists who can continue the psychoeducation process and problem-solving interventions as the recovery process evolves, particularly once the loved one is discharged home. Utilizing varied resources is useful, including referral to a social worker for aid in managing financial concerns (Bakas et al. 2004). Ultimately, when the caregiver feels more in control of his or her life, the encumbrances and emotional distress wane (Smeets et al. 2012).

Specific ways that the psychotherapist will teach the caregiver and support network to "recharge their batteries" as well as maximize their own well-being and that of the loved one are to: reinforce the carryover of the loved one's learned strategies and exercise programs to the home; employ constructive feedback with the loved one; create structured routines; maintain a busy, productive existence for everyone, including socialization experiences and cognitive stimulating enterprises; keep a positive working alliance with the treatment team; be mindful of the balance between overprotectiveness and inattention to the loved one's and others' needs; learn ways to address emotional distress and keep accord in the family system; find time for humor and laughter; show affection to one another; and remain hopeful (Elbaum 2010; Klonoff 2010; Palmer and Palmer 2011).

For spouses, fostering open dialogue with the loved one, active coping methods, and improving marital harmony are salient in the psychotherapeutic process and is indispensable, even years after the stroke onset (McPherson et al. 2010; Visser-Meily et al. 2009). Treatment venues include individual counseling for the caregiver (and loved one), marital counseling, and for the extended family (Blonder et al. 2007; McPherson et al. 2010). To the extent that conflict is lessened over the care of the stroke survivor, the caregiver's mental health is improved (Clark et al. 2004).

Spouses must be aided in adjusting to a new individual within the marital dyad. Therapy should also focus on changes in the spouses' sexual relationship (Smeets et al. 2012). Reasons for sexual disturbance post stroke include: physiological dysfunction (e.g., diminished erectile capacity, impaired sensory and/or motor functioning, reduced libido); the impact of medications; as well as reactive explanations, including lessened self-esteem, depression, fear of precipitating another stroke, and performance anxiety (see Caplan 2010, for a review). Psychoeducation, including legitimizing concerns and adaptive techniques are important components of psychotherapy (Caplan 2010). Ultimately, therapy should target self-management, coping, and mastery for both the caregiver and the loved one, so as to increase the life satisfaction of both parties (Bergström et al. 2011; Smeets et al. 2012). The psychotherapist can also point out the "silver linings" after stroke in a partner, including: renewed commitment to the marriage, with reinvestment of energy, creativity, and emotional closeness; accentuating the positive, including the valuable and enjoyable aspects of the relationship and the fact the spouse survived (Palmer and Palmer 2011; see also Chap. 3, Sect. 3.2).

Regardless of the relationship, when the psychotherapist reframes caregiving in a positive light, with attached meaningfulness, the load is easier to bear (Franzén-Dahlin et al. 2007; Gaugler 2010; Haley et al. 2009; Perrin et al. 2008; see also Chap. 10, Sect. 10.2). Meaning in the caregiver role builds self-esteem and a sense of accomplishment (Palmer and Palmer 2011). Psychotherapy can provide reminders of other sources of inspiration, including faith, hope, and optimism (Coombs 2007; Franzén-Dahlin et al. 2007; Palmer and Palmer 2011). The therapist will try to persuade the sometimes proud or private caregiver to accept input and aid from the second and third tiers of support (Niemeier and Karol 2011a; see also Chap. 1, Sect. 1.3 for a description). This can include offers from family, friends, and neighbors for respite breaks and transportation (Coombs 2007). Also, the therapists will remind the primary caregiver of compassionate and competent tier 3 community supports, including airport personnel who can facilitate travelling when the loved one has various physical and functional challenges. Community activity day-care centers can be satisfying to the loved one and a source of respite for the caregiver (Smeets et al. 2012). Emotional contacts contribute to the spouse's quality of life, as these reduce loneliness and isolation while providing reassurance, empathy, encouragement, and a feeling of being loved (Larson et al. 2005). Relatives also find support groups where they receive contact with fellow caregivers to be positive (Elbaum 2010; Klonoff and Koberstein 2010; Palmer and Palmer 2011; Schure et al. 2006; see also Chaps. 9 and 11).

6.7 Case Study

Lauren was age 65 when she suffered a left hemisphere stroke. At the time, she was living with her sister, Talia, age 60. Lauren had acute onset of right-sided weakness and the inability to communicate. Talia immediately called 911 and her sister was taken to a nearby trauma center. Neuroimaging, including a cerebral angiogram, revealed a left frontal parietal intracranial hemorrhage involving the middle cerebral artery as well as a basal ganglia hemorrhage. The doctors determined that the cause of the stroke was hypertension. Talia was distraught and terrified, as at first the neurosurgeon predicted a questionable survival, with at best profound sequelae. Talia planted herself at the bedside in a constant vigil. Lauren spent 1 week in the intensive care unit (ICU) and was then transferred to an inpatient neurorehabilitation unit. She was alert, but demonstrated a global aphasia, a right homonymous hemianopia, and right hemiparesis. She received physical, occupational, and speech therapies for 5 weeks and was discharged home.

Talia was reeling from the drastic health decline in her sister. Both Lauren and Talia were often tearful and anxious. Talia was especially worried that Lauren would suffer another stroke or fall while trying to move around, as she felt like a helpless novice in her new role as a caregiver. She met twice with a neuropsychologist who provided some emotional support by mainly answering her questions and reassuring her that Lauren had good potential to improve neurologically, based on her progress thus far and her hardworking attitude. Written materials on aphasia and hemiparesis were incorporated into the discussion. There was also a weekly support group on the unit, which Talia attended. Talia appreciated the psychoeducation and pointers, but continued to feel very overwhelmed and alarmed about Lauren's condition, especially her aphasia. At the time Lauren went home, she was ambulating using a wheelchair and required moderate assistance for all self-care activities in the home. She needed around-the-clock supervision. Talia loved Lauren dearly and loathed leaving her, even for short periods, secondary to profound fearfulness and guilt. Talia resigned from her job and succumbed to home confinement; soon, they both descended into social seclusion.

Shortly after returning home, Lauren began her outpatient therapies. She received physical, occupational, and speech therapies, each three times per week. She received psychotherapy twice monthly from a social worker because of anxiety and depression. Talia was also able to meet with the social worker for practical support, community resources, and counseling. Lauren spent three months in this setting and made progress in her language comprehension and expression, right-hand function, balance, strength, range of motion, coordination, sensation, and ambulation. At the time of discharge, she could perform basic self-care activities, including grooming, hygiene, and dressing. She still required 24/7 supervision, secondary to her aphasia and physical limitations. Given the gains in her language, her physiatrist recommended Lauren enroll in an outpatient milieu program, with emphasis on holistic treatment, group therapies, and further independence in the home and community.

Thankfully, this new program also afforded psychotherapy with Dr. Gustav for Lauren and family therapy for Talia. Dr. Gustav utilized his first couple of sessions with Talia to forge a working alliance and glean her knowledge base and subjective impressions of Lauren's status. He also began to explore Talia's emotional status, challenges, and current needs. He obtained relevant background history. Prior to this ordeal, Lauren and Talia were living together very happily in a condominium. Lauren's husband had died 10 years earlier from a cardiac arrest and Talia had divorced many years before. Lauren was a retired secretary and Talia was working part-time as a book editor. Both had enjoyed excellent health prior to this event. They were of the Jewish faith and attended a Chabad-Lubavitch synagogue. They were very active within the congregation, with a close circle of friends. Prior to her stroke, Lauren volunteered at a nearby religious school with the office secretaries. Post stroke, their rabbi wanted to visit the home and provide solace, but Lauren was far too depressed and self-conscious and adamantly declined the request. It was Dr. Gustav's impression that Talia was gaining some awareness and acceptance of the depth of her sister's struggles and needs. His perception was that Talia had remained a dedicated caregiver. Nonetheless, despite her best efforts, Talia was suffering from tier 1 caregiver strain, manifested as reduced quality of life, physical and emotional exhaustion, and financial peril (see also Chap. 2 for further discussion of early sessions).

Upon starting milieu treatment, Lauren underwent neuropsychological, speech and language, physical, and occupational therapy evaluations. A family meeting was held with the therapists, who reviewed the test findings with Lauren and Talia. The bell curve diagram was used to describe the "medium to large" cognitive and language challenges. Lauren was diagnosed with Wernicke's aphasia, verbal apraxia, as well as medium- to large-sized cognitive deficits in attention, verbal learning and recall, and executive functions (i.e., organization, problem solving, and flexible thinking). The occupational therapist reported increased spasticity and tone in Lauren's right upper extremity as well as decreased right upper extremity sensory awareness, strength, flexibility, gross motor coordination, active range of motion, and endurance. The physical therapist noted impairments in her right leg strength, ankle range of motion, coordination, motor speed, and quality of gait.

Lauren attended therapies 4 days per week, also with regular home visits. Speech therapy targeted receptive and expressive communication (including reading comprehension and writing), oral-motor speech production, memory, attention and concentration, planning and organization, use of strategies, and improving her awareness and acceptance of strengths and difficulties. Lauren was introduced to an AAC device, the Proloquo2Go on her iPad, which provided her with an extensive vocabulary, word prediction, and the capability to customize messages. Lauren practiced this in group therapy sessions, including a daily Milieu meeting and Aphasia Group. She was also taught how to develop a script for making phone calls using her AAC device. Lauren was also given homework assignments, including exercises for her speech apraxia on her iPad and home computer.

Talia attended many sessions with Lauren and the speech–language pathologist and learned how to help Lauren with her compensations. This therapist also provided a number of “helpful hints” to Talia, including to slow down her rate of speech, keep statements shorter and simpler, and limit distractions when trying to converse. Towards the end of treatment, the speech–language pathologist accompanied Lauren to the religious school to identify suitable activities and to educate her volunteer job supervisor. They determined a subset of tasks such as copying materials and preparing informational packets for prospective parents interested in the school.

At Dr. Gustav’s suggestion, Talia was proactive in discussing Lauren’s vision problems with her physiatrist. Lauren was then seen by a neurorehabilitation optometrist, who diagnosed her with a persistent right hemianopia. He also prescribed prism glasses. Her occupational therapist coordinated with the optometrist and began using the Neuro-Vision Rehabilitator (NVR) to address visual processing deficiencies. Lauren was introduced to new “high-tech” technology to address her right upper extremity deficits. This included practice with one-handed typing on her computer, iPad, and iPhone; an air splint for tone reduction; a Saebo Stretch® orthosis; the Empi®/electrical stimulation for muscle reeducation and tone reduction; and the Bioness H200® for tone management. Lauren received regular Botox injections from her physiatrist. Her occupational therapist also taught Lauren some modified yoga practices for stretching, tone reduction, and relaxation responses.

Regular home visits were performed with Talia present. The occupational therapist taught her about Lauren’s upper extremity equipment and the three of them participated in constructing a HIC with picture icons (see Fig. 6.3). Home activities were addressed, including adapting written recipes using a pictorial cookbook and the reading mode in her iPad (i.e., the Premier Talking Reader app). With guidance from the dietician, the occupational therapist developed a subset of wholesome meals and counseled Lauren and Talia how to cook them together successfully. Adaptive kitchen equipment was introduced, including a cutting board and rocker knife. A “Right Upper Extremity Use Checklist” was devised with input from Lauren and Talia. This identified all of the chores at home in which Lauren could use her right upper extremity to maximize her independence and provide her with a sense of competency.

The occupational therapist coached Lauren and Talia in modifying protocols to use their sewing machine, a hobby they both greatly cherished. After creating a grocery list in the iPad, the occupational therapist and dietician also accompanied Lauren and Talia to the grocery store to practice shopping skills in the context of Lauren's aphasia and to discuss healthier choices, given her issues with weight and blood pressure. Eventually, resources for cab vouchers were explored by the occupational therapist on behalf of Lauren to enable independent transportation. Then the occupational therapist attended the school setting where Lauren volunteered and created energy conservation systems so as to complete her daily duties in the context of her hemiparesis and hemianopia.

Lauren participated in physical therapy, including a balance group, a motor endurance group, and community outings with other patients and interdisciplinary team members to address ambulation on uneven terrain, on stairs, and the light rail system. The physical therapist performed a gym visit with Lauren, along with Talia and introduced them to some fun "Silver Sneakers" class options. She also suggested aquatic therapy and provided an exercise program they could both do.

Lauren's neuropsychologist/psychotherapist, Dr. Gustav, proposed that Lauren attend a memory group to learn more about memory challenges and fitting compensations. Lauren adopted an armamentarium of tools, including her pillbox, oven timer, color-coded labeling systems, and her iPad. He provided cognitive retraining activities to address Lauren's language and cognitive deficits (see also Klonoff 2010). Particular emphasis was placed on her attention, including how to increase her selective and divided attention with distractions and competing influences present in the sessions. He also provided her with computerized cognitive exercises (i.e., lumosity.com and happyneuron.com) which Lauren did as part of therapy sessions and for homework. Dr. Gustav recommended games for Lauren, Talia, and their friends which had cognitive benefit, including Chess and Backgammon (for executive functions); Sequence and UNO (targeting attention); Simon and Clue (to address memory); and Scrabble, Boggle, and Pictionary (to enhance language; see also Chap. 8, Table 8.5). He taught them ways to maximize Lauren's capacity to succeed in the home environment, including doing tasks in the morning when she was freshest and limiting the amount of activities per day (using her HIC list). Talia was introduced to the concept of "vanishing cues," and as Lauren became proficient at various duties, Talia diminished her prompts and supervision. This created a more normalized rapport at home.

Psychotherapy addressed Lauren's mood and adjustment, as she was prone to depression and mean utterances, emanating from her grief and vulnerabilities. Psychoeducation was utilized to improve her awareness, acceptance, and realism about her stroke and bolster her self-esteem and mastery, given her impressive skill acquisition. Her frequency of CRs also gradually reduced, especially as she became comfortable with her AAC device, which boosted her communication with Talia and the rest of her support network. Due to her depression and disrupted sleep, at the urging of Dr. Gustav, Lauren saw the program psychiatrist. She prescribed sertraline,

50 mg and trazadone, 50 mg. Once Lauren's mood and sleep were better, her daytime sustained attention and initiation improved. Talia was informed that decreased follow through emanated from Lauren's distress and reduced initiation, rather than "laziness." This was reassuring to Talia, who was feeling somewhat mistreated.

Psychotherapeutic interventions were a lifesaver for Talia. At the outset of therapy, her Sense of Self Questionnaire indicated the following statements: "Compared to before my loved one's injury, I get frustrated when I can't make everything GO RIGHT. Since the injury, when I think about the future, I feel scared and depressed. Since the injury, when I think about my role, I am Lauren's everything—her confidant, driver, friend, sister, coach, and sometimes, her enemy. Since my loved one's injury, my life is on fast forward and extremely overwhelming—sometimes, I get so fed up, I can 'lose it' with her." Dr. Gustav introduced Talia to the FEM and enlightened her about CRs by proxy and "narcissistic rage." Due to their prestroke healthy family system, Talia was devoted, warm, flexible, and accommodating, even in the face of life disruption. Through dialogue, she recognized the expected "roller coaster" of emotions from this tumultuous journey and she was able to reframe and alleviate her aggravation. Dr. Gustav also helped her resolve "second-guessing" regarding the causes of the stroke, as Talia attached self-blame for not intervening about Lauren's poor diet and lack of exercise. With his guidance, she was able to draw on her inner strength and develop a hopeful attitude about the future.

Based on the extensive training and support, also in the home environment, Talia reported feeling more confident and capable. She appreciated the new belongings in her "tool kit" she was amassing. As Lauren's mood and outlook perked up, there was a mirrored rallying in Talia. Dr. Gustav provided some tier 3 local resource websites applicable to members of their faith, including case management, support groups, and respite care (e.g., www.ajfca.org). They found the book, *One Hundred Names for Love: A Stroke, a Marriage, and the Language of Healing* by Ackerman (2011) relevant to aphasia and inspiring. Now, they were "making the best" of their predicament.

Dr. Gustav employed positive psychological techniques. Lauren was gaining self-sufficiency and Talia's battery was recharging. The two of them now yearned to get out of the house more. Dr. Gustav proffered the mantra "faith, hope, and love" (see Chap. 2, Sect. 2.4.2.5) and encouraged them to reconnect to their Jewish community. This third tier of support was robust and their friends and congregants were clamoring to provide aid. Lauren and Talia decided to return to weekly Shabbat services. Lauren found that she could participate in the religious service quite well, based on her old retained memory and the fact that she could sing many of the prayers.

Lauren was now ready to meet with the rabbi (a tier 2 support to Lauren and Talia), who frequented their home to provide revelations from Hasidism. He explained that although Lauren and Talia could not understand the cause of darkness, the best way to prevent the bleakness from prevailing was to create additional light through acts of goodness and kindness (Schwartz 2012). For example, their tier 3 synagogue friends prepared many delectable treats and meals and created a schedule for twice-weekly drop-offs, which lasted several months. The congregants also set up an email system whereby they volunteered to provide transportation for Lauren to attend her therapies and volunteer work. Talia was extremely moved by this much-needed attention and affection. Through mindful living, she was galvanized to perform her own "mitzvahs" (good deeds). She began to volunteer at the hospital, visiting with and encouraging other stroke victims' families in the ICU. She then contacted Jewish Family Services to see how she could "pay it forward" through involvement with other families encountering adversity. She was incorporating the teachings of Chabad-Lubavitch and was feeling renewed happiness and gratitude.

References

Academy of Nutrition and Dietetics. (2012). *Cooking for beginners* [Booklet]. Academy of Nutrition and Dietetics.

Ackerman, D. (2011). *One hundred names for love: A stroke, a marriage, and the language of healing*. New York: W. W. Norton.

Aniskiewicz, A. S. (2007). *Psychotherapy for neuropsychological challenges*. Lanham: Jason Aronson.

Bakas, T. (2009). Stroke and the family. In J. Stein, R. L. Harvey, R. F. Macko, C. J. Winstein, & R. D. Zorowitz (Eds.), *Stroke recovery and rehabilitation* (pp. 683–695). New York: Demos Medical Publishing.

Bakas, T., Austin, J. K., Jessup, S. L., Williams, L. S., & Oberst, M. T. (2004). Time and difficulty of tasks provided by family caregivers of stroke survivors. *Journal of Neuroscience Nursing, 36*(2), 95–106.

Baldwin, V. N., Powell, T., & Lorenc, L. (2011). Factors influencing the uptake of memory compensations: A qualitative analysis. *Neuropsychological Rehabilitation, 21*(4), 484–501.

Bauby, J. D. (1998). *The diving bell and the butterfly: A memoir of life in death*. New York: Vintage.

Benson, D. M., & Pavol, M. (2010). Neuropsychological rehabilitation: Evaluation and treatment approaches. In J. Elbaum & D. M. Benson (Eds.), *Acquired brain injury: An integrative neuro-rehabilitation approach* (pp. 122–145). New York: Springer.

Bergström, A. L., Eriksson, G., von Koch, L., & Tham, K. (2011). Combined life satisfaction of persons with stroke and their caregivers: Associations with caregiver burden and the impact of stroke. *Health and Quality of Life Outcomes, 9*(1). Jan 11;9:1. doi:10.1186/1477-7525-9-1.

Blank, A., & Rynn, M. (2012, Sept). *Aphasia treatment & technology*. Presentation at the Barrow Neurological Institute & St. Joseph's Hospital and Medical Center, Stroke Symposium, Phoenix, AZ.

Blonder, L. X., Langer, S. L., Pettigrew, L. C., & Garrity, T. F. (2007). The effects of stroke disability on spousal caregivers. *NeuroRehabilitation, 22,* 85–92.

Boles, L. (2010). *Aphasia couples therapy (ACT) workbook*. San Diego: Plural Publishing.

Bron, A. M., Viswanathan, A. C., Thelen, U., de Natale, R., Ferreras, A., Gundgaard, J., Schwartz, G., & Buchholz, P. (2010). International vision requirements for driver licensing and disability pensions: Using a milestone approach in characterization of progressive eye disease. *Clinical Ophthalmology, 4,* 1361–1369.

Brown, K., Worrall, L., Davidson, B., & Howe, T. (2010). Snapshots of success: An insider perspective on living successfully with aphasia. *Aphasiology, 24*(10), 1267–1295.

Brown, K., Worrall, L., Davidson, B., & Howe, T. (2011). Living successfully with aphasia: Family members share their views. *Topics in Stroke Rehabilitation, 18*(5), 536–548.

Brown, K., Worrall, L. E., Davidson, B., & Howe, T. (2012). Living successfully with aphasia: A qualitative meta-analysis of the perspectives of individuals with aphasia, family members, and speech-language pathologists. *International Journal of Speech-Language Pathology, 14*(2), 141–155.

Butler, D. H. (2007). *My grandpa had a stroke*. Washington, D. C.: Magination Press.

Caine, D., & Watson, J. D. G. (2000). Neuropsychological and neuropathological sequelae of cerebral anoxia: A critical review. *Journal of the International Neuropsychological Society, 6*(1), 86–99.

Cameron, J. I., & Gignac, M. A. (2008). "Timing it right": A conceptual framework for addressing the support needs of family caregivers to stroke survivors from the hospital to the home. *Patient Education and Counseling, 70*(3), 305–314.

Cao, V., Chung, C., Ferreira, A., Nelken, J., Brooks, D., & Cott, C. (2010). Changes in activities of wives caring for their husbands following stroke. *Physiotherapy Canada, 62*(1), 35–43.

Caplan, B. (2010). Rehabilitation psychology and neuropsychology with stroke survivors. In R. G. Frank, M. Rosenthal, & B. Caplan (Eds.), *Handbook of rehabilitation psychology* (2nd ed., pp. 63–94). Washington, D. C.: American Psychological Association.

Capruso, D. X., Hamsher, K. deS., & Benton, A. L. (2006). Clinical evaluation of visual perception and constructional ability. In P. J. Snyder, P. D. Nussbaum, & D. L. Robins (Eds.), *Clinical neuropsychology: A pocket handbook for assessment* (2nd ed., pp. 547–571). Washington, D. C.: American Psychological Association.

Caswell, J. (2005, Sept/Oct). When the eyes don't have it. *Stroke Connection*, 14–16.

Cherney, L. R., & Small, S. L. (2009). Aphasia, apraxia of speech, and dysarthria. In J. Stein, R. L. Harvey, R. F. Macko, C. J. Winstein, & R. D. Zorowitz (Eds.), *Stroke recovery and rehabilitation* (pp. 155–181). New York: Demos Medical Publishing.

Clark, P. C., Dunbar, S. B., Shields, C. G., Viswanathan, B., Aycock, D. M., & Wolf, S. L. (2004). Influence of stroke survivor characteristics and family conflict surrounding recovery on caregivers' mental and physical health. *Nursing Research, 53*(6), 406–413.

Cohen, R. A., Malloy, P. F., Jenkins, M. A., & Paul, R. H. (2006). Disorders of attention. In P. J. Snyder, P. D. Nussbaum, & D. L. Robins (Eds.), *Clinical neuropsychology: A pocket handbook for assessment* (2nd ed., pp. 572–606). Washington, D. C.: American Psychological Association.

Collins, L. G., & Swartz, K. (2011). Caregiver care. *American Academy of Family Physicians, 83*(11), 1309–1317.

Coombs, U. E. (2007). Spousal caregiving for stroke survivors. *Journal of Neuroscience Nursing, 39*(2), 112–119.

Copolillo, A., & Ivanoff, S. D. (2011). Assistive technology and home modification for people with neurovisual deficits. *NeuroRehabilitation, 28*(3), 211–220.

Cullum, C. M., Rilling, L. M., Saine, K., & Samson, D. (2008). Intracranial hemorrhage, vascular malformations, cerebral aneurysms, and subarachnoid hemorrhage. In J. E. Morgan & J. H. Ricker (Eds.), *Textbook of clinical neuropsychology* (pp. 392–410). New York: Taylor & Francis Group.

dePaola, T. (2006). *Now one foot, now the other*. New York: Puffin Books.

Dietz, A., Ball, A., & Griffith, J. (2011). Reading and writing with aphasia in the 21st century: Technological applications of supported reading comprehension and written expression. *Topics in Stroke Rehabilitation, 18*(6), 758–769.

Dimancescu, M. D. (2010). Neurosurgery and acquired brain injury: An educational primer. In J. Elbaum & D. M. Benson (Eds.), *Acquired brain injury: An integrative neuro-rehabilitation approach* (pp. 4–17). New York: Springer.

Douglas, K. (2003). *My stroke of luck*. New York: It Books.

Draper, P., & Brocklehurst, H. (2007). The impact of stroke on the well-being of the patient's spouse: An exploratory study. *Journal of Clinical Nursing, 16*(2), 264–271.

Duarte, R. A., & Fishman, O. (2010). The role of the neurologist in assessment and management of individuals with acquired brain injury. In J. Elbaum & D. M. Benson (Eds.), *Acquired brain injury: An integrative neuro-rehabilitation approach* (pp. 39–63). New York: Springer.

Elbaum, J. (2010). Acquired brain injury and the family: Challenges and interventions. In J. Elbaum & D. M. Benson (Eds.), *Acquired brain injury: An integrative neuro-rehabilitation approach* (pp. 275–285). New York: Springer.

Eldred, C., & Sykes, C. (2008). Psychosocial interventions for carers of survivors of stroke: A systematic review of interventions based on psychological principles and theoretical frameworks. *British Journal of Health Psychology, 13*(Pt 3), 563–581.

Esther Han, M. H. (2010). The role of the neuro-rehabilitation optometrist. In J. Elbaum & D. M. Benson (Eds.), *Acquired brain injury: An integrative neuro-rehabilitation approach* (pp. 146–175). New York: Springer.

Family Caregiver Alliance. (2004). *Fact sheet: Hypoxic-anoxic brain injury* [Booklet]. Redwood City: Family Caregiver Alliance, National Center on Caregiving.

Festa, J. R., Lazar, R. M., & Marshall, R. S. (2008). Ischemic stroke and aphasic disorders. In J. E. Morgan & J. H. Ricker (Eds.), *Textbook of clinical neuropsychology* (pp. 363–383). New York: Taylor & Francis Group.

FitzGerald, A., Aditya, H., Prior, A., McNeil, E., & Pentland, B. (2010). Anoxic brain injury: Clinical patterns and functional outcomes. A study of 93 cases. *Brain Injury, 24*(11), 1311–1323.

Fox, M. (1989). *Wilfrid Gordon McDonald Partridge*. Tulsa: Kane Miller.

Fox, S. W., Mitchell, S. A., & Booth-Jones, M. (2006). Cognitive impairment in patients with brain tumors: Assessment and intervention in the clinic setting. *Clinical Journal of Oncology Nursing, 10*(2), 169–176.

Franzén-Dahlin, A., Larson, J., Murray, V., Wredling, R., & Billing, E. (2007). Predictors of psychological health in spouses of persons affected by stroke. *Journal of Clinical Nursing, 16*(5), 885–891.

Franzén-Dahlin, A., Laska, A., Larson, J., Wredling, R., Billing, E., & Murray, V. (2008). Predictors of life situation among significant others of depressed or aphasic stroke patients. *Journal of Clinical Nursing, 17*(12), 1574–1580.

Fuchigami, D. (2012, Oct.). *Overview of attention*. Presentation at the Center for Transitional NeuroRehabilitation, Barrow Neurological Institute. Relatives' Group Presentation, Phoenix, AZ.

Garcia-Molina, A., Roig-Rovira, T., Enseat-Cantallops, A., Sanchez-Carrion, R., Pico-Azanza, N., Bernabeu, M., & Tormos, J. M. (2006). Neuropsychological profile of persons with anoxic brain injury: Differences regarding physiopathological mechanism. *Brain Injury, 20*(11), 1139–1145.

Gaugler, J. E. (2010). The longitudinal ramifications of stroke caregiving: A systematic review. *Rehabilitation Psychology, 55*(2), 108–125.

Gerrig, R. J., & Zimbardo, P. G. (2002). *Psychology and life* (16th ed.). Boston: Allyn and Bacon.

Gillen, G. (Ed.). (2011). *Stroke rehabilitation: A function-based approach* (3rd ed.). St. Louis: Elsevier Mosby.

Gillespie, A., Murphy, J., & Place, M. (2010). Divergences of perspective between people with aphasia and their family caregivers. *Aphasiology, 24*(12), 1559–1575.

Glen, A., & Hill, A. (2010, Mar.). *Technology as a tool in rehabilitation*. Presentation at the Barrow Neurological Institute & St. Joseph's Hospital and Medical Center, 5th Annual TBI Symposium, Phoenix, AZ.

Green, B. S., Stevens, K. M., & Wolfe, T. D. W. (1997). *Mild traumatic brain injury: A therapy and resource manual*. San Diego: Singular Publishing Group.

Greene, V. (2008). *Conquering stroke: How I fought my way back and how you can too*. Hoboken: Wiley.

Haley, W. E., Allen, J. Y., Grant, J. S., Clay, O. J., Perkins, M., & Roth, D. L. (2009). Problems and benefits reported by stroke family caregivers: Results from a prospective epidemiological study. *Stroke; A Journal of Cerebral Circulation, 40*(6), 2129–2133.

Heilman, K. M. (2009). Right hemispheric neurobehavioral syndromes. In J. Stein, R. L. Harvey, R. F. Macko, C. J. Winstein, & R. D. Zorowitz (Eds.), *Stroke recovery and rehabilitation* (pp. 201–212). New York: Demos Medical Publishing.

Hill, A. (2011, Aug.). *Promoting communication for a person with aphasia*. Presentation at the Center for Transitional NeuroRehabilitation. Barrow Neurological Institute. Relatives' Group Presentation, Phoenix, AZ.

Hopkins, R. O., & Bigler, E. D. (2008). Hypoxic and anoxic conditions of the CNS. In J. E. Morgan & J. H. Ricker (Eds.), *Textbook of clinical neuropsychology* (pp. 521–535). New York: Taylor & Francis Group.

Howard, R. S., Holmes, P. A., & Koutroumanidis, M. A. (2011). Hypoxic-ischaemic brain injury. *Practical Neurology, 11*(1), 4–18.

Howe, T., Davidson, B., Worrall, L., Hersh, D., Ferguson, A., Sherratt, S., & Gilbert, J. (2012). 'You needed to rehab… families as well': Family members' own goals for aphasia rehabilitation. *International Journal of Language & Communication Disorders, 47*(5), 511–521.

Johansson, M. B., Carlsson, M., & Sonnander, K. (2011). Working with families of persons with aphasia: A survey of Swedish speech and language pathologists. *Disability and Rehabilitation, 33*(1), 51–62.

Kearney, P., McGowan, T., Anderson, J., & Strosahl, D. (2010). The role of the occupational therapist on the neuro-rehabilitation team. In J. Elbaum & D. M. Benson (Eds.), *Acquired brain injury: An integrative neuro-rehabilitation approach* (pp. 215–237). New York: Springer.

Klonoff, P. S. (2010). *Psychotherapy after brain injury: Principles and techniques*. New York: Guilford Press.

Klonoff, P. S., & Koberstein, E. J. (2010). Family life. In P. S. Klonoff (Ed.), *Psychotherapy after brain injury: Principles and techniques* (pp. 150–170). New York: Guilford Press.

Klonoff, P. S., Sheperd, J. C., O'Brien, K. P., Chiapello, D. A., & Hodak, J. A. (1990). Rehabilitation and outcome of right-hemisphere stroke patients: Challenges to traditional diagnostic and treatment methods. *Neuropsychology, 4*(3), 147–163.

Klonoff, P. S., Lamb, D. G., & Henderson, S. W. (2001). Outcomes from milieu-based neurorehabilitation at up to 11 years post-discharge. *Brain Injury, 15*(5), 413–428.

Klonoff, P. S., Koberstein, E. J., Talley, M. C., & Dawson, L. K. (2008). A family experiential model of recovery after brain injury. *Bulletin of the Menninger Clinic, 72*(2), 109–129.

Ko, J. Y., Aycock, D. M., & Clark, P. C. (2007). A comparison of working versus nonworking family caregivers of stroke survivors. *Journal of Neuroscience Nursing, 39*(4), 217–225.

Kramer, P., Shein, D., & Napolitano, J. (2010). Rehabilitation of speech, language and swallowing disorders. In J. Elbaum & D. M. Benson (Eds.), *Acquired brain injury: An integrative neuro-rehabilitation approach* (pp. 238–258). New York: Springer.

Kuster, J. M. (2012). Internet: In search of the perfect speech-language app? In *The ASHA Leader*. http://www.asha.org/Publications/leader/2012/120403/Internet-In-Search-of-the-Perfect-Speech-Language-App.htm. Accessed 30 Dec 2012.

Langhorne, P., Bernhardt, J., & Kwakkel, G. (2011). Stroke rehabilitation. *Lancet, 377*(9778), 1693–1702.

Larson, J., Franzén-Dahlin, A., Billiing, E., von Arbin, M., Murray, V., & Wredling, R. (2005). Predictors of quality of life among spouses of stroke patients during the first year after the stroke event. *Scandinavian Journal of Caring Sciences, 19*(4), 439–445.

Lawrence, M., Kerr, S., Watson, H., Paton, G., & Ellis, G. (2010). An exploration of lifestyle beliefs and lifestyle behavior following stroke: Findings from a focus group study of patients and family members. *BMC Family Practice, 11,* 97–107.

Lezak, M. D., Howieson, D. B., Bigler, E. D., & Tranel, D. (2012). *Neuropsychological assessment* (5th ed.). New York: Oxford University Press.

Lillien, L. (2012). *Hungry girl to the max! The ultimate guilt-free cookbook*. New York: St. Martin's Griffin.

Lim, C., Alexander, M. P., LaFleche, G., Schnyer, D. M., & Verfaellie, M. (2004). The neurological and cognitive sequelae of cardiac arrest. *Neurology, 63*(10), 1774–1778.

Lindman, L. (2011, June). *Overview of visual difficulties post injury*. Presentation at the Center for Transitional NeuroRehabilitation, Barrow Neurological Institute. Relatives' Group Presentation, Phoenix, AZ.

Manders, E., Mariën, A., & Janssen, V. (2011). Informing and supporting partners and children of persons with aphasia: A comparison of supply and demand. *Logopedics Phoniatrics Vocology, 36*(4), 139–144.

Markus, H., Pereira, A., & Cloud, G. (2010). *Stroke medicine: Oxford specialist handbooks in neurology*. New York: Oxford University Press.

McCrum, R. (1999). *My year off: Recovering life after a stroke*. New York: Broadway Books.

McEwen, M., & Paisner, D. (2008). *Change in the weather: Life after stroke*. New York: Gotham Books.

McEwen, M., & Paisner, D. (2009). *After the stroke: My journey back to life*. New York: Gotham Books.

McPherson, C. J., Wilson, K. G., Chyurlia, L., & Leclerc, C. (2010). The balance of give and take in caregiver-partner relationships: An examination of self-perceived burden, relationship equity, and quality of life from the perspective of care recipients following stroke. *Rehabilitation Psychology, 55*(2), 194–203.

Megna, J. (2010). Balance and vestibular rehabilitation in the patient with acquired brain injury. In J. Elbaum & D. M. Benson (Eds.), *Acquired brain injury: An integrative neuro-rehabilitation approach* (pp. 200–214). New York: Springer.

National Stroke Association. (2006). *Muscle weakness after stroke: Hemiparesis* [Booklet]. Centeinnal: National Stroke Association.

Nätterlund, B. S. (2010). Being a close relative of a person with aphasia. *Scandinavian Journal of Occupational Therapy, 17*(1), 18–28.

Niemeier, J. P., & Karol, R. L. (2011a). *Overcoming grief and loss after brain injury*. New York: Oxford University Press.

Niemeier, J. P., & Karol, R. L. (2011b). *Therapists' guide to overcoming grief and loss after brain injury*. New York: Oxford University Press.

Nunn, K., Hanstock, T., & Lask, B. (2008). *Who's who of the brain: A guide to its inhabitants, where they live and what they do*. Philadelphia: Jessica Kingsley Publishers.

O'Connor, M. G., & Lafleche, G. (2006). Amnesic syndromes. In P. J. Snyder, P. D. Nussbaum, & D. L. Robins (Eds.), *Clinical neuropsychology: A pocket handbook for assessment* (2nd ed., pp. 463–488). Washington, D. C.: American Psychological Association.

Palmer, S., & Palmer, J. B. (2011). *When your spouse has a stroke: Caring for your partner, yourself, and your relationship*. Baltimore: The Johns Hopkins University Press.

Perrin, P. B., Heesacker, M., Stidham, B. S., Rittman, M. R., & Gonzalez-Rothi, L. J. (2008). Structural equation modeling of the relationship between caregiver psychosocial variables and functioning of individuals with stroke. *Rehabilitation Psychology, 53*(1), 54–62.

Perrin, P. B., Heesacker, M., Uthe, C. E., & Rittman, M. R. (2010). Caregiver mental health and racial/ethnic disparities in stroke: Implications for culturally sensitive interventions. *Rehabilitation Psychology, 55*(4), 372–382.

Peskine, A., Rosso, C., Picq, C., Caron, E., & Pradat-Diehl, P. (2010). Neurological sequelae after cerebral anoxia. *Brain Injury, 24*(5), 755–761.

Prigatano, G. P. (Ed.). (2010). *The study of anosognosia*. New York: Oxford University Press.

Prigatano, G. P., Fordyce, D. J., Zeiner, H. K., Roueche, J. R., Pepping, M., & Wood, B. C. (1986). *Neuropsychological rehabilitation after brain injury*. Baltimore: The Johns Hopkins University Press.

Rigby, H., Gubitz, G., Eskes, G., Reidy, Y., Christian, C., Grover, V., & Phillips, S. (2009). Caring for stroke survivors: Baseline and 1-year determinants of caregiver burden. *International Journal of Stroke, 4*(3), 152–158.

Rombough, R. E., Howse, E. L., Bagg, S. D., & Bartfay, W. J. (2007). A comparision of studies on the quality of life of primary caregivers of stroke survivors: A systematic review of the literature. *Top Stroke Rehabilitation, 14*(3), 69–79.

Rosenberg, C. H., Simantov, J., & Patel, M. (2010). Physiatry and acquired brain injury. In J. Elbaum & D. M. Benson (Eds.), *Acquired brain injury: An integrative neuro-rehabilitation approach* (pp. 18–38). New York: Springer.

Scheiman, M. (2011, February). *Understanding and managing visual deficits: Theory, screening procedures, intervention techniques*. Phoenix: Vision Education Seminars.

Scherer, M. J. (2012). *Assistive technologies and other supports for people with brain impairment*. New York: Springer.

Schure, L. M., van den Heuvel, E. T., Stewart, R. E., Sanderman, R., de Witte, L. P., & Meyboom-de Jong, B. (2006). Beyond stroke: Description and evaluation of an effective intervention to support family caregivers of stoke patients. *Patient Education and Counseling, 62*(1), 46–55.

Schwartz, K. (2012). *Grief and mourning begins for victims of school shooting*. www.chabad.org/news/article_cdo/aid/2075445/jewish/Grief-and-Mourning-Begins-for-Victims-of-School-Shooting.htm. Accessed 30 Dec 2012.

Senelick, R. C. (2010). *Living with stroke: A guide for families* (4th ed.). Birmingham: HealthSouth Press.

Shanmugham, K., Cano, M. A., Elliott, T. R., & Davis, M. (2009). Social problem-solving abilities, relationship satisfaction and depression among family caregivers of stroke survivors. *Brain Injury, 23*(2), 92–100.

Sherratt, S., Worrall, L., Pearson, C., Howe, T., Hersh, D., & Davidson, B. (2011). "Well it has to be language-related": Speech-language pathologists' goals for people with aphasia and their families. *International Journal of Speech-Language Pathology, 13*(4), 317–328.

Siegel, A., Bhatt, S., Bhatt, R., & Zalcman, S. S. (2007). The neurobiological bases for development of pharmacological treatments of aggressive disorders. *Current Neuropharmacology, 5*(2), 135–147.

Simmons-Mackie, N., Raymer, A., Armstrong, E., Holland, A., & Cherney, L. R. (2010). Communication partner training in aphasia: A systematic review. *Archives of Physical Medicine and Rehabilitation, 91*(12), 1814–1837.

Sinanović, O. (2010). Neuropsychology of acute stroke. *Psychiatria Danubina, 22*(2), 278–281.

Smeets, S. M., van Heugten, C. M., Geboers, J. F., Visser-Meily, J. M., & Schepers, V. P. (2012). Respite care after acquired brain injury: The well-being of caregivers and patients. *Archives of Physical Medicine and Rehabilitation, 93*(5), 834–841.

Sohlberg, M. M., & Mateer, C. A. (2001). *Cognitive rehabilitation: An integrative neuropsychological approach*. New York: Guilford Press.

Sohlberg, M. M., & Turkstra, L. S. (2011). *Optimizing cognitive rehabilitation: Effective instructional methods*. New York: Guilford Press.

Solomon, D., & Goldstein, J. E. (2009). Visual, ocular motor, and vestibular deficits. In J. Stein, R. L. Harvey, R. F. Macko, C. J. Winstein, & R. D. Zorowitz (Eds.), *Stroke recovery and rehabilitation* (pp. 227–290). New York: Demos Medical Publishing.

Starkstein, S. E., Fedoroff, J. P., Price, T. R., Leiguarda, R., & Robinson, R. G. (1993). Catastrophic reaction after cerebrovascular lesions: Frequency, correlates, and validation of a scale. *Journal of Neuropsychiatry, 5*(2), 189–194.

Stein, J. (2004). *Stroke and the family: A new guide*. Cambridge: Harvard University Press.

Stein, J., Harvey, R. L., Macko, R. F., Winstein, C. J., & Zorowitz, R. D. (Eds.). (2009). *Stroke recovery and rehabilitation*. New York: Demos Medical Publishing.

Stewart, C., & Riedel, K. (2011). Managing speech and language deficits after stroke. In G. Gillen (Ed.), *Stroke rehabilitation: A function-based approach* (3rd ed., pp. 534–552). St. Louis: Elsevier Mosby.

Taylor, J. B. (2009). *My stroke of insight: A brain scientist's personal journey*. New York: Plume.

Tröster, A. I., & Arnett, P. A. (2006). Assessment of movement and demyelinating disorders. In P. J. Snyder, P. D. Nussbaum, & D. L. Robins (Eds.), *Clinical neuropsychology: A pocket handbook for assessment* (2nd ed., pp. 243–293). Washington, D. C.: American Psychological Association.

Uchino, K., Pary, J., & Grotta, J. (2011). *Acute stroke care: A manual from the University of Texas-Houston Stroke Team* (2nd ed.). New York: Cambridge University Press.

van de Sandt-Koenderman, W. M. E. (2011). Aphasia rehabilitation and the role of computer technology: Can we keep up with modern times? *International Journal of Speech-Language Pathology, 13*(1), 21–27.

Venkatesan, A., & Frucht, S. (2006). Movement disorders after resuscitation from cardiac arrest. *Neurologic Clinics, 24*(1), 123–132.

Verfaellie, M., & Heilman, K. M. (2006). Neglect syndromes. In P. J. Snyder, P. D. Nussbaum, & D. L. Robins (Eds.), *Clinical neuropsychology: A pocket handbook for assessment* (2nd ed., pp. 489–507). Washington, D. C.: American Psychological Association.

Visser-Meily, A., Post, M., van de Port, I., Maas, C., Forstberg-Wärleby, G., & Lindeman, E. (2009). Psychosocial functioning of spouses of patients with stroke from initial inpatient rehabilitation to 3 years poststroke: Course and relations with coping strategies. *Stroke; A Journal of Cerebral Circulation, 40*(4), 1399–1404.

Waldron, B., Casserly, L. M., & O'Sullivan, C. (2012). Cognitive behavioural therapy for depression and anxiety in adults with acquired brain injury. What works for whom? *Neuropsychological Rehabilitation: An International Journal*, Nov. 5. doi:10.1080/09602011.2012.724196. Epub ahead of print.

Waldron-Perrine, B., Hanks, R. A., & Perrine, S. A. (2008). Pharmacotherapy for postacute traumatic brain injury: A literature review for guidance in psychological practice. *Rehabilitation Psychology, 53*(4), 426–444.

Warren, M. (2005, April). *Evaluation and treatment of visual perceptual dysfunction in adult brain injury part 1*. Continuing Education Seminar at visABILITIES Rehab Services, Inc., Baltimore, MD.

Weinstein, A., & Swenson, R. A. (2006). Cerebrovascular disease. In P. J. Snyder, P. D. Nussbaum, & D. L. Robins (Eds.), *Clinical neuropsychology: A pocket handbook for assessment* (2nd ed., pp. 294-317). Washington, D. C.: American Psychological Association.

Wilkinson, R., & Wielaert, S. (2012). Rehabilitation targeted at everyday communication: Can we change the talk of people with aphasia and their significant others within conversation? *Archives of Physical Medicine and Rehabilitation, 93*(1 Suppl), S70–S76.

Wilkinson, R., Lock, S., Bryan, K., & Sage, K. (2011). Interaction-focused intervention for acquired language disorders: Facilitating mutual adaptation in couples where one partner has aphasia. *International Journal of Speech-Language Pathology, 13*(1), 74–87.

Williams, O. (2010). *Stroke diaries: A guide for survivors and their families*. New York: Oxford University Press.

Wilson, B. A. (2009). *Memory rehabilitation: Integrating theory and practice*. New York: Guilford Press.

Wilson, B. A., & Kapur, N. (2009). *Compensating for memory deficits with memory aids. In memory rehabilitation: Integrating theory and practice* (pp. 52–73). New York: Guilford Press.

Chapter 7
Family Psychotherapy After a Brain Tumor

7.1 Scenario: Early Questions About Brain Tumors

This chapter provides a general overview of brain tumors, their effects on the loved one, as well as treatment options. Importantly, the focus is on the consequences for the family, as well as constructive coping mechanisms provided by the psychotherapist. Other excellent resources about brain tumors include *Living with a Brain Tumor: Dr. Peter Black's Guide to Taking Control of Your Treatment* by Black and Hogan (2006); *Orientation to Caregiving: A Handbook for Family Caregivers of Patients with Brain Tumors* by Goodman et al. (2007); http://www.abta.org/Care_&_Support/Orientation_to_Caregiving/227; "Support Organizations, Resources, and Relevant Websites" by Grenier and Gupta (2009); *100 Questions & Answers about Brain Tumors* by Stark-Vance and Dubay (2011); *Fast Facts: Brain Tumors* by Abrey and Mason (2011); and website information from the American Brain Tumor Association (www.abta.org), National Brain Tumor Society (www.braintumor.org), and Healing Exchange Brain Trust (www.braintrust.org). *Navigating Through a Strange Land* by Roloff (2010) is a unique resource which offers stories through the eyes of patients, families, and professionals.

The diagnosis of a brain tumor in a loved one is devastating and frightening for him or her, and undoubtedly the family. All parties may have some passing familiarity with various forms of cancer in other body parts, which can add to the alarm and angst. Many worries and questions arise related to the aftermath and prognosis. The family may ask questions such as: *What does it mean that my loved one has a brain tumor? What type of tumor does my loved one have? Will my loved one live? What happens next regarding treatment?*

7.1.1 Therapeutic Intervention: Neuropathology of Brain Tumors

The psychotherapist can provide a calming influence on the frantic family by reviewing fundamental educational material which will help the caregiver and relatives

P. S. Klonoff, *Psychotherapy for Families after Brain Injury*,
DOI 10.1007/978-1-4899-8083-0_7,

navigate a complex and foreign medical system. This includes the diagnostic process of brain tumors as well as brain tumor types and symptoms. This sets the stage for building awareness.

More often than not, the initial diagnosis of a brain tumor is made by a neurologist or neurosurgeon working with a team of specialists (Black and Hogan 2006). Other physicians involved in the diagnosis and treatment of brain tumors include neuro-oncologists, neuropathologists, medical oncologists, and radiation oncologists (Black and Hogan 2006; Goodman et al. 2007; National Brain Tumor Society 2010a; U.S. Department of Health and Human Services et al. 2003 [http://www.cancer.gov/cancertopics/wyntk/brain/page1]). A multidisciplinary approach optimizes the care (Abrey and Mason 2011). Brain tumors arise from cancer cells, which include those that form unnecessarily or, conversely, do not die when they are supposed to (Roloff 2010; U.S. Department of Health and Human Services et al. 2003). Brain tumors that emanate in the brain are called *primary tumors* (Black and Hogan 2006). They usually originate from glial cells (Sawrie 2006), which form the connective tissue of the brain and are the cells that support neurons (Carter et al. 2009; Hannay et al. 2004; Stark-Vance and Dubay 2011). Primary brain tumors are caused by genetic predisposition and/or an environmental trigger (Black and Hogan 2006; Lu-Emerson and Norden 2011; Palmieri 2007).

Brain tumors may also have metastasized (i.e., spread) from other cancerous locations in the body, including the breast, lung, skin, colon, or kidney (Abrey and Mason 2011; Anderson and Ryken 2008; Black and Hogan 2006; Buckner et al. 2007; see Fabi et al. 2011, for a review; Sawrie 2006; Stark-Vance and Dubay 2011; Vargo 2011). Metastatic tumors (or secondary tumors) are ten times more common than primary brain tumors (Buckner et al. 2007).

Brain tumors can affect the actual brain tissue or the surrounding coverings of the brain, called meninges (Anderson and Ryken 2008; see Hannay et al. 2004, for a review).

Risk factors for brain tumors include the male gender, Caucasians, the elderly, a positive family history for gliomas, and workers' exposure to radiation, formaldehyde, plastics, and textiles (Abrey and Mason 2011; Black and Hogan 2006; National Brain Tumor Society 2010a; Stark-Vance and Dubay 2011; U.S. Department of Health and Human Services et al. 2003). The onset of symptoms in a loved one can vary, based on the type and malignancy of the tumor. Sometimes, tumors are slow growing, resulting in the gradual emergence of symptoms (Anderson and Ryken 2008). In this case, the loved one and family may misattribute subtle deterioration as caused by depression, aging, or stress (Anderson and Ryken 2008). More rapidly growing brain tumors (including metastatic tumors) can result in the sudden onset of symptoms, including a seizure, nausea, vomiting, headaches as well as speech, vision, or motor changes (e.g., numbness or tingling; Anderson and Ryken 2008; see Hannay et al. 2004, for a review; Stark-Vance and Dubay 2011).

The diagnosis of brain tumors is usually done using some form of a magnetic resonance imaging (MRI) and computed tomography (CT) scans (Abrey and Mason 2011; Anderson and Ryken 2008; Black and Hogan 2006; Buckner et al. 2007; Chandana et al. 2008; National Brain Tumor Society 2010a; Picozzi and Kirchin 2007;

Sawrie 2006; Stark-Vance and Dubay 2011; U.S. Department of Health and Human Services et al. 2003). Other diagnostic tools are positron emission tomography (PET), single-photon emission computed tomography (SPECT), and angiography (Abrey and Mason 2011; Black and Hogan 2006). However, for a definitive diagnosis, a surgical biopsy or resection to examine the cells under a microscope is required (Abrey and Mason 2011; Black and Hogan 2006; Buckner et al. 2007; National Brain Tumor Society 2010a; Palmieri 2007; Stark-Vance and Dubay 2011; U.S. Department of Health and Human Services et al. 2003).

Brain tumors are considered either benign or malignant. *Benign* tumors are typically slow growing and once removed, usually do not recur (Roloff 2010; Stark-Vance and Dubay 2011; U.S. Department of Health and Human Services et al. 2003). Although, in general, benign tumors do not invade tissues around them or spread elsewhere, they can press on other sensitive areas of the brain (U.S. Department of Health and Human Services et al. 2003). Benign tumors can also become lethal, based on their location in the brain, ability to infiltrate brain tissue, and a potential to become malignant (e.g., malignant transformation; Palmieri 2007; Stark-Vance and Dubay 2011). In contrast, *malignant* brain tumors do recur (Picozzi and Kirchin 2007). Their rate of regrowth depends on a number of factors, including the type and malignancy of the tumor. The malignancy of primary brain tumors increases with age while the survival rate decreases (see Vargo 2011, for a review).

The World Health Organization has a four-tier system based on the features of the tumor cells (Anderson and Ryken 2008; Sawrie 2006). They are categorized as grades I–IV, with progressive malignancy (Anderson and Ryken 2008). Cells from higher grade tumors are more abnormal and generally grow faster (U.S. Department of Health and Human Services et al. 2003). Generally, a pathologist will grade the malignancy of the brain tumor (Black and Hogan 2006). Your loved one's physician may also assign a Karnofsky performance score (KPS), which rates the ability to perform daily tasks on a scale of 1–100 (100 = normal; Black and Hogan 2006). Table 7.1 describes different types of brain tumors (Abrey and Mason 2011; Anderson and Ryken 2008; Black and Hogan 2006; Buckner et al. 2007; Chandana et al. 2008; DiPatri et al. 2009; see Hannay et al. 2004, for a review; National Brain Tumor Society 2010a; Norden et al. 2011; Stark-Vance and Dubay 2011; U.S. Department of Health and Human Services et al. 2003; Vargo 2011).

Brain tumors affect function in four ways: general symptoms related to increased intracranial pressure (e.g., headaches, nausea, vomiting); seizures; focal symptoms (e.g., aphasia or hemiparesis); and secretion of hormones (Chandana et al. 2008; see Hannay et al. 2004, for a review; Palmieri 2007). Unlike a traumatic brain injury, the effects of brain tumors are typically more discrete, that is, they affect focal areas of the brain where the tumor is growing (see Hannay et al. 2004, for a review). This is especially the case at the initial stages and the tumor will produce circumscribed changes in abilities, including thinking, vision, physical, or emotional domains (Anderson and Ryken 2008; Chandana et al. 2008). Examples of focal changes are executive function deficits, expressive aphasia, and personality changes with frontal lobe tumors; memory and vision difficulties caused by temporal lobe tumors; and comprehension problems with parietal lobe tumors (Aldrich and Peterson 2010;

Table 7.1 Common types of brain tumors

Benign tumors: nongliomas
1. *Meningioma:* This tumor arises from the covering surrounding the brain between the brain and the skull (i.e., the meninges) and is the most common form of benign brain tumors. It is more common in women. It is usually slow growing and can cause relatively few symptoms until it grows large enough. A meningioma can often be removed by surgery or focused radiation
2. *Pituitary adenoma:* This tumor occurs in the pituitary and causes increased secretion of hormones. Headaches and vision symptoms are common, based on its proximity to vision centers. Treatment includes clinical observation by the physician, surgery, or radiation
3. *Acoustic neuroma:* This tumor is also called a vestibular schwannoma. It arises from cells which line the nerve that controls balance and hearing. The tumor causes dizziness and hearing loss. Other symptoms include ringing in the ears, facial weakness and numbness, headache, and double vision. This tumor tends to be slow growing and can be treated with surgery or radiation
Primary brain tumors: Gliomas
1. *Astrocytoma:* This is the most common type of primary brain tumor. It can start as a low grade one, but usually progresses to higher grades. Low-grade tumors are often diagnosed in young adults and can begin with seizures. Survival rates are approximately 5 years (but can be longer). Anaplastic astrocytomas are grade III and tend to occur in the fourth or fifth decades of life. Glioblastomas are grade IV and tend to occur in the fifth to seventh decades of life. Grade III and especially grade IV tumors are the most common glial tumors in adults and are much more aggressive. Because they infiltrate the brain, the usual treatment approach is surgical debulking, followed by radiation and chemotherapy. Survival rates for grade III tumors are approximately 2–4 years and less than 1 year to 18 months for grade IV tumors
2. *Oligodendroglioma:* This tumor is more common in men, in the age range of 20s–30s. It often occurs in the frontal or temporal lobes and arises from the cells that cover and protect nerves. A seizure, headache, or hemiparesis are often the presenting symptoms. This tends to be a slow-growing tumor, unless it becomes an anaplastic oligodendroglioma, which then becomes a more aggressive form of tumor. The typical treatment approach is surgery, followed by radiation and/or chemotherapy. The general life expectancy is about 7–10 years for an oligodendroglioma and 3–5 years for an anaplastic oligodendroglioma
3. *Ependymoma:* This tumor grows from cells that line the brain ventricles. It may present with hydrocephalus, seizures, headache, cerebellar or brainstem signs, or focal neurological symptoms. This tumor can be low or higher grade (anaplastic). Usually, surgical resection is performed and the tumor may recur. The survival rate is about 5 years

Goodman et al. 2007; Stark-Vance and Dubay 2011; see also Chap. 4, for a review of neuroanatomy). Sometimes, brain tumors occur in multiple sites in the brain and then produce multifocal changes (Anderson and Ryken 2008). This is especially common with metastatic brain tumors. There are also some associated changes in brain tissue and neurological functioning related to brain swelling (Anderson and Ryken 2008; Hannay et al. 2004).

7.1.2 Treatment of Brain Tumors

As depicted in the Family Experiential Model (FEM) of Recovery (Klonoff and Koberstein 2010; Klonoff et al. 2008; see Chap. 1, Sect. 1.5 and Fig. 1.3), predictable reactions on the part of the family and loved one at the first diagnosis of a brain tumor are disbelief, horror, and panic. Feeling on overload because of the crisis, some

Table 7.2 "Helpful hints" and considerations when seeking treatment for the loved one's brain tumor

Attend the loved one's medical appointments
Be prepared with possible questions and take notes/audio record all medical appointments
Find a physician who is trustworthy and receptive to input from your loved one and the family
Obtain a second opinion to confirm the diagnosis and compare treatment options:
Keep a complete set of records
Research possible out-of-pocket expenses in advance
Names of specialists are available through brain tumor resources
Connect with others with similar challenges for support and resources
Learn about treatment options and their side effects:
Neurosurgery
Radiation therapy
Chemotherapy
Corticosteroid medications
Anticonvulsant medications
Shunts
Be vigilant about contacting the treating physicians if the loved one's health deteriorates during treatment
Advocate for neurorehabilitation for the loved one, taking into account his or her health status and energy level

relatives may denounce the findings and retreat into denial (see Chap. 2, Sect. 2.3.4; Klonoff 2010). This can manifest as ignoring or outright rejecting recommendations and trying to "go about the normal business of the day." Not recognizing the potential ramifications of the diagnosis, the caregiver may inadvertently overtax the loved one by foisting the responsibilities of treatment upon him or her. Given the tumult and urgency, the psychotherapist should identify the best candidate to function as a tier 1 caregiver or selfobject to bolster the loved one's fragile emotions (see Chap. 1, Sects. 1.3 and 1.2.2). This individual will need guidance by the therapist to be as actively involved as possible, including when necessary, taking an advocacy role for the loved one.

Table 7.2 summarizes "helpful hints" and considerations for families when seeking treatment for their loved one's brain tumor. Once the brain tumor is diagnosed, it is crucial that a family member attend appointments with the loved one. The caregiver (and loved one) should be prepared in advance with possible questions and also take notes during the medical appointments (Goodman et al. 2007; U.S. Department of Health and Human Services et al. 2003). Other publications contain a list of topics and sample questions including the name, cause (i.e., primary versus metastatic), and grade of the tumor; whether it is benign or malignant; expected symptoms; treatment options, timelines, and side effects; prognosis; possible lifestyle changes; availability of clinical trials (or research study to evaluate the effectiveness of new drugs and procedures); how to obtain a second opinion; and how the physician can be reached (also in case of a medical emergency; Aldrich and Peterson 2010; Black and Hogan 2006; Goodman et al. 2007; National Brain Tumor Society 2011a). It may be beneficial to audio record the appointments (with the physician's permission) so as to review salient information as needed in the future. This also helps inform others in the support network who could not attend the appointment (Goodman et al. 2007).

It is paramount that the loved one and family find a physician who is trustworthy and respectful of the input from his or her patient and relatives (Black and Hogan 2006). The support network should practice open communication and share specific thoughts and questions so as to establish a collaborative relationship (Aldrich and Peterson 2010; Goodman et al. 2007). Generally, it is also advisable to obtain a second opinion to confirm the diagnosis and compare treatment options (Aldrich and Peterson 2010; Black and Hogan 2006; National Brain Tumor Society 2011b; Roloff 2010; Stark-Vance and Dubay 2011; U.S. Department of Health and Human Services et al. 2003). Obtaining a second opinion can be from another physician or through a hospital tumor board, which is a meeting of specialists who analyze the loved one's tumor status and then make a group recommendation (National Brain Tumor Society 2011b). Other reasons to consider a second opinion are when the first physician has less experience with brain tumors, especially if it is a rare type; a lack of rapport with the first physician; and/or the family and loved one are interested in clinical trial research options (National Brain Tumor Society 2011b; Roloff 2010).

The primary caregiver (and the loved one) should always keep a complete set of records for easy accessibility and to facilitate obtaining a second opinion. The physician or tumor board will need copies of the pathology reports, laboratory tests, medical records, and physician notes (National Brain Tumor Society 2011b). Of note, the family should research the possible out-of-pocket expenses for obtaining a second opinion, based on the insurance company's benefits in this regard (National Brain Tumor Society 2011b). Resources are available to obtain names of specialists for a second opinion (e.g., medical center websites; National Brain Tumor Society's Patient Services; National Cancer Institute). Connecting with other families who have a loved one with a similar type of brain tumor and treatment is another meaningful mechanism to learn more about the implications of the brain tumor diagnosis (Aldrich and Peterson 2010).

The main forms of treatment for brain tumors are neurosurgery, radiation therapy, and chemotherapy, or some combination of these (Abrey and Mason 2011; Anderson and Ryken 2008; Goldman and Turner 2009; National Brain Tumor Society 2010a; Palmieri 2007; Picozzi and Kirchin 2007; Roloff 2010; Stark-Vance and Dubay 2011; U.S. Department of Health and Human Services et al. 2003). Neurosurgery is the initial therapy for nearly all patients and can be curative for benign tumors (Black and Hogan 2006; Buckner et al. 2007; Chandana et al. 2008). Surgery also relieves the symptoms of mass effects, which constitutes the impinging of the tumor on the brain structures (Black and Hogan 2006). Metastatic tumors are typically treated using surgical interventions as well as whole brain or targeted radiation (Buckner et al. 2007; Fabi et al. 2011).

The physicians' advice about neurosurgery will take into account the location and characteristics of the tumor (i.e., its invasiveness and relation to the blood supply); its proximity to vital brain structures as well as the functional and physical status of the loved one (Anderson and Ryken 2008; National Brain Tumor Society 2010a). Sometimes, the entire tumor cannot be removed; however, the neurosurgeon will elect to remove as much of the tumor as possible and then proceed with radiation and/or chemotherapy (Anderson and Ryken 2008; Hannay et al. 2004; National

Brain Tumor Society 2010a). Side effects of surgery include damage to normal tissue, headaches, fatigue, weakness, brain swelling or edema, and infection (U.S. Department of Health and Human Services et al. 2003). Cerebral edema can result in headaches, nausea, vomiting, altered mental status, and focal neurological symptoms (Drappatz and Wen 2011). Corticosteroids (e.g., dexamethasone, prednisone) can be prescribed to reduce the effects of edema (Black and Hogan 2006; Drappatz and Wen 2011; National Brain Tumor Society 2010a; Stark-Vance and Dubay 2011; U.S. Department of Health and Human Services et al. 2003).

Radiation therapy can be a follow-up to neurosurgery or, alternatively, the treatment of choice when it is a better intervention or if the tumor is inoperable (Black and Hogan 2006; Palmieri 2007; U.S. Department of Health and Human Services et al. 2003). For a more detailed description of radiation treatment types, see information from Black and Hogan (2006); the National Brain Tumor Society (2010a); Shih et al. (2009), as well as Stark-Vance and Dubay (2011). Radiation treatment is designed to deliver higher doses of radiation to the tumor than to surrounding normal brain tissue, thereby killing cancer cells and shrinking the tumor (Abrey and Mason 2011; Buckner et al. 2007; National Brain Tumor Society 2010a; Stark-Vance and Dubay 2011; U.S. Department of Health and Human Services et al. 2003). It can be delivered externally or internally (Chandana et al. 2008).

Forms of external beam radiotherapy include involved-field radiation and stereotactic radiosurgery (e.g., Gamma Knife and CyberKnife; Black and Hogan 2006; Buckner et al. 2007; Chandana et al. 2008; National Brain Tumor Society 2010a; Stark-Vance and Dubay 2011). An external beam often consists of 25–35 daily treatments administered over a 5–7 week period (Chandana et al. 2008). Stereotactic radiosurgery uses a narrow beam of radiation directed at the tumor from various angles. Depending on the method, the loved one will wear a rigid head frame (Stark-Vance and Dubay 2011; U.S. Department of Health and Human Services et al. 2003). This technique usually delivers a single high dose of radiation in a 1-day session, although it can be given in two to three doses (Chandana et al. 2008). Interstitial radiotherapy involves surgical implantation of radioactive substances directly inside the tumor (Chandana et al. 2008).

Side effects of radiation vary according to the loved one's age, the radiation dose, and the volume and location of the irradiated brain (De Luca et al. 2009; Landier et al. 2009; Stark-Vance and Dubay 2011). They include mental "fogginess," headaches, weakness, fatigue, nausea, hair loss, ear congestion, or skin problems (Abrey and Mason 2011; Black and Hogan 2006; see De Luca et al. 2009, for a review; see Monje and Wen 2009, for a review; National Brain Tumor Society 2010a; Stark-Vance and Dubay 2011; U.S. Department of Health and Human Services et al. 2003). Other neurological sequelae include swelling and inflammation of the brain tissue, radiation necrosis (whereby healthy brain tissue dies), and sometimes memory difficulties (Abrey and Mason 2011; Black and Hogan 2006; see De Luca et al. 2009, for a review; Johnson et al. 2011; Monje and Wen 2009; Stark-Vance and Dubay 2011; U.S. Department of Health and Human Services et al. 2003).

Chemotherapy employs drugs to kill the cancer cells and is administered either by mouth or by injection into a vein, artery, cerebrospinal fluid, or tumor site (see Black and Hogan 2006, for a review; National Brain Tumor Society 2010a; see Stark-Vance and Dubay 2011, for a review; U.S. Department of Health and Human Services et al. 2003). It is often used to treat recurrent gliomas (Black and Hogan 2006). Chemotherapy is often administered by a neuro-oncologist or medical oncologist (Black and Hogan 2006; National Brain Tumor Society 2010a). Often the drug regimen occurs in cycles, with a recovery period between each cycle (Stark-Vance and Dubay 2011; U.S. Department of Health and Human Services et al. 2003). Some examples of chemotherapy drugs are BCNU (carmustine), CCNU (lomustine), and Temodar (temozolomide; Abrey and Mason 2011; see Black and Hogan 2006, for a review; National Brain Tumor Society 2010a; see Stark-Vance and Dubay 2011, for a review). Sometimes, more than one drug will be combined (Black and Hogan 2006). A neurosurgeon may also elect to place Gliadel wafers (a dissolvable wafer containing a chemotherapy drug) during neurosurgery into malignant glial tumors (Stark-Vance and Dubay 2011). For more information about types and effects of chemotherapy, see Gururangan (2009) and Abrey and Mason (2011).

Side effects of chemotherapy include fever, chills, nausea, vomiting, low blood counts (white and red cells), diarrhea, constipation, sore mouth, bleeding, appetite loss, fatigue, and weakness (Black and Hogan 2006; National Brain Tumor Society 2010a; Palmieri 2007; U.S. Department of Health and Human Services et al. 2003). Dexamethasone, ondansetron, granisetron, lorazepam, and diphenhydramine have been used to reduce nausea and vomiting (Black and Hogan 2006; Stark-Vance and Dubay 2011). The psychotherapist can encourage the family to include the input of a dietician to assist the loved one with appetite and weight-loss issues associated with nausea and vomiting (see Stark-Vance and Dubay 2011, for a review). Deficits in concentration and memory have also been reported, sometimes referred to as "chemofog" or "chemobrain" (see Monje and Wen 2009, for a review).

Myelosuppression is a complication of chemotherapy and radiation and is characterized by signs and symptoms of bleeding and infection (e.g., anemia, leucopenia or a low white cell count, or thrombocytopenia or low platelets; Palmieri 2007). Warning signs include fever, edema, easy bruising, and tarry stools (Palmieri 2007). The tier 1 caregiver should contact the loved one's neuro-oncologist immediately if these symptoms occur (Palmieri 2007).

Other treatment modalities include anticonvulsants for seizures or shunts to reduce the buildup of cerebrospinal fluid in the brain (U.S. Department of Health and Human Services et al. 2003). For a description of other newer treatment modalities, see Black and Hogan (2006).

The psychotherapist can help tier supports recognize the need for neurorehabilitation for their loved one if this is not proposed by the medical professionals. The therapeutic schedule will need to take into account the loved one's individualized needs (Anderson and Ryken 2008) in the context of his or her overall health status and energy level. However, even part-time therapies can be invaluable to address focal deficits. Consider liaisoning with a rehabilitation physician, neuropsychologist, psychiatrist, physical therapist, occupational therapist, recreational therapist, speech–language pathologist, dietician, social worker, and/or an ophthalmologist, based on the needs of the loved one (Black and Hogan 2006; Goodman et al. 2007; Palmieri 2007; Roloff 2010; Stark-Vance and Dubay 2011; see also Sects. 7.2.2, 7.3.2, and 7.4.2).

7.2 Scenario: Physical Challenges

Depending on the location of the tumor, the loved one may have physical manifestations of the brain tumor early or later on. Family members may have questions and anxieties about these symptoms and may ask questions such as: *How come my loved one has weakness on his or her right (or left) side of his or her body? How come he or she is so tired? How come his or her balance is so poor?*

7.2.1 Overview of Physical Challenges

The psychotherapist can explain that physical impairments are common with all types of brain tumors and these correspond to the location of the brain tumor. There are also general changes, including weakness, reduced energy, and increased fatigue, which can also be caused by deconditioning; depression and anxiety; sleep disturbances; pain; decreased appetite; the consequences of surgery, chemotherapy (e.g., anemia), radiation, and seizures; overexertion as well as side effects of some medications (e.g., antiepileptic drugs and steroids; National Brain Tumor Society 2011c; Palmieri 2007; Stark-Vance and Dubay 2011; see Vargo 2011, for a review). Fatigue has been reported as the most common and troubling symptom (see Drappatz and Wen 2011, for a review; see Wefel et al. 2011, for a review).

Other common physical problems include double vision, facial muscle weakness, and hemiparesis related to brainstem tumors; reduced balance, posture, coordination, and unsteady gait caused by cerebellar tumors; sensory loss due to thalamic tumors; hemiparesis or hemiplegia associated with frontal lobe tumors; reduced sensation with parietal lobe tumors; and vision impairment due to occipital lobe tumors (Aldrich and Peterson 2010; Chandana et al. 2008; Goodman et al. 2007; Palmieri 2007; Stark-Vance and Dubay 2011; see also Chap. 4, Fig. 4.3 and Chap. 6, Sect. 6.5).

As stated above, headaches are a common symptom of brain tumors; estimates are that up to 77% of patients report headaches (Abrey and Mason 2011; Goodman et al. 2007; see Loghin and Levin 2006, for a review; see Mea et al. 2011, for a review; see Vargo 2011, for a review). They are more likely with rapidly growing tumors (Purdy and Kirby 2004). Headaches can emerge from the direct effects of the brain tumor (e.g., type and site), increased intracranial pressure, aftereffects of craniotomies, brain swelling, the degree of midline shift of the brain structures, hydrocephalus, and the effects of radiation (Kirby and Purdy 2007; see Loghin and Levin 2006, for a review; see Mea et al. 2011, for a review; Purdy and Kirby 2004). The pain is usually dull, but can also be felt as pressure, pulsating, throbbing, or shooting (Kirby and Purdy 2007; see Loghin and Levin 2006, for a review; Mea et al. 2011).

7.2.2 "Helpful Hints" and Tools for Families to Cope with Physical Changes in their Loved Ones

Table 7.3 provides "helpful hints" and tools for families to cope with the physical changes in their loved ones with a brain tumor. Consultations with treating physicians

Table 7.3 "Helpful hints" and tools for families to cope with physical changes in their loved ones with a brain tumor

Consult with treating physicians to reduce fatigue by improving sleep, mood, pain levels, hormonal imbalances, exercise, diet, stress, and contributory health conditions
Explore the benefit of psychostimulants with the physician
Help the loved one keep an energy log to ascertain fatigue triggers and share this with appropriate medical professionals
Help your loved one modify activities to reduce tiredness:
Shorter and less strenuous activities
Energy conservation techniques
Adopt realistic expectations
Promote a healthy lifestyle
Work with physical and occupational therapists or a physical trainer to address physical sequelae
Incorporate home visits and assistive devices, especially when his/her health status deteriorates
Work with physicians, including possibly a pain specialist, to manage headaches

to improve sleep, mood, pain, and hormonal imbalances can reduce the debilitating repercussions of fatigue (National Brain Tumor Society 2011c; Vargo 2011). Fatigue can also be improved through exercise, a high protein diet, adequate hydration, avoidance of sugary foods, vitamin supplements, proper sleep hygiene, stress management, and treatment of other health conditions, such as anemia (National Brain Tumor Society 2011c; Stark-Vance and Dubay 2011; see Wefel et al. 2011, for a review; Vargo 2011). Some physicians will prescribe psychostimulants to reduce fatigue (see Drappatz and Wen 2011, for a review).

The psychotherapist or other therapist (e.g., a physical or occupational therapist) can provide practical suggestions to manage fatigue, including helping the caregiver develop a log of energy levels and track fatigue triggers (National Brain Tumor Society 2011c). This should be shared with treating physicians for their input. Also, the tier supports and loved one can improve their acceptance and adopt realistic expectations by modifying certain activities to reduce tiredness. These include shorter or less strenuous versions (e.g., attending social gatherings for shorter periods) and fostering energy conservation by resting, napping, self-pacing, and removing or adjusting various activities of daily living (e.g., sit to fold laundry; National Brain Tumor Society 2010a, 2011c; Palmieri 2007; Stark-Vance and Dubay 2011). The psychotherapist can reinforce a holistic approach which promotes an overall healthy lifestyle, including physical exercise, balanced nutrition (adequate consumption of fruits and vegetables), and smoking cessation, as these may reduce the risk of adverse consequences, morbidity, and mortality (Rosenthal et al. 2009; Willard et al. 2009).

Physical and occupational therapists can also address other physical sequelae (Bartolo et al. 2011; Kakuda et al. 2010), including when there is a deteriorating course (Aldrich and Peterson 2010). Under some circumstances, engaging the input of a physical trainer may also be advantageous (Rosenthal et al. 2009). Stretching, strengthening, and balance exercises as well as walking have been shown to improve activities of daily living and mobility in patients with meningiomas (Bartolo et al. 2011). Endurance training for generalized weakness and remediation of specific difficulties can enhance functionality and quality of life.

Often, the physical and occupational therapists will offer to do a functional assessment in the form of a home visit so as to better ascertain the loved one's particular needs and challenges. Safety considerations include removing objects which can increase the likelihood of accidents (e.g., rugs; Aldrich and Peterson 2010) and making modifications in the bathroom and shower to prevent slipping (e.g., grab bars). Keeping pathways well lit at night also reduces the likelihood of falls (Aldrich and Peterson 2010). Assistive devices (e.g., a cane, wheelchair) may be needed to maximize the loved one's safety in the home and community environments.

As the loved one's health status deteriorates, cognitive alterations in judgment and safety awareness can negatively impact the loved one's ability to be unsupervised or make healthy choices and decisions about ambulation, exercises, and hobbies. Therefore, close liaison with the therapists and treating physicians is essential so that the loved one does not incur some avoidable mishap. Soliciting the assistance of a visiting nurse may be warranted (Palmieri 2007).

The psychotherapist should encourage the tier 1 caregiver to work closely with the treating physicians (e.g., neurosurgeon, neuro-oncologist, radiation therapist) regarding management of headaches (Goodman et al. 2007; Loghin and Levin 2006). Treatment options include medications (corticosteroids, analgesics, opioids), whole-brain radiation, shunting for hydrocephalus, and surgery (Black and Hogan 2006; Kirby and Purdy 2007; see Loghin and Levin 2006, for a review; Vargo 2011). Relatives should also request education about underlying causes of pain and medication options (Aldrich and Peterson 2010). Sometimes, consultation with a pain specialist is warranted to identify the best medication regimen possible so as to reduce pain and increase physical and mental well-being, as well as quality of life (Aldrich and Peterson 2010).

7.3 Scenario: Cognitive, Communication, and Language Challenges

Cognitive problems are a very common occurrence with brain tumors (see Fox et al. 2006, for a review). In addition, depending on the nature of the tumor, speech, language, and communication deficits may be evident. Family members may be perplexed or troubled by these changes and may ask questions such as: *How will this tumor affect my loved one's thinking? Why is he or she having so much difficulty talking? How come my loved one's communication style is so different?*

7.3.1 Overview of Cognitive, Communication, and Language Changes

The loved one's speed of thinking, learning and memory, attention and concentration, and executive functions (e.g., initiation, planning, problem solving, flexibility, multitasking, judgment, and reasoning) are often affected by brain tumors (Calhoun-Eagan 2009; Drappatz and Wen 2011; see Fox et al. 2006, for a review; Goodman et al. 2007; National Brain Tumor Society 2011d; Palmieri 2007; Sherwood et al., 2004b; see Swartz and Keir 2007, for a review; see Chap. 4, Tables 4.2 and 4.3 and Fig. 4.6; Chap. 6, Sect. 6.4, Table 6.6). Cognitive challenges are linked to the location of the tumor, as well as other factors, including swelling and shifting/compression of the brain structures caused by the tumor, distant effects of the tumor, and the aftereffects of radiation and chemotherapy (Anderson and Ryken 2008; Drappatz and Wen 2011; see Fox et al. 2006, for a review; Talacchi et al. 2011; Wefel et al. 2011). The onset of symptoms can seem unexpectedly rapid to the caregiver (Aldrich and Peterson 2010). Typical neuropsychological and language deficits emanating from various locations in the brain are summarized in Chaps. 4 and 6.

Other causes of thinking difficulties include medications (e.g., corticosteroids) and medical complications (e.g., seizures and sleep disorders; Aldrich and Peterson 2010; Fox et al. 2006). In addition, radiation and chemotherapy may result in additional cognitive decline, sometimes evident after weeks or months (Aldrich and Peterson 2010; Anderson and Ryken 2008; see Hannay et al. 2004, for a review; Sawrie 2006).

If the brain tumor resides in the left hemisphere, patients may develop some form of aphasia, including anomia or decreased word finding (Davie et al. 2009; see Chap. 6, Sects. 6.3. and 6.4 and Table 6.3). More malignant tumors (e.g., glioblastomas) may produce more severe language impairments (Whittle et al. 1998). Language expression and comprehension, as well as reading and writing can also be affected (National Brain Tumor Society 2011d). Some researchers have proposed that the severity of aphasia may be lessened if there is linguistic reorganization in the brain during tumor growth (e.g., brain plasticity; Benzagmout et al. 2007; Davie et al. 2009). The degree of aphasia can also be reduced if presurgical imaging and intraoperative cortical mapping procedures are employed, so as to minimize damage to critical language areas during surgery (Davie et al. 2009; Duffau et al. 2009).

With frontal lobe tumor loci, the loved one may demonstrate poor communication pragmatics, including hyperverbality and tangentiality (see Chap. 4, Sect. 4.6.3 and Fig. 4.9). It is crucial for the family to understand the nature and extent of the loved one's cognitive, communication, and language difficulties, as there can be serious ramifications for his or her ability to perform self-care, activities of daily living, work, as well as actively participate in the decision-making process about medical care (Fox et al. 2006; Sherwood et al. 2004b).

7.3.2 *"Helpful Hints" and Tools for Families to Cope with Cognitive, Language, and Communication Changes in their Loved Ones*

Table 7.4 summarizes "helpful hints" and tools for families to cope with their loved one's cognitive, language, and communication changes after a brain tumor. The most effective way for tier supports to assist their loved one with cognitive, communication,

Table 7.4 "Helpful hints" and tools for families to cope with cognitive, language, and communication changes in their loved ones with a brain tumor

Pursue a neuropsychological and speech and language evaluation to gain an appreciation of the loved one's cognitive, language, and communication status
Serial evaluations will be helpful in tracking the tumor course
Share qualitative observations about cognition, language, and communication with the professionals
Be open to cognitive rehabilitation for remediation, psychoeducation, and compensation training
Be an active participant in the rehabilitation treatment process
Become well versed in the loved one's armamentarium of compensations
Be receptive, flexible, and adaptable about intensifying the need for and quality of compensations when the tumor effects worsen:
Modify tools according to the loved one's safety needs
Stick with routines
Use pictures and familiar people to help "jog" the memory
Work with the therapist to individualize compensations based on needs, preferences, functional abilities, and goals
Work with a speech–language pathologist to learn effective communication techniques:
Use short, simple, and clear phrases
Allow extra time for the loved one to process what is said and respond
Employ assistive communication devices as needed
Avoid becoming frustrated or impatient with the loved one's deficits
Avoid escalating discussions into arguments
Focus on being nonjudgmental and empathic
Use simple explanations for the unfamiliar listener when the loved one demonstrates communication pragmatic challenges
Be vigilant about the loved one's executive function problems on higher level finances and budgeting:
Work with a neuropsychologist, occupational therapist, or social worker for psychoeducation and organizational strategies
Monitor the loved one's spending habits
If appropriate, obtain a financial power of attorney
Watch for outside influences who may manipulate or exploit the loved one and take appropriate action to protect his or her property

and language limitations is to gain an appreciation of his or her relative strengths and shortcomings. As has been described elsewhere in this book, comprehensive neuropsychological and speech and language evaluations are the model means to consolidate information about the loved one's current cognitive and language status (see Fox et al. 2006, for a review; Sawrie 2006; see also Chap. 4, Sect. 4.2.1, Table 4.1 and Fig. 4.4; and Chap. 6, Sects. 6.2.1 and 6.3.1), as well as provide sound recommendations about capacity for self-care, handling finances, driving, and work (Wefel et al. 2011). Quality-of-life questionnaires are a sensible adjunct to a neuropsychological evaluation (Sawrie 2006). It is preferable to collaborate with a neuropsychologist who has experience in the field of brain tumors and can hopefully utilize test results to make cogent treatment suggestions (National Brain Tumor Society 2011d; Roloff 2010; Sawrie 2006). Oftentimes, a first (or baseline) assessment is conducted, with follow-up examinations to monitor the course of the illness (National Brain Tumor Society 2011d; Sawrie 2006).

Rehabilitation professionals will draw on the feedback from the family regarding communication changes in the loved one. Family members (and the loved one) should be educated that the neurological, communication, and language status will closely mirror that of the tumor. Specifically, if the treatment is successful in removing or decreasing the size of the tumor, there are often concomitant improvements in functional capacities. Conversely, in unfortunate instances where the tumor is increasing in size or spreading to other areas of the brain, there can be an exacerbation in existing thinking and language deficits, as well as onset of new troubles commensurate with new areas of tumor growth.

Too often, rehabilitation is considered as an afterthought for brain tumor treatment, rather than a routine option (Calhoun-Eagan 2009). When feasible, the psychotherapist will advocate for cognitive rehabilitation, which will provide remediation interventions, psychoeducation, and compensation training (Anderson and Ryken 2008; De Luca et al. 2009; Drappatz and Wen 2011; Fox et al. 2006; Gehring et al. 2011; Goodman et al. 2007; National Brain Tumor Society 2011d; Vargo 2011; Wefel et al. 2011). Cognitive rehabilitation can also address functional limitations, capitalize on preserved strengths, and enhance adaptation and quality of life (Sawrie 2006; see Wefel et al. 2011, for a review). In fact, early neurorehabilitation after surgery has been found to improve the patient's functional outcome (Bartolo et al. 2011).

Relatives should be proactive about participating in the treatment process, so as to glean as much knowledge and support as possible through "awareness training" (Klonoff and Koberstein 2010). Once the family understands the loved one's current status, they are better able to tune into the appropriate compensatory tools. This acceptance process will unearth a wealth of therapeutic tools. These are also summarized throughout this book and a prior publication (Klonoff 2010). They include a datebook system (see Chap. 4, Sect. 4.3.2 and Fig. 4.5), memory strategies (see Table 4.3), Home Independence Checklists (see Chap. 4, Sect. 4.4.4 and Fig. 4.7; Chap. 6; Sect. 6.3.2 and Fig. 6.3), other general approaches to cope with executive system deficits (see Chap. 4, Sect. 4.4.4, Table 4.4, and Fig. 4.8; Chap. 6, Fig. 6.4), and "helpful hints" for communication challenges (see Chap. 4, Sect. 4.6.4, Table 4.7). Electronic compensations are summarized in Chap. 6 and Tables 6.5 and 6.7. If available, vocational rehabilitation using a job coach at the work site can be very efficacious (National Brain Tumor Society 2011d).

What is unique to brain tumors is the requirement for the loved one and family to be flexible and adaptable about intensifying the nature and specific qualities of the compensatory strategies. If impairments are relatively focal and mild, the loved one may be trained in typical note-taking systems, a smartphone, or basic datebook entries. However, as the tumor progresses, and if vision, visuospatial, memory, or initiation skills deteriorate, the loved one may require a more comprehensive set of tools, which will be upgraded and updated by the treatment team. These may include large print datebooks, alarm systems, or eventually note taking by the family member if the loved one is unable to write or spell well enough. A core consideration is that the loved one will require increased and eventually full-time supervision as the cognitive decline progresses, as his or her safety can be in jeopardy. Sticking with routines and surrounding the loved one with familiar people and pictures is comforting when memory loss is profound (Aldrich and Peterson 2010). As with other neurological syndromes, the introduction of specific compensations by treating therapists will be individualized to the loved one, taking into account his or her needs, preferences, functional abilities, and goals. This will require receptivity and fluidity on the part of the family so that the loved one has the best tools available.

Once the tier supports glean the key symptoms, they will be able to work with the therapy team and their loved one to develop effective communication skills, so as to understand and meet their loved one's care needs. This becomes especially onerous when the loved one has cognitive and communication challenges (e.g., confusion or aphasia; see Chap. 6, Sect. 6.3.2 and Table 6.4). Speech–language pathologists are invaluable resources for tools and techniques to facilitate communication with the loved one. For example, short, simple, and clear phrases are recommended (Aldrich and Peterson 2010) as well as allowing extra time for the loved one to process and respond. Sometimes, assistive communication devices are needed. Guideposts for the caregiver include controlling the tendency to become frustrated or impatient with the loved one's behavior and reduced capacities; avoiding escalating discussions into arguments; and focusing on being nonjudgmental and empathic (Aldrich and Peterson 2010; Klonoff and Koberstein 2010).

When the loved one displays pragmatic or communication difficulties that reflect socially inappropriate or disinhibited behavior, the therapists can teach caregivers simple explanations for the overall support network or outside individuals (Aldrich and Peterson 2010). This will avoid people becoming offended or alienated. The caregiver and family will be cautioned that the utterances are a result of the brain tumor and are not meant to be hurtful (see also Sect. 7.4.2). It is strongly advised that the family liaises closely with a neuropsychologist and speech–language pathologist to gain the requisite knowledge and tools to properly assist the loved one, rather than do this in isolation with limited information and resources.

The psychotherapist will assist family members in being vigilant about the impact of math computation deficits and executive system impairments (e.g., judgment, impulsivity, problem solving) on the loved one's capacity to manage higher level finances and budgeting. A neuropsychologist, speech–language pathologist, occupational therapist, or social worker are all fitting resources to assist with psychoeducation and organizational strategies for money management and financial planning. The primary caregiver may need to be proactive about monitoring the spending habits of the loved one or obtaining a financial power of attorney (Aldrich and Peterson 2010). Also, given that the loved one can be a vulnerable adult, the extended family should be wary of outside influences who may be trying to manipulate or exploit the loved one. This would require intervention on the part of medical professionals and family members to protect the property of the loved one.

7.4 Scenario: Personality and Mood Changes

Invariably, the loved one will have personality and/or mood changes as a result of the organic effects of the brain tumor and/or understandable emotional reactions to notification about the brain tumor and the ensuing neurological aftermath. Family members may ask questions such as: *How come my loved one's personality is so different? What do I do about my loved one's irritability? I'm so worried about how depressed my loved one is—who should I contact?*

7.4.1 Overview of Personality and Mood Changes

Personality and mood changes in the loved one may seem an exaggeration of prior characteristics or emergence of new traits (National Brain Tumor Society 2011d). Common emotional problems associated with brain tumors are withdrawal, apathy, anxiety, frustration, irritability, anger, sorrow, fear, regret, impulsivity, depression, mania, and mood swings (Aldrich and Peterson 2010; see Calhoun-Eagan 2009, for a review; Drappatz and Wen 2011; Goodman et al. 2007; National Brain Tumor Society 2011d; Raver-Lampman 2010; Schubart et al. 2008; Sherwood et al. 2008b; see Sherwood et al. 2004b, for a review; see Swartz and Keir 2007, for a review; Wefel et al. 2011). The multiplicity of emotions emerge based on the size and location of the brain tumor (Swartz and Keir 2007; Wefel et al. 2011), as well as emotional reactions to the illness (Klonoff and Myles 2010; see Wefel et al. 2011, for a review). Anxiety and depression are prevalent as the loved one awaits surgery (Talacchi et al. 2011). In conjunction with the physiological consequences of the brain tumor, often strong emotional reactions emanate from catastrophic reactions (CRs), whereby the loved one becomes aware of his or her ineptitudes (see Chap. 4, Sect. 4.6.1; Klonoff 2010) and "narcissistic rage," whereby perceived failures assail the global sense of self and psychological integrity (Klonoff and Myles 2010). The loved one can be consumed with heartache and psychic pain.

As the illness progresses, the loved one's personality may alter radically, including sometimes becoming agitated, belligerent, or paranoid (Aldrich and Peterson 2010; Sherwood et al. 2008b). Usually, profound mood and personality changes correspond to increased tumor spread (Aldrich and Peterson 2010), including to the temporal lobes and limbic system (Ouma 2004). The destruction of the loved one's sense of self and identity can catalyze depression, characterized by feelings of joylessness, hopelessness, worthlessness, and emptiness (Klonoff and Myles 2010). Existential concerns also abound from loss of control; perceived burden on others; interrupted life goals; shattered hopes; fears of separation, abandonment, being forgotten, and squandering opportunities; as well as death anxieties (Klonoff and Myles 2010; Raver-Lampman 2010; see Wefel et al. 2011, for a review). Sometimes, the compound losses of deteriorating health, dependency, financial disarray, and eradication of enjoyable pastimes and future aspirations plummet the loved one into despair and serious consideration of self-harm. The family may find themselves taking care of "a stranger" insofar as the magnitude of personality and behavioral changes. Care demands and distress in the tier supports propagate.

7.4.2 "Helpful Hints" and Tools for Families to Cope with Personality and Mood Changes in their Loved Ones

Table 7.5 summarizes "helpful hints" and tools for families to cope with personality and mood changes in their loved ones with a brain tumor. A chaplain/spiritual advisor can provide emotional relief for the loved one while he or she is in the hospital (Reddick 2010; Roloff 2010). Given the complexity of the loved one's personality, behavioral, and mood changes, and the resultant distress in the caregiver (Sherwood et al. 2006), the primary recommendation is that the family be proactive about seeking psychotherapy to diminish problematic mood and behaviors in the loved one (Aldrich and Peterson 2010; Klonoff 2010; National Brain Tumor Society 2011d; Sherwood et al. 2004b, 2006; Wefel et al. 2011). Psychotherapy techniques vary widely; the loved one will need to identify a therapeutic style that is consonant for himself or herself (Roloff 2010). Many patients find that empathy, positivism, and a sense of humor in their therapeutic and support environments are key healing forces (see Roloff 2010, for a review). Sometimes, the caregiver and family may need to push for this treatment, by making sure the other treating professionals fully understand the nature and extent of the loved one's emotionality and its deleterious impact on the family system. Of course, the love and support of the caregiver and overall social network are paramount in inculcating the loved one's courage, tenacity, and hope (see Roloff 2010, for a review).

Relatives should be aware of the opportunity for pharmacologic treatment for the loved one (e.g., for depression or aggression) prescribed by a psychiatrist or neuro-oncologist (Goodman et al. 2007; Sherwood et al. 2006; Stark-Vance and Dubay 2011). Commonly used antidepressants include selective serotonin reuptake inhibitors (e.g., sertraline, fluoxetine, paroxetine, citalopram) and serotonin/norepinephrine reuptake inhibitors (duloxetine, milnacipran, and venlafaxine; Drappatz and Wen 2011; see Wefel et al. 2011, for a review). In our setting, we have seen very good results with sertraline (P. Bollam, personal communication, n.d.). Given the negative drug interactions between alcohol and chemotherapy drugs, anticonvulsants, and antidepressants, the family will need to be vigilant about encouraging the loved one to abstain completely from alcohol ingestion (Stark-Vance and Dubay 2011).

Psychotherapeutic treatment should focus not only on the loved one (Stark-Vance and Dubay 2011), but just as importantly on psychoeducation, counseling, and support services for the family (National Brain Tumor Society 2010b; Schubart et al. 2008; Sherwood et al. 2006, 2007, Tepper 2003; Wefel et al. 2011), who may be perplexed, overwhelmed, or even panicked about how to best support and handle the loved one's emotional suffering. This is especially the case if the loved one is suicidal or violent, in which case professional intervention is critical.

Other "helpful hints" that the psychotherapist and professionals will emphasize to relatives include not taking the outbursts of the loved one personally (Aldrich and Peterson 2010) and remembering that the disruptive behavior is a function of the disease, not willful acts by him or her (Schubart et al. 2008; Sherwood et al. 2007).

Table 7.5 "Helpful hints" and tools for families to cope with personality and mood changes in their loved ones with a brain tumor

Be proactive about seeking psychotherapy for the loved one as well as support and psychoeducation for the tier 1 caregiver and family
Consider chaplaincy/spiritual services at the hospital for emotional relief
Remember that empathy, positivism, and a sense of humor in the loved one's therapeutic and support environments are key healing forces
Be watchful of depression, suicidal risk, violent behavior, and alcohol use in the loved one and obtain immediate professional intervention (including psychotropic medications) by the neuro-oncologist, psychologist, and psychiatrist
Do not take outbursts personally
Remember that "out-of-character" behavior is caused by the brain tumor
Stay calm, empathic, and patient
Realize when rational discussions become futile:
Withdraw from the situation
Change the topic or setting
Work with treating professionals to understand the role of mood and cognitive factors in difficult interactions
Realize when the loved one is experiencing a CR:
Liaison with the loved one's health-care professionals to understand his/her neurological status
Look for external triggers
Be careful not to overwhelm your loved one, especially with a decline in health status
Be mindful that new deficits will reduce his/her skill set and coping capacity
Adjust expectations and approaches to meet the loved one's needs
Learn about "narcissistic rage" attacks as reactions to mortality and attempts to control the uncontrollable
Avoid overstimulation, including too many visitors
Create a visitor schedule
When the loved one has paranoid reactions:
Work with professionals to understand the underlying causes
Provide reassurance
Realize the role of helpless feelings
Help the loved one take notes to track salient information
Review financial information to allay fears
Emphasize that family members have his/her best interest at heart
Be open to psychotropic medication and coordinate with physicians (i.e., a psychiatrist)
Create a home environment that is nurturing, safe, and cheery
Engage in mutual sharing of feelings
Focus on being a good listener and don't try to "fix" every problem
Use family memorabilia to reduce feelings of loneliness and despair
Promote a multidimensional approach for the loved one to fashion new life priorities and expectations, and become "a better person"
Engage in joyful and fulfilling pastimes and stress reducing activities (e.g., through recreational therapy) that are culturally relevant
Encourage creative ways to reflect upon their sojourns (e.g., writing, drawing, etc.)
Give lots of encouragement to maximize the loved one's self-esteem and independence
Promote participation in the home and at social events
Monitor alcohol abstinence
Encourage involvement of the loved one in a support group to enable bonding with other brain tumor patients
If appropriate, support and facilitate the loved one's reintegration into the school or work setting, with the necessary accommodations

The caregiver and family may feel scapegoated, but the loved one will "hurt the one he (or she) loves" due to his or her familiarity and feelings of fright, suffering, and desperation (see Chap. 2, Sect. 2.4.2.2). In these instances, the target should remain calm, empathic, and patient, again recognizing that the loved one is perturbed with his or her predicament, not the caregiver (Aldrich and Peterson 2010). Also, the family should be cognizant of the threshold beyond which trying to reason with the loved one is productive (Aldrich and Peterson 2010); sometimes, it is better to withdraw or change the topic or setting, so as to de-escalate a situation. The treating professionals can assist the family in recognizing when the loved one is behaving irrationally or is too cognitively confused to comprehend the discussion.

The psychotherapist can instruct the family to recognize CRs so as to reduce external triggers (see Chap. 4, Sect. 4.6.2 and Table 4.6; Klonoff 2010). Collaboration with the health-care professionals to gain the optimal appreciation of the loved one's overall neurological status will help reduce the frequency and magnitude of CRs, based on not overwhelming the loved one (Klonoff 2010; Klonoff et al. 1993). This psychoeducation is indispensable when the loved one's health status is declining. New deficits will diminish his or her adeptness and coping capacity and the caregiver and family must fluidly adjust their expectations and approaches. The therapist will also educate the support network that "narcissistic rage" attacks are indicative of the stark realization of the loved one's mortality and are an attempt to gain control of the uncontrollable. Sometimes, overstimulation from excessive activities or visitors will precipitate CRs and the tier 1 caregiver will need to be mindful not to overload the loved one. Friends and visitors will also need to understand the importance of preserving the energies and privacy of the loved one (National Brain Tumor Society 2010b). Creating a visitor schedule can help to ameliorate overload and also gives the loved one and friends something to look forward to.

When temporal lobe, limbic system damage, or medication side effects (e.g., corticosteroids) cause paranoid and psychotic reactions (see Drappatz and Wen 2011, for a review; Kenna et al. 2011; Ouma 2004; Wen et al. 2006), reassurance of the loved one is important. The psychotherapist can help the loved one and caregiver understand the underlying causes of suspicious reactions, as well as how the family can lessen misperceptions. For instance, feelings of helplessness can lead to suspiciousness (Aldrich and Peterson 2010). Other strategies include helping him or her take detailed notes to recall conversations; reviewing financial information to allay fears in that sphere; and emphasizing that the support network has the loved one's best interest at heart. A number of psychotropic medications can be successful in ameliorating flagrant paranoia and psychotic reactions, including antipsychotics (e.g., risperidone, aripiprazole; P. Bollam, personal communication, 12/29/11; Drappatz and Wen 2011) and the primary caregiver should be open to physicians' input about medication to reduce these behaviors, as they can also result in safety concerns for the family. In these cases, the loved one and family are strongly advised to liaise with a psychiatrist as part of the treatment team, given the potential for drug interactions.

The psychotherapist will proffer viable suggestions to alleviate a downturn in mood, including creating a home environment that is nurturing, safe, and cheery (Aldrich and Peterson 2010). Providing communication opportunities for mutual sharing of emotions helps the loved one decompress and reinforces the realization that he or she is loved and is not an encumbrance. Focus on being a good listener (National Brain Tumor Society 2010b), without feeling the pressure to "fix problems." Easy access to family memorabilia is often soothing for the loved one and can reduce feelings of loneliness and despair. Therapy, the loved one's willpower, and the tier support networks can help the patient fashion new life priorities and expectations, with a focus on being "a better person"; one who is humane, loving, and sensitive (de Jong 2010, p. 47; Klonoff 2010).

Engaging in activities that are joyful and fulfilling should help elevate the loved one's mood. This includes creative ways to reflect upon his or her sojourns, such as writing, drawing, etc. (Klonoff and Myles 2010; Roloff 2010). A recreational therapist can identify fulfilling hobbies. Acupuncture, massage, Reiki, mind–body techniques (e.g., yoga, tai chi, meditation, hypnosis, and visual imagery), as well as music and art therapy can alleviate physical discomfort, thereby reducing the loved one's anxiety (see Rosenthal et al. 2009, for a review). The psychotherapist should also consider culturally relevant resources, for example, Native American spiritual ceremonies and healing circles (Blinn 2010). These improve mental health and quality of life (see Rosenthal et al. 2009, for a review). Lots of encouragement that maximizes self-esteem and independence will improve his or her mood (National Brain Tumor Society 2010b). This can include even simple activities (e.g., chores), as this allows the loved one to feel like an integral member of the family. Fun social events with the family and overall support network (including friends) improve the loved one's outlook and quality of life. Monitoring that the loved one does not imbibe alcohol will also reduce worrisome behavior, as this substance can increase irritability, emotional lability, and hostility (see Chap. 4, Sect. 4.6.2). Frequently, patients find consolation in interacting with other brain tumor survivors. Support groups are an invaluable way for the loved one to bond with others in a similar predicament (Roloff 2010). The primary caregiver can help orchestrate this through a number of peer mentor resources (e.g., American Brain Tumor Association www.abta.org/Care_And_Support/48; National Brain Tumor Society Peer Support Network www.braintumor.org/patients-family-friends/find-support).

Being productive and engaging in meaningful community activities is good for the loved one's mood and adjustment. It also introduces a sense of normalcy into the household. If and when the loved one is able to return to work or an academic setting, rehabilitation professionals will be cognizant of any unique needs and limitations (Calhoun-Eagan 2009; Zelko and Sorensen 2009). The caregiver and loved one should be prepared for possible modifications over time, depending on the course of the brain tumor (Zelko and Sorensen 2009). For the work setting, this can include a letter from the treating physician about possible work accommodations, including returning part-time, the opportunity for rest periods, and a quiet work space (Calhoun-Eagan 2009).

In the high school or college settings, the loved one may need special education considerations. Rehabilitation therapists and the family should be prepared to interface with the guidance counselor, disability student resources, or a school psychologist so as to implement academic adjustments and solicit assistance with career planning (Zelko and Sorensen 2009). The school personnel can write an Individualized Education Program (IEP) or a 504 plan taking into account the loved one's learning strengths and neurological limitations; this can include ancillary services in the areas of speech–language pathology, and physical and occupational therapies (Zelko and Sorensen 2009). Postsecondary settings typically require the student to be proactive in obtaining special education resources (Zelko and Sorensen 2009) and the rehabilitation therapists and family can help the loved one expedite this process. Zelko and Sorensen (2009) delineate some pragmatic academic adjustments for cognitive, physical, language, and academic deficiencies. Examples include preferential seating and test taking in a quiet room for attentional difficulties; a peer note taker or audiotaping lectures for fine motor problems; multiple-choice tests for memory impairments; and scheduling of classes in the morning for fatigue (Zelko and Sorensen 2009).

7.5 Scenario: Prognosis

As stated above in Sect. 7.1.1, brain tumors vary in their level of malignancy or rate of growth. Family members may have questions such as: *What is my loved one's prognosis? How long might he or she live? What changes might I expect over what timeline?*

7.5.1 Overview of Prognostic Factors

Regardless of the tumor grade, families describe intense emotions at the time of their loved one's diagnosis, including fright, fear, sorrow, shock, and despair (Edvardsson and Ahlström 2008; Schmer et al. 2008). Tier supports also feel in a state of chaos and on an "emotional roller coaster" (Edvardsson and Ahlström 2008; Khalili 2007; Schmer et al. 2008). The loved one and family desperately grasp for some glimmer of hope. Other universal sentiments include worry about the uncertainty of the tumor course (Roloff 2010), including what follow-up scans may show and how the loved one will fare in the future in his or her capacity for daily activities. For the relatives, this translates to "shifting sands" when administering their responsibilities (see Chap. 2, Sect. 2.4.2.3). Overarching fear can lead to the caregiver and family feeling fragile and susceptible (Edvardsson and Ahlström 2008), always anticipating new "bad news." Feelings of crisis and turbulence abound (Edvardsson and Ahlström 2008).

Some authors report an increased level of stress in tier 1 caregivers with loved ones with a lower tumor grade, especially when the caregiver is younger (Keir et al. 2006). The pressures on the family also increase when the loved one experiences distress related to the uncertainty of the tumor's prognosis, based on a study of patients with meningiomas (Kangas et al. 2007). Other themes which emerge for caregivers of loved ones with a low-grade brain tumor include the pervasive threat of tumor relapse and the concomitant functional deterioration in the context of long-term survival, sometimes, for many years (Edvardsson and Ahlström 2008). Over

Table 7.6 "Helpful hints" and tools for families to cope with tumor prognosis

Recognize that the prognosis is elusive and that doctors are reluctant to give specifics about the anticipated life span
Tier 1 caregiver needs vary according to the general course of the tumor progression—fast versus slow
Find treating professionals who are:
Sensitive to the loved one's and family's unique backgrounds and lifestyles
Compassionate and honest in their delivery style
Collaborative and respectful towards all parties
Take into account the patient's and family's readiness for feedback
Realize that denial or minimization can serve adaptive functions
Conceptualize the tumor course as a psychological transition
Employ gentle probing and psychoeducation
Allow the patient and family to take the lead in soliciting prognostic information
Willing to "lay the groundwork" to help the loved one and family cope better
For faster growing brain tumors, the caregiver and family need:
Comprehensive education and practical supports
Quick interventions when "time is of the essence"
Support in making health-care decisions
Preparation for end-of-life considerations
For slower growing brain tumors, the caregiver and family need:
Encouragement to continue with independent activities commensurate with the loved one's functional status
Reminders about self-care to preserve energies for "the long haul"
Strategies to adapt to living with uncertainty for an extended timeline

time, family members may also experience helplessness, neglect, and isolation when outside support dissipates over time (Edvardsson and Ahlström 2008), culminating in a poorer quality of life (Edvardsson and Ahlström 2009). This translates into chronic role changes, especially with the spouse caregiver transposed to a parental role, with restricted freedoms and loss of reciprocity in the relationship (Edvardsson and Ahlström 2008; Schmer et al. 2008). The caregiver and family can succumb to long-term "wear and tear."

On the other hand, caregivers with a loved one with a high-grade glioma experience abrupt stressors, sparking immediate and substantive care by the family, secondary to the rapidity of cognitive and physical decline (McConigley et al. 2010). The incidence of depression in these patients is also quite high (Catt et al. 2008), which complicates their management by the inexperienced caregiver. The family is now charged with intense requirements for accelerated coping, adjustment, and future planning.

7.5.2 "Helpful Hints" and Tools for Families Coping with Varying Prognoses

Table 7.6 provides "helpful hints" and tools for families to cope with various tumor prognoses. The prognosis of brain tumors is somewhat elusive, and relatives (and the loved one) may find that the doctors are reluctant to give specifics about the anticipated life span, in part because of the medical unknowns (Goodman et al. 2007;

Stark-Vance and Dubay 2011). Consideration factors include the type of tumor, how much is surgically removed, response to treatment, possible complications, age of the patient, and his or her overall functional status (see Chandana et al. 2008, for a review; Stark-Vance and Dubay 2011). This being said, the general prognosis affects the caregiver and family (and of course the loved one) differently. Rapidly growing tumors usually show a faster rate of deterioration and a shorter life span. Conversely, slower growing tumors correspond to a lengthier time frame with respect to impairments, punctuated by periods of decline. Therefore, caregivers and the support network are faced with differing responsibilities and stressors, based on their loved one's brain tumor malignancy (see Edvardsson and Ahlström 2008, for a review).

Treating professionals need to be sensitive to varying needs and struggles for caregivers based on the grade and course of the brain tumor. Feedback about prognosis should be couched in an understanding of the loved one's and relatives' ethnic, racial, religious, social, economic, and cultural values and practices (see Chap. 1, Sect. 1.3 and Fig. 1.1; Klonoff 2010; Moore and Wagner 2009; Tepper 2003). Patients and their families appreciate an honest, yet compassionate delivery style with intent towards collaboration and respect towards all parties (Klonoff 2010; Tepper 2003).

The therapist and other professionals should be mindful about the loved one's and family's readiness for feedback about prognosis. The timing and pacing of this is pivotal for the well-being of the loved one and family (see Chap. 2, Sect. 2.4.1.2). Often, there is a predisposition for denial or minimization of deterioration or complications. These reactions have an adaptive benefit to temporarily ward off psychological realities that are too threatening. Conceptualizing the tumor course as a psychological transition will help the therapist, loved one, and family recognize the need to abandon prior assumptions and embrace new beliefs (Khalili 2007). This becomes particularly salient with tumor reoccurrence; the loved one and family are jolted into renewed fear, uncertainty, and suffering (Khalili 2007).

In my practice, I tend to follow the lead of the loved one and family by waiting until they ask the critical questions about prognosis. This preserves the working alliance and avoids alienating the patient and family by providing information they find too jarring. Gentle probing and psychoeducation can, however, pave the way for embracing painful realities, especially when the loved one's health suddenly and profoundly deteriorates and steps need to be taken to obtain the loved one's wishes regarding medical interventions, as well as help put his or her affairs in order (see also Sect. 7.6.2). Introducing the concept of "laying the groundwork" (Norton and Bowers 2001) helps the family and loved one understand the positive intentions of the health-care professionals, including the psychotherapist.

For families of patients with faster growing, more malignant tumors, comprehensive education and practical supports (e.g., delegation of duties, professional nursing support) need to be emphasized by the psychotherapist (Catt et al. 2008; see McConigley et al. 2010, for a review), as "time is of the essence." This also includes support in making decisions regarding addressing the loved one's disabilities (McConigley et al. 2010). Professionals and the tier supports also need to engage in dialogue about end of life issues in a compassionate, yet opportune fashion (Catt et al. 2008; McConigley et al. 2010; see Chap. 10).

Because patients with lower grade tumors may be more independent and require less care, the caregivers and family members may have more freedom to pursue "extracurricular" activities. They should avail themselves of stress reduction opportunities (National Brain Tumor Society 2010b; Swartz and Keir 2007) in order to cope for the duration. Also, because there is a more extended time course for existential adjustment, some relatives of patients with benign meningiomas adapt to living with uncertainty and find psychosocial benefits from their experience as a caregiver (Kangas et al. 2011; see also Chap. 10).

7.6 Scenario: Family Members' Angst and Despair

Depending on the nature of the brain tumor, primary caregivers and the overall support network may find themselves with innumerable hurdles and emotional turmoil. This is especially the case for malignant brain tumors. The family may ask questions such as: *How can I cope with these huge stressors? Is there anybody out there who really understands what I am going through?*

7.6.1 Overview of Angst and Despair in the Caregiver

Table 7.7 summarizes the common stressors for caregivers and others involved in the care and supervision of a loved one with a brain tumor. The entire family system is typically affected (Moore and Wagner 2009; Schubart et al. 2008) and even more so as the tumor progresses, producing profound disabilities (see Schubart et al. 2008, for a review). Caregiver stress produces a variety of psychological and physiological health issues in the caregivers (Goodman et al. 2007; Swartz and Keir 2007), with rates as high as 72% (Keir 2007). As depicted in the FEM, it becomes the norm for the caregiver to overlook his or her needs, resulting in sleep deprivation, poor eating habits, and lack of exercise (Goodman et al. 2007; Klonoff and Koberstein 2010; National Brain Tumor Society 2010b). The caregiver can lapse into a frame of mind that it is unnecessary or selfish to attend to his or her own requirements (see Chap. 1, Sect. 1.5; Klonoff and Koberstein 2010; National Brain Tumor Society 2010b).

Common caregiver experiences include reduced quality of life and increased anxiety and depression (Finocchiaro et al. 2011; Goodman et al. 2007; National Brain Tumor Society 2010b). Relatives are prone to CRs by proxy, catalyzed by witnessing heartbreaking ineptitudes and disappointments in the loved one (see Chap. 2, Sect. 2.4.2.1 and Chap. 9, Sect. 9.4). Caregiver depression and distress have been found to correspond to the degree of strain from unpleasant behaviors, neuropsychiatric symptoms (e.g., depression, irritability, and apathy), and interpersonal problems in the loved one (Ownsworth et al. 2009, 2010; Sherwood et al. 2006, 2007), as well

Table 7.7 Common stressors for caregivers with a loved one with a brain tumor

Impact on the entire family system
Physiological and psychological health problems in the tier 1 caregiver
Mindset of overlooking personal needs
Reduced quality of life
Catastrophic reactions by proxy
Depression and anxiety related to emotional and interpersonal problems in the loved one
Increased care needs and dependency in the loved one
General caregiver responsibilities:
Complex medical tasks
Supervising the loved one
Providing emotional support and comfort
Researching information
Attending medical appointments
Coordinating the loved one's care
Advocating for the best care
Assisting with home exercises
Handling convoluted insurance and disability systems
Complex decision making and problem solving
Monitoring effects of new treatment regimens
"Eyes and ears" of new or worsening symptoms
Foreign responsibilities that were the purview of the loved one
Direct and indirect costs
Monetary crises
Economic hardship and debt burden
Competing demands within the family system
When, how, and what updates to share with children
Feeling overwhelmed and exhausted when needs and expectations exceed energies and capabilities
Complex emotions, including "narcissistic rage" and guilt
Reliance on physicians for guidance
Social isolation from a larger support network
Conflicting recommendations from tier 2 and 3 family and friends and "scapegoating" behavior
Uncertainty about the medical course and physiological trajectory
Confusion about the underlying etiology of the loved one's challenges
Coping with the illness for the "long haul":
Multiple hospitalizations
Insufficient training
Extensive role changes and toils
Crossing of privacy barriers
Career sacrifices
Dearth of user-friendly information
Lack of in-home physical and physiological preparation resulting in "trial-and-error" learning and crisis management

as increased care needs and dependency in the loved one (Finocchiaro et al. 2011; Ownsworth et al. 2010).

General caregiver responsibilities include performing complex medical tasks (e.g., administering medication and overseeing medical equipment); supervising the loved one; providing emotional support and comfort; researching information about the disease and treatment options; attending medical appointments; coordinating care for the loved one (including custodial care and transportation); advocating for the finest medical care; assisting with home exercises from physical and occupational therapies; handling convoluted insurance and disability systems as well as other forms of complex decision making and problem solving (Given et al. 2008; Goodman et al. 2007; Sherwood et al. 2004a; National Brain Tumor Society 2010b; Swartz and Keir 2007). They are also often in charge of monitoring the results of new treatment regimens and are the "eyes and ears" for either new or worsening of symptoms (Given et al. 2008).

Spouses may be catapulted into foreign obligations that were the purview of the loved one, including bill paying and financial decision making (Goodman et al. 2007; Sherwood et al. 2004a). There are direct costs for brain tumor treatment as well as indirect costs related to lost opportunities because of the tumor treatment (e.g., loss of income; Bradley et al. 2007). In conjunction with this are the monetary crises family members may face, due to unpaid medical bills; high medical costs and out-of-pocket expenditures (e.g., prescription drugs, co-pays, and premiums); purchase of items and equipment (e.g., bath chairs); noncovered health services; pending insurance appeals; complications qualifying for and receiving timely payments through disability insurance; and nonmedical expenses (e.g., transportation and hotel stays; Bradley et al. 2007; Patterson 2007). Economic hardship and debt load can become pervasive, especially in the context of diminished income for the loved one and/or family. This translates into emotional health concerns in the tier 1 caregiver, including frustration, depression, anxiety, fear, and unease (Bradley et al. 2007, 2009; Patterson 2007; Sherwood et al. 2008a).

Most relatives have competing demands which will increase their overload and strain (Given et al. 2008; Sherwood et al. 2004a). Spouses may have "double duty" involving the care of the partner and children; other caregivers may be "sandwiched in" by tending simultaneously to the loved one and an aging parent (Schubart et al. 2008). When there is profound neurological decline, the caregiver may feel he or she has acquired "another child" (Sherwood et al. 2004a). The parent caregiver is also faced with the difficult decision of when, how, and what to share with sons and daughters (Schubart et al. 2008). Caregivers need a myriad of talents in cognitive, psychomotor, psychological, and communication domains in order to minister to their loved one (Given et al. 2008).

Numerous caregivers report feeling overwhelmed and exhausted, as their loved one's needs and expectations often exceed their energies and capabilities (Aldrich and Peterson 2010; see Schubart et al. 2008, for a review; Sherwood et al. 2004a). Depression, anxiety, sleep disturbances, and poor physical health can propagate (see Sherwood et al. 2008b, for a review). Others become angry and resentful (Goodman et al. 2007) and may be catapulted into "narcissistic rage" attacks caused by feelings of powerlessness. Common targets encompass the loved one, treating physicians, insurance companies (e.g., limitations in care or overall costs), and the health-care system (e.g., hospital care; Schubart et al. 2008). They may then be consumed with guilt for losing patience with the loved one (Sherwood et al. 2004a). At the same time, relatives need and want to trust the physician to help guide them through the overall treatment process (Schubart et al. 2008). They feel socially isolated from a larger support network, perceiving that others cannot cope with the depressing circumstances (Schubart et al. 2008) or are too busy. Pressures mount when other tier 2 or 3 family members or friends bombard the primary caregiver with conflicting ideas (e.g., stop work versus keep working; Sherwood et al. 2004a). Sometimes, this escalates into scapegoating the primary caregiver (Sherwood et al. 2004a).

Uncertainty about the medical course and physiological trajectory of the brain tumor (e.g., onset of new disabilities) add to the caregiver's confusion and anguish (Given et al. 2008; Schubart et al. 2008). To complicate matters, relatives are perplexed and sometimes perturbed about the underlying etiology of challenges, as some deficiencies result directly from tumor growth, including seizures and actual physical, cognitive, and personality alterations (Abrey and Mason 2011). However, other troubling symptoms may emerge based on side effects of the treatments (e.g., medications; Guralnick 2006).

As stated above, for loved ones who survive many years, the family must be prepared to cope with illness and neurological deterioration for the "long haul" (see Schubart et al. 2008). Repeat hospitalizations can require caregiver nursing duties, usually with minimal to no prior training (Schubart et al. 2008). This translates into extensive role changes and toils in the home (Guralnick 2006; Khalili 2007; see Schubart et al. 2008, for a review), often crossing privacy barriers, such as toileting the loved one (Schubart et al. 2008). With this come caregiver sacrifices in their occupations, income, and quality of life (see Schubart et al. 2008, for a review).

Caregivers and the support network have reported a dearth of user-friendly information, related to the complexity and variability of the tumor diagnoses, symptom presentations, and prognosis (Schubart et al. 2008). There is also a lack of physical and psychological preparation of caregivers for in-home care for the loved one (Schubart et al. 2008). Primary caregivers may feel they are learning based on "trial and error" or after the fact, when crises subside (Schubart et al. 2008).

7.6.2 *"Helpful Hints" and Tools for the Caregivers to Cope with Stressors from a Loved One's Brain Tumor*

Table 7.8 summarizes "helpful hints" and tools for the support network to cope with their long-term stressors from a brain tumor in a loved one. Some authors have differentiated between the phases of "diagnostic quest" versus the "accommodation" or coping with the tumor reverberations on the loved one and overall social network (Schubart et al. 2008). Ongoing psychotherapy for family members is therefore integral (National Brain Tumor Society 2010b; see Sherwood et al. 2004b, for a review). Given the understandable emotional tumult, regular psychotherapy sessions (e.g., weekly to twice monthly) are recommended to provide a safe haven for the relatives to vent productively, including working through natural feelings of grief, guilt, hostility, depression, and anxiety. As one psychoanalyst wrote, "I was the repository of their hopes and fears, their secrets" (Broyard 2010, p. 97). Psychoeducation and cognitive–behavioral techniques to redefine schemas remain hallmarks of these

Table 7.8 "Helpful hints" and tools for families to cope with their stressors

Engage in supportive psychotherapy:
Schedule regular sessions
Vent understandable emotions in a safe haven
Be mindful of symptoms of depression and anxiety
Share relevant pre- and posttumor history
Consider journaling and other cathartic art forms (e.g., drawing, poetry) and share the creations
Develop a positive working alliance
Use psychiatric input as needed, including psychotropic medications
Obtain a good working knowledge of the loved one's plan of care, including hands-on training in the hospital
Pursue education and emotional solace through multiple informational resources, including brain tumor websites
Use pragmatic coping techniques to alleviate stress and cultivate resiliency:
Keep all medical records and information highly organized in a binder format
Log the loved one's medical experiences and concerns for easy access at appointments
Oversee/manage the loved one's medications using a pillbox and communicate closely with all physicians regarding polydrug treatment
Prioritize concerns, responsibilities, and what matters
Establish a "normal" yet flexible routine
Focus on short-term goals
Maintain good communication with the loved one and overall support system
Be adaptable to ever-changing circumstances
Use mindful trial and error and self-forgiveness as strategies
Be timely in putting financial and health-care matters in order
Notify relevant parties (e.g., work and school settings) and arrange for coverage
Attain knowledge, keep records, and seek outside professional assistance for practical considerations (e.g., insurance, financial management, and access to community health and support systems)
Make necessary accommodations and sacrifices to cope with treatment costs and avoid financial devastation
Be in tune with personal needs, including self-care and sustenance:
Build a sturdy tier support system
Incorporate stress-reduction techniques
Combat the tendency to isolate from others
Set realistic expectations for caregiving
Plan respite breaks
Delegate duties to willing others using an organized system
If necessary, hire an in-home health-care provider
Prioritize physical and mental health of the tier 1 caregiver(s) and the family
Realign the family's values and aspirations
Emphasize shared short-term, attainable goals
Acquire therapeutic assistance in addressing the needs of children:
Consult with a psychotherapist experienced with family therapy and child/adolescent treatment
Consider the implications of the nature, course, and manifestations of the brain tumor
Don't underestimate their perceptiveness
Expect some behavioral regression in younger children
Take the age, emotional development, personality, and specific relationship with the tumor patient into account
Allow the children to have a say-so in what is shared
Share information in a straightforward, truthful, realistic, loving, and nonthreatening manner
Use age-appropriate language
Monitor the timing of discussions
Encourage the children's self-expression and open communication

Table 7.8 (continued)

Keep teachers informed
Maintain proper discipline and expectations
Provide a comfortable and comforting ambience
Reassure the children that they are not the cause of the illness
Prepare them for worrying side effects of brain tumor treatments
Involve them in small and appropriate caregiving assignments
Role model healthy grief emotions
Multimedia resources
Books/chapters
"Support Organizations, Resources, and Relevant Websites" (Grenier and Gupta 2009)
Navigating Through a Strange Land (Roloff 2010)
Orientation to Caregiving: A Handbook for Family Caregivers of Patients with Brain Tumors (Goodman et al. 2007)
Websites
The National Brain Tumor Foundation (www.braintumor.org)
The American Brain Tumor Association (www.abta.org)
The Healing Exchange Brain Trust (www.braintrust.org)
"What You Need to Know About Brain Tumors" (U.S. Department of Health and Human Services et al. 2003) on the website http://www.cancer.gov/cancertopics/wyntk/brain/page1

sessions (see Chap. 1, Sect. 1.2). A case in point, the tier support network should be educated about typical signs of anxiety and depression so as to be mindful of deteriorating emotional symptomatology (see Chap. 4, Sect. 4.8.2 and Table 4.9).

Family members should be aware that compassionate and holistically minded professionals will evaluate the family's overall preillness functioning and current life circumstances (e.g., family composition, socioeconomic status; Moore and Wagner 2009). Also, a thorough evaluation by the treating therapist of the primary caregiver's personality attributes, strengths, beliefs, culture, availability, knowledge, other functions, and overall resources is vital (see Chap. 1, Sect. 1.3 and Chap. 3, Sect. 3.1.1 and Fig. 3.1; Given et al. 2008; Klonoff 2010; Moore and Wagner 2009). Often, the family's prior psychological health and coping patterns established with other stressful events foreshadow current coping capacities (Moore and Wagner 2009). To this end, the psychotherapist can integrate psychoanalytic constructs to better understand the interpersonal processes within the family, including their transference reactions which either breed openness or resistance to treatment suggestions (see Chap. 1, Sect. 1.2.1).

The psychotherapist may propose that the family engage in journaling or any other art form which is cathartic (e.g., drawing, poetry; Roloff 2010). These also memorialize moments of closeness and snapshots of joy, which help to alleviate some of the angst. Sharing creations with the psychotherapist can be an excellent therapeutic exercise and can assist him or her in better empathizing with the caregiver's vantage point (Klonoff and Koberstein 2010). The painful process of acceptance and adjustment to the loved one's health status and prognosis is best shepherded by a psychotherapist with whom the caregiver and family have developed a positive and comforting working alliance (Klonoff 2010; see also Chap. 2, Sect. 2.4.1 and Chap. 3, Sect. 3.1.1 and Fig. 3.1). Psychiatric intervention, including psychotropic medications, may also be warranted to help alleviate depressive and anxiety symptoms in the caregiver (Klonoff and Koberstein 2010; National Brain Tumor Society 2010b).

Mastery will enhance coping and vice versa. Therefore, the psychotherapist will suggest that tier 1 caregivers obtain a good working knowledge of their loved one's plan of care, also necessitating interfacing with nurses and social workers (Given et al. 2008; Goodman et al. 2007; Roloff 2010). In order to better prepare the primary caregiver for in-home treatment, the family should be encouraged to request hands-on training before leaving the hospital, or ideally through home health staff (Schubart et al. 2008), as well as active involvement in other relevant interventions to expand their expertise (Given et al. 2008). Family members will need to be assertive and proactive about requesting this assistance, as otherwise it is commonly omitted. Some organizations offer 1-day workshops or evening classes to teach caregiving skills (Goodman et al. 2007).

Because education is fundamental to reducing stress and enhancing coping strategies (see Sherwood et al. 2004b, for a review), caregivers also derive comfort by interfacing with other families whose loved ones have brain tumors. The psychotherapist can recommend support groups, caregiver trainings and workshops, Internet resources, or self-help books (e.g., Aldrich and Peterson 2010; Black and Hogan 2006; Goodman et al. 2007; National Brain Tumor Society 2010b). Some caregivers find Weblogs or blogs to be a beneficial way to stay connected to a support group, as well as efficiently disseminate information (Stark-Vance and Dubay 2011).

Excellent educational resources for caregivers are: the chapter, "Support Organizations, Resources, and Relevant Websites" by Grenier and Gupta (2009); the book, *Navigating Through a Strange Land* edited by Roloff (2010); and several websites, including the National Brain Tumor Foundation (www.braintumor.org), the American Brain Tumor Association (www.abta.org), and the Healing Exchange Brain Trust (www.braintrust.org). This latter website has online support groups, also for teens and young adult children of brain tumor patients. The National Brain Tumor Foundation promotes support venues through email, phone, publications, Internet resources, support groups, and regional workshops (Guralnick 2006). The support network also has access to a message board, where family members can post questions and observations (Guralnick 2006). These resources provide information, training, a sense of control about their situation, and outlets for dialogue (Guralnick 2006).

The American Brain Tumor Association provides an orientation handbook to caregiving. This association also sponsors a "connections" pen pal program (in Black and Hogan 2006). The Healing Exchange Brain Trust provides online support groups (also including various ages and relationships to the loved one), website resources, and publications. In addition, the publication, "What You Need to Know About Brain Tumors" by the U.S. Department of Health and Human Services et al. (2003) on the website http://www.cancer.gov/cancertopics/wynt/brain/page1 is very informative and includes samples of questions prior to a biopsy, initiation of treatment, surgery, radiation, and chemotherapy; informational booklets; telephone and Internet resources, including a table of links; and a glossary of terms (U.S. Department of Health and Human Services et al. 2003).

When the family receives information about symptoms, disease progression, treatment, and likely adverse events through multiple formats, the psychoeducation process is consolidated for the caregiver and overall family (Given et al. 2008;

Schubart et al. 2008). Recently, authors have identified the benefit of an informational approach that combines stories and fact-based education, as the narrative writing style encompasses more engaging and familiar language that is less threatening (Kitamura et al. 2011). Psychoeducational materials also reduce uncertainty, which in turn reduces the caregiver's stress level (Given et al. 2008).

The psychotherapist and other therapists (e.g., an occupational therapist) can teach the caregiver and other tier supports various pragmatic coping techniques to alleviate their distress and cultivate resiliency. Given the complexity of the tumor diagnosis, its treatment, and impact on the family system, it behooves the primary caregiver to keep the multitude of information highly organized. This can be done in a binder format, with various subsections identified, as in the date of diagnosis, dates of CT/MRI scans, treatment modalities and timelines, physicians' names and access information, a list of medications, support services, etc. (Black and Hogan 2006; see Goodman et al. 2007, for a review). Logging the loved one's medical experiences and concerns allows for easy access at appointments (National Brain Tumor Society 2010b). It is paramount to oversee (or when necessary manage) the loved one's medications with or for him or her, depending on his or her health status. The caregiver should be sure that the various physicians are aware of all medications that are being prescribed; the most efficient way to ensure this is to have a comprehensive list with all medications, doses, and administration schedules (Goodman et al. 2007). Use of a pillbox in the home environment is strongly recommended. The book, *Orientation to Caregiving: A Handbook for Family Caregivers of Patients with Brain Tumors* by Goodman et al. (2007) contains an appendix of very useful forms and checklists which will help to organize the caregiver (e.g., caregiving checklist; treatment log; medication log; health history form, etc.).

Other suggestions are to: prioritize concerns and responsibilities; focus on what truly matters to the process; establish a "normal" yet flexible routine; focus on short-term goals; and maintain good communication with the loved one and overall support system (Goodman et al. 2007; National Brain Tumor Society 2010b). Overall, relatives will have constantly shifting commitments and decisions, based on the course and trajectory of the loved one's health status (Schubart et al. 2008). This will necessitate a conscious mindset of being adaptable to ever-changing conditions (Aldrich and Peterson 2010). Mindful trial-and-error attempts to identify the preferred course of action and self-forgiveness when failures are encountered improve coping capacity (Aldrich and Peterson 2010).

The psychotherapist can remind the caregiver and family to be sensitive to timelines. For example, prior to neurosurgery, the primary caregiver (and loved one) should put their financial and health-care matters in order (Roloff 2010). This includes reviewing medical, disability, and life insurance policies (Black and Hogan 2006). An estate plan comprised of a will or living trust; health-care power of attorney; financial power of attorney; nomination of a conservator; letter of instruction; pour-over will with a living trust; and a property agreement should be created (Black and Hogan 2006; Roloff 2010). An example of a living will declaration is provided as an appendix in Black and Hogan (2006; see also Chap. 10, for more discussion). Notification of the work site and child care arrangements in the home should also be expedited (Black and Hogan 2006).

For practical considerations regarding insurance funding, financial management, and access to community health and support systems, it is advised that the family seek the services of a social worker, financial planner, and/or attorney with specialized knowledge in these areas (National Brain Tumor Society 2010b; see www.abta.org for other resources). Some employers may offer paid or unpaid medical leave for the caregiver (Goodman et al. 2007). The primary caregiver or assigned family member should be sure to be familiar with the loved one's insurance policy, including what medical treatments are covered, annual and lifetime limits, co-payments, deductibles, etc. (Goodman et al. 2007). Also, the caregiver should be aware of mandatory preauthorizations for treatment. Often, the family has to be persistent to receive timely input from the insurance company and may have to make follow-up phone calls to expedite services (Goodman et al. 2007). The caregiver should keep a detailed record of phone calls and copies of all paperwork (Goodman et al. 2007). If possible, request a case manager and try to build a good working relationship with this person, so that he or she understands the dire nature of the loved one's care needs (Goodman et al. 2007). Relatives should be prepared for insurance denials; a social worker or professional advocate can help liaison in these instances (see Goodman et al. 2007, for a review).

The psychotherapist can offer other strategies to families to cope with treatment costs and ward off financial devastation, such as using savings; making "trade-offs"/choices (e.g., forgoing vacations, selling assets); employing longer range conservative financial planning; taking out loans; relying on tier 2 and 3 family and friends for financial support (including sometimes fundraisers); government entitlement programs (e.g., Social Security); grant programs (e.g., hospital charity/nonprofit organizations); or assistance from drug companies (Bradley et al. 2007; Goodman et al. 2007). Often, the family system has to make sacrifices including limiting the children's extracurricular activities; selling their home or other possessions; and having teenage children engage in paid work (Bradley et al. 2007). Financial woes can also translate into marital tensions and arguments (Bradley et al. 2007), for which psychotherapy and expert financial input are advisable.

Because of the chronicity and stresses from their numerous and sometimes, arduous roles and responsibilities, the psychotherapist will try to persuade caregivers to focus on self-care and personal sustenance, as there will be a natural tendency to neglect this (Klonoff and Koberstein 2010; Moore and Wagner 2009; National Brain Tumor Society 2010b). The caregiver definitely needs a sturdy support system (i.e., tiers 1, 2, and 3), including the medical team, family and friends, support groups, peer mentors, Internet connections, local and national organizations, and counseling specialists (National Brain Tumor Society 2010b; see Chap. 1, Fig. 1.2). Research indicates that the caregivers who have a positive social support network fare better in maintaining positive psychological well-being by buffering the stress associated with caring for a loved one with functional impairments (Ownsworth et al. 2010). The therapist should also remind the family (and loved one) to seek solace through their spiritual beliefs and religious affiliations, even in the context of a harried schedule (Klonoff and Koberstein 2010). This can include chaplaincy/spiritual advisor services (Roloff 2010).

Psychotherapy should include teaching or recommending stress-reduction techniques, so that the caregiver engages in exercise, massages, meditation, yoga, deep breathing, and progressive muscle relaxation (Klonoff and Koberstein 2010; National Brain Tumor Society 2010b; Swartz and Keir 2007). Due to circumstances, the family may need or prefer to complete these in the home with their loved one (Keir 2007).

Understandably, a primary goal of psychotherapy is to help tier 1 caregivers combat the inclination to isolate from others, including a downward cycle of insisting on self-sufficiency, rebuffing the efforts of others, and then feeling overwhelmed, lonely, and depleted. Sometimes, it is advantageous for the psychotherapist to explore online support groups or other community resources during a session; this penetrates empathically the inertia from intimidation, burnout, depression, and alienation. This also eases the caregiver's intimidation by technology. Of note, exploration of the cultural and experiential background of the caregiver's family of origin is paramount to finding the most suitable milieu for the family to glean support.

Psychotherapy should help the caregiver set realistic expectations for caregiving, including a willingness to make specific requests of others (Klonoff and Koberstein 2010; National Brain Tumor Society 2010b). Caregivers should schedule regular respite breaks to pursue satisfying self-interests and unabashedly share the caregiving commitments with others (Klonoff and Koberstein 2010). Even small and simple distractions (e.g., coffee with a friend or store browsing) can be nurturing. Perceiving this as a hassle for others or a downfall of the caregiver resulting in guilty feelings should be reframed in therapy as the extension of genuine love and support from other tier supports (see Chap. 1, Sect. 1.3). Delegation of tasks between willing family members, including the extended family, as well as close friends, will help to preserve collective energies and resiliency (Goodman et al. 2007; Klonoff and Koberstein 2010; Moore and Wagner 2009; Sherwood et al. 2004a). Capitalize on the talents of the support network and consider conducting an introductory meeting to provide an overview of the loved one's needs and preferences (Goodman et al. 2007). A central calendar with everyone's schedule and a concise list of pertinent information and contact numbers are good organizational tools (Goodman et al. 2007).

Alternatively, the family may hire a health-care provider out of necessity or preference (Goodman et al. 2007; Sherwood et al. 2004a). Referrals can typically be accessed through the treating staff, the patient services department of a hospital, or by word of mouth through community contacts (Goodman et al. 2007). This is especially prudent when medical expertise is required that is beyond the scope of the relatives or when there are major behavioral problems in the loved one (Sherwood et al. 2006). In this realm, psychotherapy can also help the caregiver work through worry and remorse when shifting or abdicating undertakings and reinforce the principle that the optimal care of the patient is predicated on the physical and mental health of the caregiver and overall family (Klonoff and Koberstein 2010; Schubart et al. 2008).

Aldrich and Peterson (2010) have developed a Caregiver's Bill of Rights which delineates beneficial ways for the caregiver to be more in tune with his or her needs during such grueling times. These include the right to self-care; to seek help from others; recognize one's limits; do things for oneself; to have and express difficult emotions; to take pride in one's accomplishments; and to protect one's individuality (Aldrich and Peterson 2010). Realigning one's values and aspirations, with an emphasis on short-term concrete and attainable goals that the loved one shares also anchors the caregiver (Goodman et al. 2007).

The healthy parent will need special assistance in addressing the needs of the children due to a brain tumor in the other parent (see also Chap. 3, Sect. 3.4). Consultation with a psychotherapist trained for family therapy and child/adolescent treatment is preferable (see Aldrich and Peterson 2010, for a review; Black and Hogan 2006; National Brain Tumor Society 2010b). Children often sense that something is wrong, so parents should not underestimate their need for information (Goodman et al. 2007). The turmoil triggered by a brain tumor diagnosis in a parent may cause children to regress, act out, or show behavioral outbursts (Black and Hogan 2006; National Brain Tumor Society 2010b). In conjunction with the nature, course, and manifestations of the brain tumor, important factors to consider when disclosing to children are their age, emotional development, personality, and relationship to the family member with the brain tumor (Black and Hogan 2006; Goodman et al. 2007; Khalili 2007; National Brain Tumor Society 2010b; Stark-Vance and Dubay 2011).

Children should be given a say regarding how much information they want and for what topics (National Brain Tumor Society 2010b). General suggestions include: describe an overview of brain function and how a tumor affects this (including noticeable side effects); give sufficient information to answer basic questions in a straightforward, truthful, realistic, and loving but nonthreatening manner; use age-appropriate language; monitor timing of discussions; encourage their self-expression of emotions and open communication; keep the teachers at school informed as well as maintain proper discipline and expectations (within reason; Aldrich and Peterson 2010; Black and Hogan 2006; Goodman et al. 2007; Khalili 2007; National Brain Tumor Society 2010b; Stark-Vance and Dubay 2011).

Goodman et al. (2007) provide some apt guidelines for disclosure to children, based on their age and communication skills. Providing a comfortable and comforting ambience for children to revisit topics of concern consoles them and keeps them adequately informed. Sometimes, children need to be reassured that they did not cause the tumor (Goodman et al. 2007; National Brain Tumor Society 2010b; Stark-Vance and Dubay 2011). They also need to be prepared psychologically for side effects of the treatment (e.g., weight loss and low energy; Goodman et al. 2007). Involvement in small and appropriate caregiving assignments empowers the children (Goodman et al. 2007). It is understandable that the adult caregiver will display feelings of sadness (e.g., tearfulness) and these model healthy responses in the children (National Brain Tumor Society 2010b; Stark-Vance and Dubay 2011).

In sum, preserving and bolstering the entire family unit's emotional health is fundamental in replenishing the necessary resources to optimize care for the loved one. Psychotherapy should include preparation for end-of-life issues during the terminal phases of the illness, with respect to both realistic considerations (e.g., hospice care) as well as psychological support (Schubart et al. 2008; see Chap. 10).

7.7 Case Study

David was age 38 when he suffered a grand mal seizure while playing basketball with some neighbors. The paramedics were called and he was taken to a local hospital, where a CT scan and MRI indicated a tumor in the left frontal lobe. David's wife, Heather, was stunned at the news, at first convinced that the doctors must be mistaken, especially as David's health had been exemplary preceding the seizure. Lapsing into "automatic pilot," she agreed with the recommendation for immediate neurosurgery. Before surgery, they met with a hospital chaplain and also quickly constructed a living will. The neuropathologist's report indicated a grade 2 oligodendroglioma. Postoperatively, David had right-sided motor weakness and was initially nonverbal. He was also agitated. Medications included levetiracetam for seizure control.

As depicted in phase 1 of the FEM, Heather maintained a constant vigil at David's bedside. She frantically arranged for her sister, Susan (a tier 2 support), to come and stay with their son, Troy, age 10 and daughter, Brittany, age 13. Heather was terrified to see changes in so many areas and was plagued by questions about his capacity to recover. An inpatient neuropsychologist, Dr. Smithe, attuned to Heather's distress, met with her in consultation. Dr. Smithe presumed some wariness, as Heather asked that Susan also attend (see Chap. 2, Sect. 2.2 and Table 2.1). Heather blurted out during the first appointment that she did not trust mental health professionals. Gentle inquiry revealed that her own mother was a social worker and Heather described her as overbearing and overcontrolling. Employing psychodynamic and self-psychology frameworks, Dr. Smithe internally hypothesized that she would need to cautiously build an empathic working alliance and be watchful not to seem intrusive, so as avoid a negative transference reaction in Heather. Also, based on the initial appointment, Dr. Smithe's assessment of Heather was that she had very limited awareness of the consequences of the brain tumor diagnosis in her husband, including the life-altering ramifications. Heather was also unaware of her own need for the valuable psychoeducation and emotional support that Dr. Smithe could provide (see Chap. 2, Sect. 2.2.1 and Table 2.3). In contrast, Susan was more in tune with the gravity of the situation and was therefore keen to help both Heather and David.

Heather knew nothing about brain tumors; however, she was too terrified and distraught to take action. She was succumbing to CRs by proxy and avoidance behaviors. Susan recognized the need to intervene on Heather's behalf and Dr. Smithe suggested that she solicit as much information as possible from the nurses, neurosurgical residents, and neuro-oncologists. Susan was told that it was a slower growing tumor and that after surgery, the doctors on the tumor board recommended radiation therapy. As a way of reaching out to Heather, Dr. Smithe held a family meeting with Heather and Susan and tried empathically to support Heather. She urged them to follow the next step in David's medical management to help improve his functional status. The doctors then coordinated a transfer to the inpatient neurorehabilitation unit, where he received speech, physical, and occupational therapies for 1 week. Ten days after the surgery, much to Heather's mortification, he was discharged home.

Dr. Smithe provided Heather and Susan with contact information and encouraged them to follow up whenever needed.

Based on the advice of a social worker on the rehabilitation unit, Susan quickly began surfing the Internet to find information and resources and accessed information from the National Brain Tumor Society. Although she liked and respected David's neurosurgeon and neuro-oncologist, she felt that a second opinion for Heather and David might be advantageous before proceeding with radiation therapy. Susan assisted Heather in obtaining a complete set of records and sent a copy of these to another well-respected neuro-oncologist whose name she had obtained through the National Brain Tumor Society. Everyone went to the appointment. Susan helped Heather develop a list of pertinent questions related to treatment options and the side effects. The second opinion was identical to the first. Heather was gradually beginning to face the seriousness of the situation and she took copious notes. Afterwards, Heather and David both decided to follow up with radiation therapy with the initial neuro-oncologist, as they both felt comfortable with him and had begun to establish a good communication pattern.

Once David was home, he was still experiencing the aftereffects of the surgery. He was not able to drive or go to work and was lying around unproductively. Prior to his tumor diagnosis, David was a successful real estate developer, working lots of hours. Heather, now feeling "mateless," was frightened about the "shifting sands" of his condition and felt helpless to guide him. Susan reminded her about Dr. Smithe's offer and with some reticence, Heather called her. Dr. Smithe coordinated with the neuro-oncologist and David was referred to outpatient therapies, while finishing his 6 weeks of radiation therapy. A repeat MRI 3 months postsurgery showed no regrowth. Heather and David were extremely relieved. They decided to focus their energies on his rehabilitation to attain his maximal potential.

Physically, David was extremely tired, from both his neurosurgery as well as the radiation therapy, and Heather became acutely aware of his deconditioned state. Per the physical therapist and rehabilitation physician, Heather helped her husband keep an energy log. The physical and occupational therapists reviewed this and provided specific exercises for David in the clinic and through a home program to rebuild his endurance. They also proposed that he maintain a regulated sleep schedule, take a daily 20-minute power nap, and partition his energies by spending quality time attending his children's sports events, while temporarily limiting evening social activities. Heather was conscientious about applying these suggestions. Per a medical recommendation, Heather contacted a dietician to obtain input about healthy foods and how to supplement her husband's diet, as he had lost about 25 pounds. She gave him nutritional supplements twice daily and was diligent about having him eat more fruits and vegetables.

At Susan's urging, Heather and David continued with a couple of appointments with Dr. Smithe. David had noticed that he was slower in his processing, easily distracted, and more forgetful. Heather, on the other hand, demonstrated limited acceptance; she resorted to "yeah buts" and minimized these symptoms as normal for anyone recuperating from a major surgery. She also was vociferous about her ability to adequately cope, distrustful of Dr. Smithe's further attempts to provide her with assistance and relief (see Chap. 2, Sect. 2.2.1.2 and Table 2.3). Dr. Smithe performed a neuropsychological assessment at 3.5 months postsurgery and shared the results with David and Heather. Per this examination, David demonstrated significant challenges in complex attention, learning, and retaining verbal information, and several areas of executive functions, specifically problem solving, strategy generation, planning, and multitasking. Although David was very despondent and tearful during the feedback session, Heather became incensed at the results, refusing to acknowledge the seriousness of the situation and launching a counterattack negating the validity of the assessment tools. Dr. Smithe recognized that Heather's defiance, impatience, distrust, and unrealism were catalysts to an adversarial alliance (see Chap. 3, Sect. 3.1.1 and Fig. 3.1). She also surmised that Heather was a "hidden patient," longing for a return to normalcy (see Chap. 3, Sect. 3.2.1). Dr. Smithe judiciously monitored her own countertransference reaction, so as not to exacerbate the tensions. At Heather's insistence, David and Heather took a break from therapy; this turned out to be only temporary.

Three weeks later, Heather and David frantically contacted Dr. Smithe. They both shared with Dr. Smithe their observations that he was much more lethargic at home, spending most days on the couch, and not initiating household chores or activities with the children in the way he did prior to surgery. He was also mopey and weepy. Dr. Smithe recommended that the couple restart weekly psychotherapy sessions and that David see a local psychiatrist, Dr. Browne. At first, Heather was peeved about the referral to a psychiatrist. She expressed adamant opposition, thinking that more medication was not the answer, and that he could "snap out of it" if he only tried hard enough. Although David gave his best effort towards trying to perk up and become more active, he persisted in feeling overwhelmed and defeated. He was becoming desperate for another "tool in the tool kit." Dr. Smithe recognized that Heather was displaying FEM "yellow warning zone" behaviors (see Chap. 1, Sect. 1.5), including "narcissistic rage" attacks towards Dr. Smithe and David's other doctors, feeling they were not listening to her.

Dr. Smithe knew she needed to wear multiple hats, given their disparate realities (see Chap. 1, Sect. 1.4.2). She did not personalize Heather's negativity; instead, she validated their divergent perspectives, but cautioned Heather (and David) about the debilitating effects of chronic depression. They both hesitantly agreed for David to see Dr. Browne. David was started on sertraline, which soon greatly improved his mood and motivation. Because of sleep disruptions, the psychiatrist also prescribed trazodone. At Dr. Smithe's suggestion, he began attending a local support group to help reduce his despair and social seclusion. David had a much better outlook and demeanor. Heather's reaction was sobered and she resolved to become more amenable to therapeutic recommendations. Heather was coming to "trust the process" of therapy with Dr. Smithe (see Chap. 2, Sect. 2.4.1.1).

Dr. Smithe recommended David begin some cognitive rehabilitation exercises to improve his cognition and learn worthwhile compensations. David was reticent, but with Heather's newfound trust in Dr. Smithe, she pushed him, justifying that this would help his outlook and speed up his return to driving and work. David undertook an 8-week course of cognitive exercises and soon started to enjoy the structure and sense of accomplishment. Heather attended the sessions weekly and became familiarized with his new strategies for thinking speed and attention.

David persisted in displaying CRs, whereby he would erupt with aggravation and anger. He was cantankerous about restrictions, feeling more like a child than a husband. However, he was relatively unaware of the extent and ramifications of his behavior in the home environment. Dr. Smithe coached Heather about the precipitants of CRs and cautioned her to be mindful not to overload him with too many requests. She was asked to monitor potential triggers, such as his level of exhaustion and noisiness in their children and dogs. However, she realized that she and the children were still "walking on eggshells," and after conferring with David, she recontacted the psychiatrist. They attended an appointment together and Heather provided some specific examples of his outbursts, based on a journal that Dr. Smithe proposed she keep. Dr. Browne prescribed a low dose of risperidone and also encouraged David and Heather to continue with family therapy with Dr. Smithe. David was introduced to some stress-reduction procedures, including deep breathing and meditation, and Heather took steps to provide a calmer atmosphere in the evenings for him to practice these techniques.

Dr. Smithe encouraged David and Heather to avoid overstimulation, including too many visitors in the home, as this would also catalyze CRs. Through therapy, Heather developed an organized and titrated visitor schedule based on their children's friends, the extended family, and David's work colleagues. Dr. Smithe provided psychoeducation to Heather about the role of emotional dysregulation after the frontal lobe injury, so as to help her remain calm and compassionate. She then realized David's altered behavior was a result of the brain tumor, not factors connected to her or the children. Dr. Smithe also encouraged David and Heather to pursue enjoyable activities, including a short weekly date. Both of them abstained from any alcohol intake, to keep his spirits stable and more uplifted. Through psychotherapy, his brain tumor support group, and family discussions, David was helped to accept the need to remain off work and abstain from driving for the next few months to allow for further recuperation. Heather's kind, caring, and adaptable attitude about this was instrumental in allaying David's guilt.

In the meantime, Heather made sure to attend weekly sessions with the treating therapists to help gain knowledge and give input into treatment goals. The occupational therapist was very appreciative of her input, as she could then tailor her goals with David accordingly. Together, the three of them fashioned a Home Independence Checklist, which included David helping to set up for dinner, feeding the dogs, doing laundry once weekly, supervising the children's homework for 30 min three times per week, and scheduling "dad time" with each child, 45 min twice weekly (e.g., playing on the Wii™, shooting hoops). He was encouraged to use his right hand to do as many chores at home as possible, to rebuild his strength and hand dexterity. The occupational therapist performed some home visits to help set up routines at home, also including a pillbox system and alarm system so that Heather could oversee David's medication regimen. They were both very appreciative of the compensatory strategies. As David's mastery and energies rekindled, he asked to restart bill paying. Dr. Smithe and the occupational therapist felt this was a very good functional task to boost David's sense of self-worth and efficacy in the home. This was also a great relief to Heather, who was inundated with other duties and unfamiliar with David's computerized payment system.

David's speech and language testing indicated moderate problems with naming, language formulation, speed of thinking, fluid reasoning, and memory for verbal and written material. Although he cooperated during the testing process, his affect was flat and he did not readily initiate conversation. Once the results were reviewed with David and Heather, he embarked upon a therapy schedule of three sessions per week, with regular homework. The speech–language pathologist provided excellent compensatory tools for David, which she reviewed with Heather. David already used a smartphone to track information, but he needed a more detailed and comprehensive system, which the speech–language pathologist taught him. She suggested that Heather slow down when making requests of him in the home and also use a central calendar to track appointments and their children's activities. The speech–language pathologist also educated Heather about the neurological basis of flattened affect, so that Heather would not take David's behavior personally and interpret it as disinterest. She also encouraged Heather to use joking and humor as a way to stimulate more expressiveness in her husband.

Both David and Heather were frightened about the longer-term implications of the brain tumor diagnosis. This included finances, as David was the sole earner and the "family executive" when it had come to household decisions. Given that the tumor was a lower grade, they were hopeful that his health would maintain. They communicated a readiness to Dr. Smithe and the neuro-oncologist for more information to help with longer range planning. His neuro-oncologist stated that he had no "crystal ball," but that if David continued improving at the rate he had thus far, he could return to work in the next several weeks, albeit on a part-time basis to start. In the meantime, Dr. Smithe laid the groundwork that the prognosis was uncertain and they should seek input from a financial planner or attorney about financial management.

Thankfully, David's brother, Joseph (another tier 2 support) was very helpful in this regard, which was reassuring to Heather. Heather and David updated their estate will. Joseph volunteered to liaise with the insurance company about denied claims and also contacted David's workplace about medical leave questions. As a couple, and with Joseph's guidance, some family austerity measures were taken to ward off further financial upheaval, primarily in the form of budget tightening. Heather's sister, Susan also remained very engaged. Recognizing some of the financial hardship, she undertook to pay for some of the children's extracurricular activities. In a follow-up appointment, Dr. Smithe complimented Heather (and David) about their evolving realism for accommodating their complex circumstances and accepting outside help to reduce their strains (see Chap. 2, Sect. 2.2.1.3 and Table 2.3).

After 4 months of constant stress, Heather realized her nerves were frayed and she was overburdened by her heap of obligations (see also Chap. 2, Sect. 2.3). David's role as her companion and confidante had evaporated. She felt pulled in too many directions doing "double duty" and was afraid her children were neglected and suffering. She had stopped exercising and had numerous sleepless nights. Consumed by guilt and feelings of helplessness, she ignored her needs, feeling compelled to focus entirely on her ill husband and needy children. Susan pointed out to her that she seemed anxious and overwhelmed. Initially, Heather was in denial about the extent of her distress, but her sister persisted. With David's permission, Heather then scheduled a few private sessions with Dr. Smithe to explore ways she could rejuvenate and cope better.

Dr. Smithe first obtained more history about their marital relationship. Although Heather noted its current shakiness, there was a strong historical foundation of love and commitment. Dr. Smithe recommended some conjoint sessions employing emotionally focused couple therapy (see Chap. 3, Sect. 3.2.2), so that they could become more emotionally responsive to one another. Drs. Smithe and Browne also addressed some troubling sexual intimacy issues that had arisen related to David's physiological, self-esteem, and interpersonal challenges. Dr. Smithe provided psychoeducation about the manifestations of Heather's understandable anxiety, including edginess and muscle tension (see Chap. 4, Sect. 4.8.2 and Table 4.9). Based on exploring her family system, Heather disclosed that she came from a large Italian family, where open sharing of feelings was the norm. She liked the idea of trying a support group, as she was feeling comfortable expressing her sometimes intense emotions. Dr. Smithe counseled her about the Healing Exchange Brain Trust for ongoing education and support. Dr. Smithe also told her about a monthly support group for family members of brain tumor survivors, which she sometimes facilitated. Heather invited the friend she made at David's rehabilitation center to attend the meetings with her, as they had a lot in common. Through further dialogue, Heather was encouraged to spend a few hours weekly with her sister and/or female friends for some relaxing respite. Dr. Smithe also recommended she attend a weekly yoga class and coordinate with friends and her clearly supportive extended family to help with David's and the children's needs.

Both David and Heather were troubled about their children's emotional well-being. Troy was acting out at home, picking senseless fights with his sister, Brittany. Brittany's grades were suffering and she seemed afraid to leave her father and attend school. Troy and Brittany also had abundant questions about their father's health. At Dr. Smithe's urging, Heather contacted the schoolteachers to keep them apprised of the family stressors. Dr. Smithe then recommended they meet as a family, recognizing that the children were "at risk" (see Chap. 3, Sects. 3.4.1 and 3.4.2). Understandably, the children were mortified about the changes in their home life, including their mother's moodiness and busyness. Dr. Smithe adeptly reviewed the nature and location of the brain tumor employing user-friendly pictorial information. Dr. Smithe, David, and Heather also discussed some of the hurdles David was experiencing, including his mood, memory, and fatigue problems. Dr. Smithe normalized the changes in parenting duties, with Heather needing to "take the reins" in some areas. Dr. Smithe assured the children that their father's brain tumor diagnosis was unrelated to anything they had done. Dr. Smithe was encouraging about David's current health status, but was honest about the future unknowns. David reviewed his plans to return to work part-time and Heather discussed how everyone could support one another by being attentive and a team player. Heather and Troy were comforted that the family unit was sturdy. The need to keep up with homework and to follow behavior rules in the home was reviewed in a kindly tone by Dr. Smithe and both parents. Dr. Smithe recommended that the family resume regular attendance at their Unitarian Universalist church services on Sundays, so as to obtain community and spiritual sustenance. A nearby children's support group was recommended, as it would provide peer validation. Weekly "family fun nights" were also proposed. Each parent vowed to continue prioritizing special "quality" time with Troy and Brittany. Dr. Smithe also reinforced the benefit of the children staying involved in after-school sports and friendship activities. For Christmas, their parents promised them a dachshund puppy and they were elated. Dr. Smithe felt this would be a pleasant diversion for everyone. The dialogue was very productive and it was clear that the children felt better. Everyone agreed to continue to meet whenever needed to discuss new developments.

Fortunately, at 8 months postsurgery, David's brain tumor status was unchanged. He had returned to work and was driving. Dr. Smithe helped him make sensible accommodations at work by gradually increasing his hours and assignments and working in a quiet office to maximize his focus. He and Heather were elated with his progress, but were also cautious about the future ....

To be continued in Chap. 10.

References

Abrey, L. E., & Mason, W. P. (2011). *Fast facts: Brain tumors* (2nd ed.). Oxford: Health Press Limited.

Aldrich, J. J., & Peterson, N. M. (2010). *Connecting through compassion: Guidance for family and friends of a brain cancer patient*. United States of America: Cancer Lifeline Publications.

Anderson, S. W., & Ryken, T. C. (2008). Intracranial tumors. In J. E. Morgan & J. H. Ricker (Eds.), *Textbook of clinical neuropsychology* (pp. 578–587). New York: Taylor & Francis Group.

Bartolo, M., Zucchella, C., Pace, A., Lanzetta, G., Vecchione, C., Bartolo, M., et al. (2011). Early rehabilitation after surgery improves functional outcome in inpatients with brain tumours. *Journal of Neuro-Oncology*, Nov 29 [Epub ahead of print]. doi:10.1007/s11060-011-0772-5.

Benzagmout, M., Gatignol, P., & Duffau, H. (2007). Resection of world health organization grade II gliomas involving Broca's area: Methodological and functional considerations. *Neurosurgery, 61*(4), 741–752.

Black, P., & Hogan, S. C. (2006). *Living with a brain tumor: Dr. Peter Black's guide to taking control of your treatment*. New York: Henry Holt and Company.

Blinn, G. (2010). A different path. In T. A. Roloff (Ed.), *Navigating through a strange land: A book for brain tumor patients & their families* (pp. 31–34). Tucson: Indigo Press.

Bradley, S., Sherwood, P. R., Donovan, H. S., Hamilton, R., Rosenzweig, M., Hricik, A., et al. (2007). I could lose everything: Understanding the cost of a brain tumor. *Journal of Neuro-Oncology, 85*(3), 329–338.

Bradley, S. E., Sherwood, P. R., Kuo, J., Kammerer, C. M., Gettig, E. A., Ren, D., et al. (2009). Perceptions of economic hardship and emotional health in a pilot sample of family caregivers. *Journal of Neuro-Oncology, 93*(3), 333–342.

Broyard, A. (2010). Modern fiction on the couch: An interview with a retired psychoanalyst. In T. A. Roloff (Ed.), *Navigating through a strange land: A book for brain tumor patients & their families* (pp. 97–99). Tucson: Indigo Press.

Buckner, J. C., Brown, P. D., O'Neill, B. P., Meyer, F. B., Wetmore, C. J., & Uhm, J. H. (2007). Central nervous system tumors. *Mayo Clinic Proceedings, 82*(10), 1271–1286.

Calhoun-Eagan, R. D. (2009). Psychological and social impact of being a brain tumor survivor: Adult issues. In S. Goldman & C. D. Turner (Eds.), *Late effects of treatment for brain tumors* (pp. 309–316). New York: Springer.

Carter, R., Aldridge, S., Page, M., & Parker, S. (2009). *The human brain book: An illustrated guide to its structure, function, and disorders*. New York: DK Publishing.

Catt, S., Chalmers, A., & Fallowfield, L. (2008). Psychosocial and supportive-care needs in high-grade glioma. *Lancet Oncology, 9*(9), 884–891.

Chandana, S. R., Movva, S., Arora, M., & Singh, T. (2008). Primary brain tumors in adults. *American Family Physician, 77*(10), 1423–1430.

Davie, G. L., Hutcheson, K. A., Barringer, D. A., Weinberg, J. S., & Lewin, J. S. (2009). Aphasia in patients after brain tumour resection. *Aphasiology, 23*(9), 1196–1206.

de Jong, C. (2010). It's a cruel, crazy, beautiful world. In T. A. Roloff (Ed.), *Navigating through a strange land: A book for brain tumor patients & their families* (pp. 43–47). Tucson: Indigo Press.

De Luca, C. R., Conroy, R., McCarthy, M. C., Anderson, V. A., & Ashley, D. M. (2009). Neuropsychological impact of treatment of brain tumors. In S. Goldman & C. D. Turner (Eds.), *Late effects of treatment for brain tumors* (pp. 277–296). New York: Springer.

DiPatri, A. J., Pham, M., & Muro, K. (2009). Late effects of neurosurgery. In S. Goldman & C. D. Turner (Eds.), *Late effects of treatment for brain tumors* (pp. 7–22). New York: Springer.

Drappatz, J., & Wen, P. Y. C. (2011). Principles of supportive care. In A. D. Norden, D. A. Reardon, & P. Y. C. Wen (Eds.), *Primary central nervous system tumors: Pathogenesis and therapy* (pp. 55–84). New York: Springer.

Duffau, H., Moritz-Gasser, S., & Gatignol, P. (2009). Functional outcome after language mapping for insular World Health Organization Grade II gliomas in the dominant hemisphere: Experience with 24 patients. *Neurosurgical Focus, 27*(2), E7.

Edvardsson, T., & Ahlström, G. (2008). Being the next of kin of a person with a low-grade glioma. *Psycho-Oncology, 17*(6), 584–591.

Edvardsson, T. I., & Ahlström, G. I. (2009). Subjective quality of life in persons with low-grade glioma and their next of kin. *International Journal of Rehabilitation Research, 32*(1), 64–70.

Fabi, A., Felici, A., Metro, G., Mirri, A., Bria, E., Telera, S., et al. (2011). Brain metastases from solid tumors: Disease outcome according to type of treatment and therapeutic resources of the treating center. *Journal of Experimental & Clinical Cancer Research, 30*(1), 10–16.

Finocchiaro, C. Y., Petruzzi, A., Lamperti, E., Botturi, A., Gaviani, P., Silvani, A., et al. (2011). The burden of brain tumor: A single-institution study on psychological patterns in caregivers. *Journal of Neuro-Oncology*, Oct. 4. [Epub ahead of print]. doi:10.1007/s11060-011-0726-y.

Fox, S. W., Mitchell, S. A., & Booth-Jones, M. (2006). Cognitive impairment in patients with brain tumors: Assessment and intervention in the clinic setting. *Clinical Journal of Oncology Nursing, 10*(2), 169–176.

Gehring, K., Aaronson, N. K., Taphoorn, M. J. B., & Sitskoorn, M. M. (2011). A description of a cognitive rehabilitation programme evaluated in brain tumour patients with mild to moderate cognitive deficits. *Clinical Rehabilitation, 25*(8), 675–692.

Given, B., Sherwood, P. R., & Given, C. W. (2008). What knowledge and skills do caregivers need? *Journal of Social Work Education, 44*(3), 115–123.

Goldman, S., & Turner, C. D. (Eds.). (2009). *Late effects of treatment for brain tumors*. New York: Springer.

Goodman, S., Rabow, M., & Folkman, S. (2007). *Orientation to caregiving: A handbook for family caregivers of patients with brain tumors*. San Francisco: University of California San Francisco.

Grenier, D., & Gupta, S. (2009). Support organizations, resources, and relevant websites. In S. Goldman & C. D. Turner (Eds.), *Late effects of treatment for brain tumors* (pp. 411–425). New York: Springer.

Guralnick, E. (2006). We can all relate: Caregivers support one another. *Search, 67,* 1–2.

Gururangan, S. (2009). Late effects of chemotherapy. In S. Goldman & C. D. Turner (Eds.), *Late effects of treatment for brain tumors* (pp. 43–65). New York: Springer.

Hannay, H. J., Howieson, D. B., Loring, D. W., Fischer, J. S., & Lezak, M. D. (2004). Neuropathology for neuropsychologists. In M. D. Lezak, D. B. Howieson, D. W. Loring, H. J. Hannay, & J. S. Fischer (Eds.), *Neuropsychological assessment* (4th ed., pp. 157–285). New York: Oxford University Press.

Johnson, D. R., Ashman, J. B., Brown, P. D., Lachance, D. H., & Buckner, J. C. (2011). Complications of therapy. In A. D. Norden, D. A. Reardon, & P. Y. C. Wen (Eds.), *Primary central nervous system tumors: Pathogenesis and therapy* (pp. 103–141). New York: Springer.

Kakuda, W., Abo, M., Kobayashi, K., Momosaki, R., Yokoi, A., Hiroshi, I., & Umemori, T. (2010). Low-frequency rTMS combined with intensive occupational therapy for upper limb hemiparesis after brain tumour resection. *Brain Injury, 24*(12), 1505–1510.

Kangas, M., Williams, J., & Smee, R. I. (2007, Aug). Psychosocial functioning and support needs of adult brain tumor survivors. Conference presentation at the APA 115th Annual Covention, San Francisco, CA.

Kangas, M., Williams, J. R., & Smee, R. I. (2011). Benefit finding in adults treated for benign meningioma brain tumors: Relations with psychosocial wellbeing. *Brain Impairment, 12*(2), 105–116.

Keir, S. T. (2007). Levels of stress and intervention preferences of caregivers of brain tumor patients. *Cancer Nursing, 30*(6), E33–E39.

Keir, S. T., Guill, A. B., Carter, K. E., Boole, L. C., Gonzales, L., & Friedman, H. S. (2006). Differential levels of stress in caregivers of brain tumor patients—observations from a pilot study. *Supportive Care in Cancer: Official Journal of the Multinational Association of Supportive Care in Cancer, 14*(12), 1258–1261.

Kenna, H. A., Poon, A. W., de los Angeles, C. P., & Koran, L. M. (2011). Psychiatric complications of treatment with corticosteroids: Review with case report. *Psychiatry and Clinical Neurosciences, 65*(6), 549–560.

Khalili, Y. (2007). Ongoing transitions: The impact of a malignant brain tumour on patient and family. *Axone (Dartmouth, N. S.), 28*(3), 5–13.

Kirby, S., & Purdy, R. A. (2007). Headache and brain tumors. *Current Neurology and Neuroscience Reports, 7*(2), 110–116.

Kitamura, C., Ng, D., Chung, A., Bezjak, A., Garraway, C., Mclean, M., Nyhof-Young, J., & Wong, R. (2011). Development and evaluation of a combined story and fact-based educational booklet for patients with multiple brain metastases and their caregivers. *Palliative Medicine, 25*(6), 642–649.

Klonoff, P. S. (2010). *Psychotherapy after brain injury: Principles and techniques*. New York: Guilford Press.

Klonoff, P. S., & Koberstein, E. J. (2010). Family life. In P. S. Klonoff (Ed.), *Psychotherapy after brain injury: Principles and techniques* (pp. 150–170). New York: Guilford Press.

Klonoff, P. S., & Myles, S. M. (2010). Sense of self and identity. In P. S. Klonoff (Ed.), *Psychotherapy after brain injury: Principles and techniques* (pp. 75–99). New York: Guilford Press.

Klonoff, P. S., Lage, G. A., & Chiapello, D. A. (1993). Varieties of the catastrophic reaction to brain injury: A self psychology perspective. *Bulletin of the Menninger Clinic, 57*(2), 227–241.

Klonoff, P. S., Koberstein, E. J., Talley, M. C., & Dawson, L. K. (2008). A family experiential model of recovery after brain injury. *Bulletin of the Menninger Clinic, 72*(2), 109–129.

Landier, W., Kinahan, K. E., Shaw, S., & Bhatia, S. (2009). Screening for late effects in brain tumor survivors. In S. Goldman & C. D. Turner (Eds.), *Late effects of treatment for brain tumors* (pp. 389–409). New York: Springer.

Loghin, M., & Levin, V. A. (2006). Headache related to brain tumors. *Current Treatment Options in Neurology, 8*(1), 21–32.

Lu-Emerson, C., & Norden, A. D. (2011). Epidemiology and risk factors. In A. D. Norden, D. A. Reardon, & P. Y. C. Wen (Eds.), *Primary central nervous system tumors: Pathogenesis and therapy* (pp. 3–25). New York: Springer.

McConigley, R., Halkett, G., Lobb, E., & Nowak, A. (2010). Caring for someone with high-grade glioma: A time of rapid change for caregivers. *Palliative Medicine, 24*(5), 473–479.
Mea, E., Silvani, A., Gaviani, P., Lamperti, E., Ferrari, D., Botturi, A., et al. (2011). Headaches and brain tumors. *Journal of the Neurological Sciences*, Oct 1 [Epub ahead of print]. doi:10.1007/s10072-011-0789-8.
Monje, M., & Wen, P. Y. (2009). Neurological complications in adults. In S. Goldman & C. D. Turner (Eds.), *Late effects of treatment for brain tumors* (pp. 113–132). New York: Springer.
Moore, T., & Wagner, S. (2009). Caregiver and family issues for brain tumor survivors. In S. Goldman & C. D. Turner (Eds.), *Late effects of treatment for brain tumors* (pp. 331–339). New York: Springer.
National Brain Tumor Society. (2010a). *Understanding glioblastoma* [booklet]. San Francisco: National Brain Tumor Society.
National Brain Tumor Society. (2010b). *Coping with your loved one's brain tumor: A guide for family and friends* [booklet]. San Francisco: National Brain Tumor Society.
National Brain Tumor Society. (2011a). *10 questions to ask your doctor* [booklet]. San Francisco: National Brain Tumor Society.
National Brain Tumor Society. (2011b). *How and why to get a second opinion* [booklet]. San Francisco: National Brain Tumor Society.
National Brain Tumor Society. (2011c). *Brain tumors and fatigue* [booklet]. San Francisco: National Brain Tumor Society.
National Brain Tumor Society. (2011d). *How tumors affect the mind, emotion, and personality* [booklet]. San Francisco: National Brain Tumor Society.
Norden, A. D., Reardon, D. A., & Wen, P. Y. C. (Eds.). (2011). *Primary central nervous system tumors: Pathogenesis and therapy*. New York: Springer.
Norton, S. A., & Bowers, B. J. (2001). Working toward consensus: Providers' strategies to shift patients from curative to palliative treatment choices. *Research in Nursing & Health, 24*(4), 258–269.
Ouma, J. R. (2004). Psychotic manifestations in brain tumour patients: 2 case reports from South Africa. *African Health Sciences, 4*(3), 189–193.
Ownsworth, T., Henderson, L., Chambers, S., & Shum, D. (2009). Functional impairments and caregiver depressive symptoms in the context of brain tumour and other cancers: A mediating effect of strain. *Brain Impairment, 10*(2), 149–161.
Ownsworth, T., Henderson, L., & Chambers, S. K. (2010). Social support buffers the impact of functional impairments on caregiver psychological well-being in the context of brain tumor and other cancers. *Psycho-Oncology, 19*(10), 1116–1122.
Palmieri, R. L. (2007). Responding to primary brain tumor. *Nursing, 37*(1), 36–42.
Patterson, H. (2007). *Nobody can afford a brain tumor: The financial impact of brain tumors on patients and families* [booklet]. San Francisco: National Brain Tumor Society.
Picozzi, P., & Kirchin, M. (2007). Improving lesion detection and visualization: Implications for neurosurgical planning and follow-up. *Neuroradiology, 49*(Suppl 1), S27–S34.
Purdy, R. A., & Kirby, S. (2004). Headaches and brain tumors. *Neurologic Clinics, 22*(1), 39–53.
Raver-Lampman, G. (2010). Excerpts from magic and loss. In T. A. Roloff (Ed.), *Navigating through a strange land: A book for brain tumor patients & their families* (pp. 7–10). Tucson: Indigo Press.
Reddick, K. (2010).What is faith? Reflections of a hospital chaplain. In T. A. Roloff (Ed.), *Navigating through a strange land: A book for brain tumor patients & their families* (pp. 113–118). Tucson: Indigo Press.
Roloff, T. A. (Ed.). (2010). *Navigating through a strange land: A book for brain tumor patients & their families*. Tucson: Indigo Press.
Rosenthal, D. S., Turner, C. D., Doherty-Gilman, A. M., & Dean-Clower, E. (2009). Integrative oncology as part of the treatment for brain tumors. In S. Goldman & C. D. Turner (Eds.), *Late effects of treatment for brain tumors* (pp. 353–362). New York: Springer.

Sawrie, S. M. (2006). The neuropsychology of adult neuro-oncology. In P. J. Snyder, P. D. Nussbaum, & D. L. Robins (Eds.), *Clinical neuropsychology: A pocket handbook for assessment* (2nd ed., pp. 415–435). Washington, D. C.: American Psychological Association.

Schmer, C., Ward-Smith, P., Latham, S., & Salacz, M. (2008). When a family member has a malignant brain tumor: The caregiver perspective. *Journal of Neuroscience Nursing, 40*(2), 78–84.

Schubart, J. R., Kinzie, M. B., & Farace, E. (2008). Caring for the brain tumor patient: Family caregiver burden and unmet needs. *Neuro-Oncology, 10*(1), 61–72.

Sherwood, P. R., Given, B. A., Doorenbos, A. Z., & Given, C. W. (2004a). Forgotten voices: Lessons from bereaved caregivers of persons with a brain tumour. *International Journal of Palliative Nursing, 10*(2), 67–75.

Sherwood, P., Given, B., Given, C., Schiffman, R., Murman, D., & Lovely, M. (2004b). Caregivers of persons with a brain tumor: A conceptual model. *Nursing Inquiry, 11*(1), 43–53.

Sherwood, P. R., Given, B. A., Given, C. W., Schiffman, R. F., Murman, D. L., Lovely, M., von Eye, A., et al. (2006). Predictors of distress in caregivers of persons with a primary malignant brain tumor. *Research in Nursing & Health, 29*(2), 105–120.

Sherwood, P. R., Given, B. A., Given, C. W., Schiffman, R. F., Murman, D. L., von Eye, et al. (2007). The influence of caregiver mastery on depressive symptoms. *Journal of Nursing Scholarship, 39*(3), 249–255.

Sherwood, P. R., Donovan, H. S., Given, C. W., Lu, X., Given, B. A., Hricik, A., & Bradley, S. (2008a). Predictors of employment and lost hours from work in cancer caregivers. *Psycho-Oncology, 17*(6), 598–605.

Sherwood, P. R., Given, B. A., Donovan, H., Baum, A., Given, C. W., Bender, C. M., & Schulz, R. (2008b). Guiding research in family care: A new approach to oncology caregiving. *Psycho-Oncology, 17*(10), 986–996.

Shih, H. A., Loeffler, J. S., & Tarbell, N. J. (2009). Late effects of CNS radiation therapy. In S. Goldman & C. D. Turner (Eds.), *Late effects of treatment for brain tumors* (pp. 23–41). New York: Springer.

Stark-Vance, V., & Dubay, M. L. (2011). *100 Questions & answers about brain tumors* (2nd ed.). Boston: Jones and Bartlett Publishers.

Swartz, J. J., & Keir, S. T. (2007). Program preferences to reduce stress in caregivers of patients with brain tumors. *Clinical Journal of Oncology Nursing, 11*(5), 723–727.

Talacchi, A., Santini, B., Savazzi, S., & Gerosa, M. (2011). Cognitive effects of tumour and surgical treatment in glioma patients. *Journal of Neuro-Oncology, 103*(3), 541–549.

Tepper, S. (2003). A model for care: A transitions program designed to provide comprehensive care in treating individuals with malignant brain tumors. *Smith College Studies in Social Work, 73*(3), 337–357.

U. S. Department of Health & Human Services, National Institutes of Health, & National Cancer Institute. (2003). *What you need to know about brain tumors* [Booklet]. Washington, D. C.: U. S. Department of Health & Human Services.

Vargo, M. (2011). Brain tumor rehabilitation. *American Journal of Physical Medicine & Rehabilitation, 90*(5 Suppl 1), S50–S62.

Wefel, J. S., Armstrong, T. A., & Kohli, S. (2011). Neuropsychological function and quality of life. In A. D. Norden, D. A. Reardon, & P. Y. C. Wen (Eds.), *Primary central nervous system tumors: Pathogenesis and therapy* (pp. 143–170). New York: Springer.

Wen, P. Y., Schiff, D., Kesari, S., Drappatz, J., Gigas, D. C., & Doherty, L. (2006). Medical management of patients with brain tumors. *Journal of Neuro-Oncology, 80,* 313–332.

Whittle, I. R., Pringle, A. M., & Taylor, R. (1998). Effects of resective surgery for left-sided intracranial tumours on language function: A prospective study. *Lancet, 351*(9108), 1014–1018.

Willard, V. W., Bonner, M. J., & Guill, A. B. (2009). Healthy lifestyle choices after cancer treatment. In S. Goldman & C. D. Turner (Eds.), *Late effects of treatment for brain tumors* (pp. 343–352). New York: Springer.

Zelko, F. A. J., & Sorensen, L. G. (2009). Academic issues: Special education and related interventions. In S. Goldman & C. D. Turner (Eds.), *Late effects of treatment for brain tumors* (pp. 317–330). New York: Springer.

Chapter 8
Family Psychotherapy for Seizure Disorders

8.1 Scenario: Early Questions about Seizure Disorders

Seizure disorders are a complex entity, emanating from a multitude of etiologies, with varied manifestations. Families can be quite frightened by seizures, given their unpredictability and effect on their loved one's neurological and functional status. They may ask questions such as: *What is an epileptic seizure? What caused this in my loved one? How will a seizure disorder affect him or her? What should we do as a family to help?*

8.1.1 Therapeutic Intervention: Neuropathology of Seizure Disorders

Seizure disorders are typically treated by neurologists, internists, family physicians, or neurosurgeons, depending on the etiology and treatment needs for the loved one with epilepsy (National Institute of Neurological Disorders and Stroke 2012). If available, the loved one should be seen by an epileptologist, who is a neurologist specializing in treating epilepsy (National Institute of Neurological Disorders and Stroke 2012; Reuber et al. 2009). Clinicians, including neuropsychologists and psychotherapists, can also educate relatives about seizure disorders or epilepsy and provide emotional support and treatment resources. There are a number of very useful resources which can supplement the family's (and loved one's) knowledge about seizures. These include: *Epilepsy in our View: Stories from Friends and Families of People Living with Epilepsy* by Schachter (2008a); *Epilepsy in Our Words: Personal Accounts of Living with Seizures* by Schachter (2008b); *Epilepsy Explained: A Book for People Who Want to Know More* by Reuber et al. (2009); *Epilepsy 199 Answers: A Doctor Responds to his Patients' Questions* by Wilner (2008); *Epilepsy: Patient and Family Guide* by Devinsky (2008); *Epilepsy 101: The Ultimate Guide for Patients and Families* by The National Epilepsy Educational Alliance (2009); and *The Cleveland Clinic Guide to Epilepsy* by Wyllie (2010). Some apropos children/young adult books are *Let's Learn with Teddy about Epilepsy* by Zelenka (2008), *Mommy, I Feel*

P. S. Klonoff, *Psychotherapy for Families after Brain Injury*,
DOI 10.1007/978-1-4899-8083-0_8, © Springer Science+Business Media New York 2014

Funny! A Child's Experience with Epilepsy by Rocheford (2009), *Karen's Epilepsy* by Baltaro (2010), and *Mighty Mike Bounces Back* by Skead and Simmel (2012).

Epilepsy is considered a chronic brain disorder characterized by recurrent seizures caused by abnormal or excessive discharge of cerebral neurons (see Lee and Clason 2008, for a review; The National Epilepsy Educational Alliance 2009; Wilner 2008). Epilepsy is used synonymously with seizure disorders. These are different from a *seizure,* or a single event in which there is a sudden, excessive, and disorderly discharge of neurons which result in clinical manifestations (Lee and Clason 2008; Wilner 2008). Once focal abnormal electrical discharges spread to other areas of the brain, behavioral signs will appear (Lee and Clason 2008). Epilepsy can develop based on an abnormality in brain wiring, an imbalance in neurotransmitters, or abnormal nerve connections (National Institute of Neurological Disorders and Stroke 2012). The symptoms vary according to what parts of the brain are affected (Wilner 2008). Of note, this chapter will not focus on nonepileptic seizures, also known as nonepileptic psychogenic events (Martin et al. 2006), which is beyond the scope of this book.

Table 8.1 summarizes common types of seizure disorders (Barrett and Sachs 2006; Channing Bete Company 2008; Devinsky 2008; Hernández et al. 2010; Lee and Clason 2008; Martin et al. 2006; National Institute of Neurological Disorders and Stroke 2012; Reuber et al. 2009; Sethi et al. 2008; Stark-Vance and Dubay 2011; The National Epilepsy Educational Alliance 2009; Wyllie 2010). One category is *partial* or *focal* seizures, which occur in one part of the brain (Channing Bete Company 2008; Devinsky 2008). They account for about 60% of seizures, of which temporal lobe epilepsy is the most common syndrome (National Institute of Neurological Disorders and Stroke 2012). The other type is *generalized* seizures, which result from abnormal neuronal activity on both sides of the brain (Devinsky 2008; National Institute of Neurological Disorders and Stroke 2012). Partial seizures can progress and become generalized (Channing Bete Company 2008; Devinsky 2008; Martin et al. 2006). Some seizures are preceded by an *aura,* which is a focal seizure involving any of the five senses (e.g., funny feeling; strong odor; sharp, bitter, or sweet taste; visual spots or circles of light; Palmieri 2007; Wilner 2008; Wyllie 2010). Auras can occur alone or as a warning of onset of a stronger seizure (Wilner 2008; Wyllie 2010). For a more detailed description of many seizure types, see Devinsky (2008) and Reuber et al. (2009).

Seizure disorders affect approximately 1–4% of the population and occur across the life span (see Lee and Clason 2008, for a review). However, about half of seizures have no known cause (National Institute of Neurological Disorders and Stroke 2012). They may emerge during childhood due to prenatal injury, birth injury, anoxia, febrile convulsions, or developmental disorders (Lee and Clason 2008; National Institute of Neurological Disorders and Stroke 2012; Reuber et al. 2009; The National Epilepsy Educational Alliance 2009). Sometimes, there is a family history of seizures (Devinsky 2008; Mantoan and Kullmann 2011; National Institute of Neurological Disorders and Stroke 2012; The National Epilepsy Educational Alliance 2009). Other reasons for seizures are strokes, traumatic brain injuries, brain tumors, metabolic disorders, hydrocephalus, poisoning, overdose of alcohol or drugs, Alzheimer's disease,

Table 8.1 Common types of seizure disorders

Partial (focal) seizures
1. *Simple partial seizures*: This type of seizure begins in one cortical area, in a "focus." They have motor, sensory, autonomic, or psychic symptoms and last for several seconds to a few minutes. The loved one will remain alert and will remember the event. Symptoms match the area of the brain that is affected (e.g., motor signs of jerking in the fingers, face, or tongue related to a frontal lobe seizure focus or language difficulties related to a temporal lobe seizure focus). This seizure is sometimes a precursor to a complex partial seizure
2. *Complex partial seizures*: This type of seizure results in decreased awareness of the environment and lack of responsiveness. The loved one will not be able to recall the events which occurred during the seizure. The loved one may have an aura or signal that the seizure is coming, including a sense of déjà vu, abdominal discomfort, or olfactory hallucinations. Following that are automatisms, which are repetitive involuntary motor activities. These include picking movements, lip smacking, chewing or swallowing motions, drooling, as well as tapping or rubbing hand motions. These can last for 1 to 10 min. Amnesia for the seizure is common. Following the seizure, the loved one may be confused and, disoriented and have a headache; this is called the postictal period. This seizure occurs most often in the frontal and temporal lobes
Generalized seizures
1. *Absence (petit mal) seizures*: In this type of seizure, there is instant cessation of ongoing activity and impaired responsiveness for about 10 secs. It can look like day dreaming or lack of attention. They usually begin between ages 3 and 12 and stop during the teenage years
2. *Myoclonic seizures*: These are sudden, shock-like muscle contractions which last only a fraction of a second. They are also known as myoclonic "jerks" and may affect any group of muscles or the whole body. This type of seizure usually starts during childhood and can be accompanied by oversensitivity to light. An EEG is required to confirm the diagnosis
3. *Atonic seizures*: This type of seizure causes loss of muscle tone affecting the limb, head, neck, or entire body. The loved one becomes limp and may fall down; this is called a "drop attack." The person may also briefly lose consciousness
4. *Generalized clonic seizures*: This is a rare type of seizure and consists of rhythmic jerking movements of the arms, legs, and sometimes the face
5. *Generalized tonic seizures*: These are brief seizures that consist of sudden or gradual increased tone in muscles. This results in the loved one falling to the ground. Afterwards, the loved one may be confused, tired, or develop a headache
6. *Generalized tonic-clonic (grand mal) seizures*: This seizure may present without warning or with an aura (e.g., abdominal discomfort, dizziness, or irritable mood). It begins with a *tonic* phase. There is increased tone or stiffening across multiple muscle groups, usually with an arched back, extension of the arms and legs, an epileptic "cry," and labored breathing. There is also upward deviation of the eyes. This lasts for about 20-30 secs. and then transitions to the *clonic* phase, characterized by repeated bilateral, symmetric jerking of the arms and legs. This lasts for about 1 to 2 min. Bladder incontinence and excessive saliva production (i.e., foaming) may occur during this type of seizure. After the seizure (i.e., in the postictal period), the loved one may gradually awaken by passing through stages of coma, to confusion, to drowsiness. He or she may also fall asleep for varied time periods. Afterwards, the loved one may have muscle soreness, fatigue, or a headache

EEG electroencephalogram

anoxia, and infectious diseases (Alajbegović et al. 2009; Catt et al. 2008; Channing Bete Company 2008; Devinsky 2008; Lee and Clason 2008; Mantoan and Kullmann 2011; Martin et al. 2006; National Institute of Neurological Disorders and Stroke 2012; Reuber et al. 2009; The National Epilepsy Educational Alliance 2009; Wyllie 2010; see Chaps. 4, 6, 7, and 10 correspondingly for a more in-depth discussion of moderate to severe traumatic brain injuries, cerebrovascular accidents, and brain tumors).

The incidence of seizures after stroke is relatively low compared with other types of brain injuries and ranges from about 2.7 to 6.3% (Beghi et al. 2011; Burneo et al. 2010; Szaflarski et al. 2008). Patients with more severe hemorrhagic strokes creating cortical damage are at higher risk of developing seizures (Beghi et al. 2011; Burneo et al. 2010; Szaflarski et al. 2008). Based on the literature, the incidence of seizures in brain tumor patients ranges from approximately 20% to as high as 85% (Alajbegović et al. 2009; Aldrich and Peterson 2010; see Drappatz and Wen 2011, for a review; see Liigant et al. 2001, for a review; Mogensen 2008; van Breemen et al. 2009; Vargo 2011; Vercueil 2011). They are more prevalent in patients with low-grade, slow-growing tumors (e.g., astrocytomas, mixed gliomas, and oligodendrogliomas) commonly affecting the frontal and temporal lobes (see Drappatz and Wen 2011, for a review; see Kurzwelly et al. 2010, for a review; see Liigant et al. 2001, for a review; Palmieri 2007; Vargo 2011; see Vercueil 2011, for a review). Olfactory seizures, characterized by a foul odor, are indicative of a medial temporal lobe tumor (Krouwer et al. 2000).

After a traumatic brain injury, the incidence of seizures is about 5% if the dura of the brain (top layer of protective tissue between the brain and the skull; Carter et al. 2009) has not been penetrated. This number increases to 30–50% when the dura has been penetrated (see Luciano et al. 2011, for a review; see Tucker 2005, for a review). The risk of posttraumatic epilepsy increases with more severe traumatic brain injuries and if the loved one has a seizure during the first week after his or her traumatic brain injury (Tucker 2005). Although most posttraumatic seizures occur within the first 2 years postinjury, up to 20% of patients may experience seizure onset after 2 years. The risk of seizure remains elevated for up to 20 years after a severe traumatic brain injury (see Luciano et al. 2011, for a review). Some research shows that patients with posttraumatic epilepsy may be in remission after 15 years (see Luciano et al. 2011, for a review).

The underlying mechanisms of posttraumatic epilepsy are from physical and metabolic changes in the damaged brain, including cortical disruption, scarring, or irritation of brain tissue (Luciano et al. 2011; Tucker 2005). Commonly after a traumatic brain injury, the loved one may experience either partial seizures (often arising in the frontotemporal areas) or generalized tonic–clonic seizures (Luciano et al. 2011). A number of symptoms are associated with these seizure locations: temporal seizures present with aphasia, vertigo, sensation of déjà vu, and sometimes psychosis (e.g., auditory illusions and hallucinations, fear, agitation, and paranoia; Hernández et al. 2010; Luciano et al. 2011; Nadkarni et al. 2007). Frontal seizures can present with motor behaviors and affective expressions, including screaming or cursing (Luciano et al. 2011). Tonic–clonic seizures result from spread of the seizure from a seizure focus to other parts of the brain (Hernández et al. 2010).

The family and loved one will be educated by their treating neurologist that a seizure disorder will be diagnosed based on an abnormal electroencephalogram (EEG), which measures brain wave activity. A sleep EEG is also usually warranted (Luciano et al. 2011; National Institute of Neurological Disorders and Stroke 2012; Reuber et al. 2009; The National Epilepsy Educational Alliance 2009; Tucker 2005; Wilner 2008). However, an EEG does not always identify epilepsy and so an integral component in the diagnosis is clinical observation (Channing Bete Company 2008; Luciano et al. 2011; Mantoan and Kullmann 2011; National Institute of Neurological Disorders and Stroke 2012; Tucker 2005). The tier 1 primary caregiver's input (see Chap. 1, Sect. 1.3 and Figs. 1.1 and 1.2) in this regard is fundamental in helping the medical professional make the necessary diagnosis. He or she may be asked to time the event, carefully observe the symptomatology, write down a description, or photograph/video record the seizure event, so as to assist the doctors with a diagnostic formulation (Mantoan and Kullmann 2011; National Institute of Neurological Disorders and Stroke 2012; Reuber et al. 2009; The National Epilepsy Educational Alliance 2009; Wilner 2008). At times, the loved one will be hospitalized on an Epilepsy Monitoring Unit for video EEG monitoring in order to classify the type of seizure (The National Epilepsy Educational Alliance 2009).

Other diagnostic procedures are also employed to reveal brain abnormalities, including brain imaging. These include computed tomography (CT) scans, magnetic resonance imaging (MRI), positron emission tomography (PET), single-photon emission computed tomography (SPECT), functional MRI (fMRI), and magnetoencephalography (MEG; Devinsky 2008; Martin et al. 2006; Reuber et al. 2009; The National Epilepsy Educational Alliance 2009; Wilner 2008).

A serious complication of epilepsy is *status epilepticus*. This life-threatening condition occurs when the loved one has an abnormally prolonged seizure (e.g., longer than 5 min) or does not fully regain consciousness between seizures (National Institute of Neurological Disorders and Stroke 2012; Reuber et al. 2009). If the loved one is in status epilepticus, immediate medical intervention is warranted. This includes calling 911, transporting to an emergency room, as well as pharmacologic treatment with benzodiazepines, standard antiepileptic drugs, or general anesthetics (Geiger et al. 2011; National Institute of Neurological Disorders and Stroke 2012; Wilner 2008).

8.1.2 Treatment of Seizure Disorders

Table 8.2 summarizes "helpful hints" and considerations for families with a loved one with epilepsy. After a seizure, the loved one needs an immediate neurological evaluation (Wilner 2008) and education for the loved one and family members about how to proceed if he or she has another seizure. The family may need to be proactive in seeking a neurologist with whom a good rapport and collaboration can

Table 8.2 "Helpful hints" and considerations for families of a loved one with epilepsy

- Seek prompt neurological attention and liaison with a psychotherapist for additional support and psychoeducation
- Attend medical appointments with the neurologist or epileptologist:
  - Help provide relevant history
  - Encourage the loved one to be forthright, including substance use
  - Set an agenda
  - Bring in written questions and a calendar of seizure events
  - Take notes or audiotape
  - Ask questions about new or troubling symptoms
  - Keep up with regular appointments and assist the loved one as needed
  - Be on time and try not to bring young children
  - Bring reports from other physicians and their business cards
- If a loved one has an epileptic seizure:
  - Ask the loved one to contact an adult when he/she experiences an aura
  - Remain calm
  - Direct him/her away from harm
  - Roll him/her to one side
  - Do not place objects into his/her mouth
  - Do not restrain him/her
  - Cushion his/her head
  - Remove glasses
  - Loosen tight clothing around the neck
  - Be attuned to physical injury
  - Watch for hypoxia and cyanosis
  - Afterwards reassure and observe the loved one
  - Do not leave him/her alone or let him/her drive
  - Do not give him/her liquids or medications
  - If in status epilepticus, be sure to know the medication protocol
- Contact 911 if:
  - This is the first seizure
  - There is a second seizure
  - If full awareness does not return
  - The seizure occurred in water
  - He/she is/has:
    - pregnant
    - diabetes
    - breathing problems
    - injured oneself
  - The seizure lasts longer than two minutes
  - Confusion is longer than 15 minutes
- Update the physician about the seizure event
- Be aware of and monitor seizure triggers:
  - Menstruation
  - Address general health concerns
- Avoid:
  - Sleep deprivation
  - Stress
  - Alcohol
  - Nicotine
  - Caffeine
  - Street drugs
  - Some medications (i.e., sedating antihistamines, a few antibiotics)

Table 8.2 (continued)

Some herbs (e.g., St. John's Wort)
Flashing lights and video games
Cigarettes
Be open to anticonvulsant medication(s)
Bring all medications and other prescribing physicians' business cards to the appointments
Expect that the loved one will need periodic blood levels of some anticonvulsants
Monitor and report possible side effects from the medications to health professionals
Never:
Suspend medical appointments against a physician's advice
Lower or stop antiepileptic medications against a physician's advice
Help monitor that the loved one is taking his/her medication as prescribed
Notify the physician and psychotherapist if the loved one is noncompliant with his/her medications
Realize that there are other forms of treatment for intractable epilepsy:
Neurosurgery (with pre- and post-surgical neuropsychological evaluations)
Vagus nerve stimulator
RNS NeuroPace system
Radiotherapy and chemotherapy
Prioritize safety for the loved one by having him/her:
Wear a medical identification bracelet, locket, or tag
Carry a card with seizure related information and medications
Avoid hazardous sports or activities, especially if alone
Wear a protective helmet
Use a Home Safety Checklist
Support proper nutrition and regular exercise

be built (Devinsky 2008; The National Epilepsy Educational Alliance 2009). The psychotherapist acts as a support to the loved one and relatives and can provide informative psychoeducation to diminish the understandable trepidations.

When the loved one sees a neurologist or epileptologist, it is best for the caregiver or family member to attend. Expect that the physician will want a detailed history, which may be in a questionnaire format (Wilner 2008). This is conducted so as to try to ascertain the underlying cause of the seizure (Wilner 2008). The family should ask the loved one to be honest and accurate, including his or her use of alcohol and street drugs (The National Epilepsy Educational Alliance 2009; Wilner 2008). The neurologist and psychotherapist will encourage the loved one and family member to set an agenda and bring in written questions (The National Epilepsy Educational Alliance 2009; Wilner 2008). Examples include what to do if a dose of medication is missed or the loved one goes into status epilepticus. The psychotherapist will urge the patient and caregiver to take notes or tape-record the appointments (The National Epilepsy Educational Alliance 2009; Wilner 2008). This is especially vital if the physician changes medications and/or their doses. The family member may need to prompt the loved one to pose uncomfortable questions or report new or troubling symptoms.

The patient and family will be advised by the neurologist and psychotherapist to track the incidence of seizures. The psychotherapist and neurologist will suggest that the loved one keep a calendar and notate relevant information (e.g., the dates and number of seizures, dates of side effects, etc.; Devinsky 2008; Wilner 2008). Possible precipitating factors should be noted (e.g., missed medication doses; Devinsky 2008). The loved one and family should keep up with regular appointments with the neurologist (Wilner 2008). This may require orchestration by the relatives when the loved one has significant cognitive challenges. Arriving on time and finding alternatives to bringing young children enables the maximum benefit from all medical appointments (Wilner 2008). It is important to bring all follow-up reports from other physicians to the neurology appointments (Devinsky 2008).

The neurologist or epileptologist will enlighten the loved one and his or her tier supports about seizure interventions. If the loved one experiences an aura, he or she should be instructed to inform a nearby adult so that he or she can provide assistance (Palmieri 2007). If a family member witnesses a seizure which affects the loved one's level of consciousness, he or she should remain calm, direct the loved one away from harm (including physical hazards), and roll him or her to one side to avoid aspiration (Channing Bete Company 2008; Devinsky 2008; Hernández et al. 2010; Leppik 2007; Reuber et al. 2009; Wilner 2008). Objects should never be placed in the loved one's mouth and he or she should not be restrained (Channing Bete Company 2008; Devinsky 2008; Goodman et al. 2007; Hernández et al. 2010; Krouwer et al. 2000; Wilner 2008; Wyllie 2010). Other considerations are to cushion the loved one's head, remove glasses, and loosen tight clothing around the neck (Devinsky 2008; National Institute of Neurological Disorders and Stroke 2012; Wyllie 2010).

In cases of a tonic–clonic seizure, the relative must be attuned to a possible physical injury due to a fall or injury to the extremities, as the loved one is flailing during the event (Barrett and Sachs 2006). The relative needs to be sensitive to the emergence of hypoxia (i.e., decreased oxygen) and cyanosis (i.e., a bluish tinge around the lips, mouth, and tongue) resulting from breathing problems and inadequate oxygenation (Barrett and Sachs 2006; Devinsky 2008). After the seizure, the caregiver should reassure and observe the loved one until he or she is fully awake (Devinsky 2008; Krouwer et al. 2000; Reuber 2009). He or she should not be left alone, allowed to drive, or given liquids or medication immediately after the seizure (Channing Bete Company 2008; Devinsky 2008; Krouwer et al. 2000; Wilner 2008). If the loved one suffers from status epilepticus, informed family members and the support system should have access to preventative anticonvulsant medications (Wyllie 2010).

The family should contact 911 if: this is the first seizure that the loved one has sustained; there is a second seizure; full awareness does not return; the loved one is pregnant or has diabetes; the seizure occurred in water; the seizure lasts longer than 2–5 min; his or her confusion lasts longer than 15 min; or the loved one has breathing problems or injures himself or herself during the seizure (Devinsky 2008; Goodman et al. 2007; National Institute of Neurological Disorders and Stroke 2012; Reuber et al. 2009; The National Epilepsy Educational Alliance 2009; Wilner 2008; Wyllie 2010). If the loved one is already under the care of a physician, he or she should be notified about the event (Goodman et al. 2007; Wilner 2008).

The neurologist and psychotherapist will alert the loved one and family to a number of seizure triggers. The loved one should avoid situations producing sleep deprivation and instead maintain a regular sleep schedule (Channing Bete Company

2008; Devinsky 2008; Mantoan and Kullmann 2011; National Institute of Neurological Disorders and Stroke 2012; Reuber et al. 2009; The National Epilepsy Educational Alliance 2009; Wilner 2008). Stress, alcohol, nicotine, caffeine, drugs (e.g., cocaine, amphetamines), some medications (e.g., sedating antihistamines, a few antibiotics) and herbs (e.g., St. John's wort), as well as menstruation can also precipitate seizures (Channing Bete Company 2008; Devinsky 2008; Leppik 2007; Mantoan and Kullmann 2011; National Institute of Neurological Disorders and Stroke 2012; Palmieri 2007; Reuber et al. 2009; The National Epilepsy Educational Alliance 2009; Wilner 2008). The psychotherapist and treating physicians will provide other preventative measures, including treatment of cardiovascular disease, high blood pressure, infections, etc. (National Institute of Neurological Disorders and Stroke 2012).

Some patients are susceptible to light flashing at a certain speed; this is called photosensitive epilepsy (National Institute of Neurological Disorders and Stroke 2012). The loved one and caregiver will be instructed to be wary of this catalyst and should take the following precautions: watch television in a well-lit room; stay at least 8 feet from the television; avoid settings with flashing lights (e.g., discotheques); and wear polarized sunglasses to reduce flickering reflections (Wilner 2008). Video games should be played sparingly (Wilner 2008). Smoking cigarettes can also elicit seizures (National Institute of Neurological Disorders and Stroke 2012) and the loved one can be provided smoking cessation resources. It is sensible if the family also abstains from smoking around the loved one.

Seizure disorders are treated with antiepileptic or anticonvulsant medications. There are currently at least 20 different ones available (National Institute of Neurological Disorders and Stroke 2012). A neurologist or epileptologist will prescribe the best choice of medications by taking a number of factors into account, including the seizure type and potential side effects (Barrett and Sachs 2006; Wilner 2008). Some examples of anticonvulsants are benzodiazepines (e.g., clonazepam, diazepam, lorazepam, midazolam), carbamazepine, gabapentin, ethosuximide, felbamate, lacosamide, levetiracetam, oxcarbazepine, primidone, pregabalin, rufinamide, tiagabine, phenobarbital, phenytoin, lamotrigine, topiramate, vigabatrin, valproic acid, and zonisamide (Hernández et al. 2010; Krouwer et al. 2000; Kurzwelly et al. 2010; Luciano et al. 2011; The National Epilepsy Educational Alliance 2009; Wyllie 2010). The National Epilepsy Educational Alliance (2009); Reuber et al. (2009); and Devinsky (2008) provide a description of which medications are used for what types of seizures as well as common side effects. The loved one may need polytherapy, or more than one medication, to control his or her seizures (Geiger et al. 2011; National Institute of Neurological Disorders and Stroke 2012; The National Epilepsy Educational Alliance 2009).

The family will be educated that there are often differences in the loved one's response and tolerance to these medications (Hernández et al. 2010; National Institute of Neurological Disorders and Stroke 2012). The family should bring all medications to the neurologist's appointments (The National Epilepsy Educational Alliance 2009; Wilner 2008), as he or she may want to verify that the loved one is on the proper medication regimen. The physician will want periodic blood levels of some anticonvulsants to be sure they are in the correct therapeutic range—this includes the levels not being too low or too high (i.e., in a toxic range; Channing Bete Company 2008; Devinsky 2008; National Institute of Neurological Disorders and Stroke 2012; Tucker 2005). Bringing medications that other doctors have prescribed (and their business cards) also keeps the neurologist informed (Wilner 2008).

Anticonvulsants themselves may produce neurological side effects, including compromised attention and concentration, memory, speed of information processing, and motor speed (Devinsky 2008; Luciano et al. 2011; Tucker 2005; Wyllie 2010). Other worrisome side effects are depression, irritability, anxiety, psychosis, and a rash (Devinsky 2008; Luciano et al. 2011; National Institute of Neurological Disorders and Stroke 2012). Therefore, it is essential for the tier 1 caregiver and loved one to monitor these potential side effects and report them immediately to the prescribing physician, and if pertinent, to the rehabilitation therapists.

Because seizure recurrence is unpredictable, the neurologist may be hesitant to have the loved one stop anticonvulsant medications, especially if the EEG indicates seizure activity or if the loved one engages in behaviors which are treacherous if a seizure were to occur (e.g., driving for a living; The National Epilepsy Educational Alliance 2009; Wilner 2008). The psychotherapist will reinforce the position of the neurologist about anticonvulsant medication(s), namely, that the loved one should never suspend medical appointments or stop a medication without physician sanction (National Institute of Neurological Disorders and Stroke 2012). Stopping antiepileptic medication may precipitate a seizure or even status epilepticus (Devinsky 2008; National Institute of Neurological Disorders and Stroke 2012), which could be very dangerous, depending on what the loved one is doing at the time (e.g., driving, swimming, etc.).

Also, the psychotherapist should liaise with the neurologist and help monitor the patient's compliance with his or her medication(s). At times, the loved one (and family) do not appreciate the importance of strict adherence to the medication schedule. Noncompliance can complicate his or her health and functionality, including hospitalizations, seizure onset while driving, missed work time, decreased quality of life, and/or increased seizure frequency causing a fall or injuries (Hovinga et al. 2008). Psychoeducation and practical problem solving by the psychotherapist can rectify this dilemma. Medical professionals will recommend that the primary caregiver monitor that the loved one remembers to take his or her medication. If for any reason, he or she is resistant to taking the medication, the prescribing physician should be notified immediately. The psychotherapist can work with the loved one and, if necessary, the family, to explore underlying reasons for medication noncompliance.

Families and their loved one may be upset to find out that his or her seizure disorder does not respond to anticonvulsant medication. It is estimated that this occurs in 20–45% of cases (see Geiger et al. 2011, for a review; Martin et al. 2006; National Institute of Neurological Disorders and Stroke 2012; Tracy and Shah 2008). This is known as intractable, refractory, or uncontrolled epilepsy (National Institute of Neurological Disorders and Stroke 2012; Wilner 2008). In this case, the loved one may be eligible for surgery (Devinsky 2008; Geiger et al. 2011; Martin et al. 2006; Reuber et al. 2009; The National Epilepsy Educational Alliance 2009; see Tracy and Shah 2008, for a review). For example, surgery has been successful in patients with long-standing temporal lobe epilepsy, in which the front part of the temporal lobe is removed (Devinsky 2008; National Institute of Neurological Disorders and Stroke 2012; Reuber et al. 2009; The National Epilepsy Educational Alliance 2009; Wilner 2008).

Alternatively, the loved one may have a corpus callosotomy, in which a wide band of fibers (corpus callosum) is cut so as to decrease the electrical communication between the hemispheres (Devinsky 2008; Reuber et al. 2009; The National Epilepsy Educational Alliance 2009; Wilner 2008). Poor effectiveness of anticonvulsant medication in controlling seizures is also observed in brain tumor patients (see Kurzwelly et al. 2010, for a review). With a brain tumor, the neurosurgeon may elect to remove the "epileptogenic" zone as part of the removal of the brain tumor (Kurzwelly et al. 2010).

Often, a neuropsychologist will be asked to do a presurgical evaluation of the loved one so as to identify the specific cognitive functions of the proposed surgical area (Wilner 2008). This evaluation is often done in conjunction with an intracarotid amobarbital procedure (Wada test) and fMRI. These map the location of key abilities which are "at risk" from surgery (e.g., language and memory; The National Epilepsy Educational Alliance 2009; Tracy and Shah 2008; Wilner 2008). The loved one will likely be hospitalized on an Epilepsy Monitoring Unit (Wilner 2008). Repeat neuropsychological testing after the surgery is fundamental for identifying limitations which can guide rehabilitation and vocational planning (Tracy and Shah 2008). Psychotherapy after the surgery in combination with neurorehabilitation is often warranted to address any neurological complications and help the loved one (and family) adjust to his or her postsurgery status (National Institute of Neurological Disorders and Stroke 2012). This includes memory difficulties which can occur after anterior temporal lobectomies involving the hippocampus (Leppik 2007; Martin et al. 2006; Reuber et al. 2009; The National Epilepsy Educational Alliance 2009). Severe problems with learning and recall are known as an amnestic syndrome (O'Connor and Lafleche 2006).

Other forms of treatment for the loved one who has refractory seizures and has not responded to drug therapy are a vagus nerve stimulator and the RNS® NeuroPace system (Barrett and Sachs 2006; Devinsky 2008; Sethi et al. 2008). The vagus nerve stimulator is a battery-powered device which is surgically implanted in the chest. It delivers short bursts of electrical energy to the brain via the vagus nerve which inhibits the seizures (National Institute of Neurological Disorders and Stroke 2012; The National Epilepsy Educational Alliance 2009; Wilner 2008). The NeuroPace system is used for intractable epilepsy, and it uses electrical stimulation to stop seizures (Sethi et al. 2008; Wilner 2008). Of note, there are some preliminary data that some forms of radiotherapy (e.g., Gamma Knife) and chemotherapy may reduce seizure frequency (see Kurzwelly et al. 2010, for a review; Reuber et al. 2009).

There are a variety of safety practices that the loved one and tier supports will be coached on. For instance, the psychotherapist and neurologist will likely advise that the loved one wear a medical identification bracelet, locket, or tag or carry a card with seizure-related information, including a list of medications (Channing Bete Company 2008; Leppik 2007; Reuber et al. 2009). The family can reinforce this for safety reasons which reduce their own unease. Other suggestions to minimize risk are to avoid hazardous sports or other activities, especially if alone. These include: climbing onto ladders and heights, handling firearms, diving, swimming, motor sports, horseback riding, gymnastics, ice activities, sailing, wind surfing, sky diving, scuba diving, and skiing (Channing Bete Company 2008; Leppik 2007; Mantoan and Kullmann 2011; The National Epilepsy Educational Alliance 2009; Wyllie 2010). Sports which pose a risk of traumatic brain injury should also be avoided (e.g., boxing; Leppik 2007). Wearing protective sports helmets is also recommended (Channing Bete Company 2008) so as to reduce the likelihood of additional brain injuries.

Wilner (2008) and The National Epilepsy Educational Alliance (2009) describe a Home Safety Checklist, including: be careful when cooking (e.g., consider a microwave); use caution when bathing; carpet floors; limit stairs; keep inside doors unlocked for easy access; check in regularly with the loved one; have doctors' phone numbers accessible; be knowledgeable about correct seizure procedures; and install a home security system with a "panic" button.

Proper nutrition, including a balanced diet and a multivitamin will facilitate normal daily activities (Devinsky 2008; Leppik 2007; The National Epilepsy Educational Alliance 2009). Extra vitamin D and calcium will help offset bone weakness (The National Epilepsy Educational Alliance 2009). Neurologists may propose a ketogenic diet, especially for children with seizures (Leppik 2007). This involves avoiding carbohydrates and eating more fats (e.g., cheese, meat, butter, eggs, and oil; Reuber et al. 2009; Wyllie 2010). Regular exercise will overcome fatigue, help regulate sleep, counteract weight gain caused by antiepileptic medications, and reduce stress (Leppik 2007; The National Epilepsy Educational Alliance 2009). The program should include aerobic exercise, resistance training, and stretching (The National Epilepsy Educational Alliance 2009). Good options are walking and yoga. The loved one needs to stay well hydrated and avoid excessive exertion and overheating (The National Epilepsy Educational Alliance 2009).

8.2 Scenario: Cognitive, Communication, and Language Challenges

Cognitive and language deficits in epilepsy are somewhat amorphous. They are related to a number of factors, including what is causing the seizure disorder; age at seizure onset, seizure type and frequency; the affected parts of the brain; the effects of antiepileptic drugs; and the loved one's emotional status (see Gauffin et al. 2011, for a review; Lee and Clason 2008; The National Epilepsy Educational Alliance 2009). Family members are typically worried about these changes and may ask questions such as: *What thinking problems is my loved one having? Why are his or her language skills not as good? What can I do to help?*

8.2.1 Overview of Cognitive, Communication, and Language Changes

The neuropsychologist and treating professionals can educate the tier supports (and the loved one) that there is no specific neuropsychological "profile" that separates epilepsy from other brain disorders (Lee and Clason 2008). Because seizures are dynamic, their impact on cognition changes over time (Tracy and Shah 2008). However, typical concerns include learning and memory, especially in patients with temporal lobe epilepsy (Gauffin et al. 2011; see Lee and Clason 2008, for a review). Manifestations of memory challenges include remembering peoples' names, forgetfulness during daily activities and work tasks, as well as word-finding problems (Gauffin et al. 2011).

Overall intellectual abilities can also be affected, with poorer performance when the seizure history is more serious (e.g., earlier age of onset and higher frequency of seizures) and when there is polydrug therapy (see Lee and Clason 2008, for a review). There may be mild language deficits in patients with temporal lobe epilepsy (e.g., naming and comprehension), especially when the dominant hemisphere for language is affected (see Lee and Clason 2008, for a review). Depending on the areas of the brain involved, the loved one may experience difficulties with visuospatial or mechanical skills as well as executive functions (see Lee and Clason 2008, for a review). Anticonvulsant medications can exacerbate these limitations (see Lee and Clason 2008, for a review).

8.2.2 "Helpful Hints" and Tools for Families to Cope with Cognitive, Language, and Communication Changes in their Loved Ones

Table 8.3 summarizes "helpful hints" and tools for families to cope with their loved one's cognitive, language, and communication changes related to seizure disorders. A neuropsychological evaluation can also be beneficial in identifying the loved one's cognitive strengths and weaknesses (Martin et al. 2006). As part of this process, the clinician will conduct a detailed history. This can be useful in identifying possible precipitating events for the seizure disorder (Martin et al. 2006). The neuropsychologist will solicit historical material about the loved one, including age at the time of first seizure, possible febrile seizures during infancy, seizure frequency and symptoms, as well as past and current antiseizure medications (Martin et al. 2006). Other pertinent background includes the loved one's developmental milestones, possible learning disorders, academic and vocational obstacles, and social adjustment (Martin et al. 2006).

The neuropsychologist will review the intent and findings of the evaluation with the loved one and support network. Areas which are evaluated include: motor performance in the hands; sensation (e.g., touch, vision, auditory processing); attention; executive functions; language; memory for verbal and pictorial information; and

Table 8.3 "Helpful hints" and tools for families to cope with cognitive, language, and communication changes in a loved one with epilepsy

Consider a neuropsychological evaluation which will:
Contain a detailed medical history
Explore developmental milestones, learning disorders, academic and vocational difficulties, as well as social adjustment
Identify strengths and challenges
Consider a speech and language evaluation which will:
Assist with recommendations related to academic needs and accommodations
Be open to neurorehabilitation to:
Learn compensations
Improve functionality and quality of life
Receive psychotherapy and psychoeducation for the loved one and family
Monitor the loved one's adherence to medications through the use of helpful compensations:
Supervise medications when the loved one has cognitive hurdles
Be sure medications are taken regularly by establishing a daily routine
Be proactive about refilling prescriptions
Engage in interactive games and computer activities for intellectual stimulation and family harmony

overall intellectual abilities (Martin et al. 2006; see also Chap. 4, Sect. 4.2.1). When feasible, a speech and language evaluation is also efficacious, especially when recommendations for academic needs and accommodations are needed.

The neuropsychologist may advocate for neurorehabilitation for the loved one with a seizure disorder, based on the findings of the neuropsychological evaluation. This is especially the case when there is also a diagnosis of traumatic brain injury, brain tumor, or stroke and when the impairments require therapeutic interventions to improve the loved one's level of functionality and quality of life. As part of the neurorehabilitation process, a series of compensations for memory and executive function deficits will be taught (Klonoff 2010). The psychotherapist can reinforce the rationale and protocols for these tools and acts as a liaison with the team members, loved one, and family support system. Details of valuable compensations are found elsewhere in this book. These include the datebook (see Chap. 4, Sect. 4.3.2 and Fig. 4.5); the Home Independence Checklist (see Chap. 4, Sect. 4.4.4 and Fig. 4.7; Chap. 6, Sect. 6.3.2 and Fig. 6.3); and various types of technology, including smartphones and tablets (see Chap. 6, Tables 6.5 and 6.7). Dialogue between the loved one and caregiver is facilitated through regular "milieu meetings" to address issues and organize household responsibilities (see Chap. 4, Sect. 4.4.4 and Fig. 4.8).

As stated above, compliance with medications is vital to seizure control. Hence, the neurologist and psychotherapist will request that the loved one and family obtain compensatory devices to minimize the risk of forgetting to take anticonvulsant medications. Options include a pillbox (including those that beep), watch or phone alarms, and computerized tablets (Devinsky 2008; see Table 8.4). When the loved one has significant cognitive hurdles, the psychotherapist will appeal to the family to supervise the medications, making sure that he or she is taking them regularly. Establishing a routine of when to take medications (e.g., with meals) is most helpful

Table 8.4 Types of medication reminders

Pillboxes labeled with day and time of day
Pillboxes with pre-set alarms
Pocket pillboxes with alarms
Pill dispensers that give appropriate medication(s) at specified intervals
Alarms for the top of medicine bottles that also indicate when they were last opened
Watch alarms that are preset and either beep, vibrate, or give spoken reminders
Pagers with preset alarms
Applications for smartphones and tablets that provide reminders at specific times
Services that will call, send emails, or send text messages at designated times

(Wilner 2008). The psychotherapist can also brainstorm with the loved one and family about how to be proactive when refilling prescriptions so that he or she does not run out of medications. This includes using a calendar system and ordering medications well in advance (i.e., 7–14 days; Devinsky 2008).

The psychotherapist can suggest a myriad of games and computer activities for the tier supports to engage in with the loved one. This provides intellectual stimulation and also improves the harmony and well-being of the family unit. Table 8.5 provides a sampling of games and computer activities, categorized by executive functions, attention, speed of processing/reaction time, memory, and language domains. (Incidentally, these activities are relevant for all neurological etiologies). The psychotherapist, neuropsychologist, speech–language pathologist, and/or occupational therapist can review the benefit of these activities for the loved one from the cognitive, interpersonal, and mood perspectives. Through a collaborative dialogue, the loved one and support network can select a subset of germane therapeutic activities. Interactive games are also a great social outlet for the caregiver and his or her friends and will provide fun respite.

8.3 Scenario: Family Members' Angst

Seizure disorders affect emotions and can hinder educational and vocational achievements as well as social adjustment (Dodrill 2008; Tracy and Shah 2008). Understandably, families may be distressed about the loved one's mood and future adaptation. They may ask questions such as: *Why is my loved one struggling so much emotionally? What assistance is available at school? Will he or she be able to drive or work?*

8.3.1 Overview of Angst in the Caregiver

8.3.1.1 Emotional Problems

Table 8.6 summarizes the possible emotional difficulties associated with epilepsy in the loved one and the caregiver. A major source of worry for the caregiver and tier supports is behavioral changes. A case in point, seizures in the temporal lobe

Table 8.5 Games and computer activities to address cognitive, language, and communication challenges in the loved one

Executive Functioning:	Happyneuron.com: The Towers of Hanoi, Hurray for Change, the Bells of Notre Dame Lumosity.com: Color Match, Disconnection, Word Sort, Route to Sprout Brainmetrix.com: Arrange Game CogniFit.com: Mahjong Chess Backgammon Neuropsychonline.com executive skills tasks (for use by professionals only)
Attention:	Happyneuron.com: Pay Attention, Private Eye, Find Your Way, Catch the Ladybug, Secret Files Lumosity.com: Bird Watching, Playing Koi, Lost in Migration Positscience.com: Mixed Signals, Divided Attention Livewire Puzzles: www.puzzles.ca/wordsearch.html Spot the Difference Hidden Picture Blink Mahjong UNO Sequence Neuropsychonline.com attention tasks (for use by professionals only)
Speed of Processing/Reaction Time:	Happyneuron.com: Secret Files Lumosity.com: Speed Match, Penguin Pursuit CogniFit.com: Whack-A-Mole Positscience.com: Eye for Detail Brainmetrix.com: Brain Reflection, Reflex Test Catch Phrase
Memory:	Yahoo.com: Memory V, Concentration, Little Shop Memories, Busy Bistro Lumosity.com: Memory Matrix, Monster Garden, Familiar Faces, Memory Match Happyneuron.com: American in Paris, Elephant Memory, Restaurant Clue Simon 5 Second Rule Buzzword I Spy Neuropsychonline.com memory tasks (for use by professionals only)
Language:	Yahoo.com: Text Twist Happyneuron.com: Embroidery, the Right Word, This Story is Full of Blanks Lumosity.com: Word Bubbles, Rhyme Workout Anomia: http://www.anomiapress.com

Table 8.5 (continued)

	Last Word: http://www.buffalogames.com/vmchk/Games/Last-Word/flypage_new.tpl.html
	Password
	Boggle
	Scrabble
	Wheel of Fortune
	Word Search Puzzles
	Scattergories
	Pictionary
	Word Slinger
	Smart Mouth
	Neuropsychonline.com communication tasks (for use by professionals only)
Other Resources:	Brain Age: http://brainage.nintendo.com
	Brain Training Software: www.braintrainingsoftware.com
	MindSparke: www.mindsparke.com
	Brain Train: www.braintrain.com
	BrainBashers Puzzles and Brain Teasers: www.brainbashers.com
	MindWare: www.mindware.com/Home/HomePage.aspx
	Fun Brain: www.funbrain.com
	Set Game: www.setgame.com
	Coffee Shop: http://coolmath-games.com/0-coffee-shop
	Big Fish Games: www.bigfishgames.com
	Yahoo Games: http://games.yahoo.com
	Pogo.com: www.pogo.com
	Cut the Rope: http://www.zeptolab.com
	Where's My Water: http://games.disney.com/wheres-my-water-app
	Brainfood: http://www.rinkworks.com/brainfood
	Diner Dash: http://www.playfirst.com/home

affect the emotional centers of the brain (Dodrill 2008). However, other psychiatric indicators can include irritability, aggressiveness, impulsivity, mood swings, mania, depression, and anxiety (Devinsky 2008; Luciano et al. 2011; O'Dell et al. 2007; Tucker 2005; Wilner 2008; Wyllie 2010). Symptoms can occur for a few hours and last up to 3 days before a seizure (preictal), during (ictal), or up to 5 days after a seizure (postictal; The National Epilepsy Educational Alliance 2009). They can also occur independently of the seizure (interictal; The National Epilepsy Educational Alliance 2009). The frequency of psychiatric sequelae is greater in patients where the seizures are not well controlled (The National Epilepsy Educational Alliance 2009). Increased psychological distress has been found in males where the cultural expectation is to be the breadwinner, as well as unmarried individuals with less education and lower socioeconomic status (Khalid and Aslam 2011).

The loved one with epilepsy (commonly affecting the temporal lobes) may be prone to *psychosis.* This is defined as a mental disorder with impaired content and coherence of thought, diminished connection to reality, and paranoia (Devinsky 2008). As part of a psychosis, the loved one may experience delusions and/or hallucinations or feelings of unreality or detachment (Devinsky 2008; see Dodrill 2008, for a review; Luciano et al. 2011; Tucker 2005).

Table 8.6 Emotional problems in a loved one with epilepsy and the caregiver

Epilepsy-based emotional problems:	Irritability	Aggressiveness
	Impulsivity	Mood swings
	Mania	Depression
	Anxiety	Psychosis
	Suicidal thoughts	
Reactionary problems:	Fearfulness about recurring seizures in the community	
	Helplessness and fear of separation	
	Social isolation due to embarrassment or dread	
	Overprotectiveness of the loved one	
	Anger and guilt	
	Shame, jealousy, resentment, rage, blaming of others	
	Sense of impending doom	
	Gloomy outlook	
	Reactive depression, anxiety, and fear	

The psychotherapist can help the relatives appreciate the environmental consequences of epilepsy on the entire family unit (Weinstein 2007). Common parental worries are that a seizure will occur without adult supervision and that it will cause brain damage or cognitive changes (Weinstein 2007). Common trepidations in the loved one are death from a seizure and rejection by peers (Weinstein 2007).

The inability to control or predict seizures creates feelings of helplessness and fear of separation (Rosenbaum and Palmon 1984; Schachter 2008a; Weinstein 2007). For example, the loved one, and by extension the family, are terrified about recurring seizures, especially in public environs (Arthurs et al. 2010; Dodrill 2008; McConigley et al. 2010; Schachter 2008a). Out of embarrassment or dread, the loved one may isolate himself or herself within the comfortable confines of home (Wefel et al. 2011). Similarly, the caregiver may reinforce this behavior and become apprehensive and overprotective (Schachter 2008a; Weinstein 2007), as he or she is petrified that the loved one may be injured outside of his or her purview. Sometimes, the support network is angry about the life impediments and unfairness for the loved one and themselves, bemoaning "why them" and "why us?" (Klonoff et al. 2008; Schachter 2008a). They feel guilty about their good health and freedoms (Schachter 2008a). They can succumb to the Family Experiential Model (FEM) of Recovery "red crisis" zone behaviors of shame, jealousy, resentment, rage, and then blaming behaviors (see Chap. 1, Sect. 1.5 and Fig. 1.3; Klonoff and Koberstein 2010; Klonoff et al. 2008; Schachter 2008a). All parties can become preoccupied with a sense of impending doom which promotes a gloomy outlook (Dodrill 2008). The loved one, and thus the family, may suffer from reactive depression, anxiety, and fearfulness (Schachter 2008a). The relatives' worry is compounded if the loved one has suicidal thoughts (Luciano et al. 2011; Wyllie 2010).

8.3.1.2 "Helpful Hints" and Tools to Cope with Emotional Problems

Table 8.7 summarizes "helpful hints" and strategies for the caregiver and the family to cope with their own angst and that of the loved one. The neurologist should be contacted, as depression is common for hours or days before, during, and even after seizures (Reuber et al. 2009). The loved one and family should seek the services of a psychotherapist if they are concerned about depression; self-diagnosis is ill-advised (Reuber et al. 2009). The caregiver may need to encourage the loved one to admit to feelings of depression and/or anxiety, as he or she may be reluctant to do so, thinking that this will result in being "labeled crazy" (The National Epilepsy Educational Alliance 2009). The family (and loved one) should expect that the psychotherapist will adopt a holistic approach to the loved one's care, including assessing and discussing his or her emotional and psychosocial functioning (Dodrill 2008; Wilner 2008). Oftentimes, this is accomplished using various personality inventories and quality of life questionnaires (see Dodrill 2008, for a review; see Martin et al. 2006, for a review).

Keen observational skills and a close working alliance between the therapist and the family are integral. For instance, depression in teens may present somewhat differently, including: withdrawal from friends; poor concentration and achievement in school; eating problems; low energy and motivation; feeling scared, lonely and rejected; unusually angry or aggressive outbursts; and preoccupation with negative thoughts (Reuber et al. 2009).

When emotional difficulties are interfering with the loved one's adjustment, the psychotherapist and neurologist will likely want to coordinate their efforts to evaluate underlying causes. Emotional instability may be from the anticonvulsant medications (see Tucker 2005, for a review). In this case, the neurologist may elect to switch medications, as some antiepileptic medications also stabilize mood and reduce anxiety (e.g., carbamazepine, oxcarbazepine, gabapentin, lamotrigine, tiagabine, topiramate, and valproate; Luciano et al. 2011). Alternatively, psychotropic medications can be used to ameliorate the negative side effects of the anticonvulsants and/or to directly treat mood changes, including depression, agitation, or aggressiveness (Luciano et al. 2011).

The psychotherapist and neurologist may prefer to elicit the assistance of a psychiatrist's expertise to select the optimal mood medication. The family (and loved one) should be cautioned that it can take a period of time (e.g., 2–8 weeks) for the psychotropic medications to be noticeably effective (Reuber et al. 2009). Therefore, both parties will need to be patient with the process. The choice of medication should also take into account its sedating quality and propensity to cause seizures (Luciano et al. 2011). Currently, selective serotonin reuptake inhibitors (SSRIs) are considered safe to treat depression and anxiety (Devinsky 2008; The National Epilepsy Educational Alliance 2009). Some medical professionals feel that benzodiazepines should be avoided for treating anxiety, as they are habit forming (Devinsky 2008). Certain medications can reduce irritability, including SSRIs, buspirone, or a low dose of an antipsychotic agent (Devinsky 2008). Psychosis is typically treated with newer antipsychotic medications (e.g., quetiapine, rispiridone, and aripiprazole; Devinsky 2008).

Table 8.7 "Helpful hints" and strategies for the family to cope with angst in themselves and their loved one with epilepsy

Contact the neurologist if the loved one is depressed
Seek psychotherapy services from a psychotherapist with a holistic approach
Encourage the loved one to share emotional problems with health professionals
Note that teens may present with unique symptoms of emotional distress
Coordinate with medical professionals to ascertain underlying causes of emotional problems
Recognize that anticonvulsant medications may add to or ameliorate psychiatric symptoms
Liaison with a psychiatrist if emotional difficulties are interfering with adjustment
Consider psychotropic medications and be patient about their benefits
Expect that the caregiver and family may at times feel puzzled, aggravated, or alienated
Be open to various psychological approaches and psychoeducation about mood changes, especially depression and anxiety
Know measures to take related to suicidal risk
Develop coping strategies through psychoeducation, acceptance, realism, and balanced role revision
Learn tools to avoid conflict
Be mindful of anxiety and depression in the tier 1 caregiver:
Intensify the frequency of supportive psychotherapy
Consider adjunct pharmacologic treatment
Pursue leisure and quality of life activities
Recognize signs of burnout related to the uncertainty and chronicity of the condition
Practice self-care
Diversify interests
Participate in epilepsy support groups, meetings, conferences, Internet chat forums, blogs, and posting boards
Read books about personal accounts of epilepsy from varying points of view which are informative
Help the loved one strengthen his/her self-esteem, self-efficacy, and mastery
Avoid constant surveillance
Foster independence and self-sufficiency in the loved one
Limit excessive attention and indulgence of the loved one
Adopt an attitude of adaptability, flexibility, teamwork, and resiliency
Employ the loved one's tenacity, "heroism," humaneness, and thoughtfulness as sources of inspiration
Multimedia Resources
Websites
www.epilepsy.com
www.epilepsyfoundation.org
www.aesnet.org
www.ninds.nih.gov/disorders/epilepsy/epilepsy.htm
Books
Seizures and Epilepsy: Hope Through Research (National Institute of Neurological Disorders and Stroke, 2012)
Epilepsy 199 Answers: A Doctor Responds to His Patients' Questions (3rd ed.) (Wilner 2008)
Epilepsy: Patient and Family Guide (3rd ed.) (Devinsky 2008)
Epilepsy in Our View: Stories from Friends and Families of People Living with Epilepsy (Schachter 2008a)
Epilepsy in Our Words: Personal Accounts of Living with Seizures (Schachter 2008b)

The psychotherapist will often take the lead in providing emotional support to the caregiver and relatives when they are puzzled, aggravated, dejected, or alienated by the loved one's mood and personality changes. In fact, research has shown that when the loved one with epilepsy perceives greater social support, the degree of emotional distress wanes (Khalid and Aslam 2011). Supportive psychotherapy, behavioral interventions, psychoeducation, and coping strategies are crucial in this regard (Klonoff and Koberstein 2010; Tucker 2005; Wilner 2008). Through psychoeducation, the family (and loved one) are taught that mood changes emanate from multiple sources. This pertains to the epilepsy itself, where the brain is damaged and/or medication effects, as well as a genetic predisposition (Devinsky 2008; The National Epilepsy Educational Alliance 2009). New knowledge empowers the support network and fosters calmness, acceptance, tolerance, and empathy (Schachter 2008a, b).

The psychotherapist can help the family (and loved one) appreciate the relative contributions of endogenous or chemically based depression versus situational or reactive depression related to the loved one's troubling life circumstances (Leppik 2007; Wheless 2006). These include driving restrictions, worry about continuing seizures, cognitive deficits, work limitations, hassle of daily medication, loss of life control, etc. (Leppik 2007; Luciano et al. 2011; The National Epilepsy Educational Alliance 2009). More than likely, the loved one may experience both endogenous and reactive depression (Leppik 2007). Similarly, fear and panic may emerge during a seizure (The National Epilepsy Educational Alliance 2009) or alternatively between seizures due to anxiety about the implications of epilepsy for daily functioning (Reuber et al. 2009). Extra psychotherapeutic assistance is needed for the loved one and relatives when the seizures are uncontrolled, given their impact on quality of life (Wilner 2008).

The psychotherapist will review overt and covert signs of depression in the loved one, including feelings of hopelessness, worthlessness, pessimism, guilt, helplessness, and despair (see Chap. 4, Sect. 4.6.2 and Table 4.6). Because the rate of suicide is elevated in patients with epilepsy (Devinsky 2008; Dodrill 2008; Tucker 2005; Wyllie 2010), the psychotherapist and medical professionals will keep close tabs on the loved one's mood. If the loved one threatens self-harm, emergency measures must be initiated to preserve the loved one's safety. This includes calling 911 or taking him or her to an emergency room. The psychiatrist, neurologist, and psychotherapist should also be notified swiftly. (For further discussion on this topic, see Chap. 4, Sect. 4.6.2 and Klonoff 2010).

Patients with epilepsy and their families will benefit from cognitive–behavioral techniques which teach resourcefulness (Rosenbaum and Palmon 1984). This involves instructional material about effective coping mechanisms for stress, including a self-perception of better capacity to control the seizures (Rosenbaum and Palmon 1984). The psychotherapist can teach "self-management" which emphasizes day-to-day wellness management in the medical, life role, and emotional domains (Fraser et al. 2011). Session contents can include how to live with epilepsy (e.g., medication use, life hygiene); socializing (e.g., how to engage new friends and coping with seizures in social settings); and emotional health (stress management, self-acceptance, and mood management; Fraser et al. 2011).

Strong working alliances with professionals and thorough education about epilepsy empower the family (and loved one) to cope optimally (Schachter 2008a; Weinstein 2007). Longer-term coping strategies include accepting each other's strengths and difficulties and establishing realistic long-term goals (Klonoff 2010). Sometimes, this means relinquishing certain freedoms because of the ailing health of the loved one (Weinstein 2007). This is counterbalanced with setting appropriate boundaries and rules (including with other children) and a willingness to revise roles and duties to balance both personal needs and those of the family unit (Weinstein 2007).

The psychotherapist can provide other useful tools to the family when the loved one is upset. These include all parties agreeing on nonverbal signals to de-escalate the situation (e.g., a time-out or a cut-off sign); changing to an innocuous topic or calm environment; politely disengaging from arguments by resisting "having the last word"; and logging sensitive topics for upcoming psychotherapy sessions.

Of course, the psychotherapist will keep a watchful eye on the tier 1 primary caregiver regarding his or her overall mood to be sure he or she is not succumbing to anxiety and depression. Intensifying the frequency of supportive psychotherapy sessions; adjunct pharmacologic treatment; as well as pursuit of leisure and quality of life activities will help to offset mood downturns. The psychotherapist will also help the caregiver recognize if he or she is becoming burned out, manifested by feelings of blame and resentment towards the loved one because of the uncertainty and chronicity of his or her condition. Self-care techniques, including diversifying his or her interests away from the health of the loved one, will be emphasized. (For further discussion on burnout, see Chap. 2, Sect. 2.3.7 and Chap. 9, Sect. 9.9).

Epilepsy support groups, meetings, conferences, Internet chat forums, blogs, and posting boards (e.g., through www.epilepsy.com; www.epilepsyfoundation.org; www.aesnet.org; www.ninds.nih.gov/disorders/epilepsy/epilepsy.htm) are beneficial outlets. The loved one and the support network learn about community resources (e.g., good physicians and receptive social agencies), thereby reducing feelings of aloneness, powerlessness, and alienation because of the loved one's health concerns (Gauffin et al. 2011; Wilner 2008). A number of publications list handy resources for the loved one and family on epilepsy, including *Seizures and Epilepsy: Hope Through Research* by the National Institute of Neurological Disorders and Stroke (2012), *Epilepsy 199 Answers: A Doctor Responds to His Patients' Questions* by Wilner (2008), and *Epilepsy: Patient and Family Guide* by Devinsky (2008). These contain psychoeducational materials and publications, research literature, and a listing of national and state epilepsy associations, national epilepsy centers, and international epilepsy resources. Lastly, there are books encompassing personal accounts of epilepsy from the point of view of the individual with epilepsy, including *Epilepsy in Our Words: Personal Accounts of Living with Seizures* by Schachter (2008b) as well as by friends and families, for instance *Epilepsy in Our Words: Stories from Friends and Families of People Living with Epilepsy* by Schachter (2008a). These are informative and reduce the feeling of aloneness with the diagnosis (see also Table 8.7).

Strengthening the loved one's self-esteem, self-efficacy, and mastery will increase his or her happiness and help offset depression (Klonoff 2010). This also combats *learned helplessness,* whereby the loved one, convinced of his or her ineptitudes, loses the inner drive and confidence to tackle obstacles (Moore and Stambrook 1995). Consequently, the psychotherapist will counsel the caregiver, especially parents, to avoid constant surveillance and foster the loved one's independence and self-sufficiency. Excessive attention and indulgence should be limited, especially if this is detrimental to the needs of other siblings and family members (National Institute of Neurological Disorders and Stroke 2012; Weinstein 2007; see also Chap. 3, Sect. 3.3). Ultimately, the family unit will need to adopt an attitude of adaptability, flexibility, teamwork, and resiliency (Weinstein 2007). In fact, some outsiders have derived inspiration from the patient's tenacity, "heroism," humaneness, and thoughtfulness in the face of their adversities (Schachter 2008a).

8.3.1.3 Functional and Quality of Life Problems: Driving

Accident rates are higher for individuals with epilepsy (Devinsky 2008). One of the hardships for the loved one with a seizure disorder is the possibility of driving restrictions, particularly when seizures are poorly controlled and consciousness is affected (Wheless 2006; Wilner 2008). This leads to compromised independence (O'Dell et al. 2007). Some states will prohibit an individual with epilepsy from obtaining a commercial driver's license (Devinsky 2008).

8.3.1.4 "Helpful Hints" and Tools for the Family to Address Driving Restrictions

Table 8.8 summarizes "helpful hints" and tools for the family to address driving constraints in their loved one with epilepsy. The psychotherapist will recommend that the loved one and the caregiver consult with the neurologist regarding readiness to drive (Mantoan and Kullmann 2011; Wyllie 2010). Often, the doctor will want confirmatory input from a rehabilitation setting which assess predriving proficiencies. A list of the physical, visual/visuoperceptual, cognitive, and emotional components of driving is contained in Klonoff (2010). The occupational therapist will employ treatment exercises to improve cognitive and visual/visuoperceptual deficits which impact driving.

The neuropsychologist is also a good resource to address cognitive sequelae pertinent to driving as well as possible emotional factors (e.g., poor impulse control or low frustration tolerance). This may include up-to-date neuropsychological testing to evaluate speed of information processing, visuospatial skills, hand speed and dexterity, as well as executive functions (e.g., judgment, decision making, and multitasking). Testing is especially relevant when the loved one has seizures secondary to other types of brain injuries (e.g., traumatic brain injury and stroke). Computerized simulated driving programs are nifty interventions (e.g., Driver-ZED and

Table 8.8 "Helpful hints" and tools for the family to address driving restrictions in their loved one with epilepsy

Consult with the neurologist about driving readiness
A rehabilitation setting can assess and address pre-driving skills, using a neuropsychologist and occupational therapist
Computerized simulated driving programs are good treatment adjuncts
Consider an adaptive driving evaluation by trained professionals
The loved one should suspend driving when weaning off anticonvulsant medications
Become educated about state driving laws related to epilepsy
Consider other transportation options:
Family and friends
Hire a driver
Arrange a car pool situation
Use a local public transportation service
Notify professionals if the loved one is noncompliant with driving laws and/or his/her anticonvulsant medications
Multimedia Resources
Websites
www.epilepsy.com/epilepsy/rights_driving.html
www.epilepsyfoundation.org/resources/drivingandtravel.cfm

SmartDriver). When possible, the psychotherapist and neurologist will promote an adaptive driving evaluation, which is conducted by professionals who are specialized in assessing driving potential after a brain injury (see Klonoff 2010; Stark-Vance and Dubay 2011). All of these data are compiled to help the loved one and family gain an informed appreciation of driving capability.

The loved one should suspend driving if he or she is weaning off anticonvulsant medication. This minimizes danger to self and others, should a seizure occur (Wilner 2008). Some physicians propose this lasts for 3 to 6 months, while others may insist that the loved one be seizure free for up to 1 year before resuming driving (The National Epilepsy Educational Alliance 2009; Wilner 2008). In addition, each state has specific parameters when driving with a diagnosis of epilepsy and will regulate driver license eligibility (Leppik 2007; Wilner 2008; see also www.epilepsy.com/epilepsy/ rights_driving.html and www.epilepsyfoundation.org/resources/drivingandtravel.cfm with respect to state driving laws for epilepsy). These laws take into account possible harm to others juxtaposed with the desire to drive (Wilner 2008). Sometimes, the Motor Vehicle Department will utilize a consulting doctor or medical review board to assist with decision making (Devinsky 2008). Often, the Motor Vehicle Department will mandate periodic medical reports which document that seizure control is good (Devinsky 2008). Ultimately, it is the Department of Motor Vehicles in each state which sets the specific parameters to drive (Wilner 2008).

The psychotherapist can suggest other practical mechanisms to help with transportation needs for the loved one, especially as transporting him or her can become burdensome to the tier 1 caregiver. Ideas include: create a schedule of available drivers encompassing other tier 2 and 3 supports, for example, family members and friends; hire a driver, possibly a student or retired neighbor; or use local public transportation services (e.g., bus, light rail, subway, Dial-A-Ride, etc.). The family may also be able to arrange a car pool (Wilner 2008), whereby the caregiver alternates with other drivers to take a group of individuals to the same destination (e.g., school or work).

The family may become embroiled in a sticky predicament if the loved one with epilepsy insists on driving without state or physician clearance. In this case, the family should immediately contact the treating neurologist. He or she will then counsel the loved one regarding the obligation to report the development of epilepsy to the state (Leppik 2007). When the loved one makes the report, the physician–patient relationship is preserved (Leppik 2007). Depending on the state law, the physician may be required to report an unsafe driver to the Department of Motor Vehicles (see http://www.epilepsyfoundation.org/resources/drivingandtravel.cfm). At the very least, the neurologist and the psychotherapist can provide psychoeducation to the loved one and try to dissuade him or her from this dangerous behavior. This includes informing him or her and the family that by driving without a valid license, he or she may be civilly or criminally liable for a car accident caused by a seizure if he or she drives against medical advice or fails to notify the Motor Vehicle Department (Devinsky 2008).

8.3.1.5 Functional and Quality of Life Problems: Work, School, and Quality of Life

Having epilepsy can negatively impact the loved one's capacity to find and maintain employment, especially when seizures are poorly controlled (Schachter 2008a). Inability to drive compromises the ability to work (O'Dell et al. 2007; Reuber et al. 2009). Also, some occupations are "off-limits" due to safety concerns (Wilner 2008). These include public safety positions where others could be endangered (e.g., aircraft pilots, truck and train drivers, emergency service providers, soldiers, etc.; Reuber et al. 2009; Wilner 2008). It is estimated that 25% of individuals with epilepsy are unemployed (The National Epilepsy Educational Alliance 2009; Wilner 2008). Other conditions linked with seizures, including memory and executive function disorders from a traumatic brain injury, may also compromise the loved one's capability for gainful employment (see Chap. 4).

Quality of life is affected, including the loved one's physical, mental, and social health (O'Dell et al. 2007). The loved one (and therefore the caregiver) can feel stigmatized and marginalized by prejudice in the job market (Devinsky 2008; Khalid and Aslam 2011; Martin et al. 2006; The National Epilepsy Educational Alliance 2009). Some loved ones feel their career advancement as well as personal and professional relationships are impacted. This is related to distress in colleagues should they need to cope with a seizure (O'Dell et al. 2007). Other barriers are the employer's worries about liability or general safety concerns associated with a potential workplace seizure (Leppik 2007; Reuber et al. 2009).

Poor self-esteem in the loved one may be a product of social rebuffs, labeling, or discrimination (O'Dell et al. 2007; The National Epilepsy Educational Alliance 2009). The loved one may be subject to teasing, bullying, or avoidance in school settings (National Institute of Neurological Disorders and Stroke 2012). He or she may experience social ostracism. Societal misperceptions include beliefs that epilepsy is connected with violence, antisocial behavior, or that epilepsy is contagious (O'Dell et al. 2007). Owing to social isolation, the loved one is more dependent on family members and can feel like an encumbrance (O'Dell et al. 2007). Many see their lives as "self-limiting" with respect to their responsibilities and potential, lacking a sense of independence and fulfillment (Gauffin et al. 2011; Wheless 2006). This compounds the loved one's guilt, shame, and humiliation (Gauffin et al. 2011).

Seizure disorders create financial pressures (O'Dell et al. 2007). Direct costs include emergency medical services and emergency department fees, diagnostic tests, treatment procedures, etc. (O'Dell et al. 2007). Indirect costs relate to time away from work for the loved one and caregiver, missed school, and lessened work productivity (see O'Dell et al. 2007, for a review). Costs are exponentially increased with intractable epilepsy (O'Dell et al. 2007).

8.3.1.6 "Helpful Hints" and Tools for the Family to Cope with Functional and Quality of Life Problems

Table 8.9 reviews "helpful hints" and tools for the family to address functional and quality-of-life obstacles. When the loved one is reintegrating into the school setting, the neuropsychologist, psychotherapist, and neurologist can provide guidance about the timing and pace. Often, homebound or online courses are good stepping stones (Klonoff 2010).

Once the loved one starts attending school, it is important to access the needed tier 3 supports through an Individualized Education Program (IEP), 504 Plan, or Disability Student Resources at colleges and universities. The neuropsychologist, psychotherapist, and speech–language pathologist are valuable to the school staff (Klonoff 2010). The caregiver may need to advocate for these services to obtain the necessary accommodations, especially if the loved one has substantial cognitive or emotional challenges. Teachers will be more mindful and compassionate when they understand the loved one's disability (Reuber et al. 2009). They can also help integrate the student into the social sphere (Reuber et al. 2009). Education early on by a therapist (e.g., speech–language pathologist) or a representative from an epilepsy center can facilitate the loved one's integration and success at school (Reuber et al. 2009).

The psychotherapist is an excellent resource to guide the loved one and family about epilepsy-related social ostracism. This includes education and group discussions with teachers, student peers, and outside friends about seizure disorders so as to reduce negative or fear reactions in others. Use of small brochures (e.g., *What Everyone Should Know About Seizures* by Channing Bete Company 2008) is a user-friendly mechanism to increase social awareness and empathy.

Table 8.9 "Helpful hints" and tools for the family to address functional and quality of life problems

School:	Obtain guidance from medical professionals about the timing and pacing of returning to school Consider homebound or online courses as stepping stones Help the loved one access tier 3 supports through an Individualized Education Program, 504 Plan, or through Disability Student Resources Encourage direct involvement of a neuropsychologist, speech–language therapist, or an epilepsy specialist to support the loved one's academic and social reintegration, also through group education Small handouts are good educational tools for the teachers, student peers, and friends
Social life:	Be mindful of family overprotectiveness Foster independence, socialization, and self-esteem Provide opportunities for natural joys, challenges, and disappointments which are part of peer friendships Seek a balance between appropriate caution, versus emotional and physical confinement Pursue extracurricular sports, activities, and summer camps to enhance socialization for the loved one as well as the family Help the loved one engage in social media (e.g., Facebook) interactions wisely and if possible involve the therapists' input Get therapeutic ideas for explaining epilepsy to dating partners
Work life:	Working with neurorehabilitation staff is ideal, including a vocational counselor or occupational therapist Explore resources through Vocational Rehabilitation Services Remember that the loved one is protected by the Americans with Disabilities Act (1990) to prevent discrimination Contemplate if and how the loved one should disclose his/her epilepsy status using professional input Reasonable accommodations are required in the context of the capacity to complete essential job functions Neurorehabilitation therapists can provide onsite support and education to the employer Encourage the loved one to report any work obstacles so as to receive the necessary assistance Mechanisms are available if the loved one experiences job discrimination The workplace should be educated about first aid in case a seizure occurs, including an "Action Plan" Medical alert bracelets or necklaces keep the general public informed Other options to reduce work barriers are: Work from home Use public transportation to access work Live within walking distance of work If epilepsy develops after acquiring the job, explore accommodations Consider volunteer work as another productive work choice
Financial hardship:	Consult with the neurologist about assistance for expensive medications Work with a therapist, especially a social worker, to explore possible financial access to Social Security benefits, health insurance, respite care, or a home health aide
Multimedia resources	

Table 8.9 (continued)

Brochure:	What Everyone Should Know About Seizures (Channing Bete Company 2008)
Websites:	http://admin.disaboom.com/adaptive-sports http://www.sportsabilities.com http://www.veryspecialcamps.com/summer/epilepsy-camp https://www.facebook.com http://www.gettinghired.com http://wdcrobcolp01.ed.gov/Programs/EROD/org_list.cfm?category_ID=SVR http://www.ada.gov/cguide.pdf http://www.epilepsyfoundation.org/resources/employmenttopics.cfm http://www.epilepsyinstitute.org/faq.html www.jan.wvu.edu/links/ADAtam1.html http://janweb.icdi.wvu.edu www.rxhope.com www.needymeds.com www.access2wellness.com www.ssa.gov/disability

The psychotherapist will be vigilant about the relatives' natural inclination to be overprotective. This is especially common for parents of a loved one with epilepsy (Devinsky 2008). However, too much restrictiveness stifles the loved one's independence, socialization, and self-esteem (Devinsky 2008; see also Chap. 9, Sect. 9.6 and Tables 9.11 and 9.12). He or she needs opportunities to experience the natural joys, challenges, and disappointments inherent in peer friendships (Devinsky 2008). The psychotherapist can help the family find the balance between appropriate caution versus emotional and physical confinement. The family will need to develop a mindset of "dignity of risk" (Klonoff 2010), characterized by "inclusion, not exclusion" (Devinsky 2008). Introduction to various extracurricular activities is worthwhile, including local adaptive sports opportunities. These are exciting options to integrate the loved one into the community and can also be an excellent way for the family to meet other relatives with similar circumstances (see as examples http://admin.disaboom.com/adaptive-sports or http://www.sportsabilities.com). Summer camp experiences for those with epilepsy are also a wonderful outlet for adventure and camaraderie (see http://www.veryspecialcamps.com/summer/epilepsy-camp).

Currently, many individuals enjoy interacting through social media, including Facebook. This can be a good social outlet for the loved one and family, depending on their preferences and lifestyle. However, the loved one should be informed about potential dangers and pitfalls with Facebook (a prototype of social media), including too much self-disclosure, inappropriate interactions, and problematic relationships with unknown invitees (for more information, see Table 8.10 and http://www.pcworld.com/businesscenter/article/154374/facebook_etiquette_five_dos_and_donts.html; http://www.hongkiat.com/blog/facebook-etiquette; http://www.pcworld.com/article/169120/facebook_etiquette_10_rules_for_better_socialing.html). It is good for the loved one to work with a speech–language pathologist and/or his or her psychotherapist to set healthy boundaries when using Facebook. Postings should be shared with the family, as a designated relative may need to help oversee Facebook interactions, to be sure the loved one is using good judgment.

Table 8.10 "Helpful hints" and considerations when using Facebook

Consider reviewing contents and interactions with a speech-language therapist, psychotherapist, or responsible family member (e.g., parent or older sibling)
Remember that Facebook is in the public domain
Be vigilant about who are added as "friends:"
Make sure you know the person
Don't communicate with people you don't know
Never give out personal information (e.g., phone number, Social Security Number)
Don't overshare
Don't vent about your job
Use the same "real life" rules of etiquette as you would for person-to-person friendships
Check and monitor privacy settings, so as to limit who can see information about you
Use a "neutral" or professional profile picture
Watch that your biography does not share too much information
Don't share biographical information about other family members so as to protect their privacy
Be thoughtful about posting content, links, and personal news
Remember that messages posted on the "Wall" are seen by everyone
Monitor your tone and communication pragmatics, including appropriate language
Obtain permission before "tagging" friends and use good taste in selecting photos
Remember that Facebook can affect your reputation, future friendships, and employability
Multimedia Resources
Websites
http://www.pcworld.com/businesscenter/article/154374/facebook_etiquette_five_dos_and_donts.html
http://www.hongkiat.com/blog/facebook-etiquette
http://www.pcworld.com/article/169120/facebook_etiquette_10_rules_for_better_socialing.html

With respect to dating relationships, the psychotherapist is a great resource to help the loved one explain the consequences of epilepsy. Forthright dialogue about the symptoms is ideal (Wyllie 2010). The psychotherapist can also provide emotional support to the loved one if he or she is uneasy or embarrassed about revealing his or her medical condition.

The psychotherapist or neurologist may advise that the loved one seek neurorehabilitation services to assist with the work reentry process (Klonoff 2010). If possible, a holistic treatment approach is ideal, including a vocational counselor or occupational therapist to assess job qualifications, strengths, and weaknesses (Klonoff 2010; Reuber et al. 2009). The family should be part of a collaborative effort to identify a realistic vocational direction (Klonoff 2010). A helpful website to assist with the career search is http://www.gettinghired.com/ which specializes in available employment for individuals with disabilities.

Some states provide funds and rehabilitation through the Department of Economic Security Vocational Rehabilitation (VR) services for patients with epilepsy to seek employment (Devinsky 2008; Wilner 2008). For a list of state VR agencies, see http://wdcrobcolp01.ed.gov/Programs/EROD/org_list.cfm?category_ID=SVR. Forms of assistance include: diagnostic evaluation and establishment of a career development plan; counseling to determine and support a job direction; training to teach competencies; transportation; placement in the work force; and postemployment to help the loved one maintain the position (Devinsky 2008). The psychotherapist will council that the loved one's caregiver attends VR meetings to facilitate dialogue and advocacy. It is optimum if the neurorehabilitation setting can also coordinate efforts with VR to maximize the likelihood of success in the work setting.

The loved one with epilepsy is protected by the Americans with Disabilities Act (ADA) of 1990 to prevent discrimination (Leppik 2007; see also http://www.ada.gov/cguide.pdf). There are specific regulations about the employer inquiring about disabilities during the hiring process and it is illegal to require disclosure of disabilities on job applications or during the interview (Devinsky 2008). In my setting, however, patients are encouraged to share their medical history, insofar as it will affect work performance. This fosters a candid relationship with the employer, making it more likely that accommodations will be endorsed. However, the loved one and family support system will need to make this determination based on their specific vantage points, also taking into account possible risks of nondisclosure (Reuber et al. 2009). The Epilepsy Foundation has website information to help with this decision-making process (see http://www.epilepsyfoundation.org/resources/employmenttopics.cfm and http://www.epilepsyinstitute.org/faq.html).

Once hired, reasonable accommodations must be provided, including equal access to benefits and privileges of employment (Devinsky 2008; Leppik 2007; Wilner 2008). The psychotherapist or rehabilitation team can help the loved one and family obtain more information about reasonable accommodations (see www.jan.wvu.edu/links/ADAtam1.html and http://janweb.icdi.wvu.edu). Similarly, therapists can incorporate other teaching materials to help the loved one obtain and maintain employment and at the same time support families in their quest for knowledge.

Nevertheless, the loved one must be able to perform the essential job functions. As part of the transition process, job coaching for the tier 3 supports is utilized to develop and implement proper compensatory strategies (Klonoff 2010). Relevant professionals, including a psychotherapist, occupational therapist, speech–language pathologist, physical therapist, or vocational counselor can conduct an educational in-service and act as an advocate (Klonoff 2010). A set work schedule (rather than variable shifts) is best to be sure that the loved one does not become sleep deprived (Wilner 2008). Because epilepsy is considered by some as a hindrance to employment, the employer can also be educated that this individual will be loyal and hardworking, if given the chance (Leppik 2007).

If the loved one is noticing work insufficiencies and is hesitant to admit to this, the family may need to prompt him or her to divulge this to the rehabilitation therapists and psychotherapist so that they can intervene on his or her behalf. This should occur prior to the employer resorting to disciplinary action (The National Epilepsy Educational Alliance 2009). If the loved one feels he or she has experienced discrimination at work, a claim can be filed with government agencies, including the Equal Employment Opportunities Commission (EEOC) and Department of Justice (Devinsky 2008). The loved one may need assistance from the caregiver and an attorney in this regard.

In the workplace, the employer and coworkers can be alerted about first aid, should the individual suffer a seizure (Devinsky 2008; Leppik 2007). This can be in the form of an "Action Plan," which is made available to the worksite and lists a protocol and emergency numbers should a seizure occur. An example of an "Action Plan" format is available in Wilner (2008). As stated above, a medical alert bracelet or necklace may also be informative to the lay person. Other considerations which reduce work barriers are to work from home; use public transportation; or move close enough to walk to work (Reuber et al. 2009). Should epilepsy develop after the job is obtained, the loved one should inquire about transferring positions within the company to a more sedentary position, even if this is temporary until the seizures can become controlled (Wilner 2008).

Sometimes, the loved one's health status precludes paid work. This includes a higher grade brain tumor or severe traumatic brain injury, characterized by severe neurological, physical, cognitive, or emotional sequelae. Medical professionals, including the psychotherapist, may recommend unpaid work as another mechanism to be productive and fulfilled. Contact with a neurorehabilitation team, including a vocational counselor or occupational therapist, can help to identify suitable and fulfilling volunteer work sites.

Financial drains may be a reality for the family with a loved one with epilepsy. This includes the cost of medications. The neurologist can suggest options to reduce financial stresses, including providing free samples; enrolling in a patient assistance program with a pharmaceutical company; and connecting with a social worker to explore other forms of financial support, for instance, Medicare or Medicaid (Wilner 2008). Information on patient assistance programs is available at www.rxhope.com; www.needymeds.com; and www.access2wellness.com. A social worker or psychotherapist can guide the loved one and family to pursue Social Security benefits to offset financial struggles. Social Security Administration disability regulations can be found at www.ssa.gov/disability. Therapists, especially social workers, can also identify possible financial resources for health insurance, respite care, or home health aides (Devinsky 2008).

8.4 Case Study

Bessie was age 18 when she sustained a severe traumatic brain injury as a result of being struck by a car when she was crossing the street. She suffered loss of consciousness at the scene and her Glasgow Coma Scale score was 10. She was hospitalized and a CT scan revealed a left subdural hematoma, hemorrhage in the right frontal lobe, and edema in the left hemisphere. She remained comatose for 7 days. Two months later, she was diagnosed with epilepsy, based on intermittent seizures and a 24-hour ambulatory EEG.

Despite multiple attempts to control her seizures with different medications (including polydrug therapy), they remained intractable. Bessie resided with her parents Mary and Harry as well as her sister, Sarah, who was 2 years younger. Her family was trained by the epileptologist and a nurse practitioner regarding specific responses when Bessie was seizing. This included staying calm and helping to keep her safe. Bessie always had a postictal period of fatigue and confusion, and would need to rest for several hours. Mary was very proactive about logging Bessie's seizures, including providing videotaped recordings to her epileptologist.

Mary was in a state of constant surveillance and even insisted that Bessie sleep in her parents' bedroom, in case she had a nighttime seizure. Mary dedicated herself to Bessie's care and both of them were very compliant with the physician's instructions. Harry's emphasis was on working. He was a business executive who travelled out of town regularly. Two years later, upon the advice of her epileptologist, Bessie underwent a partial resection of the left temporal lobe, including part of her hippocampus. Unfortunately, she continued to experience intermittent complex partial seizures. She would experience an aura, characterized by a pungent odor. However, her postictal period of confusion was much shorter, only about 20 min.

After her surgery, Bessie became very disheartened, as her seizures were not cured. She had battled depression since her accident. Her physician thought this was caused by a combination of the location of her traumatic brain injury, her seizures, and her restricted lifestyle. Bessie also noticed, as did her mother, that she was much more forgetful. This deepened her angst. Her epileptologist suggested outpatient therapies, including psychotherapy with a neuropsychologist, Dr. Alti. Mary felt encouraged about possible help for Bessie and herself, as they were floundering.

When Bessie started her outpatient therapy 2.5 years postaccident, she underwent a neuropsychological examination. Dr. Alti first took a detailed history, incorporating Bessie's preaccident history. Mary attended the interview at the doctor's and Bessie's request; Harry was out of town on business at the time. Bessie had been an excellent high school student with the intention of attending college to become an interior designer. Preaccident, she had a very good relationship with her parents and sister, with no psychosocial problems.

Bessie was quite artistic prior to her accident and enjoyed painting and pottery. She was dating at the time of her traumatic brain injury, although soon after, her boyfriend ended the relationship. Bessie socialized with only a couple of girlfriends. However, this was very intermittent, as Bessie could not drive and her friends were busy with their college schedules and many hobbies. She had not attended college because of her seizures and forgetfulness. Her days were often spent watching television and running a few errands with her mother. Bessie had a seizure a few times in the community, which made leaving the house even more unnerving. Bessie felt housebound and lonely. Her mood plummeted further and she felt worthless and guilty about burdening her mother.

In follow-up, Dr. Alti met separately with Mary and Harry and conducted an intake interview, gleaning information about their own psychosocial and marital history (see Chap. 2, Sect. 2.2 and Table 2.2). They described their roles as traditional, in that Mary was a homemaker and Harry was the breadwinner. He was successful in his job and they enjoyed a comfortable middle-class lifestyle. Neither one of them had ever had psychotherapy, even after Bessie's car accident. Harry was a social drinker and reported that his intake had increased since Bessie's accident. Mary's parents lived nearby and they enjoyed a close relationship. Although they were emotionally available to Mary, they both struggled with their own health issues (e.g., her mom's diabetes and dad's dementia). Mary's reaction to the compound stresses was to move into "overdrive" to become the "super caregiver." She perceived that she was in "extended parenthood" and was prepared to make endless personal sacrifices for Bessie (see Chap. 3, Sect. 3.3.1). Harry seemed to withdraw and recede into the periphery. In listening to these narratives, Dr. Alti noted that although Mary was clearly dedicated to Bessie, she seemed on the verge of burnout. On the other hand, Harry presented as aloof and passive (see Chap. 2, Sect. 2.2 and Table 2.1). Dr. Alti also sensed emotional distance and discord between Mary and Harry and recognized that their incompatible coping styles were engendering marital turbulence (see Chap. 3, Sect. 3.3.1).

Dr. Alti explored the couple's baseline awareness, acceptance, and realism (see Chap. 2, Sect. 2.2.1). He was impressed that Mary had a good beginning handle on Bessie's difficulties. On the Family Member's Deficit Rating Scale (see Chap. 2, Table 2.4), she endorsed several cognitive and language sequelae, including memory, multitasking, and organization. Mary was able to provide some cogent examples of Bessie's forgetfulness (e.g., in taking her medications and the need for medication supervision) and was also cognizant that it was too overwhelming for Bessie to be in school. Harry's baseline awareness, acceptance, and realism were subpar. He was ill attuned to Bessie's cognitive challenges and minimized the stresses on himself. He was expecting to "prove the doctors wrong" based on an upcoming "full recovery." Therefore, he did not see much value in committing to the psychotherapy process.

Sarah was also seen by Dr. Alti as part of the intake and treatment planning for Bessie. She was attending a nearby university and worked part-time. Although Sarah loved her sister, she was rarely home because of her hectic schedule. Further exploration revealed that the totality of attention had been on Bessie since her accident and onset of her seizure disorder. Although Sarah understood her parents' predicament, she felt neglected and isolated. This alternated with guilt about her good health and liberties compared to Bessie's. Dr. Alti perceived that Sarah was a "silent victim" (see Chap. 3, Sect. 3.5.1).

Dr. Alti's clinical hypothesis was that some unhealthy family system patterns had developed (see Chap. 3, Sects. 3.1.1 and 3.3.2). Mary was utterly absorbed practically and emotionally with Bessie and they seemed enmeshed in an unhealthy dependency, thereby ignoring Harry and Sarah. Harry was deserting the marriage and the realities of Bessie's condition, instead diving into work as a diversion. Dr. Alti met with the family and proposed family interventions which would assist Bessie's functionality and repair family relations, thereby creating a new homeostasis. He sensed a potential to form a positive working alliance, although he recognized as a "red flag" that the major obstacle was Harry's reticence (see Chap. 2, Sect. 2.4.1.4). Dr. Alti decided to adopt the "companioning" approach, based on nonjudgmental coaching and collaboration.

Bessie's neuropsychological evaluation confirmed very severe memory impairment in the verbal domain. Bessie could not encode new auditory information and she was diagnosed with an amnestic syndrome. She also demonstrated mild executive system difficulties in the realms of higher level planning, decision making, mental flexibility, and multitasking. She had several residual strengths, including preserved visual and procedural memory, communication, mechanical, and fine motor skills. Given the amount of time that had lapsed since Bessie's traumatic brain injury, these findings were not surprising to her or Mary and Sarah. In fact, they all felt relieved that Dr. Alti had taken the time to do a thorough examination and share the results with such a compassionate demeanor. Harry remained skeptical, but tentatively agreed to continue with the psychotherapy process and attend some of Bessie's rehabilitation therapies to learn more about her needs and proposed compensations.

As part of her outpatient therapies, Bessie and her family took time to meet with the speech–language pathologist and occupational therapist to explore various memory compensations. Because Bessie was so forgetful, Mary felt she needed to closely supervise her medications. Sarah had bought her an iPad as a birthday present, but Bessie was flummoxed about how to use it. Bessie, her family, and the therapists decided to make this her primary memory compensation. With practice, she learned to keep track of her medication schedule, setting an alarm to remind her to take her medications.

Bessie's therapists and Mary wanted Bessie to become more functional and physically active in the home. Together, in "the spirit of partnership" (Sohlberg et al. 2001), they designed a daily calendar of events and a Home Independence Checklist, which was logged into her iPad. Her parents bought her a stationary exercise bicycle. With her physician's approval, Bessie began to ride a few times per week. She also learned to keep track of this exercise schedule in her iPad. Nonetheless, Mary remained hypervigilant and was reticent about giving Bessie any space or freedom, both at home and in the community. This also included insisting on sitting in on all of Bessie's therapy sessions, in case she had a seizure.

Dr. Alti addressed the dysfunctional patterns, characterized by Mary's stifling hypervigilance. He acquainted her with the concept of "symbiotic enmeshment," as Mary was unwittingly undermining Bessie's normal process of separation and individuation (see Chap. 3, Sect. 3.3.2). He posited the underlying dynamics of profound grief due to the initial accident, compounded by the dementing process in her father. Mary lamented that she felt "sandwiched in" by tending simultaneously to her daughter and aging parents. Up until that time, Mary had not realized the "ambiguous loss" she was still experiencing (see Chap. 3, Sect. 3.3.2). In the context of empathic relatedness, Dr. Alti facilitated Mary's exploration of her personal losses as well as feelings of powerlessness through storytelling and the sharing of pictures and mementos. He acquainted her with the "intuitive" grief style, characterized by emotional expressiveness. Through a "listening perspective," he helped Mary appreciate how the unhealthy manifestation of her own and Bessie's "spheres of influence" had emerged, based on the family events and losses (see Chap. 1, Fig. 1.1).

Dr. Alti also reviewed the subcomponents of Bessie's depression (see Chap. 4, Sect. 4.6.2 and Table 4.6). Harry was shocked at the depth of her distress and was coming to realize that his greater involvement was crucial for Bessie's well-being and community adaptation (separate from her mother). Dr. Alti also helped Mary grasp that she was compounding her daughter's feelings of ineptness, helplessness, despair, and worthlessness through her inadvertent smothering behavior. This revelation startled Mary into appreciating that she needed to reconfigure her role and relationship with Bessie. The occupational therapist collaborated with Dr. Alti and Mary to devise a "Do Not Do" checklist to curb her tendency to impede Bessie's independence (see Chap. 3, Sect. 3.3.2). Dr. Alti suggested that Bessie see a psychiatrist, Dr. Glassman, with whom he often collaborated and offered to initiate an introductory phone call. Dr. Glassman proposed that Bessie start a low dose of escitalopram. Bessie responded well to this medication and began to have a more optimistic outlook. Her anxieties about seizures in public also waned to a certain degree. This fortified the trust in the doctors' expertise and commitment to Bessie and the family.

Dr. Alti met weekly with Bessie and Mary and embarked upon cognitive–behavioral therapy, teaching both of them self-management skills. He educated them about typical seizure triggers, including an irregular sleep schedule, stress, caffeine, and alcohol. He emphasized the value of compensations, a regular exercise regime, and relaxation exercises for stress management. Psychoeducation in Family Group acquainted Mary with important concepts, including the "emotional roller coaster" of caregiving; shattering of her assumptive world; catastrophic reactions by proxy; chronic sorrow; and futuristic thinking (see Chap. 9). Mary was especially vociferous during the lesson on overprotectiveness and letting go, espousing the common tenets of "What else will go wrong?" "Things aren't safe" and "I'm waiting for another tragedy." These insights were agonizing, but also heartening. Dr. Alti then worked with Mary to gradually vacate the clinic. First, she sat in the clinic lobby; then she migrated to the cafeteria next door. Eventually, she would leave for a couple of hours.

Through regular attendance at Family Group, Mary befriended another mother whose daughter had suffered a traumatic brain injury from a skiing accident. This gave Mary a healthy opportunity for camaraderie. The two mothers recognized the perils of burnout. They started taking biweekly walks and enjoyed a light lunch before returning to the clinic. On Sundays, both mothers and their loved ones attended church together. The two mothers drew on one another's realization of life's lessons through hardships and mirrored their adaptability and future planning. Mary was progressing nicely through the FEM phases of awareness, acceptance, and realism and had developed adaptive "green coping" zone techniques (see Chap. 1, Sect. 1.5).

Dr. Alti promoted therapy to address the "marital menace." Harry could only attend individual and group meetings with Dr. Alti every couple of weeks. Dr. Alti encouraged Harry to explore his personal grief style, which was "instrumental," with an emphasis on planned action and overcoming obstacles. Dr. Alti assisted Harry in understanding the role of alcohol in numbing his feelings, which was destructive to coping and adjusting to the situation. Harry became more aware of this behavior, and greatly reduced his intake. He then felt more emotionally present. In marital sessions, Dr. Alti assisted Harry and Mary in better comprehending their unique forms of grieving, which helped to rebuild a bridge of communication and closeness. They were now able to provide more vibrant tier support to each other (see Chap. 1, Sect. 1.3 and Fig. 1.2 and Chap. 3, Sect. 3.3.2). Then, Dr. Alti assisted Mary and Harry in tackling the emotional gulf that had developed with Sarah. Conjoint sessions involving the three of them allowed Sarah to share her perspective of abandonment and guilt. The "wear and tear" on Sarah was enlightening. Cathartic tears were shed and each expressed resolve to devote quality time and attention to one another. This included one-on-one time with each parent.

Dr. Alti hypothesized that Sarah would eventually be "deputized" into the caregiving role and urged her to meet with himself and Bessie to receive psychoeducation about Bessie's long-term condition related to her physiological and cognitive deficits (see Chap. 3, Sect. 3.5.2). His input was mindful not to put her in the "pseudotherapist" role, which would engender rivalry. Instead, Dr. Alti recommended affective support in the form of encouragement and companionship and some "hands-on" help with transportation and errands. Dr. Alti also met separately with Bessie and helped her realize how her family's preoccupation with her circumstances (to the exclusion of others' needs) was detrimental to her own maturation and a richer relationship with Sarah. Bessie readily agreed and through speech–language therapy and psychotherapy began to practice the skills necessary to create a "give-and-take" relationship with Sarah.

Because Bessie felt safe in the clinic environs, she too began to cherish her independence from her mother. She started to socialize with her patient peers. A couple of times she suffered a seizure while in therapy and was relieved to see that the therapists and fellow patients were so supportive and considerate. At the invitation of her recreational therapist, Bessie began to draw. This was the first time she had undertaken artwork since her accident. Everyone was delighted to see her talent and enthusiasm.

Next, it came time for Bessie to spread her wings into the community. Dr. Alti introduced the concept of "dignity of risk." Once Mary understood the importance of further normalizing Bessie's existence, she was cautiously receptive to the rehabilitation therapists' recommendation that Bessie volunteer in a retirement setting. Here, she could use her art and communication aptitudes. They found a setting close to Bessie's home. The occupational therapist met with the setting director and explained Bessie's seizure disorder and memory challenges, also reviewing the first aid protocol. Bessie also wore a medical alert necklace and carried a copy of her medications in her wallet. Seizure problems were familiar to many of the staff, as historically, a couple of the patrons had also suffered them. Happily, there was an activities supervisor who was interested in expanding the daytime program to include more games and hobbies. She was enamored with the idea of Bessie introducing some basic drawing techniques to the patrons.

At first, Mary was too panicked to leave Bessie alone at the site. She drove her to and from the retirement center and stayed with her during her shift. Soon after starting, Bessie had a seizure. The supervisor and coworkers were comfortable with the seizure protocol and stayed with Bessie, afterwards allowing her to rest. Because she volunteered in a small and protected setting, the patrons were also compassionate. With reassuring supportive psychotherapy, Mary came to realize the saliency of fostering Bessie's community reintegration. They all agreed that Bessie would call her mother once during her volunteer shift. Bessie started taking Dial-A-Ride to and from the retirement setting. This promoted Bessie's sense of mastery and gradually her confidence improved. She made friends with a few of her coworkers and would invite them over to play games, including UNO, Buzzword, and Smart Mouth. She also befriended them on Facebook and worked with her speech–language pathologist to establish friendly, yet appropriate dialogue.

Bessie, Mary, and Harry continued with monthly sessions with Dr. Alti and all were faring better. Mary continued her attendance at the Family Group and socialized with her newfound friends in the community. Mary and Harry were devoting time to their relationship and had instituted weekly date nights. They set a rule not to discuss Bessie and instead immersed themselves in their local culture, including movies, plays, and concerts. Dr. Alti advised Bessie to expand her social pastimes and suggested she explore local adaptive sports. Galvanized by her feelings of self-efficacy and self-sufficiency, Bessie asked Sarah to accompany her to a monthly adaptive bowling event. Sarah willingly consented, savoring the prospect of partaking in community gatherings with her sister. Her self-condemnation about her own good fortune relative to Bessie's was ebbing and she exuded pride about Bessie's new courage and accomplishments. A positive feedback loop of mutual compassion, tolerance, and maturity was unfolding in both sisters. Over the course of 6 months of psychotherapy with adjunct neurorehabilitation therapies, Bessie and her family embraced the mantra of "faith, hope, and love" and achieved renewed balance, productivity, and quality of life within the family unit.

Postscript: One day at the bowling alley, Bessie meets Wally (see Chap. 4, Sect. 4.9 and Fig. 4.5). Their romance flourishes and 1 year later Bessie and Wally are betrothed.

References

Alajbegović, A., Loga, N., Alajbegović, S., & Suljić, E. (2009). Characteristics of symptomatic epilepsy in patients with brain tumours. *Bosnian Journal of Basic Medical Sciences, 9*(1), 81–84.

Aldrich, J. J., & Peterson, N. M. (2010). *Connecting through compassion: Guidance for family and friends of a brain cancer patient*. United States of America: Cancer Lifeline Publications.

Arthurs, S., Zaveri, H. P., Frei, M. G., & Osorio, I. (2010). Patient and caregiver perspectives on seizure prediction. *Epilepsy & Behavior, 19*(3), 474–477.

Baltaro, E. (2010). *Karen's epilepsy*. Omaha: WriteLife.

Barrett, R. P., & Sachs, H. T. III. (2006). Epilepsy and seizures. In L. Phelps (Ed.), *Chronic health-related disorders in children: Collaborative medical and psychoeducational interventions* (pp. 91–110). Washington, D. C.: American Psychological Association.

Beghi, E., D'Alessandro, R., Beretta, S., Consoli, D., Crespi, V., & Delaj, L., et al. (2011). Incidence and predictors of acute symptomatic seizures after stroke. *Neurology, 77*(20), 1785–1793.

Burneo, J. G., Fang, J., & Saposnik, G. (2010). Impact of seizures on morbidity and mortality after stroke: A Canadian multi-centre cohort study. *European Journal of Neurology, 17*(1), 52–58.

Carter, R., Aldridge, S., Page, M., & Parker, S. (2009). *The human brain book: An illustrated guide to its structure, function, and disorders*. New York: DK Publishing.

Catt, S., Chalmers, A., & Fallowfield, L. (2008). Psychosocial and supportive-care needs in high-grade glioma. *Lancet Oncology, 9*(9), 884–891.

Channing Bete Company, Inc. (2008). *What everyone should know about seizures* [Booklet]. South Deerfield: Channing Bete Company.

Devinsky, O. (2008). *Epilepsy: Patient and family guide* (3rd ed.). New York: Demos Health.

Dodrill, C. B. (2008). Emotional and psychosocial factors in epilepsy. In J. E. Morgan & J. H. Ricker (Eds.), *Textbook of clinical neuropsychology* (pp. 499–507). New York: Taylor & Francis.
Drappatz, J., & Wen, P. Y. C. (2011). Principles of supportive care. In A. D. Norden, D. A. Reardon, & P. Y. C. Wen (Eds.), *Primary central nervous system tumors: Pathogenesis and therapy* (pp. 55–84). New York: Springer.
Fraser, R. T., Johnson, E. K., Miller, J. W., Temkin, N., Barber, J., Caylor, L., et al. (2011). Managing epilepsy well: Self-management needs assessment. *Epilepsy & Behavior, 20*(2), 291–298.
Gauffin, H., Flensner, G., & Landtblom, A. M. (2011). Living with epilepsy accompanied by cognitive difficulties: Young adults' experiences. *Epilepsy & Behavior, 22*(4), 750–758.
Geiger, W. J., Nievera, C. C., Musil, B., & Goldstein, J. T. (2011). Managing seizures: Achieving control while minimizing risk. *Journal of Family Practice, 60*(8), 464–472.
Goodman, S., Rabow, M., & Folkman, S. (2007). *Orientation to caregiving: A handbook for family caregivers of patients with brain tumors*. San Francisco: University of California San Francisco.
Hernándezn, T. D., Levisohn, P. M., Buytaert-Hoefen, K., & Naritoku, D. K. (2010). Posttraumatic epilepsy and neurorehabilitation. In M. J. Ashley (Ed.), *Traumatic brain injury: Rehabilitation, treatment, and case management* (3rd ed., pp. 29–61). New York: CRC Press.
Hovinga, C. A., Asato, M. R., Manjunath, R., Wheless, J. W., Phelps, S. J., & Sheth, R. D., et al. (2008). Associaton of non-adherence to antiepileptic drugs and seizures, quality of life, and productivity: Survey of patients with epilepsy and physicians. *Epilepsy & Behavior, 13,* 316–322.
Khalid, A., & Aslam, N. (2011). Psychological distress among patients with epilepsy. *Indian Journal of Psychological Medicine, 33*(1), 45–48.
Klonoff, P. S. (2010). *Psychotherapy after brain injury: Principles and techniques*. New York: Guilford Press.
Klonoff, P. S., & Koberstein, E. J. (2010). Family life. In P. S. Klonoff (Ed.), *Psychotherapy after brain injury: Principles and techniques* (pp. 150–170). New York: Guilford Press.
Klonoff, P. S., Koberstein, E. J., Talley, M. C., & Dawson, L. K. (2008). A family experiential model of recovery after brain injury. *Bulletin of the Menninger Clinic, 72*(2), 109–129.
Krouwer, H. G. J., Pallagi, J. L., & Graves, N. M. (2000). Management of seizures in brain tumor patients at the end of life. *Journal of Palliative Medicine, 3*(4), 465–475.
Kurzwelly, D., Herrlinger, U., & Simon, M. (2010). Seizures in patients with low-gradegliomas—incidence, pathogenesis, surgical management, and pharmacotherapy. *Advances and Technical Standards in Neurosurgery, 35,* 81–111.
Lee, G. P., & Clason, C. L. (2008). Classification of seizure disorders and syndromes, and neuropsychological impairment in adults with epilepsy. In J. E. Morgan & J. H. Ricker (Eds.), *Textbook of clinical neuropsychology* (pp. 437–465). New York: Taylor & Francis.
Leppik, I. E. (2007). *Epilepsy: A guide to balancing your life*. New York: Demos Medical Publishing.& Saint Paul MN American Academy of Neurology Press.
Liigant, A., Haldre, S., Öun, A., Linnamägi, Ü., Saar, A., Asser, T., & Kaasik, A. (2001). Seizure disorders in patients with brain tumors. *European Neurology, 45*(1), 46–51.
Luciano, D. J., Alper, K., & Nadkarni, S. (2011). Posttraumatic Epilepsy. In J. M. Silver, T. W. McAllister, & S. C. Yudofsky (Eds.), *Textbook of traumatic brain injury* (2nd ed., pp. 265–275). Washington, D. C.: American Psychiatric Publishing.
Mantoan, L., & Kullmann, D. M. (2011). Evaluating first seizures in adults in primary care. *The Practitioner, 255*(1743), 25–28.
Martin, R. C., Bortz, J. J., & Snyder, P. J. (2006). Epilepsy and nonepileptic seizure disorders. In P. J. Snyder, P. D. Nussbaum, & D. L. Robins (Eds.), *Clinical neuropsychology: A pocket handbook for assessment* (2nd ed., pp. 318–350). Washington, D. C.: American Psychological Association.
McConigley, R., Halkett, G., Lobb, E., & Nowak, A. (2010). Caring for someone with high-grade glioma: A time of rapid change for caregivers. *Palliative Medicine, 24*(5), 473–479.
Mogensen, K. (2008). The whole picture: Addressing the diverse needs of the patient treated for a brain tumor. *Clinical Journal of Oncology Nursing, 12*(5), 817–819.

Moore, A. D., & Stambrook, M. (1995). Cognitive moderators of outcome following traumatic brain injury: A conceptual model and implications for rehabilitation. *Brain Injury, 9*(2), 109–130.

Nadkarni, S., Arnedo, V., & Devinsky, O. (2007). Psychosis in epilepsy patients. *Epilepsia, 48*(Suppl 9), 17–19.

National Institute of Neurological Disorders and Stroke. (2012). *Seizures and epilepsy: Hope through research* [Booklet]. Bethesda: National Institutes of Health.

O'Connor, M. G., & Lafleche, G. (2006). Amnesic syndromes. In P. J. Snyder, P. D. Nussbaum, & D. L. Robins (Eds.), *Clinical neuropsychology: A pocket handbook for assessment* (2nd ed., pp. 463–488). Washington, D. C.: American Psychological Association.

O'Dell, C., Wheless, J. W., & Cloyd, J. (2007). The personal and financial impact of repetitive or prolonged seizures on the patient and family. *Journal of Child Neurology, 22*(5 Suppl), 61–70.

Palmieri, R. L. (2007). Responding to primary brain tumor. *Nursing, 37*(1), 36–42.

Reuber, M., Schachter, S. C., Elger, C. E., & Altrup, U. (2009). *Epilepsy explained: A book for people who want to know more*. New York: Oxford University Press.

Rocheford, D. M. (2009). *Mommy, I feel funny! A child's experience with epilepsy*. Deadwood: Wyatt-MacKenzie.

Rosenbaum, M., & Palmon, N. (1984). Helplessness and resourcefulness in coping with epilepsy. *Journal of Consulting and Clinical Psychology, 52*(2), 244–253.

Schachter, S. C. (Ed.). (2008a). *Epilepsy in our view: Stories from friends and families of people living with epilepsy*. New York: Oxford University Press.

Schachter, S. C. (Ed.). (2008b). *Epilepsy in our words: Personal accounts of living with seizures*. New York: Oxford University Press.

Sethi, N. K., Torgovnick, J., Arsura, E., Sethi, P. K., & Labar, D. (2008). Seizure disorders: An overview. *Internet Journal of Neurology, 9*(1), 1–10.

Skead, R., & Simmel, M. (2012). *Mighty mike bounces back: A boy's life with epilepsy*. Washington, D. C.: Magination Press.

Sohlberg, M. M., McLaughlin, K. A., Todis, B., Larsen, J., & Glang, A. (2001). What does it take to collaborate with families affected by brain injury? A preliminary model. *Journal of Head Trauma Rehabilitation, 16*(5), 498–511.

Stark-Vance, V., & Dubay, M. L. (2011). *100 Questions & answers about brain tumors* (2nd ed.). Boston: Jones and Bartlett Publishers.

Szaflarski, J. P., Rackley, A. Y., Kleindorfer, D. O., Khoury, J., Woo, D., Miller, R., et al. (2008). Incidence of seizures in the acute phase of stroke: A population-based study. *Epilepsia, 49*(6), 974–981.

The National Epilepsy Educational Alliance. (2009). *Epilepsy 101: The ultimate guide for patients and families*. Leonia: Medicus Press.

Tracy, J. I., & Shah, S. (2008). Presurgical functional brain mapping and neurocognitive testing in epilepsy. In J. E. Morgan & J. H. Ricker (Eds.), *Textbook of clinical neuropsychology* (pp. 466–498). New York: Taylor & Francis.

Tucker, G. J. (2005). Seizures. In J. M. Silver, T. W. McAllister, & S. C. Yudofsky (Eds.), *Textbook of traumatic brain injury* (pp. 309–318). Washington, D. C.: American Psychiatric Publishing.

van Breemen, M. S., Rijsman, R. M., Taphoorn, M. J. B., Walchenbach, R., Zwinkels, H., & Vecht, C. J. (2009). Efficacy of anti-epileptic drugs in patients with gliomas and seizures. *Journal of Neurology, 256*(9), 1519–1526.

Vargo, M. (2011). Brain tumor rehabilitation. *American Journal of Physical Medicine & Rehabilitation, 90*(5), 50–62.

Vercueil, L. (2011). International meeting of the French Society of Neurology 2011. Brain tumor epilepsy: A reappraisal and six remaining issues to be debated. *Revue Neurologique, 167*, 751–761.

Wefel, J. S., Armstrong, T. A., & Kohli, S. (2011). Neuropsychological function and quality of life. In A. D. Norden, D. A. Reardon, & P. Y. C. Wen (Eds.), *Primary central nervous system tumors: Pathogenesis and therapy* (pp. 143–170). New York: Springer.

Weinstein, S. C. (2007). Seizures and teens: The impact of seizures and epilepsy on families. *Exceptional Parent, 37*(6), 61–62, 64–65.
Wheless, J. W. (2006). Intractable epilepsy: A survey of patients and caregivers. *Epilepsy & Behavior, 8*(4), 756–764.
Wilner, A. N. (2008). *Epilepsy 199 answers: A doctor responds to his patients' questions* (3rd ed.). New York: Demos Medical Publishing.
Wyllie, E. (2010). *The Cleveland Clinic guide to epilepsy*. New York: Kaplan Publishing.
Zelenka, Y. (2008). *Let's learn with Teddy about epilepsy*. Leonia: Medicus Press.

Chapter 9
Family Group

9.1 Overview

Family Groups are an effective therapeutic method to meet the emotional and informational needs of patients' primary caregivers and support network (Acorn 1998; Aniskiewicz 2007; Charles et al. 2007; Dell Orto and Power 2000; Klonoff et al. 2008; Klonoff and Prigatano 1987; Kreutzer et al. 2002; Ponsford and Shönberger 2010; Prowe 2010; Senelick and Dougherty 2001). Various formats and approaches have been postulated. For example, Aniskiewicz (2007) proposed 6 weekly 75–90 min sessions for 8–12 caregivers with varying roles. Each meeting focused on didactics, group discussion, experiential exercises, and weekly suggestions. The approach includes mindfulness, meditation, and active problem solving. Kreutzer et al. (2002) formulated a structured intervention model applicable to family group therapy with a curriculum of 16 topics.

With the inception of the neurorehabilitation process in my setting, family members are strongly encouraged to participate in the Family Group for caregivers and other tier supports (e.g., family members, significant others, friends, etc.). Relevant medical releases are always obtained from the loved ones (or their appropriate representative) and they are also educated regarding the intent and benefits of the Family Group. Figure 9.1 contains an introduction, including etiquette and requirements for confidentiality. It is imperative to emphasize that the personal information shared by various family members cannot be discussed with nongroup participants, so that attendees can freely express their opinions and aggravations. This includes the loved ones, as private information may migrate back to other relatives' loved ones through "word of mouth."

Previous publications have reviewed the philosophy and protocols for the Family Group (Klonoff and Koberstein 2010; Klonoff et al. 2008; Klonoff and Prigatano 1987). The format described in this chapter is open entry and open exit; therefore, new members are integrating into the group with more experienced participants. In my setting, the group is held on a weekly basis and is divided into three components. The first is a 30 min educational session; the second 30 min are a support group for attendees; and the last 30 min are spent reviewing the loved one's overall progress and current challenges to keep family members "in the loop." Generally, there are up to 20 attendees who are age 18 years and older. The group facilitators can vary,

P. S. Klonoff, *Psychotherapy for Families after Brain Injury*,

DOI 10.1007/978-1-4899-8083-0_9, © Springer Science+Business Media New York 2014

Welcome to Family Group

Purpose: To provide a forum for families of persons with brain injuries to come together to gain education, receive emotional support, and share their feelings, concerns, and triumphs.

General Information:

- Family members and significant others over the age of 18 are welcome.
- Family Group meets on Thursday afternoons (1:00 p.m. - 2:30 p.m.)
- Thursday meetings will begin with an educational component (30 min.) followed by a support group, facilitated by the Clinical Neuropsychologists (30 min.) and updates by multidisciplinary program staff (30 min.). The educational topics continually evolve, but typically address:

    1. Common emotions from the event until outpatient treatment starts
    2. Practical worries and general advice
    3. Catastrophic reactions by proxy
    4. “Why me?” and grief and loss
    5. Overprotectiveness and letting go
    6. Social isolation, loneliness, and family disruption
    7. Uncertainty about the future and “what ifs”
    8. Burnout
    9. Rites of passage and the future

Group Rules and Etiquette:

- Respect the privacy of all program patients and their families. Discussions are strictly confidential and must not be shared outside of the group.
- Respect the opinions of others.
- Leave time for others to express their thoughts and concerns – save specific discussions for individual meetings with the appropriate therapist(*)

Fig. 9.1 Introduction to Family Group

(*) Therapists are available after Family Group or at another designated time to further discuss any concerns you may have about your loved one. Please notify the therapist or front office to schedule individual appointments.

By my signature below, I acknowledge receipt of the General Information pertaining to the Family Group, including the Group Rules and Etiquette, and agree to the rules and expectations of the Group.

____________________________ __________________

Friend/Relative's Name Date

By my signature below, I agree to disclosures regarding my injury and treatment by my friend and/or family member named above as a part of their participation in Family Group, providing they are involved in my care.

____________________________ __________________

Patient Date

Fig. 9.1 (continued)

as neuropsychologists or clinical psychologists facilitate the support group. Other therapy disciplines can join for the educational component and progress updates. In fact, using the multidisciplinary approach provides a myriad of beneficial perspectives and opinions. Light snacks and beverages are served to perpetuate a nurturing ambience (Klonoff and Koberstein 2010).

The Family Group encompasses the support network from a mixture of injury etiologies, including traumatic brain injuries, strokes, seizure disorders, and brain tumors. The chronology of the injuries also varies, as does the amount of time the loved one has been receiving neurorehabilitation therapies. One parent described this as the "snowflake injury" (S. Daugharty, personal communication, 1/30/13). In my opinion, this heterogeneity greatly enhances the caregivers' experiential process. Families gain a vast perspective of the variety, severity, and complexity of neurological disorders, as well as their unique recovery course. Relatives are experiencing a "new culture" (Sherwin and O'Shanick 2000) through a robust bond of the injury repercussions, which unites them in their quest for knowledge, solace, and overall adjustment. They have life lessons to impart to one another. The story, *A Very Big Bunny* by Russo (2010) captures the essence of togetherness in a subculture embedded in a larger culture of separateness and can be shared with the group. Participants have also remarked upon the benefit of an empathic ambience which invites the sharing of stories; constructive venting; relatedness; refuge; mentorship; reflection about the commonality of losses; the contrast of viewpoints; emotional nourishment; hopefulness; camaraderie; and a sense of community. Social bonding emanates from recognizing that someone else is "in the same boat." Raw emotions, including crying, are typically bared to the group. In contrast, levity and cathartic laughter emanate from recounting humorous vignettes (Klonoff and Koberstein 2010).

Group facilitators, especially clinical and neuropsychologists, need to take a leadership role in setting the tone and treatment direction for the group. Part of this includes welcoming new members and helping them feel comfortable by not putting them in the limelight before they are ready, as well as politely redirecting the discussion when family members dominate the discussion, delve into too much detail about current worries, or become overly focused on issues tangential to their loved one's brain injury. Sensing when the caregiver needs private psychotherapy sessions or small group meetings with the loved one, family, and main treating staff is key to finding the ideal balance between a group format which is designed to allow for peer support, mentorship, and general psychoeducation versus unique and personalized needs.

In some settings, or based on a combination of the families, loved ones with the brain injury, and professional facilitators, mixed meetings with all parties are preferred (Backhaus et al. 2010; Ben-Yishay and Diller 2011; Charles et al. 2007; Fleming et al. 2009; Gan et al. 2010; Klonoff and Koberstein 2010; Kreutzer et al. 2009b). Typically, the content focuses on education, skill building, goal setting, self-management, coping skills, and emotional support (Backhaus et al. 2010; Fleming et al. 2009; Gan et al. 2010). The subject matter should be carefully orchestrated to meet the needs of the two sometimes disparate audiences. In addition, the psychological readiness of the caregivers and loved ones to integrate feedback from contrasting perspectives in the same group meeting needs to be contemplated (Klonoff and Koberstein 2010). Hence, the following protocols and ideas described in this chapter may also lend themselves nicely to conjoint dialogue between caregivers and their loved ones.

Worth mentioning is that many of the psychoeducation topics on neuroanatomy and specific symptoms and syndromes described in the earlier chapters can and should be integrated into the educational format of the Family Group. Understanding common consequences of brain injury gives an informational foundation to the family and will help reduce their confusion and distress (Klonoff and Koberstein 2010; Kreutzer et al. 2002, 2010; Sander 2005). The choice of what material to incorporate is left up to the group facilitators. It should take into account the specific Family Group's format and needs, based on injury etiology and sequelae, age, and relationship of the loved one to the caregivers, etc. Table 9.1 provides a sampling of possible educational topics. Also, many of the handouts provided in earlier chapters will lend themselves nicely to group dissemination, to help illustrate the core concepts. Providing an organized binder with related handouts and resources anchors the families in their rehabilitation journey.

To conceptualize clinical themes and content, this author also collected representative verbalizations and material based on free discussions from the past 7 years of the weekly Family Group. These have been condensed into 9 salient themes (see Table 9.2). The structure of the Family Group can be based on a 9-week rotation through the topic headings and can be extended beyond that, based on the psychological needs of the group, what psychoeducational material is to be covered, and/or how many weeks the facilitators plan to run the group. Of note, the order of any

Table 9.1 Educational topics

Neuroanatomy
Executive functions
Aphasia
Facts and myths about brain injury
Seizures and their risks
Memory
Memory compensations (e.g., datebook, tablets, checklists, and pillboxes)
Adaptive equipment for physical and vision challenges
Communication pragmatics
Mood and personality changes
Psychotropic medications
Catastrophic reactions
Family Experiential Model (FEM) of Recovery
Grief and loss
Sleep hygiene
"Brain foods"
Functions of all treatment disciplines (e.g., neuropsychology, physical, occupational, speech, and recreational therapies)
Stress management techniques

Table 9.2 Family Group themes

1. Common emotions from the event until outpatient treatment starts
2. Practical worries
3. Catastrophic reactions by proxy
4. "Why me?" and grief and loss
5. Overprotectiveness and letting go
6. Family system disruption, social isolation, and loneliness
7. Uncertainty about the future and "what ifs"
8. Burnout
9. Rites of passage and the future

subject can be shifted flexibly, based on the therapists' preferences and families' emotional status and priorities.

This chapter will be structured according to examples of relevant utterances by family members according to each theme. Following that, a treatment protocol will be presented with group exercises to facilitate peer interactions. In combination with this, examples of pertinent psychoeducation by group facilitators and instructional "helpful hints," also employing multimedia resources, are described. These techniques should maximize the caregivers' armamentarium of therapeutic knowledge and coping tools.

9.2 Common Emotions from the Event until Outpatient Treatment Starts

Table 9.3 summarizes some representative samples of families' reminiscent verbalizations during Family Group, spanning the time of notification about their loved one's injury and hospitalization until starting the outpatient neurorehabilitation

Table 9.3 Common emotional verbalizations from the event until treatment starts

Phase 1
First things first—will my loved one live or die?
Why me? Why us? Why them?
If only. . .
I'm scared, confused, upset, and angry
I feel helpless and in despair
I'm so glad my loved one is alive
The doctor said my loved one will never______
I wish the professionals had been more supportive and informative
This is surreal
Phase 2
If. . . . .then
I'm on a roller coaster
I hope to wake up from this nightmare and things will be normal
He/she has to beat the odds
I'm overwhelmed
I can't absorb all of this
Phase 3
I feel like I'm constantly "on call"
I feel so alone
I feel enslaved, victimized, and scapegoated
I'm guilt ridden
It's been a twisted journey to get help
Phase 4
I'm glad my loved one is in treatment
Will the therapists be nice?
I want him/her to have the "best of the best"
I didn't know what I didn't know
I realized there were some physical problems; I had no idea about thinking difficulties
It's hard to hear these realities
It's not like a bone
This happened to all of us, not just ______
My concept of time has radically changed
Will the future be okay?

process. This constitutes retrospective emoting, in which the attendees can feel heard and validated. The expressions are grouped according to the first four phases of the Family Experiential Model (FEM) of Recovery (see Klonoff and Koberstein 2010 and Klonoff et al. 2008 for reviews; see Chap. 1, Sect. 1.5 and Fig. 1.3). In phase 1, the horror of the situation has struck the tier 1 caregiver and reverberated within the tier supports at large. They feel vulnerable. Foremost on the family's mind is whether or not the loved one will survive, and they show great relief when he or she reaches mile markers of medical improvements. The relatives intermittently grapple with feelings of "why me, why us, why my loved one?" Emotions are intense and vacillating and include shock, anxiety, fear, confusion, guilt, and anger (Aniskiewicz 2007; Braine 2011; Dell Orto and Power 2000; Guerriere and McKeever 1997; Johnson and McCown 1997; Jumisko et al. 2007; Klonoff and Koberstein 2010; Klonoff et al. 2008; Kreutzer et al. 2002, 2010; Man 2002; Price et al. 1998; Prowe

2010; Testani-Dufour et al. 1992). Regrets emerge, with self-punishing "if onlys." Routines are disrupted, life feels surreal, and the family plummets into crisis mode (Klonoff and Koberstein 2010; Klonoff et al. 2008).

Primary caregivers and concerned parties plant themselves at the bedside, grasping for scraps of hopeful information. To their chagrin, the offerings may be meager and the professionals often seem detached. The family feels in a "no man's land," wandering without direction. When the professional's input seems overly pessimistic, the family's helplessness and despair can morph into the "blame game" towards the professionals.

As the recovery process unfolds (see phase 2), the family follows their loved one into new settings, including inpatient rehabilitation, and then eventually home. They bargain and pray their way through a hopeful progression of basic functions, with an attitude of "if . . . then . . . ." For instance, relatives may set their sights on their loved one being able to feed himself or herself, then dress himself or herself, etc., all the while telling themselves they will be satisfied if he or she makes it to the next milestone. With time, they come to realize that what they really want is for their loved one to improve rapidly and "beat the odds."

During this process, the family feels they are on an emotional roller coaster, thrust into foreign and perplexing realities. They yearn to wake up from their nightmare and return to life as it was. The complexities of their loved one's neurological condition as well as the added duties of managing health insurance, the strands of their loved one's preinjury existence, and their countless responsibilities, quickly become overwhelming. There is just too much to absorb!

As depicted in phase 3, the 24/7 hassles and obligations intensify (Klonoff and Koberstein 2010; Klonoff et al. 2008). The tier 1 caregiver feels constantly "on call" (Jumisko et al. 2007). He or she feels tied down due to the loved one's dependency (Wedcliffe and Ross 2001). Added to this are the startling changes in the loved one, with his or her angst and rage catapulted onto the caregiver, who now feels alone, enslaved, scapegoated, and victimized. This alternates with profound guilt. How can the caregiver complain when his or her loved one is suffering? No matter what the tier supports do for the loved one, they feel inadequate. They cannot do enough and there is not enough time to meet their loved one's multiplicity of needs. Worn out, the family is galvanized or often desperate to find help for their loved one and hopefully, for themselves. Often, this involves a meandering journey sometimes fraught with disappointments and worries, including fragmented medical care. Some are petrified that the "hourglass will run out" and the loved one will not get help in time.

As illustrated in phase 4, once the family finds some form of outpatient treatment for their loved one, there is a reprieve and renewed optimism. Everyone is in a honeymoon period. Some anticipation remains, as the caregiver is wondering if the therapists will be supportive and effective. The family is hoping the therapists will be "miracle workers." Admittedly, the family feels relatively ignorant of the injury consequences, stating, "I didn't know what I didn't know." Physical challenges are apparent; thinking deficits are not. However, once the therapists share evaluation findings, early realities begin to set in, including that the "brain is not like a bone." It seems the healing process is in fact convoluted and extensive. Family members express their life is in limbo, with a growing appreciation that the whole family was

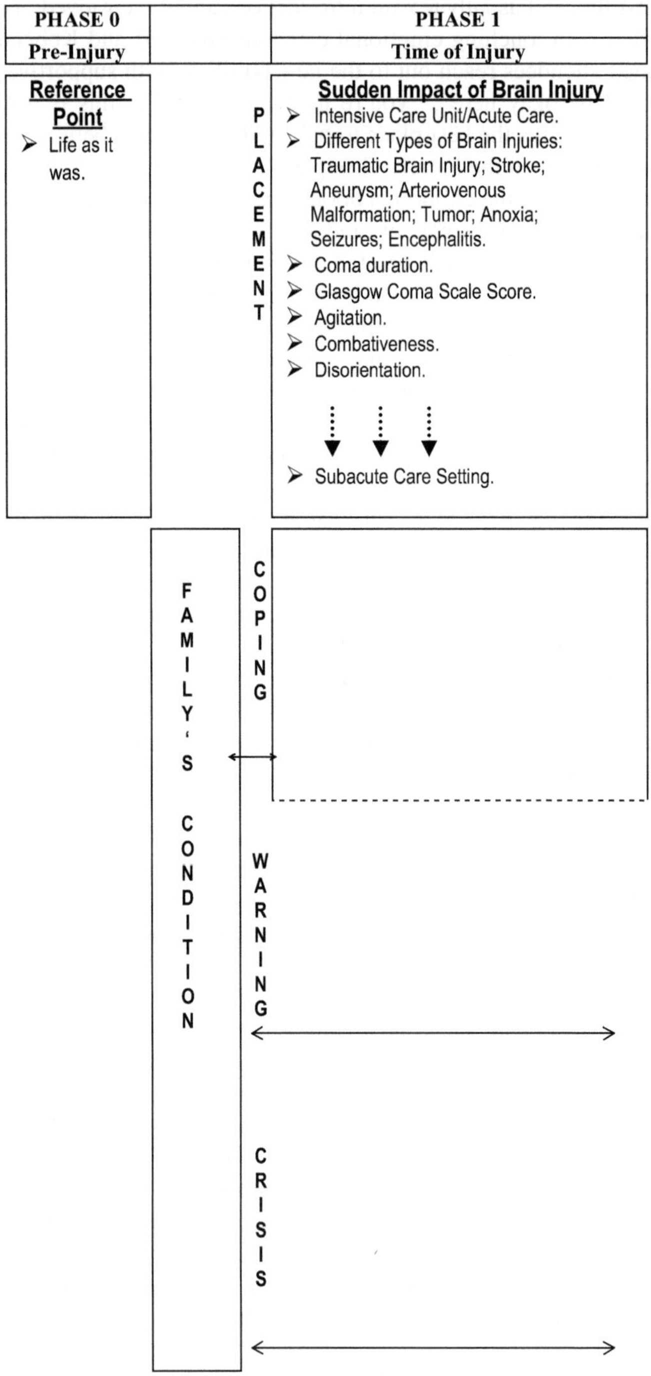

Fig. 9.2 Patient Experiential Model (PEM) of Recovery after brain injury. Psychotherapy after Brain Injury: Principles and Techniques, Pamela S. Klonoff. 2010. Copyright Guilford Press. Reprinted with permission of the Guilford Press. Principles of Neuropsychological Rehabilitation by Prigatano (1999) Fig. 8.1 p. 184. By permission of Oxford University Press/By permission of Oxford University Press, USA

PHASE 2 Early Adjustment	PHASE 3 Seeks Help	PHASE 4 Holistic Treatment Starts
		AWARENESS
Initial Problems ➢ In-Patient Neuro-rehabilitation. ➢ Post–traumatic Amnesia. ➢ Anterograde Amnesia. ➢ Retrograde Amnesia. ➢ Confusion. ➢ Agitation. ➢ Disorientation. ➢ Organic Unawareness—I see my physical problems, but not my cognitive or emotional difficulties. ➢ Physical Therapy. ➢ Occupational Therapy. ➢ Speech & Language Therapy. ➢ Recreational Therapy. ➢ Initial Neuropsychological Screening. ➢ Primary focus is on my basic activities of daily living skills (ADLs).	**Can't Cope** ➢ Rehab doctor or general physician recommends therapy. ➢ I and/or my family may refuse or cannot get the necessary treatment. ➢ Life upheaval and financial setbacks. ➢ Problems escalate at home, in the community, or at work/ school. ➢ My family becomes "stressed out" and overloaded. ➢ My family and/or I intensify the treatment search.	**Confronting Reality** ➢ I may experience a "honeymoon period." ➢ Holistic approach teaches individualized strengths and difficulties. ➢ The process is often demanding, stressful, and evokes strong emotions. ("Catastrophic Reactions;" "C.R.'s"). ➢ May feel like "Rehab Boot Camp."
	➢ I am tentative but trust that the physician and/or family have my best interest at heart. ➢ I am open to considering further rehabilitation to improve my circumstances.	➢ I have increased awareness of the effects of my injury. ➢ Enjoy the structure and feel empowered by my new knowledge. ➢ I constructively manage my anxiety, anger, frustration, and/or sadness. ➢ I become less overwhelmed and I develop better coping techniques. ➢ I develop trust in holistic therapies.
	➢ I dismiss or underestimate my problem areas. ➢ I attribute difficulties to external factors, not me. ➢ Feel I'll make a full recovery on my own without therapies.	➢ Cannot cope with feedback and I display intense and extended emotional distress. ➢ Misplaced feelings of "kill the messenger." ➢ I reject the education process and use denial or disavowal. ➢ My relationships with therapists and family are strained and deteriorate.

Period of Disintegration

Either I can't get the therapies I need/want because of insurance problems or I adamantly reject or ignore the consequences of my injury and holistic treatment recommendations. I refuse to become aware and acceptant; I negate my reality. I am filled with rage, despair, hopelessness and helplessness. (cont'd).

Fig. 9.2 (continued)

Discharge

PHASE 5 Re-training *ACCEPTANCE*	PHASE 6 Transition from Therapy *REALISM*	PHASE 7 Future ∞
Compensations ➢ Psychological introspection of injury aftermath. ➢ Development and implementation of compensations. ➢ Holistic milieu provides me a perspective on the spectrum of injury types and severities. ➢ I begin work trial and/or school courses. ➢ "Dress Rehearsal" for my new life. ➢ Opportunity for "second chance."	**Approaching Discharge** ➢ Attainable goals are identified. ➢ Therapeutic applications of new insights, skills and compensations to the "outside world." ➢ Exposed to new freedoms, independence, and meaningful activities. ➢ "Dignity of Risk." **Cake Day**	**The Real World** ➢ I have my tools learned in the program to function as independently and productively as possible in the community. ➢ My new reality sets in. ➢ Life is ever-changing and evolving. ➢ Things aren't the same, but everyone can live a meaningful and productive life.
➢ I mourn the losses. ➢ Adjust expectations and accept myself for who I am now. ➢ I embrace compensations with a "Just Do It!" attitude. ➢ I remain open to implementing feedback and strategies in multiple settings. ➢ Improved communication pragmatics enhance my interpersonal relationships. ➢ I realize that "things take time," but I am invested in compensation training. ➢ I cope with potential role changes within the family structure and in the community.	➢ Collaborate with therapists and my family towards community re-integration. ➢ I am realistic about my level of independence, productivity, and socialization skills. ➢ I constructively manage my fears and trepidations about my discharge. ➢ I develop self confidence in my skill attainment. ➢ Expand my support system. ➢ I find inner strength and courage through facing adversity. ➢ I make maximal gains in my recovery and rehabilitation.	➢ I maintain a collaborative dialogue with significant others about my compensations and life decisions. ➢ Consistently use my compensations, both at home and work/school. ➢ I modify my compensations when home/job demands change. ➢ I am successful in establishing and maintaining a "two way street" in relationships in and outside of the home. ➢ "Door is always open" for further help and support if I need it.
➢ Balk and/or rebel against my injury limitations. ➢ I am snarky, distrusting and/or resistant to feedback ("Yeah Buts"). ➢ I lack follow through; am just "going through the motions;" and/or will not cooperate. ➢ I blame others or the environment for my personal struggles. ➢ I become locked in a "power struggle" with my therapists and family. ➢ I overwhelm my family and community supports because I don't accept the changes in my roles and abilities.	➢ Insufficient personal investment negatively impacts my progress and goal attainment. ➢ I show "Flight into Health." ➢ I exhibit self-doubts, anxieties, and inadequate coping techniques. ➢ I am unwilling or unable to develop a social network. ➢ I set unrealistic goals. ➢ Experience major setbacks in my rehabilitation and recovery. ➢ Unprepared functionally or emotionally for my discharge and transition because I'm not 100% recovered.	➢ I experience "slippage" in using my compensations. ➢ I am unable to adapt to changing demands. ➢ I am unlikely to seek out help when necessary. ➢ My family members become burned out and disengage.

Period of Disintegration

(cont'd). I am suspicious and argumentative. I become socially isolated and alienated from my friends and family. I am dependent on others in the home and community. I experience work failures and financial ruin. There is fragmentation and/or dissolution of my family life. Life implodes!

Fig. 9.2 (continued)

post-acute treatment. Early on, the predominant goal is to save the patient's life. There is relatively less attention paid to possible functional changes, which are relegated to a secondary consideration.

The facilitators should encourage the tier supports about the upcoming benefits of the outpatient therapeutic process. This is best displayed within a "tapestry of teamwork," when the families feel safe and experience the treatment approach as integrated, with value placed on their input (Klonoff 2010; Kreutzer et al. 2010). The family needs to know that others appreciate their special needs, not just those of the loved one. They can be considered a key "instrument of recovery," as their drive and perseverance can help sustain their loved one. Pertinent strategies include giving real-time feedback, picking battles (see Chap. 2, Sect. 2.4.2.3), and mantras such as "you need to believe" (see Chap. 2, Sect. 2.4.1.1). Avoiding being the main bearer of bad news diminishes conflicts with the loved one (see Chap. 2, Sect. 2.4.1). This includes learning the art of keeping doors open about goal setting and/or the future prognosis or "learning to say maybe, instead of no." Facilitating the closest working alliance with the team is also based on the tier 1 caregivers being "straight shooters," avoiding "putting feelings on the back burner," and/or "keeping secrets." Sometimes, family members fall folly to the stance of "only I know my loved one." A nice symbolic representation of the potential pitfalls of this is the story of the Drug Enforcement Administration (DEA) officer (http://www.sanitaryum.com/2011/09/28/funny-written-stuff/funny-emails-and-forwards/joke-the-deas-badge/). Seasoned group mentors can confirm that allowing the therapeutic process to unfold is imperative. Although trepidations are normal, it is important to temper skepticism and avoid strife, especially if this undermines the trust-building process.

9.3 Practical Worries

Understandably, the caregiver and extended family are mostly unprepared for the complexity and chronicity of their newfound commitments and hassles. A pervasive theme is that the family feels inundated by a number of conundrums (see also Chap. 3). Table 9.5 summarizes some of the common practical worries manifested in the primary caregiver. These include their loved one's personal affairs, as well as the direct reverberations of the injury on the family system. Financial insecurity and threats to insurance coverage impede the family's adaptation (Carnes and Quinn 2005). When the loved one was the breadwinner, spouses are petrified about how to keep up with bills. Some wives have bemoaned that their husbands were in control of the finances and they feel helpless and ignorant of how to commandeer the multiple financial duties (e.g., bills, budgetary planning, and taxes). Alternatively, often the primary caregiver has to either stop work or greatly reduce his or her schedule, in order to accommodate the loved one's needs in the home, as well as provide transportation.

Adult children who were independent and launched into their own residences and careers may suddenly need to move back in with their parents or their siblings. Patients who cannot drive are even more dependent, often reliant on the generosity

Table 9.5 Examples of verbalizations about practical worries

I'm not trained to do all of this
I've never managed the household finances before
How will we keep up with the bills?
I'm afraid we will lose everything we have worked for
If I don't go to work, I'll lose my job and then where will we be?
How can I get my loved one to therapy and all of his appointments?
I thought ___ was on his/her own working and living away from home
This health insurance process is so confusing and aggravating
The lawsuit from the accident is so time-consuming and draining
What about all my other commitments to everyone else besides my loved one?
I'm lost and on overload with all of this
I feel like I'm going crazy or that I'll lose it

of the primary caregiver, extended family, and/or friends. Navigating confusing and adversarial health insurance and disability policies accentuates the caregiver's helplessness and panic. Litigation usually adds strains and drains on the caregiver's time and emotions. Amidst this, the caregiver is busily contending with his or her loved one's disabilities, often feeling largely inadequate in coping with the resultant chaos. When there are other siblings or adults in the home requiring time and energy, or additional outside stressors unrelated to the loved one, the excessive toil soon becomes unfeasible. Overall, the primary caregiver finds himself or herself juggling multiple balls, many of which are dropping.

9.3.1 Group Treatment to Cope with Practical Worries

Table 9.6 summarizes a group exercise, therapeutic "helpful hints," and general solutions, as well as multimedia resources to cope with practical worries. The movie, *Regarding Henry* (Abrams et al. 1991) is a realistic portrayal of the instantaneous and devastating impact of a brain injury on the family unit. This movie is an excellent mechanism to engender group dialogue and collaboration about the new stresses and strains after a brain injury. In addition, the richness of the group process enables the exchange of new ideas and resources between family members. The overall message is that given the array of tasks forged upon the caregiver, he or she needs to be guided to craft a personalized "survival kit."

The group facilitators should emphasize that each family's definition of practical solutions will vary, based on the specific interests and talents of the caregiver, and should also take into account pragmatic considerations (e.g., who else is willing and available to provide assistance?). Realistic group attendees advise other caregivers to both initiate and accept offers of help from the extended family as well as outsiders. This will prevent self-neglect (Cassidy 2009; Kreutzer et al. 2010; Prowe 2010; Rich 2005) and conserve their precious emotional and physical energies. A common concern is that most friends and supporters will be unsure of how best to help. Pragmatic suggestions that emerge during the discussion include that the primary caregiver should politely request specific areas of assistance (e.g., rides, meals, stints

Table 9.6 Group treatment for practical worries

Guided exercise
What resources do you all find helpful to address practical stressors?
"Helpful hints" and psychoeducation
Craft a personalized "survival kit"
Accept offers from outside supporters; make specific requests
Follow the adage of "worry about it when you need to"
Tackle the "here and now" stressors
Use organizational tools
Multimedia resources
Movie
Regarding Henry (Abrams et al. 1991)
Website
http://www.lotsahelpinghands.com
Didactics and demonstrations
Treating therapists' overview of key compensations
Guest speakers
Social worker
Local Brain Injury Alliance
Community resources
Insurance case manager
Community and/or Internet support groups
Resource manuals
Reading materials
Scientific conferences
Attorney and financial advisor input
Employer programs
Mentorship advice from other family members
Treating professionals

with the loved one, etc.). The caregiver will also need to be creative to meet his or her needs in the context of the loved one's requirements. One mother who had returned to work shared that she hired a driver to bring her son to rehabilitation; another stated she arranged car pools with parents of other patients who were in the same rehabilitation center. An impressive website is http://www.lotsahelpinghands.com, which allows the caregiver to specify what particular types of assistance are preferred so as to streamline and communicate the family's needs to their community tier 2 and 3 supports.

A helpful adage for group facilitators to promote is "worry about it when you need to," that is, set practical priorities and a realistic timeline for directing the caregiver's energies and tackle the "here-and-now" stressors. Working on what is in front of the family will alleviate a tendency to feel overwhelmed and inundated. To this end, the primary caregiver will need therapeutic assistance from all of the treating therapists to find techniques to stay organized; checklists, datebooks, smartphones, and tablets are all workable. Didactic inservices in Family Group about the available tools and compensations help to educate and inform the group participants and also reinforce that they "are not alone" in modifying their lifestyles. Not only the loved one, but also certainly the caregiver and other immediate family members, learn that they will benefit from structure, consistency, boundaries, and enforcement of the loved one's responsibilities.

Group facilitators and experienced peers can remind other family members to explore and utilize any and all community resources. Specific individuals can be invited to the group to provide input and psychoeducation, including a social worker or representatives from the local Brain Injury Alliance. Other external entities that family members can utilize include an insurance case manager; community and/or Internet support groups; resource manuals and other reading materials; scientific conferences; an attorney and/or financial advisor; the employer (regarding eligibility for the Family and Medical Leave Act); and importantly, mentorship advice from other family members savvy about convoluted health-care systems and all other common hardships. All of these outlets maximize advocacy for the loved one (Dell Orto and Power 2000; Hoffmeister 1998; Klonoff and Koberstein 2010; Prowe 2010; Rich 2005; Senelick and Dougherty 2001; Williams 1991) and reduce the families' distress. The therapists and experienced attendees counsel new joiners that when they are stumped about a particular problem, they should be proactive about consulting the treating professionals for assistance. Common issues include persistent worrisome physical symptoms (e.g., headaches) and if and when the family can take a break from therapy with the loved one without adverse medical consequences. More commentary and suggestions on these topics are contained in Sect. 9.9 on burnout.

9.4 Catastrophic Reactions by Proxy

Earlier sections of the book define *Catastrophic Reactions by Proxy* (*CRs by proxy*; see Chap. 2, Sect. 2.4.2.1 and Chap. 4, Sect. 4.8.2 and Table 4.10). In brief, these are the counterpart of CRs in the loved one, whereby the caregiver experiences an intense emotional reaction secondary to his or her appreciation of impairments and loss of potential in the loved one. Table 9.7 contains common examples of utterances by families which reflect their CRs by proxy. The tier 1 caregiver often notices a mirroring of intense emotions with the loved one, with concordance in their psychic pain. One young wife began crying during the Family Group when she (and he) first recognized her husband could no longer country dance, an activity they had enjoyed together for several years. A mother became weepy describing how her daughter was so disgusted with herself when she kept misplacing her bus pass and was eventually fined by the light rail officer for not having it with her. A father was upset when he found out about his son's discouragement over failing a final exam in algebra, an area he had excelled at pre-accident. Prior enjoyable family pastimes (e.g., hobbies and vacations) now are onerous for everyone. Both the loved one and the caregiver experience anxiety, frustration, anger, and feelings of helplessness and devastation about the ineptitudes and limitations, especially because they "can't fix them."

Relatives reflect upon the initial evaluation findings as fertile ground for CRs by proxy, especially if they had not yet seen detailed written reports delineating the limitations. The loved one's dependency on the caregiver can feel smothering to both parties. Furthermore, the medical restrictions for supervision at home as well as loss of driving and work privileges for the loved one curtail everyone's freedoms, resulting in irritation and angst.

Table 9.7 Examples of verbalizations that are catastrophic reactions by proxy

I can't believe my loved one can't ______ anymore
When my loved one is down or frustrated, so am I
It makes me so anxious that my loved one can't______
It's so hard to stand by and watch my loved one fail at things he/she was so good at before
Watching my loved one struggle is heartbreaking
I hate that I can't fix my loved one's problems
It's so upsetting to see their mishaps because of their forgetfulness
I'm angry about all of this
That initial report was a bitter pill
I feel tied at the hip to my loved one
I can't handle his/her violent outbursts
I'm always on guard that they will embarrass themselves or me
Things we used to do as a family (e.g., vacations) just aren't the same anymore
My loved one isn't like his cousins or friends anymore
He/she just isn't the same person
I can't handle everything on my plate
This is a club no one wants to be in

Temper or violent outbursts are unnerving for the patient and caregiver alike. Furthermore, when family members are continually on guard about their loved one's disinhibited or inappropriate behavior, everyone becomes resentful and exhausted. Both the loved one and family come to realize that he or she is not the same person. When the family (and loved one) compare themselves to other friends and the extended family whose lives appear "normal," the hurt and disillusionment deepen. The magnitude of the realizations can result in insights such as "I am heartbroken" or "I can't handle all of this." Some feel they are "in a club no one wants to be in."

9.4.1 Group Treatment for CRs by Proxy

Psychotherapy to advance knowledge and acquire emotional support is indispensable. The optimal antidote for reducing CRs by proxy is to understand their causes and manifestations. Because CRs so frequently occur in the loved one, it is also recommended that the support network be familiarized with this phenomenon by the group facilitators (Klonoff 2010; Klonoff et al. 1993; for an earlier discussion of CRs, see Chap. 4, Sects. 4.6.1 and 4.6.2, and Table 4.6).

Table 9.8 describes the definition, manifestations, and remedies to reduce the prevalence of CRs and CRs by proxy. Both CRs and CRs by proxy are indicative of improved awareness or the understanding of the postinjury strengths and difficulties (Klonoff 2010). Pathognomonic signs of CRs and CRs by proxy are feeling overwhelmed and snarky because of the nature and implications of the injury-related impediments. Crying is perhaps the most common outward manifestation. Typically, sadness, anxiety, fear, guilt, and shame about the disabilities and disintegration of the integrity of the self underlie CRs (Goldstein 1952; Klonoff et al. 1993; Lansky 1990) and CRs by proxy. Often, the other party (i.e., loved one or family member) is

Table 9.8 Group treatment for CRs (catastrophic reactions) and CRs by proxy

Guided exercises
Ask open-ended questions about the families' experiences with catastrophic reactions (CRs)
Explore the families' unique and shared experiences of CRs by proxy
Discuss tools and techniques that various relatives have found helpful to reduce CRs and CRs by proxy
Psychoeducation
CR: the loved one's strong emotional reaction to current difficulties in accomplishing tasks that were easy before the injury. Usually the failure is sudden and unexpected
CRs by proxy: the strong emotional reaction in the caregiver or any member of the support network, when they witness irrefutable evidence of injury-related deficits and losses in their loved one. Usually the perception of the inability is sudden and unexpected
Examples of triggers of CRs and CRs by Proxy
Memory failures
Any other cognitive, physical, or language challenge
Supervision in the home and community
Incapacity to perform hobbies and sports
Inability to drive
Poor grades
Loss of friendships

Common manifestations of CRs and CRs by Proxy	
Overwhelmed	Snarky
Frustrated/Impatient	Blaming
Angry/Rage	Defensive
Sad	Tearful
Depressed	Anxious
Guilt	Fear/Panic
Embarrassed	Withdrawn
Avoidance	Shut down
Minimizing	Concealment
Helplessness	Devastated
Hopeless	

"Helpful hints" to reduce the frequency and magnitude of CRs and CRs by proxy
Engage in psychotherapy to advance knowledge and acquire emotional support
Learn the triggers and manifestations of your loved one's CRs and your own CRs by proxy
Realize that uncooperativeness, minimizing, resistance, avoidance, withdrawal, concealment, or hostility are likely related to CRs and CRs by proxy
Do not humiliate or counter-attack, instead remain empathic
Avoid confrontations during a CR or CR by proxy, or the situation will escalate
Share and reinforce helpful tools and strategies to reduce CRs and CRs by proxy
Adjust lifestyles to reduce stress and facilitate success:
Work/study with understanding and flexible people
Simplify work and school loads so they are manageable
Delegate and pace activities
Create stepwise and best-fit goals
Make healthy life choices (exercise, rest, diet, and good friendships)
Consider psychotropic medications to ameliorate interfering mood problems
Realize that CRs and CRs by proxy may not occur in tandem
Remember that CRs and CRs by proxy produce ups and downs
Focus on disclosing "small ounces" of progress for sustenance in other group participants

the target of frustration, intense rage, and blaming. The patient or caregiver resorts to "hurting the one he or she loves" because of his or her accessibility and familiarity. Of note, frequent and intense CRs can plummet the loved one and/or family member into depression, also characterized by feelings of helplessness, hopelessness, and emotional devastation (Klonoff 2010). The family should be watchful of interactions which produce humiliation versus humility about the loved one's limitations. When the therapists reframe uncooperativeness, minimizing, resistance, avoidance, withdrawal, concealment, and hostility as symptomatic of the primary caregiver's or loved one's torment (Klonoff et al. 1993; Lansky 1990), the family remains empathic versus reacting with counter-attacks.

Once the families have a basic understanding of CRs and CRs by proxy, an excellent group exercise is to ask open-ended questions such as: *Do you see CRs in your loved one? How do CRs manifest themselves? How do you feel when your loved one is having a CR? How do you approach the situation when this happens?* Similarly, the group venue is an outstanding setting to launch a group discussion about the families' CRs by proxy. Representative questions include: *Are you having CRs by proxy? What precipitates them? How do you feel inside when this happens and what's going through your mind about your situation? How are you coping with these?* This exploration reinforces the universality of the phenomena and is very reassuring to caregivers who are otherwise flummoxed and bereft.

Family members are counseled to avoid confrontation during a CR or CR by proxy, as this typically will escalate an already emotionally charged and volatile situation. When the caregiver feels the need to discuss precipitating events, it is prudent to "strike while the iron is cold" (Yalom 2002), that is, when both parties are calm and receptive. Other therapeutic suggestions include building a communication bridge by reminding the loved one that the caregiver is his or her supporter (not the enemy) and giving him or her the requisite time and space to emotionally reconstitute after a CR.

Participants can be invited to share techniques they have discovered that reduce CRs and CRs by proxy. This includes possible tools and strategies which will ameliorate the injury-related shortcomings (see also Chap. 4, Table 4.6 for "helpful hints" for coping with CRs in the loved one). Group facilitators and educated relatives can offer their ideas and encourage their incorporation. Families can be empowered when they realize they are instrumental in helping the loved one comply with suitable strategies, rather than view them as "a ball and chain."

Another "helpful hint" is adjusting daily life to reduce stress and facilitate success. This also reduces CRs and therefore CRs by proxy. The loved one and his or her relatives should liaison with outsiders who are supportive and flexible as well as define work and school loads which are doable. This may include delegating and pacing undertakings. Overall, the community-based goals should be stepwise and the best fit for everyone involved. This will create little building blocks of success. Healthy life choices include proper exercise, rest, nutrition, and good friendships. Several medications have proved very useful in reducing the frequency and intensity of CRs and CRs by proxy (and depression), by improving frustration tolerance and coping capacity. These include selective serotonin reuptake inhibitors (SSRIs, e.g., sertraline and escitalopram; see Klonoff 2010, for a review). Numbing substances (e.g., alcohol, street drugs) should be avoided.

Group facilitators should link CRs and CRs by proxy to the awareness process. However, the caregiver should be informed that the experience of these "ah ha" moments may or may not be in tandem with revelations in the loved one or outside supports. In addition, it may feel to the caregiver that the loved one is taking "one step forward and two steps back," based on how he or she perceives and copes with injury-based impairments. This is not a straight-line process. When the family and loved are not coping well (e.g., PEM/FEM "yellow warning" zones), the support network should be tolerant and recognize that the process is arduous, with episodic setbacks. Overall, to the extent that the loved one and family are helped to "face the music" (Ben-Yishay and Diller 2011) about the challenges (including the new subsistence and goals), the longer-term adjustment is improved. Therapists can help group members appreciate "small ounces" of progress. This helps recalibrate expectations and can sustain them during CRs by proxy. Shared observations between family attendees about gains in one another's loved ones are positive eye-openers and very uplifting.

9.5 Why Me? and Grief and Loss

Tier 1 caregivers and other tier supports typically experience profound feelings of grief after a loved one suffers a brain injury (Dell Orto and Power 2000; Klonoff 2010; Klonoff et al. 2008; Prowe 2010; Rich 2005). Chapter 10 will focus on grief and loss when a loved one dies (see Sect. 10.3). This section will focus on how the Family Group helps the caregiver and relatives with their communal feelings of grief and loss related to their surviving loved one's disabilities. During the early aftermath, this is often experienced as feelings of "why me?" or "why us?" symbolizing their sudden existential perplexity (Klonoff et al. 2008). The shattering of fundamental life assumptions translates to psychological unpreparedness, with sentiments like "I never thought this could happen to me" (Janoff-Bulman 2002).

As the process unfolds, the caregiver and family become astutely aware of the multitude of losses. They grieve for their loved one, as well as themselves. Anger at the loved one or another target symbolic of life's disarray is very common. This may be precipitated by irresponsible actions on the part of the loved one and/or others associated with the brain injury. Examples include drinking while driving, resulting in a traumatic brain injury, or poor self-care resulting in a stroke. Sometimes, family members are enraged at others who were involved in the accident with the loved one, but who walked away "unscathed." The hurt is magnified when these other participants "abandon" the loved one post-accident. Some parents and spouses reluctantly admit they feel envious of their friends and peers whose loved ones are achieving impressive age- and lifestyle-appropriate aspirations, while their own loved ones contend with disabilities which have eliminated the most basic of skills.

Table 9.9 Declarations symbolic of the grief and loss process

"Why me?"
I can't stop second-guessing about what happened
What did I do to deserve this?
This is so unfair
I realize now how much I took for granted
I want to be happy for others' successes, but it is so hard when I am so miserable
Grief and loss for the loved one
My heart is broken for _____
Why my loved one, when no one else was hurt?
I can't see gains
This is like cleaning out belongings when someone dies
I want a full recovery for my loved one
I can't accept these realities
Caregiver grief and loss
I miss____
My partner vanished
My husband/wife is a child now
I have lost me-ness
I don't know when to start grieving
I am so sad some days
I turn the pillow over to get to the dry side
I'm crying endlessly
I can't bear the tragedy of the losses
I am so mad at ____ and/or the situation
I feel guilty when I'm sad or mad
My joy is always overshadowed
My grief comes in cycles
I feel stuck in grief
Altered life circumstances
I've lost my comfort zone
There is so much to grieve
This is life's hard knocks
It is such a struggle to move on
There are so many lost opportunities
I think about what is versus what could have been
Things will never be the same
I want things the way they were
I want a normal life
I want a miracle

For some families, they are befuddled as to when and what to grieve for, given the ambiguity of their loved one's condition and their recovery trajectory. Table 9.9 summarizes examples of poignant declarations symbolic of the grief and loss process. These can be divided into the perceived losses for the loved one, the family's own losses, and devastated life circumstances. Generally speaking, the grief process encompasses elements of all of these, which deepens the sorrow and hopelessness.

9.5.1 *Group Treatment for Why Me? and Grief and Loss*

Table 9.10 summarizes group exercises, psychoeducation, and "helpful hints," as well as multimedia resources for the understandable feelings of "why me?" and grief and loss. The group facilitators can conduct a round-robin discussion by asking general questions about the relatives' feelings of "why me?" or sense of loss. Participation in a safe-haven environment often facilitates the eruption of deep emotions. In what feels like a protective cocoon, there are outpourings emanating from increased awareness about the loved one's status and its ramifications for the family. Open sharing may even catalyze intense emotions in some attendees which were previously buried or constricted. This emoting in a nonjudgmental environment is essential to understanding their struggles (Patrick-Ott and Ladd 2010). A case in point, feelings of "why me?" represent the stark realization, manifested in sorrow, anger, regret, and/or bitterness, that the caregiver and family's lives are inextricably and often permanently altered from the preinjury course. Appreciation of the far-reaching consequences of the brain injury on the family system creates global feelings of powerlessness and incapacitation. This can precipitate "narcissistic rage" attacks against unsuspecting targets, including health-care professionals, other tier supports, innocent bystanders trying to assist, and unfortunately, even the loved one (see Chap. 1, Sect. 1.2.2). Unexpected revelations about the nature and magnitude of various injury-related sequelae in the loved one, especially in the more elusive cognitive, emotional, and interpersonal realms, will also precipitate in-the-moment CRs by proxy (see Sect. 9.4). To this end, the psychotherapist can legitimize the relatives' overarching and episodic emotional angst.

The group facilitators and attendees will observe various grief styles and reactions. Some members are "emoters," while others are "doers." Education can be provided about grieving styles, all of which are personal and legitimate. One classification is a tendency towards experience and expression of the affective components, or *intuitive* grievers (Doka and Martin 2010). Another style is the instrumental griever, who uses the cognitive, problem-solving, and "action plan" approach (Doka and Martin 2010; see also Chap. 3, Sect. 3.3.2). A good inroad into exploring grief styles is to explain the concepts and ask the participants questions such as: *Where do you fall on the continuum of instrumental versus intuitive grieving? What styles have you and your relatives used to handle various crises?* One husband referenced the movie, *Rocky* (Chartoff et al. 1976) as his inspiration for a more instrumental grieving style, while a mother described a daily phone call to her sister to lament her circumstances as her intuitive approach. Psychoeducation will reinforce that these approaches span a continuum within the family system and that often these complement one another, especially in the face of crises.

One of the epiphanies which emerges from the group discussion is that there is no answer to "why me?" In fact, one family member countered in a moment of clarity, "why not me?" The support network finds some way through spiritual or existential beliefs to make sense of the seemingly nonsensical. With the aid of the therapists, these convictions fashion a road towards acceptance and adjustment. It also helps

Table 9.10 Group treatment for "Why me?" and grief and loss

Guided exercises
Ask general questions about the relatives' feelings of "why me?" and their sense of loss
Where do you fall on the continuum of instrumental versus intuitive grieving?
How do you feel about the theories of "chronic sorrow" and "ambiguous loss?"
What are your own stories of grief and mourning?
Which FEM placement phase and coping zone are you in?
"Helpful hints" and psychoeducation
When comfortable, use the support group as a safe haven to explore and express painful feelings
Feelings of "why me?" and grief and loss emanate from increased awareness about the loved one's predicament and its ramifications for the family
"Narcissistic rage" towards outsiders emanates from global feelings of powerlessness and incapacitation about the far-reaching, deleterious effects of the brain injury
Unexpected episodic revelations about the loved one's deficits will also precipitate CRs by proxy and emotional angst
Grief styles fall across continuums of instrumental and intuitive approaches
The group consensus is there are no answers to "why me?"
Spiritual and existential beliefs as well as reading materials help families accept the feelings about "why me?" and cultivate forgiveness
"Chronic sorrow" and "ambiguous loss" are helpful constructs to understand grief and loss after brain injury
"Chronic sorrow" is a process which will be triggered episodically based on real-world reminders of losses
Understand the role of "reference points" of the "day before" versus the "day of" in grief reactions
Remember that grief and loss have many manifestations, layers, and causes
The caregiver's/family's grief and loss process is likely different in manifestation and timing from their loved one
Anger is a common byproduct of chronic sorrow
Differentiate between the process of grief and mourning
There is dynamic oscillation between the loss and restoration process
The group process helps the families gain a better perspective and can stimulate thoughts about the "silver linings"
The FEM is a helpful model to differentiate "adaptive grief" from "stuck grief"
When a family member is mired in grief, he or she should supplement Family Group with individual psychotherapy and psychiatric care
Pursue treatment for other members of the family system (e.g., siblings)
Over time, families gradually adapt to their "chronic sorrow" but often still experience "lingering sadness"
As family members grapple with acceptance and realism, their grief and loss transforms through an adjustment and mastery process to increased hope, optimism, and futuristic thinking
Multimedia resources
Movie
Rocky (Chartoff et al. 1976)
Books
When Bad Things Happen to Good People (Kushner 1981)
Man's Search for Meaning (Frankl 1984)
A Decade of Hope (Smith and Smith 2011)
Model
Family Experiential Model (FEM) of Recovery (Klonoff and Koberstein 2010; Klonoff et al. 2008)

families cultivate forgiveness towards those directly or indirectly involved in the injury mayhem, who themselves are immature and often consumed with guilt and fear. Resources for group dialogue about this quandary include various materials or books, such as *When Bad Things Happen to Good People* by Kushner (1981), *Man's Search for Meaning* by Frankl (1984), or *A Decade of Hope* by Smith and Smith (2011).

The group facilitators should introduce the concept of *chronic sorrow* (Olshansky 1962, as cited in Roos 2002a) to spark discussion about the grief and loss process after brain injury. "Chronic sorrow" is considered a specialized type of grief reaction to a loss, which is not final and is ever present (Roos 2002a). It is a pervasive sadness that is permanent, periodic, and potentially progressive from a "living loss" (Olshansky 1962 as cited in Lee et al. 2001 and Roos 2002a). Some have termed this "nonfinite loss" (Bruce and Schultz 2002; see Collings 2008 for a review). Loss of a normal future as well as the hopes and dreams associated with normal development are considered central components of chronic loss (Collings 2008). The family suffers greatly over the relinquishment of life as it was planned (Jumisko et al. 2007; see Chap. 3, Sect. 3.3.2 for more discussion about chronic sorrow). There is also *ambiguous loss*, when a loved one is fundamentally different, but has not died; the loss is chronic, amorphous, and unfinished (Boss 2006; Guerriere and McKeever 1997; Kean 2010). A state of limbo also adds to the experience of grief and loss (Smith and Godfrey 1995; Testani-Dufour et al. 1992).

This "ambiguous loss" also affects the family system, based on how the loved one's obstacles affect everyone's position in the family (Boss 2006). The patient becomes the principal focus of the family system's attention and resources. Siblings must cope with a "different" family and often feel sad, displaced, forgotten, or even guilty about their own accomplishments (Roos 2002b; see Chap. 3, Sect. 3.5). Postinjury sorrow in the caregiver is often most intense at the time of the event, and although it typically diminishes, it can continue for months or years postinjury (Lee et al. 2001). "Chronic sorrow" or "episodic loss reactions" are triggered intermittently whenever real-world reminders underline the negative disparity between the loved one's preinjury potential and postinjury losses (Teel 1991). To this end, some family members report that they do not want to view pictures or video tapes of the early injury aftermath, as they are too upsetting. Others feel this is a good "report card" of how far their loved one has progressed. Similarly, some attendees state they do not look at preinjury pictures or videos, as they create too much heartache. These varying preferences reflect the difference between the family members' "reference points" of the day before the injury compared with the day after. As part of the group exchange, the group facilitator can comment upon the validity of different coping strategies with a reminder that no "one size fits all."

Because the grief and loss process for the primary caregiver and family has many layers of bleakness, the group facilitators must use keen listening skills to unearth the breadth and depth of the anguish between different attendees. Gently probing the participants' feelings about new theories (e.g., "chronic sorrow" and "ambiguous loss") can spark meaningful group discussion. Families often compare and contrast their specific circumstances and sources of grief, at the same time noticing their commonalities. Acknowledging the duality of grief related to concrete causes (e.g., patients' loss of function versus the family's own addition of new, sometimes unwanted responsibilities) is important (Aniskiewicz 2007; Johnson and McCown 1997). Other hardships include loss of freedoms, pleasures, intimacy, and a sense of security (Braine 2011; Johnson and McCown 1997; Rich 2005). Some have lamented the loss of the "essence" of their loved one (Kean 2010). In addition, the manifestations and timing of grief reactions in family members are likely different from those of their loved one, especially when he or she is struggling with unawareness of the injury-effects (Roundhill et al. 2007).

A powerful realization in the group is that agitation or mad reactions are common by-products of "chronic sorrow" after a brain injury. Sometimes, the group members' fury represents blaming behavior and is an attempt to counteract feelings of helplessness, guilt, or personal regrets. A therapeutic review of contributory factors helps dissipate the anger, including the role of a more severe injury; unconstrained behavioral problems (e.g., social disinhibition, poor insight, mood swings); and older aged loved ones who show regressed behavior, especially towards mothers who are tier 1 caregivers (Zinner et al. 1997).

As part of the group education process, the facilitators can discuss the difference between grief, defined as a process of self-dissolution into a deep emotional well (Klonoff and Myles 2010), versus mourning, or "the metamorphosis of raw affect into a reconstitution process" (Klonoff and Myles 2010, p. 77). Understandably, there is a dynamic oscillation between the loss and restoration orientations (Roundhill et al. 2007); the group dialogue allows the traversal into and between these states. Intrinsic to this process are periods of disavowal or denial, which when temporary, are usually adaptive stepping stones to titrate otherwise overwhelming emotions and realities (Klonoff 2010; see Chap. 2, Sect. 2.3.4).

Storytelling is an agent of the therapeutic process (see Rossheim and McAdams 2010 for a review) and is very conducive to the support group format. A useful group exercise is for the therapists to encourage families to explore their personal journeys of grief and mourning. Then, as part of the reconstitution process and collective sharing, families are assisted in appreciating subtle discrepancies between the strengths and challenges in various loved ones (e.g., better physical recovery in one loved one versus better memory functioning in another). This breeds an enhanced perspective and also engenders thinking about the "bright side" of what to be grateful for in individual circumstances.

The psychoeducation process in the group is also a positive venue for relatives to discuss the different ways to cope with grief and loss. To this end, the FEM is an enlightening tool, specific to styles of coping, ranging from adaptive ("green coping" zone) to the warning ("yellow warning" zone) to the Period of Disintegration ("red crisis" zone; Klonoff 2010; Klonoff et al. 2008). The "green coping" and "yellow warning" zones can be considered representative of a healthier grieving process, whereby the family mourns losses but also incrementally adjusts expectations and learns to accept the patient for who he or she is. When relatives have descended into a deep well of rage and even self-defeating behavior, in the "red crisis" zone, they may be struggling with the deleterious consequences of maladaptive grief. They may be "stuck in grief" and are unable to use productive coping skills over the course of many months or even years. There is a predominance of retrospective rumination and an inability or unwillingness to accept and adapt to their new circumstances. Caregivers are consumed with nihilistic and "doom-and-gloom" thoughts about the future. Stuck grief may also be an indicator of family burnout (see Sect. 9.9), preexisting depression and anxiety, and lack of outside supports (see Boerner and Schulz 2009, for a review). Once relatives are familiar with the nomenclature, a thought-provoking exercise is to ask attendees to identify which FEM placement phase and coping zone they see themselves in.

Group facilitators must be mindful of when it becomes evident during the group exchange that the caregiver is mired in grief. Telltale signs are when he or she is constantly dominating the group exchange, with an enduring depressive and hopeless perspective. Neither the group facilitators nor other family members can help the "stuck" caregiver shift his or her outlook, despite their best efforts. In these cases, individual psychotherapy is strongly suggested as a supplement to the Family Group. Often, it is a combination of the facilitators' observations and peer input that helps the individual realize they are suffering greatly. Private sessions then afford the necessary individualized attention to underlying issues. As an example, cognitive behavioral therapy can address cognitive distortions privately, so that the caregiver can progress to believing that a rich life is possible, despite the loved one's illness (Rossheim and McAdams 2010). In addition, psychiatric consultation may be warranted, with consideration of psychotropic medication, especially if the family member cannot face his or her daily assignments and/or is experiencing an incapacitating mood disorder. Sometimes, adjunct family therapy for the immediate family is required to help with "chronic sorrow" in siblings and other members. This validates their grievous state, yet gives "permission" to pursue their own needs and aspirations.

Through the group's mentorship, relatedness, and healthy venting, in the context of empathic responsiveness in the therapists, families come to realize that "chronic sorrow" is a process (rather than stages), with difficulty attaining closure (Collings 2008; Kean 2010). The relational and psychoeducational processes help attendees realize that grief is fluid and dynamic, ameliorating over time, without necessarily reaching an endpoint (Collings 2008; Doka and Martin 2010). The group members will learn that their gradual adaptation to "chronic sorrow" requires adjustment of existing schemas; reformulating who they are and what was lost; attachment of a meaningful framework to loss; and learning to function with the loss (Collings 2008; Doka and Martin 2010).

Despite the understandable sorrow and grief, with time, the tier 1 caregiver and tier supports travel through and between the FEM phases 5 and 6 where they grapple with acceptance and realism in a revolving manner, visiting different coping styles (Klonoff and Koberstein 2010; Klonoff et al. 2008). Sometimes, they describe coping well, while other times they dip into the "yellow warning" zone, characterized by disgruntlement, anxiety, and self-doubts. Psychoeducation and supportive interventions help to gradually improve the relatives' innate capacity to cope with "bad news." The psychotherapists foster the participants' sharing of improvements, portraying these as "big little things." This is heartening to the relatives that small and gradual improvements are key building blocks and "mile markers." Even though the situation cannot be "fixed," through resilience, mastery, and a gradual adjustment process, some participants become more comfortable with ambivalence and emerge more flexible, open, hopeful, and optimistic (Boss 2006; Klonoff and Koberstein 2010). They adapt to the realization that things are, and will be different. They grasp the value of prioritizing the "cans" versus "wants" of life.

Some group contributors have described the progression towards "picking up the pieces," "turning the corner," adopting a "glass half full attitude," "finding bright spots," and "deciding to be happy." Some have even progressed to a position of "counting their blessings" (Klonoff et al. 2008) based on redefining their potential, recreating fulfillment, searching for goodness in themselves and others, as well as cherishing togetherness with their loved one and overall family. Active coping through involvement in diversionary personal interests and hobbies also counteracts some of the sorrow (Lee et al. 2001). Overall, despite the *lingering sadness*, the caregiver and family learn to reframe their experiences and find new meanings (Patrick-Ott and Ladd 2010). More of this will be described in Sect. 9.10.1, which addresses futuristic thinking and Chap. 11.

9.6 Overprotectiveness and Letting Go

Family members are often preoccupied with their loved one's health and safety because of the dramatic deficits caused by the brain injury. This is compounded because they lived through every terrifying moment, including at "death's doorstep" while the loved one was oblivious, due to the neurological compromise (e.g., coma, disorientation, amnesia; Elbaum 2010). Through clinical observation and their self-report, mothers seem especially prone to hypervigilance, hypersensitivity, and consequently hovering, controlling, and/or mollycoddling their sons and daughters after brain injuries (see Chap. 3, Sect. 3.3 for more discussion on this topic). Table 9.11 summarizes some common verbalizations from families indicative of overprotectiveness and difficulty "letting go" of their loved one after the brain injury. Emerging themes include a keen awareness of the fragility of life and trepidation about another catastrophe, characterized by "waiting for the other shoe to drop." Also, the primary caregiver may lean towards micromanaging and scrutinizing his or her loved one to combat plaguing feelings of guilt and powerlessness, emanating from his or her incapacity to prevent the first accident. One relative characterized the pervasive dread as the "family fear factor."

Other reasons for overprotectiveness stem from the loved one's propensity to make poor judgments and act impulsively, secondary to sizeable memory and executive function deficits (see Chap. 4, Sects. 4.3 and 4.4). Also, when the loved one is oblivious to his or her weaknesses due to organic unawareness, the caregiver may try to overcompensate for poor planning and decision making (see Chap. 4, Sect. 4.5). Common concerns are that the loved one will: make poor financial decisions; forget to take medications; make unsafe decisions in the home environment; and have

Table 9.11 Common verbalizations about overprotectiveness and letting go

Overprotectiveness
You (the loved one) weren't "there," so you don't realize how terrifying this was
What else will go wrong?
Things aren't safe
I'm afraid of another tragedy
It's like raising him/her all over again
I'm holding my breath
It's the calm before the storm
I feel like a drill sergeant
Will he/she have another car accident?
I'm a nag
I used to be "hip mom;" now I'm "crotchety mom"
He/she is on a "choke chain"
He/she is not competent to make these choices
I'm a policeman/woman
Letting go
I'm afraid to let go
How and when should I back off?
What happens if I'm not there?
It's so hard to step back
It's just easier and quicker if I do it
I don't want to micromanage, but if I don't...
I want him/her to "succeed' in rehab, so I better jump in and do....
If I back off, he/she will fail in school
What will happen if he/she moves out?
It's so hard to leave him/her and go back to work
What if his/her friends don't understand and something bad happens?
What if he/she drinks alcohol?
He/she is so vulnerable, other people will take advantage if I am not there
How can I learn not to live in fear?

problems driving safely (Kreutzer et al. 2009a). When the caregiver perceives the loved one as gullible or suggestible, there is an intensified need to police his or her social interactions.

Sometimes, practicalities spur the primary caregiver to intervene on behalf of the patient and do more than he or she should for him or her. For example, it is quicker and easier for the caregiver to do chores in the home than the loved one, especially if he or she has prominent memory or physical incapacities (e.g., hemiparesis or ataxia). Alternatively, the family's strong desire for the loved one to recover maximally and "succeed" in his or her rehabilitation also translates into the perceived need to micromanage or meddle with schoolwork or other daily assignments. With an attitude of "more is better," the family becomes the drill sergeant of rehabilitation in the home and community. Some family members have described the need to "fix the problems," as they cannot bear to see their loved one struggle and/or fail. Although the caregiver's behavior is derived from wanting the best for the loved one, it can be perceived as stifling, nitpicking, and therefore disempowering to the patient. It also reflects great underlying anxiety, which can be very incapacitating to the caregiver.

9.6.1 Group Treatment to Counteract Overprotectiveness and Facilitate Letting Go

Typically, a popular topic is how caregivers can reduce their overprotectiveness and learn to "let go." This is especially relevant to mothers, who can commiserate that their primal instinct to care for their children is reawakened to a point of "overdrive." The group therapists can propel the discussion by asking broad questions such as: *How are you doing with letting your loved one do for himself or herself? How is this similar or different for spouses versus parents? What gets in the way of backing off? How can group input and experiences help you with this paradox?* In conjunction with the emoting process, Table 9.12 lists therapeutic ideas, "helpful hints," psychoeducation, and multimedia resources to spawn discussion about how tier 1 caregivers should gauge how and when to intervene on behalf of the loved one, so as to recede into more of an advisory role. As such, group members will gain a healthier perspective, enabling them to reduce overprotectiveness and gradually transition into a constructive stance of letting go. Given the uniqueness and complexity of issues associated with the loved one's resumption of functional independence and autonomy, the group is encouraged to collaborate closely with the treating therapists, including the neuropsychologist (Klonoff 2010; Moberg and Kniele 2006). Experienced participants can reinforce the value of trusting their professionalism and at times deferring to their expertise, despite understandable reticence. The important resource of medical guidance by physiatrists, neurologists, and psychiatrists is shared to protect the loved one, family, and even the community from behavior that is hazardous to the welfare of the loved one or others.

Depending on the cognitive, language, and/or emotional status of the loved one, family members are shocked or perturbed that he or she may demonstrate the inability to manage his or her affairs. This is a huge source of worry to families. The Family Group is an excellent outlet for constructive venting and the group facilitators should engage the participants in a discussion of their observations and fears. The group venue is also a good way to disperse an informative overview of methods to protect the loved one's interests. Guest speakers may be helpful in this regard, including a social worker or a lawyer. One option is guardianship, whereby the court identifies an individual or agency to be a substitute decision maker and supervisor for day-to-day decisions, including living arrangements, health care, finances, and other basic needs (Moye 2003). Alternatively, the individual may need a conservator, whereby the court appoints a substitute decision maker and manager only for finances as it pertains to the estate (Moye 2003). This will involve evaluation of the loved one's overall competency or the ability to exert decision-making skills, so as to act on his or her own behalf (Moberg and Kniele 2006). There are a number of steps in this process; relevant resources for families in this regard are *When the Mind Fails: A Guide in Dealing with Incompetency* by Silberfield and Fish (1994); "Assessment of Mental Capacity" by Newby and Ryan-Morgan (2013); and www.ehow.com/how_5122660_declare-someone-mentally-incompetent.html. The protocol includes contacting the probate court where the loved one resides to obtain the correct forms. Typically, some form

Table 9.12 Group treatment for families to reduce overprotectiveness and facilitate letting go

Guided exercises
Ask broad questions about the caregiver's challenges with overprotectiveness and letting go
Compare and contrast tier support reactions based on their roles (e.g., parent versus spouse)
Obtain the participants' observations and fears related to the loved one managing his or her affairs
Explore the attendees' experiences and concerns about the spectrum of decision making deficits in their loved ones
"Helpful hints" and psychoeducation
Trust the therapists and professionals when discussing appropriate goals and limits
Learn ways and access outside resources to protect the loved one's financial interests and monitor day-to-day decision making: mental competency determines autonomy
Use safety as the gauge for the loved one's independence
Help the loved one become self-directed with incremental resumption of duties along a simple to difficult continuum
Support and reinforce the use of compensations and home programs
Address how to overcome fears through individual and group therapy
Adjust expectations realistically
Conceptualize independence as a wavering transition
Focus on improving awareness, acceptance, and realism
"Cue, not do"
Do not bombard the loved one
Strive for healthy vigilance versus over control
"Raise the bar" to encourage self-sufficiency
Work with the psychotherapist to orchestrate "planned failures" that constitute life lessons
Apply concepts of "hindsight is 40/40" and the "dignity of risk"
Watch for dependency and learned helplessness
Separate "slippage" and "flight into health" from "spreading one's wings"
Remember, it's their life, not yours
Multimedia resources
Guest speakers
Social worker
Attorney
Writings
When the Mind Fails: A Guide to Dealing with Incompetency (Silberfield and Fish 1994)
"Assessment of Mental Capacity" (Newby and Ryan-Morgan 2013)
Website
www.ehow.com/how_5122660_declare-someone-mentally-incompetent.html
Poem
"The Friend Who Just Stands By" (Williams 2004)

of psychological interview, also including collateral informants, is obtained. A neuropsychological and functional ability evaluation should be performed by a qualified professional (Moberg and Kniele 2006). The paperwork is then submitted to the court. Sometimes, it is helpful to solicit the input of a mental health or guardianship attorney to assist with this process (Moye 2003). Of note, given the intricacy of these issues, families should be cautioned that the loved one's and caregiver's specific needs should be followed up in private sessions (see Chap. 10, Sect. 10.1.2).

Even if the loved one is deemed mentally competent to make independent decisions, family members bemoan that there are a number of nuances related to a "gray area" of decision-making deficits. This is complicated by such wide variation in the rate and course of recovery after brain injury, as the loved one's overall condition can seem like a "moving target" that the family wrestles to keep up with. They need time and space in the group to compare and contrast their experiences. The group facilitators can emphasize that safe judgments and behavior should be considered the hallmark when ascertaining if and how to provide more space for the loved one. Direct observations by the tier 1 caregiver, tier supports, and treating therapists of the loved one being self-directed in the clinic, home, and community environments are invaluable indicators of readiness for increased independence. Successful resumption of duties should be incremental, with accomplishment of easier tasks (e.g., self-care), preceding more complex ones (e.g., bill paying, financial management, driving).

Seasoned group members often espouse the empowering value of compensations in their loved one's mission for independence (Ben-Yishay and Diller 2011; Klonoff 2010). The group didactics and dialogue can review integral memory and executive function tools (see Chap. 4, Sects. 4.3.2 and 4.4.4; Chap. 6, Sect. 6.4.2), so as to support and reinforce their utilization. Similarly, the caregivers are educated that prescribed home programs will further the physical and visuoperceptual recovery and enhance the loved one's functionality (see Chap. 6, Sect. 6.5.2). Of note, the families' shared observations of any disappointments and failures help fine-tune the rehabilitation endeavors.

Even in the face of good evidence of the loved one's capabilities, due to the family's predisposed entrenched anxiety and fear, typically they will require the Family Group and individual sessions to help them adjust their expectations realistically and "let go of the reigns." As depicted in phases 5 and 6 of the PEM and FEM (see Fig. 9.2 and Chap. 1, Fig. 1.2), this will entail the loved one and family members traversing the twisty path of awareness, acceptance, and realism, with an emphasis on a shared understanding of strengths and difficulties, utilization of compensations, and demonstration of good judgments and choices for community reintegration (Klonoff 2010; Klonoff et al. 2008). Many families have shared within the group the sensation of having to raise their loved one again through the developmental and maturational phases. They have to fight the urge to constrict the loved one's freedoms, even when the patient pressures them with "hurry up and let me. . . ." Some relatives have lamented needing many months or a couple of years to acclimate into separating from the loved one. They need to "relax into the process." If they feel pressured to "steamroll the process," their angst will only escalate.

Certain caveats aid the caregiver and other tier 1 and 2 supporters in reducing overprotectiveness, including recognizing the benefits of the loved one returning to the societal mainstream. The group facilitators can reinforce that it is not realistic or fair to the family or loved one to protect him or her 24/7; control must be relinquished to facilitate healing in all parties. To this end, the caregiver should take a position of cueing and guiding versus bombarding and doing the tasks for the loved one (Klonoff 2010). Healthy vigilance will necessitate legitimate concern or "not turning a blind eye" (G.A. Lage, personal communication, n.d.), while also encouraging "raising the bar" of challenges for the patient so as to blossom into self-sufficiency (Klonoff 2010). Finding the right balance and letting go is especially difficult for parents.

Some find that it is helpful to imagine that they are a "work supervisor" versus a parent, and calibrate the amount of self-sufficiency and accountability that will be expected on the job. Framing interactions in the home with the loved one in this manner assists all parties in recognizing the benefits of gradations of autonomy.

"Letting go" will lead to inevitable failures. Psychotherapy can guide the family to create "planned failure" opportunities. These are thoughtfully constructed scenarios whereby the loved one "is allowed" to fail as a way to improve awareness and acceptance of his or her limitations (Klonoff 2010). Ideally, "planned failures" should be therapeutic "life lessons" versus demoralizing and unproductive (see also Chap. 4, Sect. 4.5.2). In conjunction with the therapist, relatives may want to conduct a "cost–benefit" analysis of enabling versus prohibiting the loved one from undertaking certain challenges. Also, often the loved one may need therapeutic and family guidance to appreciate how his or her choices have led to derailments, as this may be difficult for him or her to grasp, given memory and/or executive function difficulties. Without this, the loved one is bound to repeat a cycle of failures.

Another therapeutic concept in this regard is "hindsight is 40/40," which reminds the families that second-guessing and overanalysis of past actions is counterproductive (Klonoff 2010). Instead, the support network may need to embrace the idea of "dignity of risk" (M. Pepping, personal communication, n.d.), whereby the family comes to terms with their own trepidations through focus on the loved one's inherent right to self-determination (Klonoff and Koberstein 2010). The poem, "The Friend who Stands By" by Williams (2004), can be a source of group solace during these nerve-racking occasions. When members share their positive experiences in letting go both for themselves and their loved ones, other group members are enticed to do the same.

The group members (in conjunction with treating therapists) should be wary of the two extremes. One is dependency and "learned helplessness" (Maier and Seligman 1976) whereby the loved one (and caregiver unit) becomes comfortable in overindulgence. The other pole is "slippage" and "flight into health," wherein the loved one is overestimating his or her capabilities and abandons crucial tools and compensations (Klonoff 2010). At any rate, although painful to accept, the primary caregiver and other tier supporters must remember the adage that ultimately "it's their life, not yours." This creates healthy separation of roles and obligations, and can be of consolation when the loved one veers in a counter-direction that unnerves the relatives. Ideally, with time, trial and error, and practice, the loved one will embark upon a life characterized by renewed independence, meaning, and fulfillment.

9.7 Family System Disruption, Social Isolation, and Loneliness

Related to the enormity of the caregiver burden and the ensuing emotional upheaval in the family, many times the primary caregiver and the immediate family experience loneliness and social isolation (Boyle and Haines 2002; Braine 2011; Cassidy 2009; Inzaghi et al. 2005; Jumisko et al. 2007; Kreutzer et al. 2010; Patrick-Ott and Ladd 2010; Pepping 1998; Prowe 2010; Rich 2005; Wedcliffe and Ross 2001). This can be the case even many years postinjury (Boyle and Haines 2002). As depicted in phases 1 and 2 of the FEM, this can begin with social seclusion whilst the loved one is in the intensive care unit (ICU) or acute care setting, and persist throughout the hospitalization process (Klonoff et al. 2008). Once the loved one is discharged home (phase 3), the caregiver and the immediate family become even more preoccupied with the all-encompassing needs of the loved one, as the hospital nursing and medical supports have now terminated (Klonoff et al. 2008; Kreutzer et al. 2002). This usually fragments the family system, with skewed and foreign roles and commitments thrust upon the members. Spouses miss their preinjury partner. Siblings are often ignored, due to the predominant needs of the injured loved one. Bickering and adversarialism erupt due to the excessive strains. Sometimes, divorce ensues from the irreparable strains on the marriage (Johnson and McCown 1997; Patrick-Ott and Ladd 2010; Senelick and Dougherty 2001; see Chap. 3 for more discussion).

Because the caregiver and family's new predicament is so removed from their previous life-style, they soon become alienated and detached from their extended family, as well as their prior friends and pastimes. It is as if people who have never experienced the aftereffects of brain injury cannot fathom the intricacies and stressors. Other times, the caregiver chooses to limit disclosures, so as to preserve the privacy of the loved one and the family. Regardless of the reasons, the caregiver puts up walls and retreats into a solitary, often miserable existence.

Behavioral problems in the loved one (e.g., childlike behavior, disinhibition, aggressiveness, impulsivity) can result in social ostracism or social isolation (see Klonoff 2010, for a review). Depending on cultural norms and expectations, stigma and shame about brain injury lead to the family's social withdrawal (Simpson et al. 2000). Table 9.13 depicts some of the family's opinions when they are experiencing social isolation, loneliness, and overall family disruption.

9.7.1 Group Treatment for Family System Disruption, Social Isolation, and Loneliness

Table 9.14 summarizes guided exercises, psychoeducation, "helpful hints," and multimedia resources to reduce the family system disruptions, social isolation, and loneliness. Pivotal to therapeutic support for caregivers is the opportunity to socialize and commiserate with the support network of other patients who truly identify with their hurdles (Charles et al. 2007; Dell Orto and Power 2000; Klonoff and Koberstein 2010; Wedcliffe and Ross 2001). Face-to-face contact with their comrades in the group is perhaps the ideal way to share inner longings, and the group facilitators can softly tread into this arena through inquiry. Sometimes, relatives prefer other outlets or want to supplement their group experience. Butera-Prinzia et al. (2010) describe a "Link-Up Program," which facilitated peer connections and mentoring between families with a loved one with a brain injury in person, by phone, teleconferencing, or Skype. Benefits included sharing and validation of their common experiences; empowerment; resourcing; giving to others; increased compassion and understanding; and building a sense of community (Butera-Prinzia et al. 2010).

Table 9.13 Common verbalizations about family system disruption, social isolation, and loneliness

Family system disruption
I'm tied down 24/7
There is so much tension and fighting at home
Will my family be the same?
The door is closed on my past life
Social isolation
I can't bear to see anyone right now
It's too hard to explain everything that is going on
I don't want to reveal the details of everything. . . .this is private to our family
I feel like I am living in a bubble
I know I am putting up walls
Friends and family have stopped calling
I can't relate to people who don't have an injured loved one
It's "easy for you to say"
Outsiders have "no clue"
The injury is invisible to everyone but me
I'm so vigilant and embarrassed in social situations because of my loved one's behavior
It's a jungle out there
I feel alienated from my prior social network
Loneliness
I can't lean on _____ like I used to
Misery does not like company
Friends and family "don't get it"
It drives me crazy when they say "he'll/she'll be fine"
They don't get it
Outsiders listen, but they can't relate
I feel abandoned
I'm longing for how it was
I feel so alone

The primary caregiver and overall family will likely need specialized counseling (outside of the Family Group; see Chap. 3, Fig. 3.1) to help them adapt to the unavoidable reverberations of the brain injury within the family system. However, Family Group is an excellent chance for the primary caregivers to explore and compare their individual and collective family needs with others facing the same troubles. The group is also a worthwhile domain in which to receive constructive feedback from the facilitators and other caregivers to be sure that the delicate balance between the loved one, primary caregiver, and other relatives is "on the radar." Therefore, the primary caregiver should make a concerted effort to nurture balanced relationships with other members of the immediate and extended family, including emphasis on others' needs and preferences. This will take preplanning and forethought, to be sure that adequate time and attention are provided for enriching activities. Family "milieu meetings" (see Chap. 4, Sect. 4.4.4) are an excellent way to plan for these activities and solicit the commitment of potential participants. Special attention will need to be paid to younger children/siblings, in order to integrate them into comfortable interactions and activities, especially when they are perplexed or upset about the injury aftereffects (see Chap. 3, Sect. 3.5).

Table 9.14 Group treatment to cope with family disruption, social isolation, and loneliness

Guided exercises
Ask about the family's social support network and explore if they are feeling isolated and lonely
Encourage group attendees to announce weekly any upcoming social and educational events
Have families commit and be accountable about undertaking community pursuits
"Helpful hints" and psychoeducation
Socialize and commiserate with like-minded caregivers using therapeutic mediums
If necessary, pursue specialized family counseling
Explore and compare individual and collective family needs to find a fluid balance
Focus on nurturing all family relationships
Use "milieu meetings" to plan family social events
Pay attention to the unique social needs of youngsters
Engage in family social activities inside and outside of the home
Solicit the professional guidance of a recreational therapist
Supplement the group process with other resources (e.g., Internet, books)
Participate in paid or volunteer work, hobbies, and other appealing community pursuits
Find new friendships and leisure interests
Cultivate liaisons with "true blue" old friends
Be forgiving of outsiders' platitudes
Be genuine in your disclosures
Multimedia resources
Journal article
"Family-to-Family Link Up Program: A community-based initiative supporting families caring for someone with an acquired brain injury" (Butera-Prinzia et al. 2010)
Internet options
Facebook
Online support groups
Meetup.com
Books: Family-authored books about brain injury
Someone Stole Yesterday (Wright 2000)
Smile and Jump High (Lloyd and Kehoe 2001)
Where is the Mango Princess (Crimmins 2001)
Being with Rachel: A Story of Memory and Survival (Brennan 2002)
Coping with Brain Injury: How to Help after Accidents, Stroke and Illness (Rich 2005)
Brain Injury Survivor's Guide: Welcome to Our World (Jameson and Jameson 2007)
In an Instant: A Family's Journey of Love and Healing (Woodruff and Woodruff 2007)
Climbing the Mountain: Stories of Hope and Healing after Stroke and Brain Injury (Fancher et al. 2008)
Successfully Surviving a Brain Injury: A Family Guidebook (Prowe 2010)
Gabby: A Story of Courage and Hope (Giffords et al. 2011)
One Hundred Names for Love: A Stroke, a Marriage, and the Language of Healing (Ackerman 2011)
The Vow: The True Events that Inspired the Movie (Carpenter et al. 2012)
Book: Children's story
The Eagle and the Wren (Goodall 2000)

Group therapists can facilitate the dissemination of information about community activities by taking time at the outset of the group to solicit "community news" from the attendees. In our group, typically, one or more caregivers take the initiative to announce upcoming social and educational events, and will even bring in advertisements to be posted in the clinic lobby. Other therapeutic suggestions to reconstruct a cohesive family unit are coordinating family activities with the loved one present, including attending community events (sports games, movies, restaurants, etc.). The family may also enjoy attending and participating in conjoint social groups for patients and families, participating in Parks and Recreation programs, or coordinating games at home (e.g., a Wii^{TM} system). Sometimes, mingling with like-minded tier 1 caregivers and loved ones in a community social group without therapists' involvement can be very rewarding and enjoyable (Klonoff and Koberstein 2010). When possible, liaison with recreational therapists is strongly advised, as their wealth of knowledge about hobbies, games, and community leisure activities can be extremely valuable in infusing pleasure and togetherness into the family unit (Klonoff 2010).

Group members express that when they are housebound, their social isolation and loneliness are amplified. In cases where they cannot attend Family Group, supplemental Internet options may be indispensable, including Facebook or other online support groups. Reading books from the perspective of other families with a brain injury survivor (e.g., Brennan 2002; Jameson and Jameson 2007; Woodruff and Woodruff 2007) also eases the feeling of aloneness. (For a more complete list, see Table 9.14).

Once the loved one is sufficiently capable and ensconced in his or her own activities, group facilitators and peers can gently "pressure" attendees to undertake their own community pursuits, including paid or volunteer work, hobbies, and/or any other appealing community interests. This is an excellent exercise to propel the relatives to "take action," as they know they will be held accountable in upcoming meetings. Given the often profound changes in the lifestyle of the caregiver, he or she may need to develop new friendships or leisure interests of his or her own. Websites such as Meetup.com are fun resources to provide new ideas. Family members should be optimistic that there are compassionate "good Samaritans" in the community who will take a sincere interest in their woes. In these cases, it is important to be genuine about the strains the family is facing. Phrases such as "things are fine" should be replaced with more real sentiments, such as "it's a long haul," or "it's a challenge." So as not to breed resentment, caregivers should be reassured that some of the old platitudes by outsiders that "everything will be okay" reflect the cultural norm or naïveté, rather than intentional insensitivity. Other participants have expressed appreciation for the loyalty of "true blue" old friends who, based on their historical perspective, are empathic towards the adversity the family is coping with (Pepping 1998). The children's book, *The Eagle and the Wren* (Goodall 2000) is a poignant rendition of the power of togetherness.

9.8 Uncertainty about the Future and What Ifs

A recurring topic during Family Group is the sense of unknown about the loved one's and ergo, the caregiver's and overall family's future prospects. They have many uncertainties and "what ifs" (Braine 2011; Dell Orto and Power 2000; Jumisko et al. 2007; Keenan and Joseph 2010; Klonoff et al. 2008; Price et al. 1998; Prowe 2010).

Table 9.15 Common verbalizations related to uncertainties about the future and "what ifs"

Will he/she have any medical complications?
What if he/she dies?
How long will this process take?
How close to where he/she was preinjury will my loved one come?
Is it true he/she won't improve after the 6 month window?
Why didn't we find therapy sooner?
Is it too late for my loved one to get the help from therapy?
What happens if he/she refuses to cooperate?
Will my loved one work/go back to school?
Will he/she support me and the family?
What if I die or become incapacitated?

Table 9.15 summarizes some examples of attendees' verbalized worries and uncertainties. The family is frightened about medical complications. Recurrent themes are the risk of seizures (De Reuck 2011; Ferguson et al. 2010) or additional brain injuries caused by poor judgment, impulsivity, and risky behavior (including substance abuse; Corrigan et al. 1995). In the back of their minds, they agonize about "what if" the loved one dies.

Other sources of unease surround the unpredictable and uncontrollable unfolding of the recovery process, including its unknown rate and outcome. The caregiver also frets about the ill-effects of an extended delay in the loved one receiving intensive therapy in the context of a supposed finite window of time for healing. Added to this is ire with the loved one's perpetual noncompliance with therapeutic recommendations, with a legitimate concern that this may negatively impact the eventual degree of recovery.

Longer-range apprehensions revolve around the loved one's ultimate level of productivity in the community, as it pertains to succeeding in school and at work. Spouses stew over whether or not their significant other can return to the same level of work and income. Compounded angst surfaces about "what if" the caregiver dies or becomes incapacitated, and cannot continue with the burden of responsibility for the loved one and the rest of the family.

9.8.1 Group Treatment for Family Members to Cope with Uncertainty and "What Ifs"

Table 9.16 summarizes guided exercises, psychoeducation, "helpful hints," and multimedia resources for families to cope with injury-based uncertainties and "what ifs." A beneficial inroad to this topic is to ask the participants to review their personalized "what if?" worry list. Common subjects to launch a discussion are angst about the loved ones' futures and who else can provide for their needs. The first step for the group facilitators is to respond empathically to the family's perspective and put themselves in their shoes (Hojat 2007). Group turmoil and fearfulness interlinked with the unknowns can be diminished by affirming statements such as "this is a long, hard road," or "recovery is a work in progress." Reminding the three tiers of support to take a "wait-and-see" attitude can offset preoccupations with the long-term outcome

Table 9.16 Group treatment for coping with uncertainty and "what ifs?"

Guided exercises
What is your personalized "what if" worry list?
What are your techniques to guide your loved ones, yet maintain your own mental health?
What is your "plan A" versus "plan B" etc. for your loved one?
What is your own "plan A" versus "plan B" etc.?
What concrete steps have you taken for the future to reduce your anxieties?
"Helpful hints" and psychoeducation
Utilize the group process for empathy and affirmation about the families' angst
Rely on mantras such as "this is a long, hard road," "recovery is a work in progress," and "wait and see"
Gain relevant knowledge about medical complications
Avoid second-guessing and self-blame about prior decisions for your loved one, including about treatment opportunities
Learn every tool in the "tool kit" to encourage the loved one to stay in treatment
Remember that the ultimate decision to embrace therapy is made by your loved one
Review research evidence to bolster the advantages of compensations
Focus on short-term goals, practicality, and realism
Identify "plan A" versus "plan B," etc. for all parties
Recognize that coping with uncertainty becomes easier over time
Engage in sensible problem solving; be proactive about longer range planning to protect you and your loved one's health needs
Let the process unfold and deal with challenges and setbacks as they transpire
Multimedia resources
Model
Family Experiential Model (FEM) of Recovery (Klonoff and Koberstein 2010; Klonoff et al. 2008)
Handouts
Seizure pamphlet (Channing Bete Co. 2008)
Article abstracts about recovery and outcome (e.g., Klonoff et al. 2007, 2010)
Guest speakers
Social worker
Financial planner
Group home owner

of specific deficiencies (see Chap. 4, Sect. 4.5.2). Similarly, as depicted in the FEM (see Fig. 1.3), framing the recovery process as fluid and evolving has a calming effect.

Addressing relatives' specific "what if" worries about medical complications helps abate them. To this end, they should be given handouts and psychoeducation about seizure risk and interventions after brain injury (Channing Bete Co. 2008; see Chap. 8) and factors which increase the likelihood of additional brain injuries (see Chap. 5, Sect. 5.1.3.1). This builds confidence and lessens their feelings of helplessness.

With respect to self-reproach over delays in finding optimal therapeutic interventions for the loved one, this author finds it heartening to reassure the families that they eventually come to the right treatment setting "when they are meant to." Family members with this historical perspective of the meandering course of recovery will often chime in and agree with this assertion. This sustaining thought counteracts their tendency towards second-guessing and self-recrimination. When the loved one is noncompliant, the family member should be given every "tool in the tool kit" to encourage him or her to maximize investment in the treatment process. The group facilitators pose relevant queries to encourage group input from other caregivers regarding their chosen techniques to guide their loved ones, yet maintain their own mental health. Often, the conclusion is that the ultimate responsibility for cooperation and follow through rests with the loved one. This disentangles the family from an undue burden of responsibility and a "no win" dilemma (see Chap. 2, Sect. 2.4.1.3).

Other "helpful hints" include the emphasis on the "process of recovery," including developing and using compensations to increase functionality. Sometimes, research findings are encouraging to the support network, so as to corroborate these notions with scientific evidence. For instance, a relationship has been established between advanced use of compensations and better outcome with respect to driving and work/school at the time of discharge from neurorehabilitation (Klonoff et al. 2007, 2010). This is reassuring and invigorating to family members, who can then exert their efforts proactively and productively.

Group discussion reveals that juxtaposed with the waves of unpredictability and helplessness are temporary reprieves through pursuing short-term objectives and "keeping their eyes on the prize." Along these lines, the caregiver and family can focus on pragmatism and realism, by conceptualizing possible alternative goals as "plan A" versus "plan B," etc., not only for their loved one but also just as importantly for themselves. This will promote a hopeful, yet flexible approach (Klonoff 2010).

Through the sharing and healing processes, the group attendees gradually adapt to new uncertainties and "what ifs," resulting in "learning to live with it." A guided exercise to compare and contrast practical solutions and longer range plans for known variables reduces anxieties. Options include guest speakers (e.g., a social worker, financial planner, or group home owner) to present information on: a revised financial plan if income decreases long term; a living will for the loved one and caregivers; and contingency plans if anyone's health status worsens, including local group homes (see Chap. 11, Sect. 11.5). As one family member exclaimed, "We are where we are and that's the way it is"; another chimed in with "I'm clipping a few branches, but maintaining altitude." Yet another repeated the mantra "this too shall pass," when she became derailed by new frights and "what ifs." These expressions reflect a willingness to let the process unfold and deal with their challenges and setbacks as they transpire. Oftentimes, this is the best advice and support that can be offered at the time.

9.9 Burnout

Burnout in the primary caregiver, and by extension often for the entire family, is a grave hazard after brain injury; this has been replicated in other cultures (Simpson et al. 2000). Chapter 2, Sect. 2.3.7 provides an overview of the research literature about subjective caregiver burden or burnout. Signs include emotional exhaustion, sleep disturbance, weight loss, feeling worn down, anxiety, and depression (Simpson et al. 2000). Often, primary caregivers sleep with "one eye open" linked to worries about their loved one's health. Others report disrupted sleep and insufficient rest secondary to their excessive workload, or the bonus of personal time once everyone else goes to bed.

Table 9.17 Common lamentations related to caregiver burnout

Burden of multiple responsibilities

I can't sleep—I'm so worried about _____ and everything else on my "to do" list
I feel like I am governing two lives
I feel like a babysitter
I'm tired of being a chauffeur
I'm in a pressure cooker at home and at work
This 24/7 is too much
I'm exhausted and pulled in too many directions
There isn't enough time in the day
My plate is overflowing
I feel pelted by life's hassles

Patient behavior

I'm tired of hearing ____'s complaining
I hate being the target of his/her wrath
I'm exasperated with _____ never using his/her compensations
I'm exhausted pushing _____ to get things done
I'm fed up policing ______
I'm tired of it being "all about ______"

General exhaustion and depletion of resources

I feel like a shrew
It's a grind
I feel like I'm damned if I do and damned if I don't
This process is grueling
No matter what I do, it won't be enough
Everyone and everything is stressing me out
I hate how I am handling all of this
The best-laid plans, but I can't do it anymore
I need a break from all of this
I'm at my wit's end
What about me and my needs?
I'm in the "red" zone

Table 9.17 summarizes examples of primary caregivers' lamentations when they have fallen victim to burnout. A number of premises emerge from these expressions. First, is the unrelenting and overpowering burden of responsibilities for the loved one (Machamer et al. 2002; Siegert et al. 2010; Simpson et al. 2000), many of which seem either physically taxing or unpleasant. Several examples are illuminated in Sect. 9.3, which describes common practical worries and demands on the primary caregiver. Other factors include the loved one's dependency (Machamer et al. 2002; Marsh et al. 1998), with the caregiver having to assist with the loved one's personal self-care long term, and/or having to monitor safety concerns in the home and community, secondary to the loved one's compromised memory, judgment, impulse control, and decision making. This has been referred to as the "reversed empty nest syndrome," with parents having to oversee their loved ones in the home indefinitely (Collings 2008).

Burnout is magnified when there is impingement of other outside stressors on an already precarious family system. Examples include health issues (e.g., ailing elderly parents), psychiatric illness in other family members, and unsupportive or dysfunctional work environments. The movie, *What's Eating Gilbert Grape* (Blomquist et al.

1993) depicts the emptiness and uncontrollable frustrations that can beset even the most devoted tier 1 caregiver with unrelenting demands. Like Gilbert, the stresses are compounded in chaotic family systems; in his case, his mother suffers from agoraphobia and paralyzing depression due to the father's sudden abandonment.

Severe behavior problems and personality changes in the loved one can exhaust and overburden even the most motivated and tolerant of families (see Blake 2008, for a review; see Carnevale et al. 2006, for a review; Wells et al. 2005). This is especially the case when the patient is argumentative, "mean," explosive, demanding, or self-centered. Similarly, the loved one's struggles with apathy and initiative nullify the primary caregiver's capacity to attend to his or her own needs (Marsh et al. 1998). Repeated episodes of "killing the messenger," when the family provides what they feel are caring offerings, deplete the support system's energy and patience. When patients refuse to embrace rehabilitation efforts and compensation training, the brunt of daily toils falls on the caregiver's shoulders. He or she then lugs an even greater burden and the pressures escalate.

The overwhelmed or scapegoated primary caregiver can end up scapegoating other members of the support network, who although may be naïve, are typically well meaning. Guilty feelings can exacerbate caregiver burden (Dell Orto and Power 2000; Klonoff and Koberstein 2010; Kreutzer et al. 2002, 2010; Prowe 2010; Rich 2005; Siegert et al. 2010), producing a vicious cycle. The main character, Gilbert, in *What's Eating Gilbert Grape* (Blomquist et al. 1993) is initially torn between catering to the infinite needs of his family, yet pursuing his own emotional needs. This results in self-flagellation when he inadvertently sacrifices his brother's safety. Alternatively, when the caregiver personalizes the loved one's shortcomings as indicative of his or her own ineptitudes, he or she can become despondent (Hanks et al. 2007).

Chronic and pervasive fear about the loved one's impairments often contributes to burnout. Internalized dread can cause depressive symptomatology; externalized worry can manifest as rage reactions. Exhaustion also leads to focusing on the negative and blaming others (Kreutzer et al. 2010). An absence of medical, emotional, and practical support for the caregiver also breeds burnout (Smith and Smith 2000). As depicted in the "red crisis" zone, the burnt-out family becomes consumed with resentment, anguish, despair, or rage (Klonoff and Koberstein 2010; Klonoff et al. 2008). Overall, the caregivers (and family) feel squeezed out of their own meaningful existence, with all efforts and energies usurped by the loved one. They feel hopeless about the loved one's recovery and prognosis, and view life's obstacles as never ending.

9.9.1 Group Treatment for Burnout

Table 9.18 summarizes group exercises, psychoeducation, "helpful hints," and multimedia resources to combat the families' burnout. Thwarting burnout is a requirement for long-term sustenance in the caregiver role. In fact, to counteract burnout, the tier 1 caregiver and tier supports need to be proactive about maintaining emotional and

Table 9.18 Group treatment for burnout

Guided exercises

Are you experiencing burnout and how would you know?
What steps are/can you take to alleviate burnout in you and other family members?

"Helpful hints" and psychoeducation

- Consider self-care a priority and be proactive
- Recognize signs of burnout and be receptive to lifestyle modifications
- Monitor and work on the negative mindset and the guilty complex
- Incorporate stress management techniques
- Take time for yourself
- Delegate to others
- Create a reciprocal sustaining relationship with other tier supports
- Balance work and other demands
- Abstain from stressful and low-priority external demands
- Become attuned to good sleep and eating habits as well as regular exercise
- Stay up to date with your own medical appointments/needs
- Get involved in and schedule pleasurable and productive quality of life activities:
  - Hobbies
  - Friendships and confidantes
  - Games
  - Movies and concerts
  - Outdoor activities
  - Baths
  - Spa days
  - Pets
  - Home projects
  - Humor and fun
  - Vary the daily routine
  - Work (paid or volunteer)
- Relaxation Exercises:
  - Meditation
  - Diaphragmatic breathing
  - Imagery
  - Yoga
- Take respite breaks:
  - Vacations without the loved one
  - Retreats with like-minded caregivers
- Work with the therapists to understand the underlying reasons for your loved one's behavioral problems
- Learn behavioral interventions and conflict resolution strategies
- Remember the role of normal developmental processes
- Focus on the loved one's gains
- Avoid "losing battles" and/or needless power struggles
- Foster the loved one's independence
- Teach the loved one sensitivity and the "two way street"
- Be the "good enough" caregiver

Multimedia resources

Guest speakers

Dietician

Table 9.18 (continued)

Didactics and demonstrations
Stress reduction techniques (e.g., yoga, diaphragmatic breathing)
Members':
Journal entries
Spiritual outlets
Inspirational movies, songs, and books
Proverbs
T.T.T. (Things Take Time) (Hein 2003)
Take it day by day
Never give up
Wait and see
"Patience, trust, and collaboration" (Klonoff 2010)
Time heals

physical resources, rather than reactive, once the exhaustion and overload have become entrenched. The concept of "placing the oxygen mask on yourself first" (Pais 2002) is an apt metaphor for promoting self-care. Conversing about the complexities of burnout is a "must do" in a Family Group setting. An added bonus of the Family Group is the opportunity for attendees to hold each other responsible for avoiding, acknowledging, and addressing burnout (Klonoff and Koberstein 2010).

Of vital importance is the caregiver learning to recognize the indicators of burnout, and being receptive to outside help as well as modifications of his or her routine. Because burnout is often self-perpetuating, family members must be mindful of "being stuck in a rut" with a negative, "nothing-can-help" attitude. Succumbing to a guilty complex of refusing to find enjoyment and relief is very prevalent, but only furthers the trapped and miserable sentiments (Klonoff and Koberstein 2010).

Group facilitators and better-adjusted families are proponents of stress management techniques as instrumental for preventing emotional collapse (Kreutzer et al. 2002, 2010). One of the prime antidotes to burnout is for the caregiver to take much needed time for himself or herself (Cassidy 2009; Klonoff and Koberstein 2010; Kreutzer et al. 2002, 2010; Senelick and Dougherty 2001). This will entail delegating chores to others (Klonoff and Prigatano 1987; Kreutzer et al. 2002). This may be other family members; trusted friends; or hired caregiver(s) (Klonoff and Koberstein 2010). In fact, other tier 1, as well as tier 2 and 3 supports can create a reciprocal relationship of sustaining each other in the quest for peace of mind and emotional and physical well-being (for more discussion, see Chap. 1, Sect. 1.3).

Self-care will also mean being vigilant about balancing other demands (e.g., work), so that any free time is not consumed by other equally stressful commitments. Life priorities need to be determined and the caregiver needs to learn the art of politely abstaining from lower priority and/or stressful outside requests (Klonoff and Koberstein 2010; Kreutzer et al. 2002). Part of self-care requires healthy life habits, including diet, sleep, and exercise (Kreutzer et al. 2002; Prowe 2010; Senelick and Dougherty 2001). Inviting a dietician as a guest speaker is helpful in this regard. Often, the family will postpone regular medical appointments, placing a bigger priority on others' needs. This can backfire with the primary caregiver's compromised health negatively impacting his or her overall energy and effectiveness.

Group participants can share examples of pleasurable activities and quality of life which "broaden horizons" and replenish much-needed emotional and physical resources. Options include hobbies, sharing in friendships (and when possible with confidantes), games, movies, concerts, outdoor activities, baths, spa days, pets, and home projects (Cassidy 2009; Klonoff and Koberstein 2010; Prowe 2010). Seeking entertainment and humor also promotes brighter outlooks (Braine 2011; Prowe 2010). Varying the daily schedule also adds novelty. Some have found that meaningful work in some capacity, even on a part-time or volunteer basis, is a worthy diversion and a normalizing enterprise (Klonoff and Koberstein 2010). Moving outside of one's confined realm may also help to create a renewed personal perspective in the context of others' woes.

Other calming and soothing pastimes include relaxation exercises, meditation, diaphragmatic breathing, imagery, and yoga (Klonoff and Koberstein 2010; Kreutzer et al. 2002; Prowe 2010). These are very handy when the caregiver has had a particularly unpleasant day. Although the primary caregiver is often reticent, restful vacations without the loved one are an ideal way to decompress and obtain a bolus of reinvigoration. Leaving behind the routine prevents the caregiver from supplanting one type of drudgery with another. Some family members have found weekend getaways with other caregivers to be a positive source of camaraderie and respite.

Group facilitators can encourage the attendees to share multimedia representations of their journeys. These include journal entries, spiritual outlets, inspirational movies, songs, and books which offset the wear and tear stemming from constant obligations and worries. Proverbs, such as "T.T.T." (Things Take Time; Hein 2003); "take it day by day;" "never give up;" "wait and see;" "patience, trust, and collaboration" (Klonoff 2010); and "time heals," offset tough stages and inspire the caregiver to forge onward.

When families are baffled or disturbed by the loved one's behavioral problems, clarification from the treating therapists about the underlying causes of troublesome behavior is necessary. Caregiver burden can breed oversensitivity; it is as if the loved one's conduct is purposefully or even intentionally targeted towards the caregiver just to aggravate him or her. As an example, caregivers bemoan the "mean" retorts from their loved ones. Family education about the role of organic factors in behavior is warranted. This clarifies how, why, and when the loved one's behavior is outside of his or her conscious control. The group facilitators can explain other salient contributions, including unhealthy family dynamics, CRs, and grief and loss reactions. These insights reframe the aberrant behavior and assuage the hurt (see also Chap. 6, Sect. 6.4.2). The support network also benefits from guidance about conflict resolution. Figure 9.3 summarizes basic considerations when managing complex and disruptive behaviors (Myles 2008). For more severe behavioral problems, educational groups, in conjunction with individualized behavior plan training by trained professionals, are advisable (Carnevale et al. 2006). Part of this involves therapeutic guidance about the role of the brain injury in contrast with normal developmental rebellion.

Facilitators and group members discuss the value of a patient, optimistic, and hopeful mindset as indispensable to the families' well-being. Emphasis on the loved one's gains provides peace of mind. Avoiding "losing battles" and/or needless power

Basic Principles for Managing Behavior Conflicts after Brain Injury

Behavior conflicts can be defined as disagreements, arguments, or conflicts with your loved one about how he or she is behaving. Examples include resistance to input and "acting out."

Several factors contribute to behavior problems after brain injury, including cognitive impairments, emotional difficulties, personality changes, and amplification of preinjury characteristics.

The following summarize ways to avoid and manage behavior conflicts:

Avoiding Behavior Conflicts

1. Make sure there is "money in the bank" or credit that the caregiver can draw on later. This translates to a positive trusting relationship with the loved one. "Deposits" can be made by doing enjoyable activities together so as to strengthen the relationship. This reduces the likelihood of behavioral conflicts.

2. Reduce vulnerability to behavior conflicts by everyone meeting their basic needs, including addressing physical illness, pain, fatigue, hunger, and safety. Ensuring that the loved one is taking his or her medications and not misusing psychoactive substances is also important.

3. Agree on expectations and set limits in advance. Uncertainty is stressful and increases the likelihood of behavior conflicts. The caregiver should agree in advance and document with the loved one as to what are considered appropriate/inappropriate behaviors.

Managing Behavior Conflicts

1. *"Water the roses, not the weeds."* Although problems tend to dominate our attention, it is more important to praise what the loved is doing correctly. Consider giving ten times more attention to appropriate behaviors than to inappropriate ones (as long as the loved one is not putting himself or herself in harm's way).

2. *"Don't sweat the small stuff."* Many minor behavior problems can be managed effectively though ignoring (e.g., giving minimum attention) and redirection toward appropriate, on-task behavior. Do not succumb to battles over minor issues; focus on the "big picture." Little arguments can quickly escalate into big disagreements.

3. *Be timely and specific with praise.* Any small sign of progress should be recognized and commended.

Fig. 9.3 Basic concepts for managing behavior conflicts after brain injury

4. *Set the ball rolling* by first having the loved one do easy tasks, before introducing more challenging or daunting undertakings.

5. *Look to the future* when anticipating improvements in behavior problems. Today's efforts will pay off down the road.

6. *Consistency* is the key to managing your loved one's behavior.

7. *Stay cool, calm, and collected* as your loved one will mirror the caregiver's stress and inappropriate reactions.

8. *Don't let the solution become part of the problem.* When the caregiver is giving corrective feedback or consequences, he or she should avoid discussing the behavior plan itself. The caregiver should explain only once why the behavior is problematic and then divert further dialogue to the treating therapist.

9. *It takes a village when managing behavior conflicts.* Usually this means not only the family's commitment, but also a treatment team's skill in developing a behavior management plan; monitoring problematic behaviors; following through with consequences; and recording relevant incidences.

10. *Don't let the weeds grow.* If the patient is showing the behavior problem and it is not addressed, the behavior is strengthened and more resistant to change. One option is to designate a "peace table" (P. Bugg, personal communication, 9/8/11), whereby conflicts are immediately addressed in a roundtable format.

11. *Communication is vital.* All parties should be communicating about the effectiveness of the strategies. Often this requires written behavior logs, which should be developed and implemented by a neuropsychologist in conjunction with the loved one, family, and other treating professionals. Behavior plans and tools should be modified as needed.

12. *Take breaks from difficult situations* so that the caregiver does not display maladaptive reactions, which the loved one might mirror.

(modified from Myles, October, 2008)

Fig. 9.3 (continued)

struggles preserve the caregiver's emotional reserves. A proactive approach to the loved one's recovery should encourage his or her independence, as well as teach sensitivity and "two-way" communication. These accomplishments benefit all parties and build nourishing and sustainable relationships. When the caregiver reminds himself or herself that he is providing "good enough" care (Bettelheim 1987; Winnicott 1994), emanating from love, concern, and healthy boundaries, he or she is liberated from debilitating anxiety, self-doubts, and/or recriminations.

Table 9.19 Common verbalizations related to rites of passage and therapy termination

Injury anniversaries
I relive the accident every anniversary
Anniversaries are a "re-birthday"
Anniversaries are bittersweet
It's a time to reminisce and then let go
My feelings about anniversaries have changed as the years have gone on
Every year, I look at mile markers of success
Anniversaries reset my perspective
I'm grateful for another chance
Therapy termination
I'm excited, but also scared about discharge
It turns out discharge is determined by reaching goals, not the date on the calendar
There are still lots of maybes in life
Compensations are life long
I feel like we beat the odds
I found a silver lining: I am closer to my loved one now than before the injury
This has been a learning experience
I have accepted a new path
I have grown and adapted through this process
I have expanded from being here and coping with the injury
He's/she's discharged, but not cured
It's a second chance, and maybe the second choice
It's a second path and a new way of life
Discharge is a huge rite of passage for my loved one and us
We've learned to be the best we can be
Setting goals has paid off
I found light at the end of the tunnel
I have learned to love this new person
Our family is closer
I can do this now
I have a "new me" in conjunction with my "new loved one"

9.10 Rites of Passage and the Future

As families witness first their loved ones' survival and then their gains, they come to appreciate various milestones, often including functional independence in the home; return to driving, school, and/or work; and completion of formal therapies. The tier 1 caregiver and other tier supports also experience various rites of passage and with time, evolve towards futuristic thinking. Two common themes which families focus upon are: their feelings about injury anniversaries and their feelings about termination of neurorehabilitation. Table 9.19 includes a series of common verbalizations allied with each topic.

Injury anniversaries bring the injury into acute focus. It is common for the loved one and many families to think of the injury date as a "re-birthday." This is especially the case when the caregiver has to relive the redevelopment of basic skills in the loved one, including eating, toileting, walking, etc. Many group participants describe the injury anniversaries as "bittersweet." On the one hand, they are acutely aware of the magnitude of the injury losses; on the other hand, they are grateful that their loved one is alive.

Further discussion has revealed a progression of feelings as anniversaries occur. At the time of the first anniversary, many caregivers describe reliving in a "moment-by-moment" scenario the terrifying events of the accident day. Sometimes, family members want to celebrate the survival and the gains in their loved one. This is done in the form of a party or social get-together with friends and families. By year 2, as some of the more chronic realities set in, families have described a phase of realization and resignation. There is sometimes less interest in large parties or celebrations; often, the family has a smaller get-together with key members of tiers 2 and 3. By year 3 and onwards, the relatives find a more hopeful stance, finding their own path, and witnessing the accomplishments of their loved one. Anniversaries become more about contemplation, and occur more privately within and between the caregivers and loved ones. Each year, however, the anniversary date becomes a time for reflection and then recalibration of a new existence. One uplifting approach is to assess mile markers of success, with appreciation for new opportunities.

Therapy termination is another rite of passage. There are usually mixed feelings in the family. There is excitement about reintegration into the community, but some trepidation about the change in routine, and phasing out of therapy supports. Realities have set in due to the long-term benefit of compensations. The family also realizes some of the uncertainties still facing their loved one, and consequently, themselves (Aniskiewicz 2007; Klonoff 2010). Thus, as depicted in phases 4, 5, and 6 of the FEM, the family has typically attained substantial learning and insights, as well as growing acceptance and adjustment to their loved one's injury, and a different lifestyle for themselves. Even so, there are some natural disappointments as the caregiver recognizes that the injury is not cured and that sacrifices have and will be made by all parties. Overall, the family sees a light at the end of the tunnel and has learned to love a "new person." Very often, priorities have shifted, with more value placed on closer family relationships. The family sees themselves as a "new us," and feel empowered to move forward, doing the best they can.

9.10.1 Group Treatment for Coping with Rites of Passage and Therapy Termination and to Promote Futuristic Thinking

Table 9.20 summarizes a number of the family's articulations, conceptualizations, and interventions which promote futuristic thinking, including rites of passage and therapy termination. Guided inquiries are the best vehicle for self-reflection and peer perspectives. One useful conversation starter is to share the poem, "Welcome to Holland" by Kingsley (1987) and ask family members to identify whether they are in Holland or Italy. Interestingly, some relatives reminisce that at first they thought they (and the loved one) were in a war-torn country, or Antarctica, fighting to survive. Family members who are struggling to cope with the existential dilemmas imposed by their loved one's brain injury search ardently for ways to reconstruct their shattered existence. Patients' adjustment has been referred to as *existential assimilation*, or defining one's new life philosophy, including values (Klonoff 2010). A parallel

Table 9.20 Group treatment for promoting futuristic thinking

Guided exercises
What does your loved one's injury mean to your life?
What is your outlook now for yourself, your family, and your loved one?
Is there a "silver lining" or any positives associated with where you are now in this journey?
Conceptualizations and interventions
Encourage group discussion about existential dilemmas
Assist families in reconstructing their shattered worlds
Help with an adjustment process to define a new life philosophy and values
Help with reformulating new attitudes about assumptive words, using new schemas
Look to "senior" group members and facilitators to provide solace and guidance to the "rookies"
Employ positive reframing to develop an optimistic perspective
Remember the power of the educational process
Foster mindfulness, courage, inner motivation, resiliency, and mastery
Realize that struggles produce posttraumatic growth, thriving, and personal transformation
Articulations about futuristic thinking
This process is a marathon, not a sprint
I've made peace with what I have
I have learned to go on in life
Whatever is—is
There is a "new normal"
We are blossoming
The pluses outweigh the minuses
I now focus on quality of life
I have found meaning in life
I have new priorities, dreams, and aspirations
Hope is all I have
I see new frontiers
I am a better person because of all of this
I'm striving for joy, patience, and kindness in my own life
I feel grateful and I want to give back
I had to find myself again
This process was transformational
I am happy with life
I believe in faith, hope, and love
This was a triumph of the will
Multimedia resources
Poem
"Welcome to Holland" (Kingsley 1987)
Book
The Carrot Seed (Krauss 1945)
Journal article
"Hope" (Buchholz 1990)
Movie
Pay It Forward (Abrams et al. 2000)
Song
"Soak up the Sun" (Crow and Trott 2002)

process unfolds for the relatives, who like the loved one, will need to rebuild relationships and attitudes about their assumptive world (Corr 2002; Landsman 2002). Some family members view postinjury life as precarious, unpredictable, and dominated by fate (Dell Orto and Power 2000; Guerriere and McKeever 1997). As with other forms of traumatic loss, new schemas are formed in the domains of control, justice, and nonrandomness of the universe (Landsman 2002).

Sharing is integral to this existential journey. More "senior" participants who have coped with the injury for longer periods usually help to shepherd "rookie" caregivers immersed in earlier phases of despair. Group facilitators can also employ positive reframing, by facilitating optimistic perspectives (Kreutzer et al. 2010) and reminding veteran attendees how much they have learned about brain injury as well as themselves. Realism requires rethinking the injury recovery and the family's state as a marathon, not a sprint (S. Myles, personal communication, n.d.). Connected to this, the caregiver and tiers of support focus on creating a "new normal," with the realization that "whatever is... is." Therefore, self-reflection and self-appraisal recast adaptation as "playing the hand you're dealt" (Guerriere and McKeever 1997). Nevertheless, through positive psychology, many families are coping with loss by embracing new meaning, quality of life, priorities, dreams, and aspirations (Aniskiewicz 2007; Dell Orto and Power 2000; Klonoff 2010). They are drawing on mindfulness and their reserves of compassion, devotion, courage, inner motivation, resiliency, perseverance, and mastery (Aniskiewicz 2007; Ben-Yishay and Diller 2011; Boss 2006; Braine 2011; Jumisko et al. 2007; Man 2002; Perlesz et al. 1999; Prowe 2010; Smith and Smith 2011). The children's book, *The Carrot Seed* by Krauss (1945) is a touching depiction of these qualities and is a wonderful tool to galvanize discussions.

The therapist can suggest that struggling with adversity can produce "adversarial growth" (Linley and Joseph 2004) or "posttraumatic growth" (Joseph 2011; Triplett et al. 2011; see also Chap. 10, Sect. 10.4.2). "Deliberate rumination" about the disrupted assumptive world spurs posttraumatic growth in the areas of personal strength, relationships with others, as well as appreciation and meaning of life (Joseph 2011; Triplett et al. 2011). Part of thriving is valuing change with a reconfiguration of sense of self, life views, priorities, and future goals (Joseph 2011). When families are adjusting positively, there is renewed hope, happiness, and faith in new frontiers (Dell Orto and Power 2000; Jumisko et al. 2007; Klonoff et al. 2008; Price et al. 1998). The group facilitator can introduce the article, "Hope" (Buchholz 1990), which is a lovely and creative description of the power of hope. With a "pay it forward" (Abrams et al. 2000; Heinlein 1951) orientation of giving to others, actual manifestations include pride, pleasure, and confidence in the caregiving role (Jumisko et al. 2007); mentorship relationships with other families with an injured loved one; charitable community service to others in need (e.g., fund raising); and/or other life pursuits which foster self-actualization. The process involves personal transformation. Many families feel they have grown into kinder, more grateful, patient, and loving individuals. Personal suffering has spawned triumph of the will. Ultimately, it is the grasp of "it's not having what you want; it's wanting what you've got" (Crow and Trott 2002).

References

Abrams, J. J., Greenhut, R., MacNair, S., Nichols, M., Rudin, S. (Producers), & Nichols, M. (Director). (1991). *Regarding Henry* [Motion picture]. United States: Paramount Pictures.

Abrams, P., Carson, P., Levy, R., McLaglen, M., Reuther, S., Treisman, J. (Producers), & Leder, M. (Director). (2000). *Pay it forward* [Motion picture]. United States: Warner Bros. Entertainment.

Ackerman, D. (2011). *One hundred names for love: A stroke, a marriage, and the language of healing*. New York: W. W. Norton.

Acorn, S. (1998). The family as caregiver. In S. Acorn & P. Offer (Eds.), *Living with brain injury: A guide for families and caregivers* (pp. 155–162). Toronto: University of Toronto Press.

Aniskiewicz, A. S. (2007). *Psychotherapy for neuropsychological challenges*. Lanham: Jason Aronson.

Backhaus, S. L., Ibarra, S. L., Klyce, D., Trexler, L. E., & Malec, J. F. (2010). Brain injury coping skills group: A preventative intervention for patients with brain injury and their caregivers. *Archives of Physical Medicine and Rehabilitation, 91*, 840–848.

Ben-Yishay, Y., & Diller, L. (2011). *Handbook of holistic neuropsychological rehabilitation: Outpatient rehabilitation of traumatic brain injury*. New York: Oxford University Press.

Bettelheim, B. (1987). *A good enough parent: A book on child-rearing*. New York: Alfred A. Knopf.

Blake, H. (2008). Caregiver stress in traumatic brain injury. *International Journal of Therapy & Rehabilitation, 15*(6), 263–271.

Blomquist, A. C., Hallström, L., Matalon, D., Ohlsson, B., Teper, M. (Producers), & Hallström, L. (Director). (1993). *What's eating Gilbert Grape* [Motion picture]. United States: Paramount Pictures.

Boerner, K., & Schulz, R. (2009). Caregiving, bereavement and complicated grief. *Bereave Care, 28*(3), 10–13.

Boss, P. (2006). *Loss, trauma, and resilience: Therapeutic work with ambiguous loss*. New York: W. W. Norton.

Boyle, G. J., & Haines, S. (2002). Severe traumatic brain injury: Some effects on family caregivers. *Psychological Reports, 90*(2), 415–425.

Braine, M. E. (2011). The experience of living with a family member with challenging behavior post acquired brain injury. *Journal of Neuroscience Nursing, 43*(3), 156–164.

Brennan, K. (2002). *Being with Rachel: A story of memory and survival*. New York: W. W. Norton.

Bruce, E., & Schultz, C. (2002). Non-finite loss and challenges to communication between parents and professionals. *British Journal of Special Education, 29*(1), 9–13.

Buchholz, W. M. (1990). A piece of my mind: Hope. *JAMA: The Journal of the American Medical Association, 263*(17), 2357–2358.

Butera-Prinzia, F., Charles, N., Heine, K., Rutherford, B., & Lattin, D. (2010). Family-to-Family Link Up Program: A community-based initiative supporting families caring for someone with an acquired brain injury. *NeuroRehabilitation, 27*(1), 31–47.

Carnes, S. L., & Quinn, W. H. (2005). Family adaptation to brain injury: Coping and psychological distress. *Families, Systems, & Health, 23*(2), 186–203.

Carnevale, G. J., Anselmi, V., Johnston, M. V., Busichio, K., & Walsh, V. (2006). A natural setting behavior management program for persons with acquired brain injury: A randomized controlled trial. *Archives of Physical Medicine and Rehabilitation, 87*(10), 1289–1297.

Carpenter, K., Carpenter, K., & Wilkerson, D. (2012). *The vow: The true events that inspired the movie*. Nashville: B & H Publishing Group.

Cassidy, J. W. (2009). *Mindstorms: The complete guide for families living with traumatic brain injury*. Philadelphia: Da Capo Press.

Channing Bete Co., Inc. (2008). *What everyone should know about seizures* [Booklet]. South Deerfield: Channing Bete Company.

Charles, N., Butera-Prinzi, F., & Perlesz, A. (2007). Families living with acquired brain injury: A multiple family group experience. *NeuroRehabilitation, 22*(1), 61–76.

Chartoff, R., Kirkwood, G., Winkler, I. (Producers), & Avildsen, J. G. (Director). (1976). *Rocky* [Motion picture]. United States: United Artists.

Collings, C. (2008). That's not my child anymore! Parental grief after acquired brain injury (ABI): Incidence, nature and longevity. *British Journal of Social Work, 38*(8), 1499–1517.

Corr, C. A. (2002). Coping with challenges to assumptive worlds. In J. Kauffman (Ed.), *Loss of the assumptive world: A theory of traumatic loss* (pp. 127–138). New York: Brunner-Routledge.

Corrigan, J. D., Rust, E., & Lamb-Hart, G. L. (1995). The nature and extent of substance abuse problems in persons with traumatic brain injury. *Journal of Head Trauma Rehabilitation, 10*(3), 29–46.

Crimmins, C. (2001). *Where is the mango princess? A journey back from brain injury*. New York: Vintage.

Crow, S., & Trott, J. (2002). *Soak up the sun* [recorded by Sheryl Crow]. *On c'mon c'mon* [CD]. Los Angeles: A & M.

De Reuck, J. (2011). Risk factors for late-onset seizures related to cerebral contusions in adults with a moderate traumatic brain injury. *Clinical Neurology and Neurosurgery, 113*(6), 469–471.

Dell Orto, A. E., & Power, P. W. (2000). *Brain injury and the family: A life and living perspective* (2nd ed.). Boca Raton: CRC Press.

Doka, K. J., & Martin, T. L. (2010). *Grieving beyond gender: Understanding the ways men and women mourn* (Revised ed.). New York: Routledge.

Elbaum, J. (2010). Acquired brain injury and the family: Challenges and interventions. In J. Elbaum & D. M. Benson (Eds.), *Acquired brain injury: An integrative neuro-rehabilitation approach* (pp. 275–285). New York: Springer.

Fancher, C., McDivitt, L., & Fletcher, J. B. (Eds.). (2008). *Climbing the mountain: Stories of hope and healing after stroke and brain injury*. Minneapolis: Fairview Press.

Ferguson, P. L., Smith, G. M., Wannamaker, B. B., Thurman, D. J., Pickelsimer, E. E., & Selassie, A. W. (2010). A population-based study of risk of epilepsy after hospitalization for traumatic brain injury. *Epilepsia, 51*(5), 891–898.

Fleming, J., Kuipers, P., Foster, M., Smith, S., & Doig, E. (2009). Evaluation of an outpatient, peer group intervention for people with acquired brain injury based on the ICF 'Environment' dimension. *Disability & Rehabilitation, 31*(20), 1666–1675.

Frankl, V. E. (1984). *Man's search for meaning* (3rd ed.). New York: Simon & Schuster.

Gan, C., Gargaro, J., Kreutzer, J. S., Boschen, K. A., & Wright, F. V. (2010). Development and preliminary evaluation of a structured family system intervention for adolescents with brain injury and their families. *Brain Injury, 24*(4), 651–663.

Giffords, G., Kelly, M., & Zaslow, J. (2011). *Gabby: A story of courage and hope*. New York: Scribner.

Goldstein, K. (1952). The effect of brain damage on the personality. *Psychiatry, 15*(3), 245–260.

Goodall, J. (2000). *The eagle and the wren*. New York: North South Books.

Guerriere, D., & McKeever, P. (1997). Mothering children who survive brain injuries: Playing the hand you're dealt. *Journal of the Society of Pediatric Nurses, 2*(3), 105–115.

Hanks, R. A., Rapport, L. J., & Vangel, S. (2007). Caregiving appraisal after traumatic brain injury: The effects of functional status, coping style, social support and family functioning. *NeuroRehabilitation, 22*(1), 43–52.

Hein, P. (2003). T. T. T. In *PoemHunter.com*, poems by Piet Hein. http://www.poemhunter.com/poem/t-t-t/. Accessed 3 July 2011.

Heinlein, R. A. (1951). *Between planets*. New York: Charles Scribner's Sons.

Hoffmeister, A. L. (1998). The role of the social worker. In C. D. Sturm, T. R. Forget Jr., & J. L. Sturm (Eds.), *Head injury information and answers to commonly asked questions: A family's guide to coping* (pp. 229–246). St. Louis: Quality Medical Publishing.

Hojat, M. (2007). *Empathy in patient care: Antecedents, development, measurement, and outcomes*. New York: Springer.

Inzaghi, M. G., De Tanti, A., & Sozzi, M. (2005). The effects of traumatic brain injury on patients and their families: A follow-up study. *Europa Medicophysica, 41*(4), 265–273.

Jameson, L., & Jameson, B. (2007). *Brain injury survivor's guide: Welcome to our world*. Denver: Outskirts Press.

Janoff-Bulman, R. (2002). Foreword. In J. Kauffman (Ed.), *Loss of the assumptive world: A theory of traumatic loss* (pp. xi–xii). New York: Brunner-Routledge.

Johnson, J., & McCown, W. (1997). *Family therapy of neurobehavioral disorders: Integrating neuropsychology and family therapy*. New York: Haworth Press.

Joseph, S. (2011). *What doesn't kill us: The new psychology of posttraumatic growth*. New York: Basic Books.

Jumisko, E., Lexell, J., & Söderberg, S. (2007). Living with moderate or severe traumatic brain injury: The meaning of family members' experiences. *Journal of Family Nursing, 13*(3), 353–369.

Kean, S. (2010). The experience of ambiguous loss in families of brain injured ICU patients. *Nursing in Critical Care, 15*(2), 66–75.

Keenan, A., & Joseph, L. (2010). The needs of family members of severe traumatic brain injured patients during critical and acute care: A qualitative study. *Canadian Journal of Neuroscience Nursing, 32*(3), 25–35.

Kingsley, E. P. (1987). Welcome to Holland. http://www.our-kids.org/Archives/Holland.html. Acessed 11 Feb 2013.

Klonoff, P. S. (2010). *Psychotherapy after brain injury: Principles and techniques*. New York: Guilford Press.

Klonoff, P. S., & Koberstein, E. J. (2010). Family life. In P. S. Klonoff (Ed.), *Psychotherapy after brain injury: Principles and techniques* (pp. 150–170). New York: Guilford Press.

Klonoff, P. S., & Myles, S. M. (2010). Sense of self and identity. In P. S. Klonoff (Ed.), *Psychotherapy after brain injury: Principles and techniques* (pp. 75–99). New York: Guilford Press.

Klonoff, P., & Prigatano, G. P. (1987). Reactions of family members and clinical intervention after traumatic brain injury. In M. Ylvisaker & E. M. R. Gobble (Eds.), *Community re-entry for head injured adults* (pp. 381–402). Boston: College-Hill Publication.

Klonoff, P. S., Lage, G. A., & Chiapello, D. A. (1993). Varieties of the catastrophic reaction to brain injury: A self psychology perspective. *Bulletin of the Menninger Clinic, 57*(2), 227–241.

Klonoff, P. S., Talley, M. C., Dawson, L. K., Myles, S. M., Watt, L. M., Gehrels, J., & Henderson, S. W. (2007). The relationship of cognitive retraining to neurological patients' work and school status. *Brain Injury, 21*(11), 1097–1107.

Klonoff, P. S., Koberstein, E. J., Talley, M. C., & Dawson, L. K. (2008). A family experiential model of recovery after brain injury. *Bulletin of the Menninger Clinic, 72*(2), 109–129.

Klonoff, P. S., Olson, K. C., Talley, M. C., Husk, K. L., Myles, S. M., Gehrels, J., & Dawson, L. K. (2010). The relationship of cognitive retraining to neurological patients' driving status: The role of process variables and compensation training. *Brain Injury, 24*(2), 63–73.

Krauss, R. (1945). *The carrot seed*. New York: HarperCollins Publishers.

Kreutzer, J. S., Kolakowsky-Hayner, S. A., Demm, S. R., & Meade, M. A. (2002). A structured approach to family intervention after brain injury. *Journal of Head Trauma Rehabilitation, 17*(4), 349–367.

Kreutzer, J. S., Livingston, L. A., Everley, R. S., Gary, K. W., Arango-Lasprilla, J. C., Powell, V. D., & Marwitz, J. H. (2009a). Caregivers' concerns about judgment and safety of patients with brain injury: A preliminary investigation. *PM & R, 1*(8), 723–728.

Kreutzer, J. S., Stejskal, T. M., Ketchum, J. M., Marwitz, J. H., Taylor, L. A., & Menzel, J. C. (2009b). A preliminary investigation of the brain injury family intervention: Impact on family members. *Brain Injury, 23*(6), 535–547.

Kreutzer, J. S., Marwitz, J. H., Godwin, E. E., & Arango-Lasprilla, J. C. (2010). Practical approaches to effective family intervention after brain injury. *Journal of Head Trauma Rehabilitation, 25*(2), 113–120.

Kushner, H. (1981). *When bad things happen to good people*. New York: Avon Books.

Landsman, I. S. (2002). Crises of meaning in trauma and loss. In J. Kauffman (Ed.), *Loss of the assumptive world: A theory of traumatic loss* (pp. 13–30). New York: Brunner-Routledge.

Lansky, M. R. (1990). Escalation of trauma in the family of the patient with organic brain disease. *Family Systems Medicine, 8*(3), 231–240.

Lee, A. L., Strauss, L., Wittman, P., Jackson, B., & Carstens, A. (2001). The effects of chronic illness on roles and emotions of caregivers. *Occupational Therapy in Health Care, 14*(1), 47–60.

Linley, P. A., & Joseph, S. (2004). Positive change following trauma and adversity: A review. *Journal of Traumatic Stress, 17*(1), 11–21.

Lloyd, D. J., & Kehoe, S. L. (2001). *Smile and jump high!: The true story of overcoming a traumatic brain injury*. Monroe: Starlight Press.

Machamer, J., Temkin, N., & Dikmen, S. (2002). Significant other burden and factors related to it in traumatic brain injury. *Journal of Clinical and Experimental Neuropsychology, 24*(4), 420–433.

Maier, S. F., & Seligman, M. E. (1976). Learned helplessness: Theory and evidence. *Journal of Experimental Psychology: General, 105*(1), 3–46.

Man, D. W. K. (2002). Family caregiver's reactions and coping for persons with brain injury. *Brain Injury, 16*(12), 1025–1037.

Marsh, N. V., Kersel, D. A., Havill, J. H., & Sleigh, J. W. (1998). Caregiver burden at 1 year following severe traumatic brain injury. *Brain Injury, 12*(12), 1045–1059.

Moberg, P. J., & Kniele, K. (2006). Evaluation of competency: Ethical consideration for Neuropsychologists. *Applied Neuropsychology, 13*(2), 101–114.

Moye, J. (2003). Guardianship and conservatorship. In T. Grisso, R. Borum, J. F. Edens, J. Moye, & R. K. Otto (Eds.), *Evaluating competencies: Forensic assessments and instruments* (2nd ed., pp. 309–389). New York: Kluwer Academic/Plenum Publishers.

Myles, S. M. (2008, Oct.). Basic principles for managing behavior conflicts after brain injury. Presentation at the Center for Transitional NeuroRehabilitation, Barrow Neurological Institute. Relative's Group Presentation, Phoenix, AZ.

Newby, H., & Ryan-Morgan, T. (2013). Assessment of mental capacity. In G. Newby, R. Coetzer, A. Daisley, & S. Weatherhead (Eds.), *Practical neuropsychological rehabilitation in acquired brain injury: A guide for working clinicians* (pp. 179–207). London: Karnac Books Ltd.

Pais, S. (2002). Remember to place the oxygen mask on yourself first.... *Journal of Clinical Activities, Assignments & Handouts in Psychotherapy Practice, 2*(4), 109–115.

Patrick-Ott, A., & Ladd, L. D. (2010). The blending of Boss's concept of ambiguous loss and Olshansky's concept of chronic sorrow: A case study of a family with a child who has significant disabilities. *Journal of Creativity in Mental Health, 5*(1), 73–86.

Pepping, M. (1998). Long-term adjustment following significant brain injury. In S. Acorn & P. Offer (Eds.), *Living with brain injury: A guide for families and caregivers* (pp. 56–69). Toronto: University of Toronto Press.

Perlesz, A., Kinsella, G., & Crowe, S. (1999). Impact of traumatic brain injury on the family: A critical review. *Rehabilitation Psychology, 44*(1), 6–35.

Ponsford, J., & Schönberger, M. (2010). Family functioning and emotional state two and five years after traumatic brain injury. *Journal of the International Neuropsychological Society, 16*(2), 306–317.

Price, E., Johnston, A., & Kirsch, G. (1998). Emotional reactions and coping strategies. In C. D. Sturm, T. R. Forget Jr., & J. L. Sturm (Eds.), *Head injury information and answers to commonly asked questions: A family's guide to coping* (pp. 209–228). St. Louis: Quality Medical Publishing.

Prowe, G. (2010). *Successfully surviving a brain injury a family guidebook: From the emergency room to selecting a rehabilitation facility*. Gainesville: Brain Injury Success Books.

Rich, M. (2005). *Coping with brain injury: How to help after accidents, stroke and illness*. London: Sheldon Press.

Roos, S. (2002a). *Chronic sorrow: A living loss*. New York: Brunner-Routledge.

Roos, S. (2002b). Chronic sorrow: Siblings of children with disabilities have needs too. *The Brown University Child and Adolescent Behavior Letter, 18*(11), 1, 6–7.

Rossheim, B. N., & McAdams III, C. R. (2010). Addressing the chronic sorrow of long-term spousal caregivers: A primer for counselors. *Journal of Counseling & Development, 88*(4), 477–482.

Roundhill, S. J., Williams, W. H., & Hughes, J. M. (2007). The experience of loss following traumatic brain injury: Applying a bereavement model to the process of adjustment. *Qualitative Research in Psychology, 4*(3), 241–257.

Russo, M. (2010). *A very big bunny*. New York: Random House.

Sander, A. M. (2005). Interventions for caregivers. In W. M. High Jr., A. M. Sander., M. A. Struchen, & K. A. Hart (Eds.), *Rehabilitation for traumatic brain injury* (pp. 156–175). New York: Oxford University Press.

Senelick, R., & Dougherty, K. (2001). *Living with brain injury: A guide for families* (2nd ed.). Birmingham: HealthSouth Press.

Shannon, G. (2007). *Rabbit's gift*. Orlando: Harcourt.

Sherwin, E. D., & O'Shanick, G. J. (2000). The trauma of paediatric and adolescent brain injury: Issues and implications for rehabilitation specialists. *Brain Injury, 14*(3), 267–284.

Siegert, R. J., Jackson, D. M., Tennant, A., & Turner-Stokes, L. (2010). Factor analysis and Rasch analysis of the Zarit Burden Interview for acquired brain injury carer research. *Journal of Rehabilitative Medicine, 42*(4), 302–309.

Silberfield, M., & Fish, A. (1994). *When the mind fails: A guide to dealing with incompetency*. Toronto: University of Toronto Press.

Simpson, G., Mohr, R., & Redman, A. (2000). Cultural variations in the understanding of traumatic brain injury and brain injury rehabilitation. *Brain Injury, 14*(2), 125–140.

Smith, L. M., & Godfrey, H. P. D. (1995). *Family support programs and rehabilitation: A cognitive-behavioral approach to traumatic brain injury*. New York: Plenum Press.

Smith, J. E., & Smith, D. L. (2000). No map, no guide. Family caregivers' perspectives on their journeys through the system. *Care Management Journals, 2*(1), 27–33.

Smith, D., & Smith, D. (2011). *A decade of hope: Stories of grief and endurance from 9/11 families and friends*. New York: Viking Penguin.

Teel, C. S. (1991). Chronic sorrow: Analysis of the concept. *Journal of Advanced Nursing, 16*(11), 1311–1319.

Testani-Dufour, L., Chappel-Aiken, L., & Gueldner, S. (1992). Traumatic brain injury: A family experience. *Journal of Neuroscience Nursing, 24*(6), 317–323.

Triplett, K. N., Tedeschi, R. G., Cann, A., Calhoun, L. G., & Reeve, C. L. (2011). Posttraumatic growth, meaning in life, and life satisfaction in response to trauma. *Psychological Trauma: Theory, Research, Practice, and Policy,* Advance online publication. doi:10.1037/a0024204.

Wedcliffe, T., & Ross, E. (2001). The psychological effects of traumatic brain injury on the quality of life of a group of spouses/partners. *South African Journal of Communication Disorders, 48,* 77–99.

Wells, R., Dywan, J., & Dumas, J. (2005). Life satisfaction and distress in family caregivers as related to specific behavioural changes after traumatic brain injury. *Brain Injury, 19*(13), 1105–1115.

Williams, B. Y. (2004). The friend who just stands by. In J. Cotner (Ed.), *Looking for God in all the right places: Prayers and poems to comfort, inspire, and connect humanity* (p. 125). Chicago: Loyola Press.

Williams, J. M. (1991). Family Support. In J. M. Williams & T. Kay (Eds.), *Head injury: A family matter* (pp. 299–312). Baltimore: Brookes Publishing.

Winnicott, D. W. (1994). The building up of trust. In C. Winnicott, C. Bollas, M. Davis, & R. Shepherd (Eds.), *Talking to parents* (pp. 121–134). Cambridge: Perseus Publishing.

Woodruff, L., & Woodruff, B. (2007). *In an instant: A family's journey of love and healing*. New York: Random House.

Wright, H. (2000). *Someone stole yesterday*. Franklin: Providence House Publishers.

Yalom, I. D. (2002). *The gift of therapy: An open letter to a new generation of therapists and their patients*. New York: HarperCollins Publishers.

Zinner, E. S., Ball, J. D., Stutts, M. L., & Philput, C. (1997). Grief reactions of mothers of adolescents and young adults with traumatic brain injury. *Archives of Clinical Neuropsychology, 12*(5), 435–447.

Chapter 10
Loved Ones' End-of-Life and Existential Considerations as a Caregiver

10.1 Scenario: Questions about End of Life

This section will explore the role of caregiving for loved ones in the later phase of neurological deterioration, ending in death. It will include practical and existential considerations. A user-friendly definition of *existential* is "pertaining to existence" (Yalom 2009). Given the breadth of this field and the multiplicity of possible terminal diagnoses (e.g., late effects/complications of stroke or traumatic brain injuries, dementias, etc.), the prototype of the discussion will be brain tumors, with an emphasis on how psychotherapy can guide the tier 1 caregiver and other tier supports through this tumultuous journey. Of note, Chap. 7 has addressed earlier caregiver roles for a loved one with a brain tumor.

When the loved one with a brain tumor is worsening in his or her function and is approaching death, the caregiver and family may ask questions such as: *Is my loved one dying? How long will he or she live? How should I prepare myself, my loved one, and my family for this? How will I survive this loss?*

10.1.1 Overview of End-of-Life Issues Related to Brain Tumors

Coping with the loved one's chronic terminal illness and nearing death from a brain tumor can be excruciatingly painful and overwhelming for the primary caregiver and overall support network (Sherwood et al. 2004a; Tepper 2003). Tumor recurrence restarts the roller coaster of emotions, including dashed hopes for survival (see Khalili 2007, for a review). Profound declines in the loved one's physical, cognitive, and emotional status are exceedingly stressful (Adelbratt and Strang 2000; Aldrich and Peterson 2010; Khalili 2007; Sherwood et al. 2004a, b). Common difficulties involve speech, swallowing, walking, lethargy, and incontinence (Black and Hogan 2006). This progresses to drowsiness, loss of appetite, coma, and labored breathing (Black and Hogan 2006). As the dying process unfolds, the family can feel like the loved one is dying twice—once through a loss of personhood and the other through a physical demise (Sherwood et al. 2004a; Strang and Strang 2001).

P. S. Klonoff, *Psychotherapy for Families after Brain Injury*,
DOI 10.1007/978-1-4899-8083-0_10,

Physical and psychological assistance by the primary caregiver is necessitated and there are marked lifestyle changes for everyone, affecting roles, self-care, daily activities, finances, and schedules (see Bainbridge et al. 2009, for a review; Hebert et al. 2009; see Kutner and Kilbourn 2009 for a review; see Sand et al. 2010, for a review; Schmer et al. 2008; see Sherwood et al. 2004b, for a review). Role discontinuity related to the totality of extra duties emerges, especially with a cognitive decline in the loved one (Sherwood et al. 2004a). Role conflict stems from competing obligations and role overload is catalyzed by insufficient coping energies and resources (Sherwood et al. 2004a).

Stressors greatly impact the family unit's equilibrium and typical routines, often producing exhaustion in the caregiver (Khalili 2007). The understandable constant demands create loneliness, social isolation, his or her own health issues, and decreased life satisfaction (see Kutner and Kilbourn 2009, for a review). Caregivers in poor health and/or younger ones with competing responsibilities are particularly vulnerable to caregiver strain (Bainbridge et al. 2009). Many feel like they are unprepared for the loved one's impending death, which exacerbates their emotional distress (see Hebert et al. 2008a, for a review).

The relatives are often engulfed in anxiety, dread, frustration, edginess, guilt, helplessness, hopelessness, and numbness, especially when the loved one is suffering (Aldrich and Peterson 2010; Kitamura et al. 2011; see Kutner and Kilbourn 2009, for a review; Schmer et al. 2008; see Sherwood et al. 2004b, for a review). These emotions mirror those of the loved one, who may also be experiencing *death anxiety,* characterized by loss of autonomy, fear of the unknown, his or her inevitable annihilation, and separation from family and friends (Adelbratt and Strang 2000; Yalom 2009).

Some families choose to channel their energies into finding life-saving care options (Tepper 2003). The caregiver is also inundated with daily concerns when pressured to put personal affairs in order (Aldrich and Peterson 2010; Tepper 2003). The relatives may self-isolate, desiring to spend every waking moment with the loved one (Schmer et al. 2008). Regardless of the chosen path, the loved one and support network are transitioning, with a hallmark of change from curative treatment possibilities to palliative care (see Khalili 2007, for a review). Some have described this as "entering the unknown" (Khalili 2007). Fear of abandonment emerges when the caregiver realizes the treatment team will be shifting (Khalili 2007).

Certain relatives are more easily able to accept the loved one's terminal stages of illness (Adelbratt and Strang 2000). For others, it feels preferable to avoid facing topics, such as death, end-of-life wishes, and after-death preparation (Aldrich and Peterson 2010; Tepper 2003). There can be denial of the seriousness of the condition (Schubart et al. 2008). Tier 1 caregivers may be torn about who to share the realities of the diagnosis with for privacy reasons and/or fear of worrying or upsetting others, especially children (Khalili 2007; Schmer et al. 2008; Smith 2007). Subsequently, the caregiver and support network (and also the loved one) may be ill-prepared for death (Aldrich and Peterson 2010; Schubart et al. 2008; Tepper 2003). Overall, the caregiver is juggling the total disruption of his or her life while keeping some semblance of family order (see Schmer 2008, for a review). He or she must also balance a myriad of desires, expectations, feelings, and needs emerging from the loved one, other family members, the health-care system, society, and, importantly, within himself or herself (see Sand et al. 2010, for a review).

Norton and Bowers (2001) identify elements of a *bad death* for the loved one as unrealistic treatment decisions, "unfinished business," unresolved conflict, difficulty grieving, and poor symptom and pain management. Based on research with other terminal illnesses, often the relatives have questions for health-care professionals about what the dying process will entail; how to access medical services; ways to share information with other family members (especially in conflict-ridden situations); and existential questions connected to spirituality and the meaning of life (Hebert et al. 2008a; Strang et al. 2001). However, frequently caregivers are reluctant to make inquiries, sometimes due to being stumped as to what to ask but also because of perceptions that the health-care professional is unavailable, untrustworthy, or will judge the family for "ignorant" questions (Hebert et al. 2008b).

10.1.2 "Helpful Hints" and Tools for Families to Cope with End-of-life Issues Related to Brain Tumors: Practical Aspects

Table 10.1 summarizes "helpful hints" and tools for families to cope with the practical aspects of end-of-life issues caused by a brain tumor in the loved one. It is advisable to begin the discussion of treatment considerations and the dying process with a brain tumor diagnosis as early as possible, as there is often a shorter illness trajectory (Khalili 2007; Tepper 2003). Time estimates are not foolproof and the loved one is susceptible to complications, including infections, blood clots, pneumonia, and malnutrition (Stark-Vance and Dubay 2011). Once a crisis occurs, the opportunities for meaningful discussions about values, goals, and choices are forfeited (Moore 2005).

Therapy should, of course, take into account the preferences and requirements of the family (and loved one; Power and Dell Orto 2004; Tepper 2003). A psychologist, social worker, or counselor can provide brief or more extensive treatment, including crisis intervention, psychoeducation, and resource referrals (Power and Dell Orto 2004; Tepper 2003). However, this discourse must be at the time and pacing that the family unit is comfortable with (Khalili 2007; see Chap. 2, Sect. 2.4.1.2). Advance care planning should be revisited during the course of the terminal illness, as needed, based on the loved one's prerogatives (Moore 2005). The psychotherapist can be a good spokesperson for having the family (and loved one) initiate this process proactively as well as advocate for intercommunication between specialists (American Psychological Association 2012).

Feedback from health-care professionals should also take into account individualized needs, including familial, societal, and cultural factors, as these dictate response styles (see also Chap. 1, Sect. 1.3 and Fig. 1.1; American Psychological Association 2012; Hebert et al. 2008b; Power and Dell Orto 2004; Tepper 2003; Wong and Tomer 2011). Other therapeutic strategies are to cultivate a working alliance or

Table 10.1 "Helpful hints" and tools for families to cope with end-of-life issues related to brain tumors: practical aspects

Begin discussion of treatment considerations and end-of-life issues as early as possible
Remember that time estimates about longevity are not foolproof
Therapies include crisis intervention, psychoeducation, and resource referrals from a psychologist, social worker, or counselor
Discourse should proceed at the time and pacing that is comfortable for the tier 1 caregiver and support network
Interventions with the psychotherapist and health-care professionals should be individualized to the loved one's and support network's unique needs and circumstances by:
Incorporating familial, societal, and cultural factors
Fostering a working alliance
Laying the groundwork of trust, protection, and rapport
Providing the "big picture" to facilitate informed decisions
Educating the family and loved one about prognosis and treatment choices
Planting the seeds about survival
Reframing the situation from chronic illness to imminent death
Working together in the best interest of the loved one
Be proactive about meeting with the neurosurgeon about options and possible complications and audiotape appointments, if possible
Utilize the psychotherapist to help structure questions and concerns in advance of medical appointments
Consider second opinions and research what interventions the insurance company covers
Help your loved one make an informed decision about when to stop active treatment
Utilize other specialists for guidance and education, including physicians, nurses, chaplaincy services, hospital ethics committees, social workers, psychologists, and psychiatrists
It is optimal to address advance care planning while the loved one is mentally competent, which may necessitate a separate competency evaluation
Become educated about what advance directives entail and share paperwork with relevant family members and physicians
Make sure that the loved one's personal business is managed by a trusted individual and keep copies of all documents
Family meetings with the psychotherapist are a good forum to discuss the loved one's wishes, including when to initiate palliative care
Promote preparation for a "good death"
The family should research hospice options in advance to allow for an informed choice
Utilize the available hospice services, including respite opportunities and grief counseling
Multimedia resources
Book
100 Questions & Answers about Brain Tumors (Stark-Vance and Dubay 2011)
Website
For end-of-life resources and hospice: http://kspope.com/hospices/index.php

"lay the groundwork" with trust, protection, and rapport; provide the "big picture" regarding the loved one's condition so that the caregiver, patient, and family make more informed decisions; educate the relatives (and patient) vis-à-vis prognosis and treatment choices; plant seeds about limited survival; shift the picture by reframing the situation from chronic illness to imminent death; and work together in the best interest of the loved one (Hebert et al. 2008b; Norton and Bowers (2001). Some have termed the process as "hoping for the best, but preparing for the worst" (Klonoff 2010; Stark-Vance and Dubay 2011).

The psychotherapist should encourage the caregiver, family, and loved one to meet with treating physicians and explore avenues and possible consequences of various interventions, including additional neurosurgeries. The therapist can provide assistance to the parties in developing salient questions such as the possible surgical outcomes and complications, potential pain level, and effect on functionality and quality of life (Black and Hogan 2006). If possible, audiotaping medical appointments is ideal (see Chap. 7, Sect. 7.1.2). Obtaining a second opinion is often worthwhile (Stark-Vance and Dubay 2011). When other treatments are advised (e.g., chemotherapy), the primary caregiver or his or her designee will need to investigate what types of interventions the insurance company will support (Black and Hogan 2006).

A major consideration is when to stop treating the tumor versus addressing symptoms, so as to improve quality of life (Black and Hogan 2006). This will be based on the natural progression of the brain tumor; personal preferences concerning duration versus quality of life; and the outcome of various interventions (Black and Hogan 2006). When a decision is being considered to stop treatment, the loved one and caregiver need emotional support from the therapist and continued encouragement to seek education and guidance from treating physicians, nurses, chaplaincy services, hospital ethics committees, social workers, psychologists, and psychiatrists (American Psychological Association 2012; Black and Hogan 2006; Connor et al. 2006).

As stated above, serious decisions are time sensitive, so it is imperative to address advance care planning while the loved one is mentally competent (Black and Hogan 2006; Goodman et al. 2007; see also Chap. 9, Sect. 9.6.1). The psychotherapist may recommend that the loved one undergo a competency examination by an outside skilled professional, to be sure he or she can give informed consent to be involved in the discussion as well as make health-care decisions (American Psychological Association 2012). Topics include understanding life-sustaining treatments; alternatives for life-threatening conditions; personal values, existential considerations, and spiritual beliefs about death and dying; identifying who would make decisions once the loved one cannot; and discussing and preparing documentation about end-of-life preferences (American Psychological Association 2012; Goodman et al. 2007; Norton and Bowers 2001).

Advance directives, including a living will and/or a health-care proxy (or durable power of attorney for medical care), should be identified early to ensure the voice of the loved one is heard and followed (Black and Hogan 2006; Smith 2002; Stark-Vance and Dubay 2011). The health-care proxy is often a spouse or relative and this person should be asked if he or she is comfortable with this role (Goodman et al. 2007). The name and contact information of this individual should be provided to the physician and incorporated into the medical records (Goodman et al. 2007; Moore 2005; Stark-Vance and Dubay 2011).

Advance directives are legal documents that specify end-of-life decisions. These include what kinds of supportive care the individual wants and for how long (Black and Hogan 2006; Stark-Vance and Dubay 2011; Tepper 2003). Specific examples include: withholding food and water; withdrawing a breathing and/or feeding tube;

abstaining from the use of antibiotics; choosing not to resuscitate; and increasing the dose of morphine (Black and Hogan 2006; Stark-Vance and Dubay 2011). A living will protects the loved one's rights to accept or refuse care (Goodman et al. 2007). This reduces the burden of responsibility of life and death decisions for the caregiver (Goodman et al. 2007). Typical components include: do not resuscitate (DNR) orders (e.g., instructions to refuse cardiopulmonary resuscitation if breathing or heartbeat stops); choices about artificial hydration, nutrition, and life-saving equipment (e.g., ventilators and respirators); comfort care (e.g., pain medications); and education on organ and tissue donation (Goodman et al. 2007). A copy of this should be given to relevant relatives and treating physicians (Smith 2002).

The loved one's personal business will also need to be managed by a trusted individual (Goodman et al. 2007). The loved one should identify a durable power of attorney for finances, who is often the primary caregiver. Financial data regarding the loved one that should be accessible include: bank accounts; safety deposit boxes; life insurance policies; health insurance policies; deeds and property titles; stocks and bonds; the birth certificate; military papers; social security papers; benefit forms; loan papers; vehicle registrations; and income tax returns (Goodman et al. 2007). Given the complexity of these issues, the designee is counseled to consult with an attorney, bank associate, hospital patient relations department, a social worker, or reputable sources on the Internet (Goodman et al. 2007). Other important documents include: a will; estate executor; trust funds; rights of survivorship on all financial accounts; burial or cremation wishes; and preferences for funeral services (Aldrich and Peterson 2010; American Psychological Association 2012). Estate planning can also be complex and consultation with an attorney and a social worker is advisable (Goodman et al. 2007). Key family members should have a copy of all significant documents (Aldrich and Peterson 2010; Moore 2005).

A constructive forum is family meetings with the psychotherapist, centered on the loved one's wishes, especially when there is a pending decline in his or her status (Hebert et al. 2008b; Norton and Bowers 2001). This enables clarification about the expected progression of the brain tumor, which increases everyone's acceptance and collaboration. These factors promote a *good death,* in which the loved one and family can direct energies toward the optimal interventions, including pain control, openness to social workers and spiritual counselors, cherishing time together, and when appropriate, discontinuing questionably curative treatments (Aldrich and Peterson 2010; Norton and Bowers 2001; Palmieri 2007; Tepper 2003). The loved one and relatives can then psychologically entertain palliative care opportunities, including hospice (Palmieri 2007).

The term hospice traces back to the root words of hospitality and host (Connor et al. 2006). It strives to treat the whole person by addressing the psychosocial, spiritual, and emotional needs (Connor et al. 2006). It caters to the patient and his or her family system (Connor et al. 2006). Hospice care is skilled nursing care at home or in a facility and must be certified by a physician with the understanding that the diagnosis will limit the loved one's life span to less than 6 months (Black and Hogan 2006; Goodman et al. 2007; Stark-Vance and Dubay 2011). Other criteria are that the loved one and patient are no longer seeking curative measures and that a DNR order has been supplied by the physician (Stark-Vance and Dubay 2011). The aim of hospice is to minimize suffering through comfort and alleviate symptoms through physical, psychological, and spiritual care; it does not hasten death (Black and Hogan 2006; Connor et al. 2006; Goodman et al. 2007; Stark-Vance and Dubay 2011).

Research on hospice care should be done well enough in advance to allow sufficient time for calm decision making (Stark-Vance and Dubay 2011). When identifying the finest hospice care, the relatives may want to obtain an endorsement from others who had personal experience with the care (Stark-Vance and Dubay 2011). Finding the most suitable palliative care for the loved one reduces the relatives' anguish, which in turn preserves their own emotional and physical resources, so as to enhance their supportive care of the loved one (Kutner and Kilbourn 2009). Inquiry should also be conducted to be sure the hospice is contracted with the loved one's health-care plan and that the ambience is compassionate and competent (Goodman et al. 2007; Stark-Vance and Dubay 2011). More guidelines for selecting a hospice are available in the book, *100 Questions & Answers about Brain Tumors* by Stark-Vance and Dubay (2011).

When hospice care is provided in the home, the primary caregiver will also be trained in relevant techniques (Stark-Vance and Dubay 2011). Hospice nurses will coordinate closely with the physician to address the loved one's symptoms, such as seizures, headaches, fever, shortness of breath, and pain (Stark-Vance and Dubay 2011). Some hospice facilities provide volunteer programs or inpatient stays so that the caregiver can obtain some much-needed respite (Empeño et al. 2011; Stark-Vance and Dubay 2011). Grief counseling is also available for the loved one and family (Goodman et al. 2007). The website http://kspope.com/hospices/index.php provides handy information about hospice and end-of-life resources.

10.1.3 "Helpful Hints" and Tools for Families to Cope with End-of-life Issues Related to Brain Tumors: Emotional Aspects

Table 10.2 summarizes "helpful hints" and tools for families to cope with the emotional aspects of end-of-life issues for the loved one with a brain tumor. The grief and loss process is usually intense and all-consuming (Power and Dell Orto 2004). Besides practical considerations, the psychotherapist is central in addressing the caregiver's and relatives' angst. This is instrumental not only for them but also for the loved one (Kutner and Kilbourn 2009; Richman 1995). A positive therapeutic relationship which emphasizes the listening perspective is fundamental to this process, so as to inculcate a "respectful death" (Power and Dell Orto 2004; Richman 1995; Wasserman 2008). The tier 1 caregiver and family should seek a therapist whom they relate well to, including that he or she takes time to build rapport; gives undivided attention; maintains good eye contact (when culturally applicable); is compassionate, genuine, and nonjudgmental; facilitates emotional expression; and validates strong

Table 10.2 "Helpful hints" and tools for families to cope with end-of-life issues related to brain tumors: emotional aspects

Remember that the grief and loss process is usually intense and all-consuming

Find a psychotherapist who is easy to relate to and addresses the angst and agony through skills of:

- Emphasizing the listening perspective
- Taking time to build rapport
- Giving undivided attention
- Maintaining good/appropriate eye contact
- Exuding compassion, genuine, and nonjudgmental qualities
- Facilitating emotional expression
- Validating strong emotions
- Balancing information dispensing with emotional support and encouragement

Expect to learn pertinent nomenclature, including "anticipatory grief," avoidance, and denial

Anticipatory grief does not replace postdeath grief

Realize that avoidance of topics of death and dying may occur because of fear, embarrassment, ambivalence, awkwardness, or an attempt to protect the loved one

Psychotherapy can assist with "emotional preparedness" for the loved one's death, including cognitive, affective, and behavioral factors

Expect to think about how life will be without the loved one

Utilize the psychotherapist to assist children in their grieving process:

- Remember that children are perceptive
- Obtain support based on their developmental phase and emotional readiness
- Give them clarifying information and do not exclude them from the dying and ritual process

The family may warrant therapy to reframe the loved one's decision to stop aggressive treatment, in the context of cultural diversities

If needed, involve a psychotherapist, social worker, and/or hospital ethics committee members to resolve questions and conflicts about stopping aggressive treatment

Realize the instrumental role of the caregiver and tier supports in providing comfort to the loved one through a process of "presencing"

Draw on inner patience and courage to cope with the loved one's deteriorated health and life quality

Accept the help from the second and third tiers of support who want to:

- Attend medical appointments
- Help with chores at home
- Drop off meals or food gift cards
- Assist with transportation
- Arrange for short visits
- Spend scheduled time with the loved one
- Set up additional paid respite care
- Send cards, notes, banners, and other uplifting items
- Include the family in a prayer list
- Band together and pay for house/yard work
- Help offset other financial burdens
- Conduct a fundraiser

Realize that sometimes the loved one will want to end his/her life and obtain the necessary psychological and psychiatric interventions for him/her and the family so as to keep him/her safe

Utilize therapy to be proactive about end-of-life preparation, including "bucket lists," "unfinished business," resolving family tensions, and saying "good-byes"

Help the loved one establish a personalized legacy

Remember to incorporate self-care and adjustment strategies to cope with the impending death of a loved one:

- Minimize personal health risks
- Engage in a healthy lifestyle

Table 10.2 (continued)

Use problem-focused and emotion-focused coping skills
Avoid maladaptive coping techniques
Obtain mastery of the caregiving role
Establish social connections with others
Take respite breaks
Use personal therapy to establish meaning in life and find spiritual supports
Consider a support group, especially if relatives are struggling emotionally
Multimedia resources
Movies
My Life (Lowry et al. 1993)
Under the Piano (Grant et al. 1996)
What's Eating Gilbert Grape (Blomquist et al. 1993)
Poem
"The Friend Who Just Stands By" (Williams 2004)
Book
Final Gifts (Callanan and Kelley 1997)
Song
"Wishlist" (Vedder 1998)

emotions (American Psychological Association 2012; Moore 2005; Power and Dell Orto 2004; see Chap. 2, Sect. 2.4.1). Psychoeducation should be balanced with encouragement and emotional support, so as to avoid anxiety and numbness (Buchholz 1990).

One useful tactic for the therapist is to introduce the primary caregiver and support network to pertinent nomenclature about their complex emotional responses. This boosts the insight and appreciation of the commonality of their experiences. Some authors have described *anticipatory grief,* whereby the bystander support network witnesses and expects the death of the loved one (Aldrich and Peterson 2010). It constitutes sorrow and mourning before the actual death, heightened concern for the loved one, rehearsal of the death, and sometimes attempts to adjust to the ramifications (Aldrich and Peterson 2010; Worden 2009). This is a complex phenomenon, yet does not take the place of postloss grief (Aldrich and Peterson 2010; Worden 2009).

With anticipatory grief, acceptance commonly alternates with denial of the realities (Worden 2009). Psychotherapy can assist the caregiver and relatives in exploring this phenomenon. It helps families to understand that denial is a refusal to accept change, loss, and finality in reaction to feelings of vulnerability and powerlessness (see Power and Dell Orto 2004, for a review). Communication about the death and dying process may also be actively avoided by the loved one and support network for a variety of reasons, including fear, embarrassment, ambivalence, or awkwardness (see Planalp and Trost 2008, for a review). Many opt not to discuss the reality of the situation in an attempt to protect the loved one from bereftness (Planalp and Trost 2008). However, the concept of denial is complex. Some have proposed that hope is a coping strategy that can be mistaken as denial (Benkel et al. 2010). It provides a temporary mental refuge from the grieving process (Benkel et al. 2010). Others have cautioned that denial can be a misdiagnosis for normative grief and conflict, severe psychological fragility, as well as cultural and religious practices that focus on curative hope and/or prohibit discussion of death and dying (Weiner and Roth 2006).

The relatives also need assistance with *emotional preparedness,* defined as the degree the support network is ready for the loved one's death (Hebert et al. 2006, 2008a). Health-care professionals may be remiss in preparing the support network (and loved one) for the impending death and the bereavement process (Barry and Prigerson 2002). Separation anxiety, emotional detachment, or overinvolvement in anticipation of losing the loved one can be prominent (Kutner and Kilbourn 2009; Worden 2009). Understandably, the caregiver may wish that the loved one would die so as to minimize his or her pain, but then feel guilt ridden that he or she is abandoning him or her (Aldrich and Peterson 2010; Worden 2009). There are psychological wanderings and wonderings about how life will be without the loved one (Aldrich and Peterson 2010; Khalili 2007; Worden 2009). Afterwards, the caregiver may be overcome with survivor's guilt (Adelbratt and Strang 2000).

Therapists, including social workers, are adept at assisting in this regard, including teaching adaptive coping methods to manage debilitating emotions and acting as a liaison between different health-care providers (Hebert et al. 2008a). Subcomponents of emotional preparedness are the *cognitive* or knowledge dimension, which encompasses the medical (e.g., prognosis), practical (e.g., community resources), psychosocial (e.g., family conflict), and religious/spiritual information; the *affective* aspect (e.g., mental and emotional preparation); and *behavioral* factors (e.g., specific tasks that need to be completed; Hebert et al. 2009). Again, cultural beliefs and practices influence emotional preparedness (Hebert et al. 2006). In essence, good communication concerning dying and bereavement helps the support network manage their uncertainties and prepare for the approaching death of the loved one (Hebert et al. 2006, 2009).

The psychotherapist can play an integral role in assisting the children of the loved one in the grieving process, whether using his or her clinical skills or involving a properly trained mental health specialist. The adult relatives should not underestimate their children's perceptiveness about impending death (Goodman et al. 2007). The therapist and family should provide support and education based on the children's developmental phase and emotional readiness (Goodman et al. 2007; Khalili 2007; Smith 2007). Nonetheless, they may need clarification about the permanency of the loved one's condition and eventual death, as well as the normalcy of painful feelings of loss (Black and Hogan 2006; New York University Child Study Center 2006). Excluding children from the dying and ritual process can result in their own creation of potentially inaccurate and destructive explanations (Smith 2007).

The family (and patient) may want supportive counseling that the loved one's decision to stop aggressive treatment is not "giving up," but instead is an understandable appraisal of his or her medical status (Stark-Vance and Dubay 2011). There may be tensions or conflicts between the loved one and various family members about the treatment possibilities (Black and Hogan 2006). In this case, a trained psychotherapist, social worker, or hospital ethics committee members are fitting resources to consult with to work through feelings of sadness, guilt, or blame (Black and Hogan

2006). A reassuring tenet for Western cultures is to follow the wishes of the loved one, who is entitled to personal choices and dignity in dying (American Psychological Association 2012; de Pentheny O'Kelly et al. 2011; Kutner and Kilbourn 2009). In other societies (e.g., Latino, Asian, and Muslim), the family has more input and decision making and tends to shield the loved one; thus, treating professionals should be mindful of cultural diversities (American Psychological Association 2012; de Pentheny O'Kelly et al. 2011; Kreling et al. 2010).

Psychotherapy can help the primary caregiver and tier supports appreciate their influential role in providing comfort to the loved one, merely with their presence (Aldrich and Peterson 2010; Sherwood et al. 2004a). This is vital given that dying is considered the loneliest life event (Yalom 2009). This has been termed *presencing* or "fellow travelers," whereby the support network's unwavering company and sensitivity provides comfort, connection, security, hope, and spiritual support (Nixon and Narayanasamy 2010; Olsson et al. 2010; Yalom 2009). The movie, *My Life* (Lowry et al. 1993) depicts the primary caregiver's (Bob's wife, Gail) and his parents' unwavering presence and support as the loved one nears the end of his life. The same principle applies to the psychotherapist who is assisting the loved one and family face the illness and dying process. The poem, "The Friend Who Just Stands By" by Williams (2004) symbolizes being at peace with the helpless feeling of sideline support, yet fulfilling the role of active listening (Khalili 2007).

The family will have to draw on their inner patience and courage to cope with the loved one's deteriorated health and life quality (Aldrich and Peterson 2010). Relatives also provide physical comfort, for example, keeping the loved one at home and creating a serene ambience (Sherwood et al. 2004a). The patient will require reassurance that his or her immediate needs will be addressed by the loyal caregiver, including minimizing pain and discomfort (Aldrich and Peterson 2010). The book, *Final Gifts* (Callanan and Kelley 1997) is a valuable resource which conveys how the loved one prepares the support network for his or her death. The authors stress the importance of gaining "nearing death awareness" through an attuned kinship, so as to decipher the loved one's communications, feelings, and requests (Callanan and Kelley 1997).

The second and third tier of supports, namely extended family, friends, connections through religious affiliations, and even coworkers, are important companions and sounding boards, also to one another (Black and Hogan 2006; Power and Dell Orto 2004; Schmer et al. 2008; see Chap. 1, Sect. 1.3). In the movie, *Under the Piano* (Grant et al. 1996), the brother-in-law, Nick's and nanny, Mrs. Syms' compassionate support of Rosetta's autistic behaviors relieves some of the load for Franny, her dedicated primary caregiver. This is significant, as Rosetta's mother, Regina, cannot remain attuned, succumbing to disillusionment and depression. The loved one and primary caregiver should realize that there could be surprises in who steps up; at times close allies become too overwhelmed and seemingly "strangers" will be more responsive (Black and Hogan 2006). The character, Becky, in the film, *What's Eating Gilbert Grape* (Blomquist et al. 1993) is a newcomer who accepts Arnie's autism by respecting and ultimately joining Gilbert's consuming requirements as a tier 1 caregiver.

There are a number of ways that second and third tiers of support can provide critical backup, including to: attend medical appointments as an advocate; help with chores around the house; drop off meals or food gift cards; assist with transportation; arrange for short visits; spend scheduled time with the loved one; set up additional paid respite care; send cards, notes, banners, and other uplifting articles; include the family in a prayer list; band together and pay for house and/or yard cleaning and home maintenance projects; pay for certain household needs when financial strain arises; conduct a fundraiser to help pay for expensive treatments, etc. (Aldrich and Peterson 2010; Black and Hogan 2006; Bradley et al. 2007; Sherwood et al. 2004a).

One potentially startling realization is when the loved one's fear of the unknown manifests as imploring the caregiver to assist in ending his or her life (Aldrich and Peterson 2010). The wish for suicide can also be caused by fear of encumbering the family; anxiety concerning uncontrollable pain; loss of personhood, life meaning, and dignity; and depression (Aldrich and Peterson 2010; see the American Psychological Association 2012, for a review). Psychotherapy can assist the caregiver in explaining to the loved one that this is not a viable option, with an emphasis on reassuring him or her that he or she is not an onus, but a gift, and restating that the priority will be to help with a tranquil transition (Aldrich and Peterson 2010; Sherwood et al. 2004a). The relatives may also need to take precautions if they are worried that the loved one is suicidal due to distress over his or her impending demise (Aldrich and Peterson 2010). Keeping the environment safe (e.g., controlling medications and access to weapons) as well as immediately notifying health-care professionals (including psychiatry) are necessary precautions in these instances (Aldrich and Peterson 2010; see also Chap. 4, Sect. 4.6.2).

Ideally, if the family is in treatment with the psychotherapist during the terminal phases of the illness, he or she can assist them in being proactive about end-of-life preparation. A case in point, the psychotherapist and other professionals should appeal to the support network to address "unfinished business," resolve family tensions, and say "good-byes" (American Psychological Association 2012; Barry and Prigerson 2002; Kutner and Kilbourn 2009; Worden 2009). Without this, there can be a festering of hostility and self-blame, creating a "double burden" (Power and Dell Orto 2004). This includes not postponing crucial conversations related to gratitude and forgiveness, as well as the sharing of joyful experiences, especially as there is no clear timeline or advance warning as to when the loved one will lose the capability to communicate (Aldrich and Peterson 2010; Khalili 2007; Kutner and Kilbourn 2009). Therapy can guide the loved one and support network to create and accomplish their respective "bucket lists" of dreams, specifically related to personal and familial values. The song, "Wishlist" (Vedder 1998) aptly symbolizes this process. The movie, *My Life* (Lowry et al. 1993) poignantly portrays the loved one (i.e., Bob Jones) fulfilling a "bucket list" item of making amends with his parents and brother, thereby "putting his house in order" and finding love, forgiveness, well-being, gratitude, and peace. Ultimately, he proclaims, "dying is a hard way to learn about life" (Lowry et al. 1993).

Helping the loved one establish a legacy is vital and can take various forms, based on the preferences of the loved one. Psychotherapy can support the primary caregiver (and loved one), so that personalized and meaningful mediums are chosen and implemented. These can include photographs, video recordings, letters, etc. This expression becomes especially salient when the loved one is leaving behind children and close family members (e.g., a heart-broken spouse). The movie, *My Life* (Lowry et al. 1993) illustrates the power of videography both for working through the cancer victim's existential issues and for leaving a tangible self-representation for his young baby and wife. The loved one can also share his or her legacies with the support network (American Psychological Association 2012). Positive communication has a salutary effect and diminishes postdeath conflict and regrets (Barry and Prigerson 2002; Worden 2009). Acceptance of the inevitability of death is liberating, humanizing, and life enhancing and galvanizes the relatives (and loved one) into living authentically (Wong and Tomer 2011).

As reflected throughout this book, self-care and adjustment strategies for the tier 1 caregiver are mandatory for maximizing his or her capacity to tend to the loved one. Specific guidance in the context of coping with the terminal aspects of illness include: minimize personal health risks (e.g., lifting or moving the patient); engage in a healthy lifestyle (e.g., exercise, balanced diet, regular sleep, and following medical advice); use problem-focused coping skills (e.g., psychoeducation, setting attainable goals, requesting help as needed) and emotion-focused coping skills (e.g., cognitive behavioral methods, humor, appropriate outlets for a range of emotions, such as journaling, art, prayer, and meditation); avoid maladaptive coping techniques (e.g., substance abuse); master the caregiving role; connect socially with others (including the loved one); take respite breaks; and engage in personal psychotherapy to address meaning and spirituality (Collins and Swartz 2011; Khalili 2007; Kutner and Kilbourn 2009).

The psychotherapist may suggest a support group (in person, phone, or Internet) for relatives struggling with impending death of a loved one (Barry and Prigerson 2002; Collins and Swartz 2011; Schubart et al. 2008; Sherwood et al. 2004a). These venues provide options for trouble shooting; emotional solace; and a shared experience in the face of deep losses (Sherwood et al. 2004a; also see Chaps. 9 and 11).

10.2 Scenario: Positive Aspects of Caregiving

This section will summarize positive aspects of caregiving, whether or not the loved one has a short or long life span due to his or her neurological condition. Families may ask questions such as: *How can I learn to appreciate my role as a caregiver? How can I (and my loved one) benefit from this process?*

10.2.1 Overview of the Positive Aspects of Caregiving

Although considerable clinical and research material is devoted to the strains of caregiving, there are indications of positivity, enhanced growth, and empowerment linked to this praiseworthy undertaking (Kutner and Kilbourn 2009; Wells et al. 2005). A more in-depth analysis indicates that usually there is dissonance from coexisting positive and negative thoughts and feelings (Ayalong 2004; Goodman

Table 10.3 "Helpful hints" and tools in fostering the positive aspects of caregiving

The psychotherapist will assist relatives in identifying and cherishing the positive aspects of caregiving by:
Using an attitude of mindfulness
Creating a "mattering list"
Recognizing the positive and sustaining aspects of their mission
Remembering that sensitive and compassionate caregiving counteracts reciprocal suffering
Cultivating adjustment as well as personal and existential growth through good values, wisdom, purpose, meaning, and fulfillment
Seeing how contributing to something larger than oneself breeds happiness
Noticing how giving hones the relatives' sense of self and identity
Appreciating the admirable attributes that develop, including:
Increased drive
Self-reliance
Coping skills
Resourcefulness
Mastery
Confidence
Empowerment
Problem-solving skills
Competency
Self-esteem and pride
Emotional satisfaction and well-being
Grittiness
Realigning and prioritizing values and life goals
Grasping that tending to the loved is an honor and privilege
Witnessing their richer spirituality
Appreciating the concept of "rippling" on the societal level
Multimedia resources
Movies
My Life (Lowry et al. 1993)
What's Eating Gilbert Grape (Blomquist et al. 1993)
Marvin's Room (Brody et al. 1996)
Under the Piano (Grant et al. 1996)
Book
A Farewell to Arms (Hemingway 2012)

et al. 2007; Strang and Strang 2001). Predeterminants of a positive adjustment to caregiving include role modeling and early experiences with providing informal care (Ayalong 2004).

10.2.2 "Helpful Hints" and Tools in Fostering the Positive Aspects of Caregiving

Table 10.3 delineates "helpful hints" and tools in fostering the positive aspects of caregiving. The therapist can assist the relatives in identifying and cherishing the positive aspects of caregiving through an attitude of *mindfulness*. This entails meeting and intentionally attending to each moment of life with full awareness and without judgment of self and others (Napoli 2011; Sanderson 2010). Mindfulness promotes acceptance, flexibility, and the ability to notice our experiences (Napoli 2011; see also Chap. 1, Sect. 1.2.9). In this vein, some advocate the creation of a "mattering list" defining the beliefs and values that nourish the caregiver as well as daily reflections about positive moments (Goodman et al. 2007). Love, attachment, commitment, togetherness, finding humor, and deepened family connections with the loved one are sustaining factors in shouldering the caregiver's enormous responsibilities (Goodman et al. 2007; Khalili 2007; Linge 1990; Sand et al. 2010; Sherwood et al. 2004a). Spouses and families note improved communication and intimacy (Black and Hogan 2006; Goodman et al. 2007; Moore and Wagner 2009). The movie, *My Life* (Lowry et al. 1993) is representative of a pregnant wife's enduring love and dedication to her husband who is dying from cancer, which then spreads to the brain.

Therapy reinforces that sensitive and compassionate caregiving counteracts reciprocal suffering in the family and loved one (Goodman et al. 2007; see Kutner and Kilbourn 2009, for a review; Sand et al. 2010). Inculcation of good values, wisdom, purpose, meaning, and fulfillment furthers adjustment as well as personal and existential growth in the family (Acorn 1998; Goodman et al. 2007; see Kutner and Kilbourn 2009, for a review; Sand et al. 2010). Contributing to something larger than oneself breeds happiness (Harvard Health Publications 2011). Sense of self and identity are honed through the giving role. Some tier 1 caregivers have expressed: "I now understand the crushing pain that many people endure; it's taught me compassion and humility." "I truly understand tragedy and gratitude." "Nowadays, life has more purpose. I focus on family, doing what's right, and living each day to the fullest." "I am reforming and evolving." "God, kindness, mankind, and world peace, are what matter."

Psychotherapy can pinpoint how admirable attributes evolve, including an increase in drive, self-reliance, coping skills, and resourcefulness; mastery and confidence in skill attainment; empowerment, problem solving, and competency related to facing challenges; self-esteem and pride in accomplishments; as well as emotional satisfaction and well-being (Black and Hogan 2006; Finocchiaro et al. 2011; Goodman et al. 2007; Hassan et al. 2011; Khalili 2007; Klonoff et al. 2008; Kreutzer et al. 2010; see Kutner and Kilbourn 2009, for a review; Schmer et al. 2008; Sherwood et al. 2004b, 2008; Wells et al. 2005). "Grittiness," or the unrelenting combination of high persistence and deep passion, propels extraordinary achievement (Seligman 2011). Notably, potentially overwhelming feelings of passivity, shame, torment, guilt, loneliness, and resignation are ameliorated by embracing the roles and duties (Sand et al. 2010). The lead characters in the movies, *What's Eating Gilbert Grape* (Blomquist et al. 1993) and *Marvin's Room* (Brody et al. 1996) typify how devotion and kindness outweigh taxing commitments and self-sacrifice. Likewise, in the film, *Under the Piano* (Grant et al. 1996), Franny's loving watchfulness, vibrancy, and stick-to-itiveness optimize her autistic sister's (Rosetta's) well-being and productivity. Without her self-object, Rosetta withers and becomes suicidal.

Psychotherapy can guide the primary caregiver and family in realigning and prioritizing value-driving life aspirations (see Black and Hogan 2006, for a review;

Goodman et al. 2007). These should be formalized, including in a list form (Goodman et al. 2007). Tending to the needs of the loved one becomes an honor and privilege and the relatives feel grateful, especially when they can feasibly care for the loved one at home (Acorn 1998; Sherwood et al. 2004a). Families often report richer spirituality in the context of their strivings (Goodman et al. 2007). In essence, the caregiver benefits through forces of both altruism (i.e., attending to the loved one's well-being) and egoism (i.e., his or her own benefits, including receiving praise and respect; Sand et al. 2010).

On the societal level, positive caregiving produces *rippling* (Yalom 2009). The loving support network creates circles of good deeds which positively influence others, also expanding to future generations. Enlarging the life of others is a wonderful existential byproduct, even beyond the primary caregiver's demise (Yalom 2009). In *A Farewell to Arms,* Ernest Hemingway captured the essence of personal and communal growth in these instances, as "the world breaks everyone and afterward many are strong at the broken parts" (Hemingway 2012, p. 318).

10.3 Scenario: Grief and Mourning Reactions after the Death of the Loved One

A previous publication has defined *grief* as a process of self-dissolution related to feelings of loss and suffering (see Klonoff and Myles 2010, for a review). The counterpart of this is *mourning,* which is the reconstitution process (Klonoff and Myles 2010). The bereaved oscillate between the loss and restoration orientations (see Worden 2009, for a review). This subsection will first address grief reactions and treatment for tier 1 caregivers and other relatives after the death of a loved one. Although very applicable to brain tumor patients, the concepts and treatment recommendations are considered pertinent to coping with the loss of a loved one because of other neurological disease states or complications. The mourning process involving reconstitution will be addressed in Sects. 10.3.3 and 10.3.4. After the death of the loved one, the relatives may ask questions such as: *Why did this happen? How can I cope with this intense grief? What will happen to me and the rest of my family? How can I go on?*

10.3.1 Overview of Grief and Loss associated with Bereavement

Clearly, the emotions associated with caregiving persist after the death of the loved one (Sherwood et al. 2004a). Grief reactions are unpredictable, fluid, and vary widely for the caregiver and tier supports during the bereavement period (Connor et al. 2006; Power and Dell Orto 2004; Worden 2009).

Grief and loss reactions are predicated on a number of factors, including the kinship (i.e., the loved one's relationship with the surviving relatives—parent, spouse, etc.); strength and security of the attachment; possible ambivalences and conflicts in the relationship; and the degree of interdependency (Worden 2009; see also Chap. 3, Sect. 3.1 and Fig. 3.1). With central, strong, close, and positive relationships, the grief and loss reaction may be heightened (Power and Dell Orto 2004; Worden 2009). Coping with feelings of preventability influences the bereaving process (Power and Dell Orto 2004). The surviving family members' prior experiences with death and coping styles affect the grief and loss process, especially when there is prior entrenched depression or unresolved issues (Worden 2009). Social variables also affect grief reactions, as isolation and alienation can intensify the grief process (Worden 2009). Other factors which influence the grief and loss process are the degree of diversified role involvements as well as ethnic and religious subcultures which have predetermined rituals (Klass and Chow 2011; Worden 2009).

10.3.2 "Helpful Hints" and Tools for Families to Cope with Grief and Loss during Bereavement

Psychotherapy can be integral to the family's ability to cope with grief and loss throughout the illness continuum, including after the death of the loved one (Tepper 2003). Table 10.4 summarizes "helpful hints" and tools for families coping with grief and loss during bereavement. Grief and loss therapy can be provided in an individual or group format, including peer support and the Internet (Gilbert and Horsley 2011; Worden 2009). One model advocates sending a sympathy card to the family, signed by all team members (Tepper 2003). Objectives of counseling include increasing the reality of the loss; helping with the psychic pain; assisting with readjustment; and finding the balance of a bond with the deceased loved one while reinvesting in life (Worden 2009). This includes a joint therapeutic exploration of the nature of the relationship and emotional reactions in the primary caregiver and various family members toward the deceased loved one. For instance, often there is unreality regarding the death, resulting in numbness (Worden 2009). This is exemplified in the movie, *The Descendents* (Boyd et al. 2011), whereby the husband, Matt, expresses alarm and dismay at the unexpected death of his wife from a traumatic brain injury, especially as he is now thrust from the role of the "backup understudy" into the role of the primary parent.

Some family members fight the belief that the loved one has died (Worden 2009). This denial usually pertains to the facts or meaning of the loss (Worden 2009). Manifestations of denying the facts include holding onto the loved one's physical belongings or environs for the long term (Worden 2009). Perceiving the loss of the individual as less valuable than it was is a form of denial of meaning, as minimizing the impact becomes a form of self-protection (Worden 2009). This latter form of denial is often linked to conflicted relationships (Worden 2009). Not feeling can also be a form of self-protection to avoid overly painful and disturbing emotions (Worden 2009). Denial is a form of avoidant emotional coping which provides only temporary solace (Worden 2009). The caregiver and support network will need time to accept the loved one's death on both the intellectual and emotional level and can be characterized by alternating between belief and disbelief (Worden 2009).

Table 10.4 "Helpful hints" and tools for families to cope with grief and loss during bereavement

Therapy can be provided in an individual or group format with the goals of:
Increasing the reality of the loss
Helping with psychic pain
Assisting with readjustment
Finding the balance of a bond with the deceased loved one while reinvesting in life
Sometimes, family members may deny that the loved one has died due to emotional struggles
Therapy can help the relatives actualize the loss and cope with multiple emotions, including sadness, anger, blame, helplessness, withdrawal, loneliness, guilt, self-hatred, and regrets
When the death is unexpected, there may be a sense of "unfinished business" and meaninglessness:
Expect heightened anxiety and helplessness
Second and third tiers of support can feel powerless and relations may become strained
Helpful therapy tools for complex emotions and to encourage the family to:
Share meaningful symbols
Engage in journaling and writing
Role-play anxiety-provoking situations
Use cognitive restructuring
Compile a memory book
Resolve issues through direct imagery
Work through feelings using metaphors
Expect feelings of desolation about the whereabouts of the loved one and helpful strategies are to:
Use stories or other resources to carve a personal view of life after death
Envision how the loved one would want the surviving relatives to find a forward course
Rely on support networks of friends, coworkers, extended family members, and religious leaders
Explore the role of faith and spirituality
Grief reactions reverberate throughout the entire family system and family therapy will address its unique factors:
Employ positive sharing to change dysfunctional patterns
Recognize and respect diverse grief reactions
Reorganize roles
Reinvest in a new family constellation while connecting to the deceased loved one
Create and value personalized group rituals, ceremonies, and legacies
Children have multiple reactions and specialized needs related to the death of a loved one and the therapist will propose ideas:
Foster a sharing environment
Use careful listening and honest responding
Encourage the expression of feelings in a safe, quiet, and private place
Grant permission to grieve without unnecessary boundaries
Normalize their concerns
Provide reassurance about stable parenting
Reinforce adhering to regular routines
Promote friendships and social activities
Teach coping skills
Help to construct positive memories of the loved one
Tune into their distress
Correct misunderstandings
Expect temporary behavioral problems and regressions
Watch "adult" discussions about death
Be proactive about professional guidance

Table 10.4 (continued)

Use age-appropriate multimedia resources that take into account the children's intellectual capacity, emotional readiness, and distress level
Utilize spiritual and religious traditions as a reassuring framework
Sometimes, selected caregivers or family members experience symptoms of complicated grief, including delayed, masked, or exaggerated grief reactions
Seek in-depth psychotherapy and possibly psychiatric interventions for complicated grief with the goals of:
Identifying underlying extended grief factors
Reviving memories of the deceased loved one
Addressing affective reactions (or lack thereof)
Changing unhelpful negative thought patterns
Acknowledging the finality of and integrating the loss
Designing a new life
Improving social relationships
Multimedia resources
Movies
The Descendents (Boyd et al. 2011)
P.S. I Love You (Finerman et al. 2007)
We Bought a Zoo (Deason et al. 2011)
Play
Rabbit Hole (Lindsay-Abaire 2006)
Books
ABC's of Healthy Grieving (Smith 2007)
A Decembered Grief: Living with Loss While Others are Celebrating (Smith 2011)
The Next Place (Hanson 1997)
Where Did Papa Go? (Laufer 2012)
I Don't Have an Uncle Phil Anymore (Pellegrino 1999)
Samantha Jane's Missing Smile (Kaplow and Pincus 2007)
Black Jack Jetty (Carestio 2010)
Complicated Grief: Scientific Foundations for Health Care Professionals (Stroebe et al. 2012)
Grief and Bereavement in Contemporary Society: Bridging Research and Practice (Neimeyer et al. 2011)
Grief Counseling and Grief Therapy (Worden 2009)
Songs
"Sweetness Follows" (Berry et al. 1992)
"If You Could See Me Now" (Kipner et al. 2012)
Website
Pertaining to children's grief and loss: www.aboutourkids.org/families/helping_kids_cope

For the family to actualize the loss, the therapist will counsel them to delve into the specifics of the loss and the aftermath (Worden 2009). The relatives may need to be encouraged to visit the gravesite or wherever the remains are housed to reduce the feeling of unreality (Worden 2009). Common emotions in the survivors are sadness, anger, guilt, helplessness, and loneliness (Power and Dell Orto 2004; Worden 2009). Expression and experience of sadness, including crying, should be validated as part of the psychotherapeutic process (Worden 2009). Anger may be turned inward and become depression or displaced outwards as blame. There can be rage toward outsiders as a counteraction to feelings of powerlessness and disorder (Worden 2009). The psychotherapist can help the family explore these feelings by asking open-ended questions, for example: *What do you miss about your loved one?* (Worden 2009).

Some caregivers and relatives struggle to adapt to the loss of the loved one (Worden 2009). This can manifest as helplessness, withdrawal, and abdication of daily responsibilities (Worden 2009). The play, *Rabbit Hole* (Lindsay-Abaire 2006) conveys the layers, untidiness, senselessness, and uncertainties during the grief and loss process for a mother whose young son was killed. The role of profound guilt and self-condemnation in creating self-hatred, misery, loneliness, and estrangement from other friends and family is dolefully portrayed in this storyline and can be a useful resource to share with families who are experiencing the same anguish.

Feelings of guilt may be exacerbated as the caregiver torments himself or herself with questions of "if only," feeling that somehow he or she should have done more on behalf of the loved one. Talk therapy can unearth irrational expectations (Worden 2009). Another helpful concept for addressing paralyzing guilt is "hindsight is 40/40," underlining the energy depletion associated with nonproductive self-recriminations (Klonoff 2010).

Regrets often abound after the death of the loved one. This is another form of "what ifs" and "if onlys" (Aldrich and Peterson 2010). Research indicates that often caregivers are remorseful about not being adequately prepared to manage their loved one's symptoms (Schubart et al. 2008). Due to stresses, time may be spent in the latter stages of the loved one's life in acrimonious exchanges with him or her or select members of the support group. The song, "Sweetness Follows" (Berry et al. 1992) captures the individual's inner conflict when grudges and alienation contaminate end-of-life communications. The family may also be regretful about not expressing enough of their love and appreciation for the loved one before he or she became too ill to grasp the sentiments (Aldrich and Peterson 2010). Alternatively, the caregiver may be disappointed about not fulfilling his or her last wishes (Aldrich and Peterson 2010). The film, *P.S. I Love You* (Finerman et al. 2007) captures a wife's feelings of desolation, loneliness, alienation, regret, and life disarray after her husband dies from a brain tumor. It also reflects how deep grieving is accentuated when others in one's environment are enjoying life achievements and joy, including weddings and births.

The relatives may have a sense of "unfinished business" and meaninglessness of the event due to the unexpectedness of the death (Worden 2009). This can cause heightened anxiety and helplessness (Worden 2009). The second and third tiers of support can feel powerless to comfort the primary caregiver, who because of his or her deep suffering, may be easily infuriated, defensive, and sometimes envious of others' fortunes. Relations become strained and outsiders may withdraw, avoid, or conceal news, especially if they feel guilty regarding positive experiences in their own lives. This tendency is captured in the play, *Rabbit Hole* (Lindsay-Abaire 2006), whereby the grieving mother's sister is reticent to share that she is pregnant.

Therapy tools to address the complex emotions of grief and loss include: encouraging the family to share special symbols (e.g., pictures, letters, audiotapes, etc.); engaging in journaling and writing, including a farewell letter; drawing pictures; role-playing anxiety-provoking occurrences; cognitive restructuring to reduce distortions and overgeneralizations; compiling a memory book of memorabilia; resolving issues through directed imagery; and working through feelings using metaphors (Worden 2009). The book, *ABC's of Healthy Grieving* (Smith 2007) is a user-friendly tool encompassing many usable adages for the grieving process. A few pithy examples include: respect individual differences in grieving within the family; take baby steps; expect tough days and nights; find a safe place to grieve; finish unfinished business; know one's limitations; and remember, ritualize, and symbolize the grief process, together with cherishable memories (Smith 2007). Another beneficial resource for grief and loss is *A Decembered Grief: Living with Loss While Others are Celebrating* by Smith (2011).

The bereaved family's distress may be from desolation concerning the whereabouts of the loved one. The book, *The Next Place* (Hanson 1997) gives the relatives solace that the loved one is in a place of serenity, comfort, and peace. Other therapeutic reminders to diminish grief reactions are to envision how the loved one would want the surviving relatives to find a forward course; reliance on support networks of friends, coworkers, extended family members, and religious leaders; and exploration of the role of faith and spirituality (Aldrich and Peterson 2010; Park and Halifax 2011; Schmer et al. 2008). The song, "If You Could See Me Now" (Kipner et al. 2012) communicates the imagined dialogue with the deceased loved one (selfobject) bestowing delight about the surviving relatives' achievements (see also Chap. 1, Sect. 1.2.2 for a discussion of self-psychology concepts).

Grief reactions reverberate within the entire family system and can disrupt family functioning (Kissane and Hooghe 2011; Power and Dell Orto 2004; Worden 2009). Factors affecting the family system's homeostasis include the functional significance, position, and role of the deceased relative as well as the degree of emotional integration of the family (Worden 2009). Other positive antecedents are cohesiveness in the family as well as supportive family members and outside networks (see Worden 2009, for a review). Family therapy is advantageous for assisting families grappling with a deepened understanding of themselves, based on their unique constellations (Kissane and Hooghe 2011). Dysfunctional patterns can be addressed with an intent of positive sharing (Kissane and Hooghe 2011). The family unit will need to recognize and respect diverse grief reactions; reconfigure roles; and reinvest in a new family constellation while staying connected to the deceased (see Worden 2009, for a review). Creating and valuing personalized and group rituals and ceremonies as well as legacies unify the family in their grief (Lewis and Hoy 2011; see Worden 2009, for a review).

For children, the death of a loved one creates a "primary loss" because of the physical absence and "secondary losses" or "ripple effects," including a reduced sense of security; a shaken sense of purpose and faith; and an altered self-view and family position (New York University Child Study Center 2006). Childhood reactions to the death of a loved one are plentiful and include: sadness, crying, irritability, acting out, bullying, academic difficulties, decreased interest and withdrawal from daily activities, longing for the loved one, fears, anxiety, panic, sleep disturbance, denial, resentment, self-blame, guilt, physical concerns and complaints, sensitivity to failure or rejection, and the need to protect and help the family and minimize conflicts (Black and Hogan 2006; New York University Child Study Center 2006). The movie, *We Bought A Zoo* (Deason et al. 2011) captures many of the above signs of emotional turbulence in two children whose mother has recently died.

The therapist will propose certain ideas to the parents so as to enhance the children's coping capacity, which include: develop a sharing environment, based on careful listening and honest responding; encourage the open expression of feelings by providing a safe, quiet, and private place; grant permission to grieve without unnecessary boundaries; normalize their concerns; provide reassurance about a stable parenting presence; continue routines; promote their friendships and social involvements; teach coping skills, including avoiding "taking out" negative feelings on others; help to construct positive memories of the deceased loved one; tune into the child's distress; correct misunderstandings; and expect temporary behavioral problems and regressions (Black and Hogan 2006; New York University Child Study Center 2006; Smith 2007; Worden 2009). In the movie, *We Bought a Zoo* (Deason et al. 2011), the father, Benjamin, gradually inculcates these practices, which are reinforced by the friendships and "new story" created at this unique setting. They all learn that "the secret to talking is listening."

The therapist will caution the parent and relatives to monitor the nature and amount of adult conversations on the subject of death; resist expecting children to fulfill adult roles; and monitor unhealthy coping behaviors (e.g., substance abuse and risky behaviors; New York University Child Study Center 2006). Professional input should be accessed whenever warning signs arise (New York University Child Study Center 2006).

Potential resources for grief-struck children are picture books, doll play, simple analogies (e.g., pets or flowers), and soothing actions (e.g., cuddling, singing) for very young children (aged 2–3); explanation of objects and concepts in relation to the loved one's medical status, including play using a "doctor kit" in children aged 4–5; interactive communication that is concrete using diagrams, books, movies, and a family album for children aged 6–7; and reality-based dialogue, including their questions and feelings concerning the expected outcome with children aged 8 and older (Goodman et al. 2007; New York University Child Study Center 2006). Several books are useful adjunct therapeutic tools, including: *Where Did Papa Go?* by Laufer (2012); *I Don't Have an Uncle Phil Anymore* by Pellegrino (1999); *Samantha Jane's Missing Smile* by Kaplow and Pincus (2007); and *Black Jack Jetty* by Carestio (2010).

All interventions should take into account the children's intellectual capabilities, emotional readiness, and distress level (Goodman et al. 2007). Spiritual and religious traditions can be a reassuring framework to address their ambiguous thoughts and emotional distress (Black and Hogan 2006; Goodman et al. 2007). For more information on age-specific reactions and guidelines for children coping with the death of a loved one, see New York University Child Study Center (2006) and www.aboutourkids.org/families/helping_kids_cope.

At times, the caregiver or selected family members experience complicated grief (Kutner and Kilbourn 2009; Shear et al. 2011; Worden 2009). A detailed discussion of this phenomenon is beyond the scope of this book. In essence, *complicated grief* is a complex and controversial entity and has also been referred to as prolonged grief (Worden 2009). It tends to be connected to extended duration and difficulty with the mourning or reconstitution process (Kutner and Kilbourn 2009; Shear et al. 2011; Worden 2009). It has been associated with a "fixation" in grief and an inability to "let go" (see Roos 2002, for a review). An impasse occurs between the intellectual acknowledgment of the loss and an emotional denial of its reality (see Roos 2002, for a review). The relative often feels overwhelmed and "frozen" (see Roos 2002, for a review). Other signs and symptoms of complicated grief are intense longing, preoccupation with thoughts and memories of the loved one, entrenched sorrow, bitterness, joylessness, life stagnation, withdrawal, abdication of daily obligations, moodiness, distrust, and suicidal thoughts (Kutner and Kilbourn 2009; Shear et al. 2011).

Possible contributors to complicated grief are profound loss, usually manifested as depression, hopelessness, and worthlessness; preexisting psychiatric dysfunction; ambivalent feelings about the loved one; and high dependency needs (Kutner and Kilbourn 2009; Worden 2009). Sometimes, there are delayed grief reactions; a contributing factor is being too overwhelmed by the loss to grieve sufficiently (Worden 2009). Other times, the caregiver may experience masked grief, whereby feelings of loss are not expressed overtly (Worden 2009). The grief may then be manifested in physical illness. The relatives may also experience exaggerated grief reactions which can lead to profound depression and despair; anxiety disorders (e.g., panic attacks or phobias); posttraumatic stress disorder; as well as serious alcoholism or other substance abuse (Worden 2009).

In these situations, in-depth psychotherapy and possibly psychiatric interventions are urged (see Kutner and Kilbourn 2009, for a review; Shear et al. 2011; Worden 2009). Treatment goals involve: identifying underlying factors for extended grief; reviving memories of the deceased; addressing affective reactions (or lack thereof); changing unhelpful negative thought patterns; acknowledging the finality of and integrating the loss; designing a new life; and improving social relationships (Shear et al. 2011; Worden 2009). Therapeutic procedures include the Gestalt technique of "empty chair" (whereby the survivor speaks to the deceased by imagining he or she is sitting in the chair); role-playing psychodrama (where the relative plays himself or herself and the deceased loved one in order to resolve a conflict); homework (e.g., letters to the deceased); dream analysis; and seeking ways to honor the legacy of the loved one (Shear et al. 2011; Worden 2009). For a more in-depth discussion of this phenomenon and treatment methodologies, see *Complicated Grief: Scientific Foundations for Health Care Professionals* by Stroebe et al. (2012); *Grief and Bereavement in Contemporary Society: Bridging Research and Practice* by Neimeyer et al. (2011); and *Grief Counseling and Grief Therapy* by Worden (2009).

10.3.3 Overview of Mourning and Adjustment after the Death of a Loved One

Mourning or emotional reconstitution encompasses the assimilation of new feelings into an altered worldview, self-redefinition, life reintegration, transcendence, self-transformation, and reconstruction of meaning (see Klonoff 2010, for a review). It is a healing and rebuilding process (Power and Dell Orto 2004). Worden (2009) postulates three areas of adjustment after the death of a loved one. *External adjustment* refers to different living arrangements, roles, and skills that the family embraces due to the death of the loved one (Worden 2009). *Internal adjustments* pertain to the tier 1 caregiver's sense of self, including self-definition, self-esteem, and self-efficacy

Table 10.5 "Helpful hints" and tools for families to cope with mourning and adjustment after the death of a loved one

Psychotherapy will facilitate finding an enduring connection with the deceased loved one while embarking on a new life course
The psychotherapist will assist with "emotional relocation," or creating an appropriate and healthy place for the deceased loved one in their lives, including reminiscing about him/her
The therapist can assist with practical problem solving and decision making
The survivor may benefit from outside resources for education and support
Be careful about making sudden major life changes
Realize that the mourning process doesn't "finish"
With time, there is a gradual adjustment to a life without the loved one
The family will have to create meaning in the loss
The mourning process will enable a "lightening" of the grief
Multimedia resources
Movies
P.S. I Love You (Finerman et al. 2007)
We Bought a Zoo (Deason et al. 2011)
Books/stories
The Dance (Evans 1999)
The Invisible String (Karst 2000)
"Birthday Box" (Yolen 1997)
Grief Recovery Handbook (James and Friedman 2009)
Play
Rabbit Hole (Lindsay-Abaire 2006)

(Worden 2009). This is understandable, especially when there was a strong and secure tie to the loved one (Worden 2009). *Spiritual adjustments* pertain to a subjective view of the world, life assumptions, personal values, and philosophical beliefs (Worden 2009). The surviving family member may initially feel that he or she is being punished for being unworthy and/or that the world is void of benevolence (Worden 2009). Over time, the relatives reformulate a perspective that incorporates the fragility of life and limits of their control (see Worden 2009, for a review).

10.3.4 "Helpful Hints" and Tools for Families to Cope with Mourning and Adjustment after the Death of a Loved One

Psychotherapy for the caregiver and support network can be a salvation to assist with the mourning and adjustment process after the death of the loved one. Table 10.5 summarizes "helpful hints" and tools for families to cope with mourning and adjustment after the death of a loved one. On occasion, the caregiver and close family members will be desperate to find an enduring connection with the deceased loved one, while still trying to embark on their new lives (Worden 2009). Examples include speaking to, thinking and dreaming about, as well as feeling watched by the loved one who has died (Worden 2009). For children, this can be particularly reassuring.

The psychotherapist will guide the bereaved relatives in creating an appropriate and healthy place for the deceased loved one in their lives, yet live an effective and meaningful life (Worden 2009). This is called *emotional relocation* (Worden 2009). It includes integrating the deceased loved one's influences, values, and inspirations into existing lifestyles and relationships (Worden 2009). Contextualizing loss creates a familial, cultural, and human continuity (McGoldrick 1991).

One psychotherapeutic process for integrating the loved one's death is to invite the family to reminisce about the deceased loved one, as this allows a divestment of the emotional energy (Worden 2009). The stories, *The Dance* by Evans (1999), *The Invisible String* by Karst (2000), and *Birthday Box* by Yolen (1997) adeptly and touchingly illustrate this process of the metamorphosis from absence, emptiness, paralyzing fear, and heartache to a promising future which still encompasses fond memories and heartening influences of the deceased loved one. In the film, *P.S. I Love You* (Finerman et al. 2007), Holly's husband functions as her internalized and sustaining self-object in the face of overwhelming sorrow. There is a gradual and eventual letting go of this strong attachment that had precluded her capacity to truly live in the present, including forming new relationships. Sharing these resources with the mourning caregiver and family can be healing.

As part of the coping process, the psychotherapist may need to assist with day-to-day problem solving and decision making with the surviving caregiver (Worden 2009). This is especially necessary when the survivor is a spouse who was not responsible for complex daily decisions (Worden 2009). The survivor may need referrals to outside resources for education and support (e.g., a social worker, financial planner, etc.). The family should be cautioned regarding making sudden major life changes soon after the death of a loved one (New York University Child Study Center 2006; Worden 2009).

Often, the caregiver, other relatives, or outsiders are impatient for the mourning process to "be over with." The therapist can inform the bereaving family that mourning is never "finished." Instead, wrenching pain evolves into the dull ache of missing the loved one. There is a regained interest in life activities, the experience of hope and gratification, and gradual adjustment to a life without the presence of the loved one (Worden 2009). The play, *Rabbit Hole* (Lindsay-Abaire 2006) also depicts the metamorphosis of the mourning process. The metaphor of the "brick in the pocket" exemplifies the transformation process of desolation into something more bearable, yet ever present.

Inherent in the mourning process is creating meaning in the loss. The therapist can assist in this process by encouraging the bereaved relatives to find their personal answers to the loved one's death. Unanswerable "whys" must be explored (Power and Dell Orto 2004). There is exploration of their sense of the loss and creation of fresh directions and aspirations (Worden 2009). Looking backwards facilitates moving forwards (Power and Dell Orto 2004). When the therapist encourages the sharing of mementos and vignettes, the working relationship is bolstered and the therapist better comprehends the family's phenomenological stance (Klonoff and Koberstein 2010). In the movie, *We Bought a Zoo* (Deason et al. 2011), Benjamin purchases a zoo as an adventure and diversion to lessen the pain associated with his wife, Katherine's untimely death. He also memorializes Katherine by pondering over pictures and divulging stories to his children.

The *Grief Recovery Handbook* by James and Friedman (2009) provides techniques and vignettes to assist with recovering from grief. Overall, the mourning process enables a "lightening" of the grief, with some recalibration of expectations and hopes about the loved one (Roos 2002). The relationship with the deceased loved one is recasted, with a shifting focus to positive and comforting memories (Roos 2002). With outside emotional support, customs and traditions, and a memorialization process, the surviving family members ultimately achieve emotional calm and peacefulness (Roos 2002). For further discussion of the existential aspects of the caregiving and grief and loss process, see also Sect. 10.4.

10.4 Scenario: Existential Considerations for the Caregiver and Support Network after Brain Injury

Illness and death pose multiple existential and practical considerations with which the patient must contend (Olsson et al. 2010). It is empowering for the loved one to exert influence over his or her state of affairs, including communicating about life and death, finding meaning, striving for normality, preparing for death, and taking responsibility for the future of his or her family (Olsson et al. 2010). Examples include: the loved one preparing for his or her own funeral, composing thoughts and sentiments, and viewing pictures (Olsson et al. 2010). Hope is preserved through a dual process of sustaining life and preparing for death (Olsson et al. 2010). Tier 1 caregivers and the other tier supports undergo a tandem process and may be propelled into an existential crisis related to the loved one's illness, injury, or death, which also reverberates through the whole support network. Soul searching may raise many questions such as: *Why is this happening? Isn't life supposed to be fair? What is the meaning of my life now? Where has my hope gone?*

10.4.1 Overview of Existential Considerations for the Caregiver and Family after Brain Injury

Caregiving transforms the family in numerous ways existentially when the assumptive world of justice, predictability, comfort, and security vanish (Janoff-Bulman 2002; Landsman 2002; Roos 2002). The "taken-for-granted" realities are uprooted (Neimeyer and Sands 2011). Through fate, the relatives are beset with pervasive sorrow, due to an existence characterized by unfairness, betrayal, and alienation (Roos 2002). Life-altering traumas catalyze anguish, confusion, and life disorientation (Roos 2002). Specifically, the support network battle with: disappointment and disillusionment about cherished expectations and dreams; core aloneness and disconnection (including from the loved one); dyscontrol and helpless fragility; inequity (based on the myth that fairness and goodness will prevail); personal obscurity and insignificance; and personal mortality (Roos 2002). Lifestyle collapse can engender a sense of meaninglessness (Sand et al. 2010; Triplett et al. 2011). One relative described her plight as "I feel cheated. I remember the comfortable arrogance of thinking I could protect my kids—I was so naïve. My world will never quite be the same. It's filled with real darkness and real suffering, not just imagined."

The caregiver and family will contend with *ambiguous loss,* symbolized by the profound alterations in the loved one which are apparent for the long term (Boss 2006; Boss et al. 2011). There is a lack of closure and others may not officially acknowledge the loss (Boss et al. 2011). *Chronic sorrow* or pervasive sadness emanates from living losses (Boss et al. 2011; see also Chap. 3, Sect. 3.3 and Chap. 9, Sect. 9.5.1 for more discussion of these topics). Strains cause family members to suffer from *soul sickness* or demoralization, characterized by existential despondency, hopelessness and helplessness, as well as loss of meaning and purpose in life (Clarke and Kissane 2002; Perakis 2010). The caregiver can feel psychologically impotent, trapped, and generally incompetent (Clarke and Kissane 2002; Perakis 2010). Internal and external stresses seem exorbitant and there is a proclivity to "check out" of life (Perakis 2010). Self-esteem and coping skills wane and life seems pointless (Clark and Kissane 2002).

Engel (1968) described a "giving-up–given-up" condition, which captures many of the above symptoms, as well as a depreciated self-image; impoverished relationships and roles; and fractured continuity between the past, present, and future. When the current pressures reactivate prior unresolved crises, the caregiver can feel at his or her "last straw" of accumulated stressors (Engel 1968).

10.4.2 "Helpful Hints" and Tools for the Caregiver and Family to Cope with Existential Challenges after Brain Injury

Table 10.6 summarizes "helpful hints" and tools for the caregiver and family to cope with existential challenges after a loved one's brain injury. Through psychotherapy, efforts should be undertaken with the family to make sense of the loved one's neurological illness, predicated on a restructuring of daily life and core beliefs (Roos 2002; Schubart et al. 2008). This holistic therapeutic process should incorporate existential and spiritual considerations (Clarke and Kissane 2002; Strang et al. 2001). The therapist will need to be mindful of the depth of turmoil (Roos 2002; Strang et al. 2001) and gently guide the family through this psychologically perilous journey using a multiplicity of techniques and tools, individualized to the relatives' predicament. Given the gravity of this process, the clinician should be heedful of his or her countertransference reactions, which can manifest as becoming dismissive and avoidant of such deep introspections (Clarke and Kissane 2002; Klonoff 2011).

Families will inevitably grapple with abundant existential questions such as the role of G-d, punishment, and randomness in the universe as causal agents in the loved one's and family's suffering (Roos 2002; Strang and Strang 2001). Triplett and colleagues (2011) describe a metacognitive process of *deliberate rumination,* whereby the individual reflects on his or her position, reconstructs an assumptive world, and experiences posttraumatic growth. In actuality, death of a loved one

Table 10.6 "Helpful hints" and tools for the caregiver and family to cope with existential challenges after a loved one's brain injury

The psychotherapist will assist relatives in making sense of the loved one's neurological illness
The turmoil can be deep and the predicament is unique to each individual
Existential questions include the:

- Role of G-d
- Punishment
- Randomness in the universe

Psychotherapy consists of "deliberate rumination," incorporating social and cultural beliefs as well as values
An "unlived" life can be transformed into an enriched and fulfilled existence
Venting of fears and worries helps with feelings of vulnerability
Adaptive and practical coping strategies include:

- "One day at a time"
- "Enjoy the moment"

Legal proceedings may counteract feeling unfairly wronged
Accept that suffering and unfairness abound
Feelings of insignificance can be reframed based on the vital role of caregiving
Sometimes, pursuing other life interests boosts self-worth and life satisfaction
Structured daily routines are beneficial
Strive for a purpose-driven existence
Therapy can address feelings of mortality and also provides effective resources for the loved one's well-being
Finding meaning in life requires reorientation and reconstruction of the family's existence
Therapy can combat feelings of aloneness
Explore religion and spirituality as possible sources of guidance
"Ambiguous loss" and "chronic sorrow" can be addressed by the techniques of:

- Encouraging the narrative or storytelling process
- Treating the family system
- Teaching dialectical thinking
- Seeking forgiveness for root causes of loss
- Doing small good works
- Incorporating social rituals
- Finding positive attributions for events
- Recognizing sacrifices for the greater good

The search for meaning is predicated on embracing life values, including togetherness, quality of life, and hope
Therapy can assist the family in adopting a revision of hope by:

- The search for "silver linings"
- The therapist's empathic presence and resonance
- Symptom relief
- Reminders for good physical and mental health
- Collaborative discovery of new possibilities
- Teaching personal power and mastery through creativity, spirituality, and positive relations
- The support network developing patience and being realistic about the loved one's circumstances

Misery is ameliorated by rebuilding self-esteem through incremental victories and mastery of the stressors using:

- Psychoeducation
- Behavioral changes
- Coping skills training
- Cognitive restructuring techniques

Table 10.6 (continued)

Principles of positive psychology that are instrumental to the existential transformation are to:
Focus on positive emotions and strengths of character, including hope, love, passion, gratitude, curiosity, and resiliency
Promote wisdom, knowledge, competency, courage, justice, temperance, and transcendence
Display a cheerful disposition, positivity, and autonomy
Belong to a community
Discover "learned optimism" for reaching potentials and living boldly
Find a "new normal"
Take personal responsibility for actions
Reframe guilt and shame
Reduce feelings of stigma
Enhance problem-solving and decision-making skills
Apply tenets of positive psychology to children and to societal endeavors
Develop positive morale in the family unit
Construct a worthwhile future predicated on celebrating rites of passage (versus crisis markers of past devastating events)
Inculcate a fighting spirit to increase the family unit's coherence, comprehensibility, and manageability of their situation
Multimedia resources
Film/television broadcast
"Helping Others" chapter in the documentary, *Happy* (Shadyac et al. 2011)
"Separated" (Goldberg 2012)
Books
What Doesn't Kill Us (Joseph 2011)
Posttraumatic Growth in Clinical Practice (Calhoun and Tedeschi 2013)
When Bad Things Happen to Good People (Kushner 1981)
Flourish (Seligman 2011)
Learned Optimism (Seligman 2006)

catalyzes the survivors' soul searching, in part to fill the void (Jacobson 2004). The family's social and cultural beliefs and values are often instrumental in providing a life compass (Roos 2002; Triplett et al. 2011). Yalom (2009) suggests that the awareness of urgent life events and death catalyze an awakening for the possibility of constructive life modifications. For the support network (and loved one), an "unlived life" can be transformed into an enriched and fulfilled existence (Yalom 2009). The adage "If you wait until you find the meaning in life, will there be enough life left to live meaningfully?" (Lubavitcher Rebbe 2012) beautifully expresses the principle of cognitive reframing to optimize "living life." The consequence can be embracing a more purposeful and meaningful existence filled with goodness (Jacobsen 2004). The books, *What Doesn't Kill Us* by Joseph (2011) and *Posttraumatic Growth in Clinical Practice* by Calhoun and Tedeschi (2013) are excellent resources to further explore the transformational constructs associated with posttraumatic growth.

Coping with feelings of vulnerability is a challenge. The therapist should endorse healthy "venting" of fears and worries, which naturally originate from uncertainty about the future (Roos 2002). Adaptive and practical coping strategies to preserve the caregiver's emotional resources for the long haul are paramount (Roos 2002), such as promoting the attitude of "one day at a time" and "enjoying the moment" (Khalili

2007; Klonoff 2010). Possible antidotes for feelings of being unfairly wronged are legal proceedings, although these are not always successful (Roos 2002). Therefore, justice must be redefined (Boss 2006). In truth, suffering and unfairness abound, and the therapeutic process can assist the family in integrating this harsh reality or else bitterness can become entrenched (Boss 2006; Roos 2002). The story of the Chinese woman seeking the mustard seed to assuage her grief and misfortune in *When Bad Things Happen to Good People* (Kushner 1981) is a fine reminder of this painful realization.

The therapeutic process can assist the caregiver in combating feelings of insignificance by reframing his or her central role as a caregiver, including his or her compassion, courage, and devotion when ministering to the loved one (Roos 2002). Protective instincts are galvanized, so as to manage the pressures, reduce powerlessness, and preserve the loved one's dignity (Sand et al. 2010; Strang and Strang 2001; see also Sect. 10.4 on Positive Aspects of Caregiving). Alternatively, when needed, the primary caregiver should be induced to pursue other life interests and callings to boost his or her self-worth and life satisfaction (Roos 2002). Creating daily routines becomes important life symbols (Sand et al. 2010). A purpose-driven existence promotes psychological well-being and life satisfaction (Seligman 2011; Triplett et al. 2011).

The loved one's illness or death is a reminder of everyone's mortality. The therapist should explore the worries and fears in this regard with the caregiver. Oftentimes, the primary caregiver is petrified about the loved one's care needs if he or she outlives this lifeline (Roos 2002). The therapist can be a key source of resource information and referrals to be sure that the loved one's best interests will be accounted for outside of current arrangements. (For more discussion on this topic, see Chap. 11, Sect. 11.5.1).

To regain meaning in life, the tier 1 caregiver and tier supports will need to accept their circumstances, adapt to a novel reality, and transcend suffering (Klonoff and Koberstein 2010; Klonoff et al. 2008; Neimeyer and Sands 2011; Perakis 2010). Reorientation and reconstruction of the family's existence creates emotional satisfaction (Klonoff et al. 2008; Lezak 1986). Therapeutic dialogue can facilitate the internal search for a redefinition of hopes, dreams, and expectations, as well as core beliefs and values (Bowen et al. 2010; Roos 2002; Sand et al. 2010; Triplett et al. 2011). Facing illness and death imbues a zest for life and hence strivings for a more authentic existence (Adelbratt and Strang 2000). Primary caregivers have the conscious free will to take active responsibility, which entails putting self-interests aside, surmounting fears, and doing their best for the family unit (see Sand et al. 2010, for a review).

To combat aloneness, therapy can help the family address feelings of abandonment and cruelty by a higher power and hopefully fashion new spiritual connections (Roos 2002). Fortified and special relationships with others and a sense of belonging are also crucial, especially when frivolous preoccupations are abandoned (Clarke and Kissane 2002; Roos 2002). The chapter, "Helping Others," in the documentary, *Happy* (Shadyac et al. 2011) beautifully conveys how a banker, Andy, rejects an empty career and moves to Calcutta to help the dying. He eloquently describes his enlightenment of acceptance and tolerance through joining a mission so much bigger than himself.

Relearning life's dimensionality requires accepting the loss of the prior assumptive world and acquiring new constellations (Attig 2002). The psychotherapist can respectfully suggest religion and spirituality as possible sources of guidance for this renewed life vision. Familiar religious traditions inherent in formal organized faith reduce chaos through providing structure and comfort (McColl et al. 2000; Strang and Strang 2001). Spirituality means "looking outwards at the world, upwards at a higher power and inwards at the self" (McColl et al. 2000, p. 555). Worthy manifestations of this broader connection are meditation, retreats, communing with nature, chanting and singing, and listening to music (Attig 2002). From these spiritual endeavors flows an abundance of positive emotions, including joy, forgiveness, compassion, and gratitude (Vaillant 2008).

Rediscovering meaning in life usually necessitates accepting ambiguous loss and chronic sorrow (Boss 2006; Boss et al. 2011). Therapy should validate the losses; strengthen the capacity to live with loss and uncertainty; normalize mixed emotions; and reconstruct identity (Boss et al. 2011). Psychotherapeutic activities include: encouraging the narrative or storytelling process; treating the family system (including group therapy); teaching dialectical thinking (i.e., the person is gone, yet present); seeking forgiveness of root causes of loss; doing small good works; incorporating social rituals; finding positive attributions for events; and recognizing sacrifices "for the greater good" (Boss 2006).

The search for meaning means truly embracing life values, including togetherness, quality of life, and hope (Boss 2006; Klonoff et al. 2008; Linge 1990; Sand et al. 2010; Strang and Strang 2001). *Hope* can be defined as the belief in a future good, with the expectation that suffering will cease (Boss 2006). After a brain injury, hope represents longing for better things (Linge 1990). As Martin Gray said, "The secret of life is the power of hope" (Gray 2006, p. v). Integral to the reconstitution process is the reinstallation of hope (Clarke and Kissane 2002; Linge 1990; Perakis 2010). However, the family system will have to adopt a revision of hope and relinquish the status quo (Boss 2006; Boss et al. 2011; Bowen et al. 2010). Relatives will need to project themselves into the future and imagine more opportunities than currently exist (Buchholz 1990). Hope means transforming and transcending bleakness (Boss 2006). It creates purposeful behavior for coping with dark times, including pessimism, anxiety, aloneness, and fear (Buchholz 1990).

The psychotherapist's task is to help the caregiver without hope find it (Boss 2006). For some, meaning reconstruction is personified in a quest for "silver linings" (Neimeyer and Sands 2011; see also Chap. 2, Sect. 2.4.2.4). The practitioner can facilitate this process through empathic presence and resonance, symptom relief, reminders for proper physical and mental care, collaborative discovery of new possibilities, as well as teaching personal power and mastery through creativity, spirituality, and positive relations (Boss 2006; Buchholz 1990; Clarke and Kissane 2002; Hassan et al. 2011; Neimeyer and Sands 2011; Perakis 2010). Other guidelines include the support network developing patience and being realistic about one's circumstances (Boss 2006). This has also been described as "moving forward in the fog" (Boss 2006), as the caregiver must imagine new alternatives and become comfortable with ambiguity (Boss 2006).

Misery is also ameliorated by rebuilding self-esteem through incremental victories and overcoming stressors; personal morale is then restored (Clarke and Kissane 2002; Perakis 2010). Psychoeducation; behavioral interventions (e.g., problem solving and goal setting); coping skills training toward adaptation (e.g., role and activity diversification); and cognitive restructuring techniques (e.g., addressing cognitive distortions and exploring global meaning) are essential (Clarke and Kissane 2002; Klonoff and Koberstein 2010; Perakis 2010). Gradually, with time, healing, and psychotherapeutic guidance, this psychological crossroad is navigated and a psychological equilibrium can be reestablished (Engel 1968).

The therapist can draw from positive psychology, as this field contributes prominent constructs related to existential transformation in the face of life traumas associated with the caregiving role (see also Chap. 1, Sect. 1.2.9). For the relatives, it focuses on positive emotions (e.g., happiness and fulfillment) as well as strengths of character, including hope, passion, gratitude, and curiosity (Kobau et al. 2011; Peterson 2009). The attributes of engagement, vitality, and self-determination will also engender a flourishing life (Seligman 2011). Ultimately, tier supports can create a more gratifying existence, recognizing that there are unlimited personal paths to choose from (Peterson 2009). Therapy should reiterate the centrality of other people, giftedness, life satisfaction, and optimism (Peterson et al. 2008b). The resource, *Flourish* by Seligman (2011) thoughtfully explores the vital elements that enable positive well-being and human flourishing.

Resiliency has been defined as the ability to "stretch," "flex," or "thrive" in the face of life's strains and adversities (Boss 2006; Yalom 2009). It is typified in Nietzsche's adage "that which does not kill me makes me stronger" (see Yalom 2009, for a review). Resiliency applies to the personal level as well as to the family system, and even the community (Boss 2006). Instilling resiliency is imperative, as this quality underlies posttraumatic growth; allows improved relationships with others; creates openness to new possibilities; accesses a deeper appreciation of life; and enhances personal strength and spirituality (Joseph 2011; see Peterson et al. 2008a, for a review; Seligman 2011). The positive dispositions of creativity, bravery, kindness, tenacity, and optimism feed resiliency (Kobau et al. 2011). For children, the therapeutic objective of increasing resiliency is predicated on reinforcing close attachment relationships for youngsters as well as encouraging sharing of feelings, beliefs, and reactions in older offspring (New York University Child Study Center 2006). The family environment should be supportive, attentive, and safe with consistent parenting styles and an emphasis on strong values and a positive outlook (New York University Child Study Center 2006).

Other strengths that the therapist can reinforce are wisdom, knowledge, competency, courage, justice, temperance, and transcendence (Seligman and Peterson 2003). These are manifested in a cheerful temperament, positivity, interest in and belonging to a community, as well as autonomy (Perakis 2010). Personal narration or storytelling, with an emphasis on a sense of agency (versus victimhood), is an effective strategy to identify and build personal strengths (Seligman and Peterson 2003). The story of Jen Bricker in the broadcast, "Separated" (Goldberg 2012), who was born with no legs, is one such example. It depicts her inner qualities of drive, authenticity, perseverance, and purpose in the face of her life predicament.

The psychotherapist can also promote *learned optimism,* so that the family avoids "thinking traps," remains calm, focused, and keeps things in perspective (Kobau et al. 2011). Learned optimism sustains the caregiver and family in their quest and dismantles depressive and anxious reactions (Seligman and Peterson 2003). The psychotherapist can help the caregiver transform feelings of helplessness, hopelessness, and amassed regrets into personal responsibility, choices, preferences, accomplishments, and efficacy (Seligman and Peterson 2003; Yalom 2009). This breeds self-realization of reaching potentials and living boldly (Yalom 2009). The book, *Learned Optimism* by Seligman (2006) skillfully delves into the practice of this construct as a fundamental underpinning of quality of life.

For family members with a loved one with a serious neurological diagnosis or terminal illness, resiliency spawns a "new normal" (see Moore and Wagner 2009), enabling different roles, lifestyle modifications, newfound coping and advocacy strategies, and also survivorship skills (Moore and Wagner 2009). The psychotherapist can assist the caregiver and family in taking personal responsibility for their actions; reframing guilt and shame; reducing feelings of stigma; and enhancing problem-solving and decision-making skills to augment family pride (Boss 2006). The psychotherapist can also incorporate similar tenets from positive psychology for the parents to apply to children coping with grief and their own existential disquiet. This includes building resiliency through teaching persistence as well as achievement-directed behavior (Peterson 2009). On the societal level, therapy can encourage family members to find social connections and build community bonds through shared endeavors (Boss 2006; Judd and DeBoard 2009; Klonoff and Koberstein 2010). This includes the second and third tiers of support (see also Chaps. 9 and 11 for positive group experiences).

The psychotherapist can introduce the concept of morale, based on positive psychological principles, as this relates to the cognitions, emotions, and motivations of a group (Peterson et al. 2008b), including a family unit. It subsumes qualities of confidence, optimism, enthusiasm, loyalty, resiliency, trust and respect, moral rightness in one's undertakings, and common purpose (Peterson et al. 2008b). In troubled times, assisting the family in understanding and building its strengths and virtues becomes even more of a priority (Seligman and Peterson 2003). One effective exercise is to encourage family members to journal and/or discuss daily sources of gratitude, as this fosters a mindful approach to positivity. Consequently, helping the family develop and maintain positive morale in the context of the many threats and stressors is a product of therapeutic interventions.

Overall, psychotherapy can help the primary caregiver and family construct a worthwhile future, which is predicated on celebrating rites of passage which are progress based, rather than crisis markers of past devastating life events (Roos 2002). This requires a positive and forward-thinking mindset. A "fighting spirit" is cultivated, which increases the family unit's sense of coherence, comprehensibility, and manageability of the circumstances and existential dilemmas (Linge 1990; Strang and Strang 2001).

10.5 A Continuation of the Chap. 7 Case Study

David's neurological health was stable for approximately 18 months. He was followed up by his neuro-oncologist who conducted regular magnetic resonance imagings (MRIs) every 4 months. However, gradually, both Heather and David noticed increased symptoms. He began having more seizures. A repeat MRI showed new tumor growth in the frontal gyri, extending into the thalamus. Heather and David both contacted Dr. Smithe and a consultation was arranged in short order.

David was aware of memory lapses, citing forgetting to listen to voice mails on his phone. Both he and his wife provided a severity rating of 4–5/10 (1 = small; 10 = large; see also Chap. 2, Sect. 2.2.1.1 and Table 2.4). Other difficulties and severity ratings stated by them were: attention and concentration (= 6/10); multitasking (= 7/10); preplanning (= 4/10); and feeling overwhelmed (= 5/10). During the interview, David admitted to some periods of depression and helplessness. He had been instructed by his neuro-oncologist to stop driving and staying alone with his children, Troy and Brittany, due to the increased frequency of seizures. Heather also described her own observations of worrying changes in David, including lack of initiative, poor judgment and problem solving, as well as increased "snarkiness" and insensitivity to her needs. She also felt he was withdrawing from her and the children, spending more time isolated in his bedroom and sleeping. With respect to work, David had noticed sizeable ineptitudes. He felt physically and mentally exhausted after 2 h of work in his office handling real estate deals. He also saw an increase in his errors on spreadsheets. He had created a large backlog of work and he was placed on medical leave by his employer.

Dr. Smithe could empathically sense the distress and panic in David and Heather. She posed several ideas, including restarting marital psychotherapy and repeat neuropsychological testing, in order to gain an up-to-date appraisal of David's cognitive and emotional status. Dr. Smithe proposed that the emphasis of treatment be on monitoring mood and adjustment; functionality in the home; and quality of life, with a pragmatic emphasis. Both David and Heather were very relieved to reengage the therapeutic process with Dr. Smithe, shedding simultaneous tears of joy for the support and sorrow over the frightening circumstances.

Repeat neuropsychological testing confirmed a decline in David's neuropsychological profile compared with prior testing approximately 2 years before. Affected areas were verbal learning and recall as well as executive functions, including complex attention, planning, problem solving, and multitasking. Dr. Smithe carefully reviewed the test findings, again using the bell curve (Chap. 4, Sect. 4.2.1). Personality testing revealed that David was much more depressed than on his previous examination. He was tense, irritable, and very preoccupied with his situation. He was pessimistic about the future and fearful about the uncertainty of his health and life span.

Although this confirmatory evidence was unsettling, all parties realized the benefit of this new feedback in helping David and Heather cope with their new dilemmas. A decision was made to stop work entirely and David was placed on short-term and then long-term disability. Dr. Smithe assisted David and Heather in recalibrating compensations, including closer monitoring of medications and increased note taking in his smartphone to keep track of daily events. Both David and Heather were very amenable to twice-weekly "milieu meetings" at home together, given all of the stressors (see Chap. 4 Sect. 4.4.4). Given David's angst, his psychiatrist, Dr. Brown, advised an increase in his sertraline dose to 150 mg per day. At David's request, the family took a long weekend vacation to a beach house. This afforded crucial and meaningful time together, alternating between heartfelt discussions and lighthearted family events, including board games and water sports for the children.

As David's health worsened, Heather initially assumed substantial duties as his tier 1 caregiver. This included all of the transportation and extracurricular program needs of Troy and Brittany; carrying the bulk of the responsibility for disciplining the children; assuming the totality of household bill paying and finances; and closer physical monitoring of him in the home (from increased seizures and fall risk). Heather found herself needing to oversee some of his email correspondence, due to difficulty with thought formulation and bluntness. She was experiencing an overwhelming combination of role discontinuity, role conflict, and role overload! However, "milieu meetings" proved to be beneficial in helping David structure productive time with Troy and Brittany, secondary to his increasing struggles with decision making, judgment, "black-and-white" thinking, and cognitive rigidity. This included making sure that Troy completed all of his homework before playing video games with his father and identifying mutually enjoyable activities to share with Brittany, including scrapbooking their recent vacation.

Although Heather had lived for months in a constant apprehensive state of "when the tumor regrows," she found herself experiencing considerable dread and feelings of powerlessness now that the day had come. Susan, Heather's sister, urgently began researching possible cures, some of which entailed long-distance travel for second opinions at other hospitals. David oscillated between "death anxiety," characterized by moroseness and fear versus hopefulness that a last-minute miraculous cure would be found. A follow-up appointment with the neuro-oncologist just 3 weeks later indicated that the tumor was spreading rapidly and was now affecting the corpus callosum and brainstem. The doctor recommended a biopsy, which David consented to.

Prior to this procedure, at the suggestion of Dr. Smithe, David and Heather called a "family meeting," which Susan and David's brother, Joseph, attended as they were both strong tier 2 supports of David and Heather. Troy and Brittany witnessed a portion of the discussion, especially related to an update of David's health and his stated desires of how to prioritize quality-of-life activities with them. During the dialogue, Susan was advocating transfer of care to another facility which was doing experimental research. However, Heather and David took a more conservative approach, preferring to stay with the current treatment team and remain in town to be available to their children. On behalf of Troy and Brittany, they wanted to keep routines and a semblance of order in the household. At Dr. Smithe's urging, she set up outside counseling for Troy and Brittany, as their perceptiveness was catalyzing emotional distress and an inability to focus on homework.

Fortunately, based on the prior psychotherapy with Dr. Smithe when David was first diagnosed, Joseph had assisted David and Heather in constructing advance directives. A living will was in place, including a DNR and a desire for no life-saving equipment, opting for comfort care. Heather had been identified as the durable power of attorney for finances, and with Joseph's assistance, some preparation had occurred, including life insurance policies and lucrative investments. Based on the counseling with Dr. Smithe and their embracement of the realities of the situation, they were preparing for a "good death."

Postprocedure, the neuro-oncologist and neurosurgeon met with the family and at Dr. Smithe's urging, they audiorecorded the discussion for later reference. The findings of the biopsy were sobering as the tumor was now considered a grade 4 and had tripled in size from June to July. The physicians reviewed options, including radical surgery, restarting chemotherapy, or radiation. A fourth possibility was also proposed—not doing any invasive treatment and transferring to palliative care. The name of a competent and compassionate social worker was provided to David and Heather, should they decide to pursue this path. David and Heather were of course devastated by the news. In the interim, Dr. Smithe had initiated dialogue with the neuro-oncologist so that she could be well informed regarding David's tumor regrowth prognosis.

In their next session with Dr. Smithe, they reviewed the "big picture" of David's condition and grappled with choices. Dr. Smithe had already gingerly laid the groundwork of candid dialogue and the session was productive with respect to David and Heather understanding the reality of his limited life span and imminent death. They constructed "best and worst" case scenarios of treatment and prolonging David's life. Everyone was working together in the best interest of David. Thankfully, David and Heather had considered this path and both of them knew they did not want to pursue any more aggressive treatment at the point he could not communicate his needs or feed himself. They wanted to involve hospice and allow David to die within the loving ambience of his own home. They contacted the social worker and also reached out to the pastor of their Unitarian Universalist church, both of whom were extremely accommodating and supportive. David was also followed up by Dr. Browne during this transition, who carefully monitored his mood. After brainstorming with Dr. Smithe, David and Heather called another "milieu meeting" with the children and shared the news. Susan and Joseph were also informed and Susan reluctantly abandoned her search for life-saving remedies.

David and Heather still had a strong church and friend support network. They jumped into action, helping with transportation for Troy and Brittany; dropping off meals; running errands; and constructing a prayer list. At Dr. Smithe's suggestion, people took turns sending small cards and letters to David with inspirational sayings. These tokens were also very meaningful to Heather. With encouragement, Heather also pursued other personalized spiritual outlets, including meditation and consoling music.

Heather continued to meet with Dr. Smithe and she alternated between empathic responsiveness and psychoeducation. Together they explored Heather's "anticipatory grief," which encompassed the spectrum of denial to urgent anguish when imagining a future without David. Dr. Smithe assisted with emotional preparedness, including helping Heather with practical decision making concerning David's needs, particularly with his physicians vis-à-vis pain management. Sessions also focused on coping mechanisms for Heather's emotional distress, including relaxation therapy, private meetings with her church pastor, and reliance on her extended family for emotional and hands-on support. Themes of the appointments were "presencing, dignity, meaning, quality of life, and legacy," which helped Heather carve a role and purpose. Dr. Smithe commented to David and Heather how impressed she was with their tenacity, humor, heart, grace, and courage in the face of such troubling circumstances. Throughout David's dying process, Dr. Smithe reinforced the importance of Heather's self-care, encouraging her to continue her yoga exercises and attendance at a family support group, as well as eat healthfully, and not run herself ragged. Together with her closest friends, Heather created a quilt (i.e., healing blanket) embedded with pictures of family and friends. This provided huge solace to David and by extension for Heather. They both drew on the love and compassion from their support network. Heather's friendships and connection to Dr. Smithe also helped sustain her through this perilous journey.

David's status was going downhill. At his request, he met privately with Dr. Smithe, asking that afterwards his wife join the appointment. At that time, David oscillated between vague hopefulness and "what ifs," ultimately deciding he wanted to be sure to complete the remaining items in his "bucket list." With supportive guidance, he was able to tearfully articulate to Heather that he wanted to emphasize quality time with his family and to die with dignity. Dr. Smithe referenced the song, "Wishlist" (Vedder 1998) as symbolic of this opportune process. David desired to begin sharing his feelings with those people who mattered most to him. However, he was befuddled as to how to accomplish this, given his fatigue and cognitive deficits. He was also emotionally overwrought. Dr. Smithe recommended that David and Heather collaborate to accomplish this together. Calmly and lovingly, they reviewed some mediums, including writing letters, as well as creating photo albums and videos. David and Heather quickly got this process underway, both realizing that time was slipping away.

David was suffering from excruciating headaches, vomiting, and numbness in his left leg. Hospice nurses began in-home services, including training Heather and respite assistance so that she could attend to more of the children's needs. That included meeting with the school counselors with Troy and Brittany present to update the school personnel regarding David's neurological deterioration. Extended family and close friends encompassing additional second and third tiers of support were invited over for short, yet genuine exchanges and good-byes. David spontaneously expressed feeling so indebted to Heather for giving him the opportunity to reminisce and express his gratitude to those he valued. He even resolved some old regrets and conflicts, which now seemed so incidental. He felt he was getting his life in order and was preparing to die in a manner that felt authentic, liberating, and peaceful.

At home, Heather facilitated dialogue between David and their children. She wanted to be sure there was no "unfinished business" related to parting sentiments. She helped David write cards to their children, including for their upcoming and future birthdays. They also created "messages in a bottle" by putting endearing expressions of meaning and love into paper towel tubes which would be dispensed in later times after David's death. Heather made sure to find time in the day when David was strong and alert enough to interact with the children. Heather often overheard David giving advice, yet conveying his eternal love. She was completely devoted to providing comfort, love, and security for David. This helped to combat her feelings of inadequacy and misery.

As a tangible symbol of empathy, Dr. Smithe gave Heather a copy of the poem, "A Friend Who Just Stands By" by Williams (2004), which she read to David and the children. As David's state worsened, Dr. Smithe offered to make home visits. During one of the last visits, with Heather's permission, Dr. Smithe gave Troy and Brittany a copy of the book, *The Next Place* by Hanson (1997). Heather reported she often saw her children reading this book together, sometimes to David. Two weeks later, David lapsed into a coma. Dr. Smithe continued to visit the home, providing comfort to Heather, Troy, and Brittany. Susan and Joseph were often present, providing for the family's needs by running errands and making meals. Three days later, David died. His immediate family was by his side.

Heather and her family launched into preparing the memorial service, which she called "a celebration of life." Given her Italian heritage, relatives came from all over and provided immense emotional and culinary sustenance. She reported she found this heartening, as it gave her an outlet for her grief energies. At the same time, she could become overwhelmed, as the totality of the decisions fell on her. She was grounded during this process by asking herself, *What would David want?* and *What's best for Troy and Brittany?* Dr. Smithe provided her with a copy of *The ABC's of Healthy Grieving* by Smith (2007), for which she was extremely appreciative.

Heather wrote the following to everyone on the memorial invitation: "Our lives will never be the same, but with much needed love and support, we will find a way to mend. Thank you for loving us." At the time of the church service, Heather invited the attendees to write any notes, memories, etc. on special note cards that were placed in a "memory box." The closing songs were "Live Like You Were Dying" (Nichols and Wiseman 2004) and "Timeless" (Jollett 2013), which were two of David's favorites. After the service, balloons were released; Troy and Brittany conceived of this idea. Everyone was discouraged away from flowers and instead to make donations to a brain tumor fund in David's name. Immediately after the service, Heather and the support network planted a tree in the backyard, with a bench and stone nearby.

After David's funeral, Heather wrote Dr. Smithe a letter with an enclosed picture of herself, David, and their children. She shared:

> Dearest Dr. Smithe:
> I want to thank you for all of the years of compassion and support for David, myself, and our family. With life's ups and downs, you were always there for us. I know David really appreciated your coming to visit him at home during his last few weeks and he smiles down on you every time we now meet. You are a blessing to our dear family.

Hospice resources were vital at that time. The children and Heather each began attending grief support groups. Susan wrestled some with regrets and second guessing, still contemplating that further treatment may have extended David's life span. Heather arranged for a conjoint meeting with Dr. Smithe involving Susan. The sisters explored their feelings about David's death, revealing stories and spilling tears. Thoughts of self-blame and "would have-should have" were reframed as respecting David's last wishes (including the family trip) and allowing him to die by his own terms and with decorum. Dr. Smithe reminded Heather and Susan of the multitude of positive attributes they had as tier 1 and 2 caregivers, including their mindfulness about David's choices; the serene ambience they had provided at home to reduce David's and the children's fears and despair; and their burgeoning sense of resourcefulness, coping, and self-reliance. Movie resources were proposed by Dr. Smithe, including *Marvin's Room* (Brody et al. 1996), illustrating the principles of devotion and kindness. The danger of "hindsight is 40/40" was portended and this also reduced Susan and Heather's guilt. Upon Dr. Smithe's advice, they met with the neuro-oncologist to resolve some of their questions. He reiterated that there was "uncontrollable growth" at the late stages of David's disease. These discussions greatly helped to alleviate their misgivings.

Incrementally, Heather was traversing the mourning and adjustment process. She considered moving versus renovating her home and Dr. Smithe cautioned her to postpone any large financial decision. She was making external adjustments and was well ensconced in the totality of her role as a parent. Her internal accommodations included feeling more secure and a sense of mastery in independently providing for the needs of her children. Her spiritual adjustment was evolving. She continued to attend church and started going to a weekly bible study group. In addition to group grief therapy, Heather engaged in several other healing activities, including journaling. This provided an outlet to grapple with the "whys" and she began to fashion a new existence without David's physical presence.

Dr. Smithe reminded Heather of the "ripple effect" of David's death on the children. Heather remained vigilant about the coping styles of Troy and Brittany. Both alternated between crying and crankiness. She constructed a book of pictures for her son and daughter, portraying special events and memories. Each child also had a collection of memorabilia and keepsakes on a shelf in their bedrooms to which they regularly returned. In order to further address their well-being, Heather met with the schoolteachers and counselor, as well as their child therapist (also with the children present) to be sure they received the requisite emotional support and boundaries. Joseph volunteered to attend Boy Scouts with Troy and play X-box with him as his father had done. Heather made sure to encourage Brittany to continue with her peer friendships and extracurricular dance activities. These "surrogate helpers" were essential to ameliorating Troy's and Brittany's deep sorrow and lonesomeness for David.

Many evenings, Heather sat with Troy and Brittany in the backyard near David's tree, sharing and exchanging thoughts and sources of grief, as well as reading stories, including "Birthday Box" by Yolen (1997) and *The Invisible String* by Karst (2000). They would read cards from the memory box and write "letters to heaven." They poured their grief into an imaginary bowl of "tear soup," which was bonding and cathartic. These experiences constituted the emotional relocation process of David and were sustaining rituals for the foreseeable future.

Heather shared with Dr. Smithe that she was "in and out of grief." She felt a void and was especially lonely for David's companionship. She was at loose ends, craving more meaning in life. Psychotherapy, attendance at her hospice grief group, and long walks with close friends helped her begin to fashion a new assumptive world. Through "deliberate rumination," she concluded that she wanted a fulfilled existence for herself and realized this was an important model for her children's posttraumatic growth. Heather began to imagine a new future, characterized by hopefulness and value-driven purpose. She contemplated returning to school to obtain an early education degree; something she could do fairly quickly, given her educational background. She was attracted to this vocation, as she loved children and recognized her natural nurturing qualities. In the spirit of the "rippling" effect (Yalom 2009), she chose to do good deeds for her community, in repayment for their generosity to her.

Dr. Smithe employed principles of positive psychology, reinforcing Heather's many admirable personality characteristics, including her patience, grit, empathy, resiliency, and optimism. Heather and her family's morale were reconstituting. They were discovering their "new normal," one that honored and memorialized David. She had faith in her "fighting spirit" to move forward and manage her challenges to the best of her abilities, while embracing new opportunities.

References

Acorn, S. (1998). The family as caregiver. In S. Acorn & P. Offer (Eds.), *Living with brain injury: A guide for families and caregivers* (pp. 155–162). Toronto: University of Toronto Press.

Adelbratt, S., & Strang, P. (2000). Death anxiety in brain tumour patients and their spouses. *Palliative Medicine, 14*(6), 499–507.

Aldrich, J. J., & Peterson, N. M. (2010). *Connecting through compassion: Guidance for family and friends of a brain cancer patient*. United States of America: Cancer Lifeline Publications.

American Psychological Association. (2012). End-of-life issues and care. http://www.apa.org/topics/death/end-of-life.aspx. Accessed 13 July 2012.

Attig, T. (2002). Questionable assumptions about assumptive worlds. In J. Kauffman (Ed.), *Loss of the assumptive world: A theory of traumatic loss* (pp. 55–68). New York: Brunner-Routledge.

Ayalong, L. (2004). Cultural variants of caregiving or the culture of caregiving. *Journal of Cultural Diversity, 11*(4), 131–138.

Bainbridge, D., Krueger, P., Lohfeld, L., & Brazil, K. (2009). Stress processes in caring for an end-of-life family member: Application of a theoretical model. *Aging & Mental Health, 13*(4), 537–545.

Barry, L. C., & Prigerson, H. G. (2002). Perspectives on preparedness for a death among bereaved persons. *Connecticut Medicine, 66*(11), 691–696.

Benkel, L., Wijk, H., & Molander, U. (2010). Using coping strategies is not denial: Helping loved ones adjust to living with a patient with a palliative diagnosis. *Journal of Palliative Medicine, 13*(9), 1119–1123.

Berry, B., Buck, P., Mills, M., & Stipe, M. (1992). *Sweetness follows* [Recorded by R.E.M.]. *On Automatic for the people* [CD]. New York: Warner Bros./WEA.

Black, P., & Hogan, S. C. (2006). *Living with a brain tumor: Dr. Peter Black's guide to taking control of your treatment*. New York: Henry Holt and Company.

Blomquist, A. C., Hallström, L., Matalon, D., Ohlsson, B., Teper, M. (Producers), & Hallström, L. (Director). (1993). *What's eating Gilbert Grape* [Motion picture]. United States: Paramount Pictures.

Boss, P. (2006). *Loss, trauma, and resilience: Therapeutic work with ambiguous loss*. New York: W. W. Norton.

Boss, P., Roos, S., & Harris, D. L. (2011). Grief in the midst of ambiguity and uncertainty: An exploration of ambiguous loss and chronic sorrow. In R. A. Neimeyer, D. L. Harris, H. R. Winokuer, & G. F. Thornton (Eds.), *Grief and bereavement in contemporary society: Bridging research and practice* (pp. 163–175). New York: Routledge.

Bowen, C., Yeates, G., & Plamer, S. (2010). *A relational approach to rehabilitation: Thinking about relationships after brain injury*. London: Karnac Books.

Boyd, T., Burke, J., Parra, G., Payne, A., Taylor, J. (Producers), & Payne, A. (Director). (2011). *The descendants* [Motion picture]. United States: Fox Searchlight Pictures.

Bradley, S., Sherwood, P. R., Donovan, H. S., Hamilton, R., Rosenzweig, M., Hricik, A., et al. (2007). I could lose everything: Understanding the cost of a brain tumor. *Journal of Neuro-Oncology, 85*(3), 329–338.

Brody, T. S., De Niro, R., Gering, C., Guare, J., Palef, B., Rosenthal, J., Rudin, S., et al. (Producers), & Zaks, J. (Director). (1996). *Marvin's room* [Motion picture]. United States: Miramax Films.

Buchholz, W. M. (1990). A piece of my mind: Hope. *JAMA: The Journal of the American Medical Association, 263*(17), 2357–2358.

Calhoun, L. G., & Tedeschi, R. G. (2013). *Posttraumatic growth in clinical practice*. New York: Routledge.

Callanan, M., & Kelley, P. (1997). *Final gifts: Understanding the special awareness, needs, and communications of the dying*. New York: Bantam Books.

Carestio, M. A. (2010). *Black Jack Jetty: A boy's journey through grief*. Washington, D. C.: Magination Press.

Clarke, D. M., & Kissane, D. W. (2002). Demoralization: Its phenomenology and importance. *Australian & New Zealand Journal of Psychiatry, 36*(6), 733–742.

Collins, L. G., & Swartz, K. (2011). Caregiver care. *American Academy of Family Physicians, 83*(11), 1309–1317.

Connor, S. R., Lycan, J., & Schumacher, J. D. (2006). Involvement of psychologists in psychosocial aspects of hospice and end-of-life care. In J. L.Werth Jr & D. Blevins (Eds.), *Psychosocial issues near the end of life: A resource for professional care providers* (pp. 203–217). Washington, D. C.: American Psychological Association.

Deason, P., Gordon, M., Harlacker, J., Herzberg, I., Panek, M., Porter, A. L., Yorn, J. (Producers), & Crowe, C. (Director). (2011). *We bought a zoo* [Motion picture]. United States: Twentieth Century Fox Film Corporation.

de Pentheny O'Kelly, C., Urch, C., & Brown, E. A. (2011). The impact of culture and religion on truth telling at the end of life. *Nephrology, Dialysis, Transplantation, 26*(12), 3838–3842.

Empeo, J., Raming, N. T. J., Irwin, S. A., Nelesen, R. A., & Lloyd, L. S. (2011). The hospice caregiver support project: Providing support to reduce caregiver stress. *Journal of Palliative Medicine, 14*(5), 593–597.

Engel, G. L. (1968). A life setting conducive to illness. *Annals of Internal Medicine, 69*(2), 293–300.

Evans, R. P. (1999). *The dance*. New York: Simon & Schuster Books for Young Readers.

Finerman, W., Flynn, J., Hollond, J., Huntsinger, J., Johnson, B., Kosove, A. A., O'Sullivan, M., et al., (Producers), & LaGravenese, R. (Director). (2007). *P. S. I love you* [Motion picture]. United States: Warner Bros. Pictures.

Finocchiaro, C. Y., Petruzzi, A., Lamperti, E., Botturi, A., Gaviani, P., Silvani, A., et al. (2011). The burden of brain tumor: A single-institution study on psychological patterns in caregivers. *Journal of Neuro-Oncology*, Oct. 4. [Epub ahead of print]. doi:10.1007/s11060-011-0726-y.

Gilbert, K. R., & Horsley, G. C. (2011). Technology and grief support in the twenty-first century: A multimedia platform. In R. A. Neimeyer, D. L. Harris, H. R. Winokuer, & G. F. Thornton

(Eds.), *Grief and bereavement in contemporary society: Bridging research and practice* (pp. 365–373). New York: Routledge.
Goldberg, B. (Reporter/Host). (2012, July 17). *Separated* [Television broadcast]. In Perskie, J. (Producer), *Real sports with Bryant Gumbel*. New York: Home Box Office.
Goodman, S., Rabow, M., & Folkman, S. (2007). *Orientation to caregiving: A handbook for family caregivers of patients with brain tumors*. San Francisco: University of California San Francisco.
Grant, T., Gray, N. J., Sullivan, K. (Producers), & Scaini, S. (Director). (1996). *Under the piano* [Motion picture]. Canada: Sullivan Entertainment.
Gray, M. (2006). *For those I loved: 35th anniversary expanded edition*. Charlottesville: Hampton Roads Publishing Company.
Hanson, W. (1997). *The next place*. Golden Valley: Waldman House Press.
Harvard Health Publications. (2011). *Positive psychology: Harnessing the power of happiness, mindfulness, and personal strength*. Boston: Harvard Health Publications.
Hassan, S. T., Khaw, W. F., Rosna, A. R., & Husna, J. (2011). Traumatic brain injury: Caregivers' problems and needs. *Journal of Nepal Medical Association, 51*(181), 53–55.
Hebert, R. S., Prigerson, H. G., Schulz, R., & Arnold, R. M. (2006). Preparing caregivers for the death of a loved one: A theoretical framework and suggestions for future research. *Journal of Palliative Medicine, 9*(5), 1164–1171.
Hebert, R. S., Copeland, V. C., Schulz, R., & Amato, C. A. (2008a). Preparing family caregivers for the death of a loved one: Implications for hospital social workers. *Journal of Social Work in End-of-Life & Palliative Care, 4*(4), 269–285.
Hebert, R. S., Schulz, R., Copeland, V., & Arnold, R. M. (2008b). What questions do family caregivers want to discuss with health care providers in order to prepare for the death of a loved one? An ethnographic study of caregivers of patients at end of life. *Journal of Palliative Medicine, 11*(3), 476–483.
Hebert, R. S., Schulz, R., Copeland, V. C., & Arnold, R. M. (2009). Preparing family caregivers for death and bereavement. Insights from caregivers of terminally ill patients. *Journal of Pain and Symptom Management, 37*(1), 3–12.
Hemingway, E. (2012). *A farewell to arms: The Hemingway library edition*. New York: Scribner.
Jacobson, S. (2004). *Toward a meaningful life: The wisdom of the Rebbe Menachem Schneerson* (new ed.). New York: HarperCollins Publishers.
James, J. W., & Friedman, R. (2009). *The grief recovery handbook: The action program for moving beyond death, divorce, and other losses, including health, career, and faith* (20th anniversary expanded ed.). New York: HarperCollins Publishers.
Janoff-Bulman, R. (2002). Foreword. In J. Kauffman (Ed.), *Loss of the assumptive world: A theory of traumatic loss* (pp. xi–xii). New York: Brunner-Routledge.
Jollett, M. (2013). *Timeless* [Recorded by The Airborne Toxic Event]. *On The secret* [CD]. Santa Monica: Island Records.
Joseph, S. (2011). *What doesn't kill us: The new psychology of posttraumatic growth*. New York: Basic Books.
Judd, T., & DeBoard, R. (2009). Community-based neuropsychological rehabilitation in the cosmopolitan setting. *Neuropsychological Rehabilitation, 19*(6), 841–866.
Kaplow, J., & Pincus, D. (2007). *Samantha Jane's missing smile: A story about coping with the loss of a parent*. Washington, D. C.: Magination Press.
Karst, P. (2000). *The invisible string*. Camarillo: DeVorss & Company.
Khalili, Y. (2007). Ongoing transitions: The impact of a malignant brain tumour on patient and family. *Axone (Dartmouth, N. S.), 28*(3), 5–13.
Kipner, S., Frampton, A., O'Donoghue, D. J., & Sheehan, M. A. (2012). *If you could see me now* [Recorded by The Script]. On *#3* [CD]. US: Epic.
Kissane, D. W., & Hooghe, A. (2011). Family therapy for the bereaved. In R. A. Neimeyer, D. L. Harris, H. R. Winokuer, & G. F. Thornton (Eds.), *Grief and bereavement in contemporary society: Bridging research and practice* (pp. 287–302). New York: Routledge.
Kitamura, C., Ng, D., Chung, A., Bezjak, A., Garraway, C., Mclean, M., Nyhof-Young, J., & Wong, R. (2011). Development and evaluation of a combined story and fact-based educational

booklet for patients with multiple brain metastases and their caregivers. *Palliative Medicine, 25*(6), 642–649.

Klass, D., & Chow, A. Y. M. (2011). Culture and ethnicity in experiencing, policing, and handling grief. In R. A. Neimeyer, D. L. Harris, H. R. Winokuer, & G. F. Thornton (Eds.), *Grief and bereavement in contemporary society: Bridging research and practice* (pp. 341–353). New York: Routledge.

Klonoff, P. S. (2010). *Psychotherapy after brain injury: Principles and techniques*. New York: Guilford Press.

Klonoff, P. S. (2011). A therapist experiential model of treatment for brain injury. *Bulletin of the Menninger Clinic, 75*(1), 21–45.

Klonoff, P. S., & Myles, S. M. (2010). Sense of self and identity. In P. S. Klonoff (Ed.), *Psychotherapy after brain injury: Principles and techniques* (pp. 75–99). New York: Guilford Press.

Klonoff, P. S., Koberstein, E. J., Talley, M. C., & Dawson, L. K. (2008). A family experiential model of recovery after brain injury. *Bulletin of the Menninger Clinic, 72*(2), 109–129.

Klonoff, P. S., & Koberstein, E. J. (2010). Family life. In P. S. Klonoff (Ed.), *Psychotherapy after brain injury: Principles and techniques* (pp. 150–170). New York: Guilford Press.

Kobau, R., Seligman, M. E. P., Peterson, C., Diener, E., Zack, M. M., Chapman, D., & Thompson, W. (2011). Mental health promotion in public health: Perspectives and strategies from positive psychology. *American Journal of Public Health, 101*(8), e1–e9.

Kreling, B., Selsky, C., Perret-Gentil, M., Huerta, E. E., & Mandelblatt, J. S. (2010). 'The worst thing about hospice is that they talk about death': Contrasting hospice decisions and experience among immigrant Central and South American Latinos with US-born White, non-Latino cancer caregivers. *Palliative Medicine, 24*(4), 427–434.

Kreutzer, J. S., Marwitz, J. H., Godwin, E. E., & Arango-Lasprilla, J. C. (2010). Practical approaches to effective family intervention after brain injury. *Journal of Head Trauma Rehabilitation, 25*(2), 113–120.

Kushner, H. (1981). *When bad things happen to good people*. New York: Avon Books.

Kutner, J. S., & Kilbourn, K. M. (2009). Bereavement: Addressing challenges faced by advanced cancer patients, their caregivers, and their physicians. *Primary Care, 36*(4), 825–844.

Landsman, I. S. (2002). Crises of meaning in trauma and loss. In J. Kauffman (Ed.), *Loss of the assumptive world: A theory of traumatic loss* (pp. 13–30). New York: Brunner-Routledge.

Laufer, J. E. (2012). *Where did papa go*? Phoenix: Little Egg Publishing Company.

Lewis, L., & Hoy, W. G. (2011). Bereavement rituals and the creation of legacy. In R. A. Neimeyer, D. L. Harris, H. R. Winokuer, & G. F. Thornton (Eds.), *Grief and bereavement in contemporary society: Bridging research and practice* (pp. 315–323). New York: Routledge.

Lezak, M. D. (1986). Psychological implications of traumatic brain damage for the patient's family. *Rehabilitation Psychology, 31*(4), 241–250.

Lindsay-Abaire, D. (2006). *Rabbit hole*. New York: Theatre Communications Group.

Linge, F. R. (1990). Faith, hope, and love: Nontraditional therapy in recovery from serious head injury, a personal account. *Canadian Journal of Psychology, 44*(2), 116–129.

Lowry, H., McDermott, K. J., Netter, G., Rubin, B. J., Zucker, J. (Producers), & Rubin, B. J. (Director). (1993). *My life* [Motion picture]. United States: Columbia Pictures.

Lubavitcher, R. (2012). Daily Quote. In Chabad.org TODAY IN JUDAISM: Thursday. http://www.chabad.org/. Accessed 11 Oct 2012.

McColl, M. A., Bickenbach, J., Johnston, J., Nishihama, S., Schumaker, M., Smith, K., Smith, M., et al. (2000). Spirtiual issues associated with traumatic-onset disability. *Disability and Rehabilitation, 22*(12), 555–564.

McGoldrick, M. (1991). Echoes from the past: Helping families mourn their losses. In F. Walsh & M. McGoldrick (Eds.), *Living beyond loss: Death in the family* (pp. 50–78). New York: W. W. Norton.

Moore, C. D. (2005). Communication issues and advances care planning. *Seminars in Oncology Nursing, 21*(1), 11–19.

Moore, T., & Wagner, S. (2009). Caregiver and family issues for brain tumor survivors. In S. Goldman & C. D. Turner (Eds.), *Late effects of treatment for brain tumors* (pp. 331–339). New York: Springer.

Napoli, M. (2011). React or respond: A guide to apply mindfulness for families and therapists. *Families in Society: The Journal of Contemporary Social Services, 92*(1), 28–32.

Neimeyer, R. A., Harris, D. L., Winokuer, H. R., & Thornton, G. F. (Eds.). (2011). *Grief and bereavement in contemporary society: Bridging research and practice*. New York: Routledge.

Neimeyer, R. A., & Sands, D. (2011). Meaning reconstruction in bereavement: From principles to practice. In R. A. Neimeyer, D. L. Harris, H. R. Winokuer, & G. F. Thornton (Eds.), *Grief and bereavement in contemporary society: Bridging research and practice* (pp. 9–22). New York: Routledge.

New York University Child Study Center. (2006). *Caring for kids after trauma, disaster and death: A guide for patents and professionals* (2nd ed.). New York: New York Child Study Center.

Nichols, T., & Wiseman, C. M. (2004). *Live like you were dying* [Recorded by Tim McGraw]. *On Live like you were dying* [CD]. Nashville: Curb Records.

Nixon, A., & Narayanasamy, A. (2010). The spiritual needs of neuro-oncology patients from patients' perspective. *Journal of Clinical Nursing, 19*(15–16), 2259–2270.

Norton, S. A., & Bowers, B. J. (2001). Working toward consensus: Providers' strategies to shift patients from curative to palliative treatment choices. *Research in Nursing & Health, 24*(4), 258–269.

Olsson, L., Östlund, G., Grassman, E. J., Friedrichsen, M., & Strang, P. (2010). Maintaining hope when close to death: Insight from cancer patients in palliative home care. *International Journal of Palliative Nursing, 16*(12), 607–612.

Palmieri, R. L. (2007). Responding to primary brain tumor. *Nursing, 37*(1), 36–42.

Park, C. L., & Halifax, R. J. (2011). Religion and spirituality in adjusting to bereavement: Grief as burden, grief as gift. In R. A. Neimeyer, D. L. Harris, H. R. Winokuer, & G. F. Thornton (Eds.), *Grief and bereavement in contemporary society: Bridging research and practice* (pp. 355–363). New York: Routledge.

Pellegrino, M. W. (1999). *I don't have an uncle Phil anymore*. Washington, D. C.: Magination Press.

Perakis, C. R. (2010). Soul sickness: A frequently missed diagnosis. *Journal of the American Osteopathic Association, 110*(6), 347–349.

Peterson, C. (2009). Positive psychology. *Reclaiming children and youth, 18*(2), 3–7.

Peterson, C., Park, N., Pole, N., D'Andrea, W., & Seligman, M. E. (2008a). Strengths of character and posttraumatic growth. *Journal of Traumatic Stress, 21*(2), 214–217.

Peterson, C., Park, N., & Sweeney, P. J. (2008b). Group well-being: Morale from a positive psychology perspective. *Applied Psychology: An International Review, 57,* 19–36.

Planalp, S., & Trost, M. R. (2008). Communication issues at the end of life: Reports from hospice volunteers. *Health Communication, 23*(3), 222–233.

Power, P. W., & Dell Orto, A. E. (2004). *Families living with chronic illness and disability: Interventions, challenges, and opportunities*. New York: Springer.

Richman, J. (1995). From despair to integrity: An Eriksonian approach to psychotherapy for the terminally ill. *Psychotherapy: Theory, Research, Practice, Training, 32*(2), 317–322.

Roos, S. (2002). *Chronic sorrow: A living loss*. New York: Brunner-Routledge.

Sand, L., Olsson, M., & Strang, P. (2010). What are motives of family members who take responsibility in palliative cancer care? *Mortality, 15*(1), 64–80.

Sanderson, C. (2010). Mindfulness for clients, their friends, and family members. http://ebookbrowse.com/mindfulness-for-clients-and-family-members-pdf-d28312970. Accessed 19 Aug 2012.

Schmer, C., Ward-Smith, P., Latham, S., & Salacz, M. (2008). When a family member has a malignant brain tumor: The caregiver perspective. *Journal of Neuroscience Nursing, 40*(2), 78–84.

Schubart, J. R., Kinzie, M. B., & Farace, E. (2008). Caring for the brain tumor patient: Family caregiver burden and unmet needs. *Neuro-Oncology, 10*(1), 61–72.

Seligman, M. E. P. (2006). *Learned optimism: How to change your mind and your life*. New York: Vintage.

Seligman, M. E. P. (2011). *Flourish: A visionary new understanding of happiness and well-being*. New York: Atria.

Seligman, M. E. P., & Peterson, C. (2003). Positive clinical psychology. In L. G. Aspinwall & U. M. Staudinger, (Eds.), *A psychology of human strengths: Fundamental questions and future directions for a positive psychology* (pp. 305–317). Washington, D. C.: American Psychological Association.

Shadyac, T., Reid, F., Shimizu, E. H., Belic, R. (Producers), & Belic, R. (Director). (2011). *Happy* [Motion picture]. United States: Wadi Rum Productions.

Shear, M. K., Boelen, P. A., & Neimeyer, R. A. (2011). Treating complicated grief converging approaches. In R. A. Neimeyer, D. L. Harris, H. R. Winokuer, & G. F. Thornton (Eds.), *Grief and bereavement in contemporary society: Bridging research and practice* (pp. 139–162). New York: Routledge.

Sherwood, P. R., Given, B. A., Doorenbos, A. Z., & Given, C. W. (2004a). Forgotten voices: Lessons from bereaved caregivers of persons with a brain tumour. *International Journal of Palliative Nursing, 10*(2), 67–75.

Sherwood, P., Given, B., Given, C., Schiffman, R., Murman, D., & Lovely, M. (2004b). Caregivers of persons with a brain tumor: A conceptual model. *Nursing Inquiry, 11*(1), 43–53.

Sherwood, P. R., Given, B. A., Donovan, H., Baum, A., Given, C. W., Bender, C. M., & Schulz, R. (2008). Guiding research in family care: A new approach to oncology caregiving. *Psycho-Oncology, 17*(10), 986–996.

Smith, H. I. (2002). *Finding your way to say goodbye: Comfort for the dying and those who care for them*. Notre Dame: Ave Maria Press.

Smith, H. I. (2007). *A B C's of healthy grieving: A companion for everyday coping*. Notre Dame: Ave Maria Press.

Smith, H. I. (2011). *A decembered grief: Living with loss while others are celebrating*. Kansas City: Beacon Hill Press.

Strang, S., & Strang, P. (2001). Spiritual thoughts, coping and 'sense of coherence' in brain tumour patients and their spouses. *Palliative Medicine, 15*(2), 127–134.

Strang, S., Strang, P., & Ternestedt, B. M. (2001). Existential support in brain tumour patients and their spouses. *Supportive Care in Cancer: Official Journal of the Multinational Association of Supportive Care in Cancer, 9*(8), 625–633.

Stark-Vance, V., & Dubay, M. L. (2011). *100 Questions & answers about brain tumors* (2nd ed.). Boston: Jones and Bartlett Publishers.

Stroebe, M., Schut, H., & van den Bout, J. (Eds.). (2012). *Complicated grief: Scientific foundations for health care professionals*. New York: Routledge.

Tepper, S. (2003). A model for care: A transitions program designed to provide comprehensive care in treating individuals with malignant brain tumors. *Smith College Studies in Social Work, 73*(3), 337–357.

Triplett, K. N., Tedeschi, R. G., Cann, A., Calhoun, L. G., & Reeve, C. L. (2011). Posttraumatic growth, meaning in life, and life satisfaction in response to trauma. *Psychological Trauma: Theory, Research, Practice, and Policy*. Advance online publication. doi:10.1037/a0024204.

Vaillant, G. E. (2008). Positive emotions, spirituality and the practice of psychiatry. *Medicine, Mental Health, Science, Religion, and Well-being, MSM, 6*, 48–62.

Vedder, E. (1998). *Wishlist* [Recorded by Pearl Jam]. *On Yield* [CD]. US: Sony Records.

Wasserman, L. S. (2008). Respectful death: A model for end-of-life care. *Clinical Journal of Oncology Nursing, 12*(4), 621–626.

Weiner, J. S., & Roth, J. (2006). Avoiding iatrogenic harm to patient and family while discussing goals of care near the end of life. *Journal of Palliative Medicine, 9*(2), 451–463.

Wells, R., Dywan, J., & Dumas, J. (2005). Life satisfaction and distress in family caregivers as related to specific behavioural changes after traumatic brain injury. *Brain Injury, 19*(13), 1105–1115.

Williams, B. Y. (2004). The friend who just stands by. In J. Cotner (Ed.), *Looking for God in all the right places: Prayers and poems to comfort, inspire, and connect humanity* (p. 125). Chicago: Loyola Press.

Wong, P. T. P., & Tomer, A. (2011). Beyond terror and denial: The positive psychology of death acceptance. *Death Studies, 35*(2), 99–106.

Worden, J. W. (2009). *Grief counselling and grief therapy: A handbook for the mental health practitioner*. New York: Springer.

Yalom, I. D. (2009). *Staring at the sun: Overcoming the terror of death*. San Francisco: Jossey-Bass.

Yolen, J. (1997). Birthday box. In J. Hurwitz (Ed.), *Birthday surprises: Ten great stories to unwrap* (pp. 27–33). New York: Beech Tree.

Chapter 11
Aftercare Group for Long-Range Needs

11.1 Overview

Research and clinical observation reveal that caregiver burden and adjustment to life alterations are pervasive phenomena, even in the chronic postinjury period (Brooks et al. 1986; Hassan et al. 2011; Klonoff and Koberstein 2010; Klonoff et al. 2008; Minnes et al. 2010; Smeets et al. 2012). However, there is a dearth of organized care systems after discharge from rehabilitation facilities (see Minnes et al. 2010, for a review). A *Family Aftercare Group*, for the purposes of this discussion, is defined as a posttreatment support group for the family members of the loved one with an acquired brain injury. The goals are to provide ongoing emotional sustenance and peer mentoring after formal neurorehabilitation ends (Klonoff 2010). It embodies a process of "collaborative self-examination," whereby attendees share perspectives, develop skills, and cultivate self-care (Kreutzer et al. 2010). Beneficial subcomponents include psychoeducation, counseling, strategizing, socialization, and practical resource provision (Klonoff 2010; Rodgers et al. 2007).

This chapter describes relevant topics for families of patients with moderate to severe brain injuries in which functional abilities are not expected to deteriorate markedly. This includes traumatic brain injury, cerebrovascular accidents, and seizure disorders, but excludes higher-grade brain tumors. The longer range issues associated with recurring brain tumors are unique and outside the range of this particular conceptualization.

The family Aftercare Group is modeled after the Family Group (see Chap. 9), but with topics germane to the long-range challenges and acquired wisdom. Participation is of course voluntary, and upon treatment discharge, the support network is invited to attend. There is no charge for the group and this facilitator volunteers her time. However, participants are invited to make a nominal donation (US $10) towards a patient "scholarship" fund to assist patients in obtaining rehabilitation services who otherwise would be unable to. Proper medical releases are always obtained from the loved ones (or their representative) and attendees are educated regarding the intent and benefits of the Aftercare Group. Figure 11.1 is an introductory document, which includes group etiquette and requirements for confidentiality. As with the Family Group, the group facilitator reiterates that the personal information shared

P. S. Klonoff, E. Koberstein, *Psychotherapy for Families after Brain Injury*,
DOI 10.1007/978-1-4899-8083-0_11,

Welcome to the Family Aftercare Group

Purpose: To provide a longer-term support group for families of persons with brain injuries to come together to gain education, receive emotional support, and share their feelings, concerns, and triumphs.

General Information:

- Family members and significant others over the age of 18 are welcome.
- Aftercare Group meets monthly on Tuesday evenings (5:00 p.m. – 6:00 p.m.).
- The group is facilitated by a Clinical Neuropsychologist. The group promotes open sharing. Typical topics include:

  1. Slippage and Flight into Health
  2. Evolutionary changes
  3. Longer term practical worries
  4. Emotions and sense of self
  5. Adjustment
  6. Social reintegration

Group Rules and Etiquette:

- Respect the privacy of all program patients and their families. Discussions are strictly confidential and must not be shared outside of the group.
- Respect the opinions of others.
- Leave time for others to express their thoughts and concerns – save specific discussions for individual meetings with an appropriate therapist/resource.

By my signature below, I acknowledge receipt of the General Information pertaining to the Aftercare Group, including the rules and etiquette, and agree to the expectations of the group.

______________________________ ____________________
Friend/Relative's Name Date

By my signature below, I agree to disclosures regarding my injury and treatment by my friend and/or family member named above as a part of their participation in the Family Aftercare Group, providing they are involved with my care.

______________________________ ____________________
Patient Date

Fig. 11.1 Introduction to Family Aftercare Group

by various relatives cannot be divulged to the loved ones or nongroup participants. This creates a confidential and safe environment for candid expression.

Previous publications have described the philosophy and protocols for Aftercare Group (Klonoff 2010; Klonoff et al. 2008). As with the Family Group, the format is open entry and open exit. As such, new members merge into the group with more experienced participants. The group comfortably accommodates 12–16 family members or other tier 1 or tier 2 supports (e.g., significant others and friends), 18 years and older. Of course, the group facilitators can vary, including neuropsychologists, clinical or rehabilitation psychologists, or social workers. In our setting, a dinner is served for 30 min before the group, and continues afterwards for up to 60 min (without the facilitator present). This encourages an unfettered socialization experience in a nurturing setting (Klonoff 2010).

As stated above, the Aftercare Group encompasses a mixture of injury etiologies, for which the chronic picture reflects at least neurological stability, if not gradual improvement. The chronology of the injuries varies, ranging from approximately 1 year to many years (sometimes 15+ years) postinjury. The amount of time the loved one attended neurorehabilitation is also variable, but usually ranges from 3–12 months. As with the Family Group, common constructs emerge regardless of the patient mix, yet the heterogeneity provides a rich landscape by which to acquire a unique and multidimensional perspective. Generally, the tier supports attending Aftercare Group know some of the group members, based on the relationships forged during the rehabilitation process. However, new enrollees also meet "veterans" whose loved ones "graduated" from their treatment weeks, months, or possibly years ago. Embedded in the Aftercare Group is a feeling of inclusion, warmth, and camaraderie for the "long haul." As a facilitator, it is always gratifying to observe the seamless integration of newcomers into the group milieu surrounded by likeminded and hearty cohorts.

This author's Aftercare Group has a number of "regulars" or caregivers who have attended the group since its inception and have developed a strong emotional bond. Obviously, the group makeup may change in other settings, based on the needs and availability of family members, or the preferences of the group facilitators. Even if the format is different (e.g., closed entry and time-limited attendance), it is felt that many of the ideas described within this chapter are applicable to the chronic effects of brain injury and can be modified at the discretion of the facilitator and group participants. In addition, when the support network has not attended a Family Group, the group facilitators can easily amalgamate the topics of Chap. 9 (Family Group), and/or any other content from other chapters so as to create a customized therapeutic family support group. This includes organizing handouts provided in earlier chapters into a binder to fortify the collaborative dialogue. Table 11.1 provides a sampling of educational topics. Another worthwhile venue is occasional conjoint meetings with the loved ones and family members. Psychoeducational lectures, short films, and inspirational speakers are especially effective.

Because our Aftercare Group members are generally seasoned, this group is typically more self-operating. The group facilitator generally takes a background listening role, with intermittent guiding questions or reflective summations. The group begins with brief introductions for the new attendees, with a description of the loved one's injury. The overall flow of the group can be conceptualized as a fluid

Table 11.1 Educational topics about brain injury

The Patient Experiential Model (PEM) of Recovery
The Family Experiential Model (FEM) of Recovery
Common cognitive, language, physical, emotional, and interpersonal problems after brain injury and their impact on independence, school, and/or work
Typical patient challenges post-discharge
Relevant compensations
Benefits of psychotropic medications
Contraindications for alcohol use postinjury
Limit setting versus facilitating independence
Changes in sense of self
Grief and loss
Relationships after brain injury
Coping strategies
The value of values
Existential adjustment postinjury
Retrospective perspective of recovery and rehabilitation with a family presentation
Career information systems
Driving
Community transportation options
Adaptive sports in the community
Adaptive tai chi
Family-oriented therapy activities
Computer cognitive tasks
Motion control gaming systems (e.g., Wii System™)
Adaptive recreational sports equipment
Community resources for brain injury
Caregiver information

exchange encompassing a revolving and reverberating process of sharing, venting, and recalibration. One family member described the ambience as "tears and cheers" (S. Barcus, personal communication, 3/5/13). As with the Family Group, the facilitator remains attuned to when the caregiver needs individualized attention because of urgent or overwhelming concerns. Pertinent resources are then provided at the conclusion of the meeting, with appropriate follow-up, as required.

To conceptualize clinical trends, this author gathered representative verbalizations and material based on free discussion of chronic considerations from the past 7 years of the monthly Aftercare Group. These have been condensed into six salient themes and topics (see Table 11.2). These subjects can span several weeks, or can be fused into a meeting. Because our group is ongoing, there is no need to structure the discussion. Instead, the emphasis is on free-flowing conversations, with introduction of didactic psychoeducation, when warranted.

As with Chap. 9 (Family Group), each theme will be illustrated using family members' descriptive utterances. In this chapter, responses from a Sense of Self Questionnaire will be highlighted. This will be followed by a therapeutic protocol with exercises to spark peer interactions. In combination with this, examples of "helpful hints," psychoeducation, and multimedia resources are presented. These techniques will guide the group facilitator in maximizing the group experience. The next section will first briefly review phase 7 of the Family Experiential Model (FEM)

Table 11.2 Aftercare Group themes

1.	Slippage and flight into health
2.	Evolutionary changes
3.	Longer term practical worries
4.	Emotions and sense of self
5.	Adjustment
6.	Social reintegration

of Recovery and the Patient Experiential Model (PEM) of Recovery (Klonoff 2010; Klonoff and Koberstein 2010; Klonoff et al. 2008) to provide a context for the thematic discussions.

11.2 The FEM of Recovery and PEM of Recovery: Phase 7

Earlier chapters have reviewed the constructs in the FEM and PEM (see Chap. 1, Sect. 1.5 and Fig. 1.3 and Chap. 9, Sect. 9.2.1 and Fig. 9.2). Phase 7 of these models articulates the expected accomplishments and potential dilemmas for the loved one and family, as well as possible coping styles (Klonoff 2010; Klonoff and Koberstein 2010; Klonoff et al. 2008). Note the placement phase depicts "future" with an infinity sign (i.e., ∞), indicating the ongoing and likely lifetime struggles and adjustments facing each party. With respect to the patients, they are hopefully functioning independently and productively in the community, using an array of personalized compensatory tools. There is a "new reality" and an acknowledgment that over time life will evolve. They recognize that things are different postinjury, but their existence is meaningful. Similarly, the caregiver and family are adjusting to their "new realities." Their role is to continue collaborative dialogue with the loved one regarding injury ramifications and the value of compensations. Everyone is coming to terms with the enduring impact of the brain injury on the family unit, and is cultivating an optimistic life view.

The FEM and PEM coping ("green" zone), warning ("yellow" zone), and crisis ("red" zone) reflect relative coping styles. As identified in prior publications, undoubtedly, there will be natural fluctuations between healthier and problematic coping strategies and a strong interconnection between how the loved one and family are relating and functioning (Klonoff 2010; Klonoff and Koberstein 2010; Klonoff et al. 2008). The groundwork of rehabilitation and psychotherapy in phases 1–6 has been to assist the loved one and family members in immersing themselves into a balanced lifestyle, including adaptive community pursuits, as well as positive family and social liaisons. For the loved one in PEM phase 7, a positive adjustment ("green coping" zone) means embracing tools and adeptly modifying them when needed. Relationships are valued and nurtured, and he or she willingly recognizes when and how to reach out for therapeutic and family assistance. Coping struggles ("yellow warning" zone) are manifested as a gradual disuse of compensations, an inability or unwillingness to evolve strategies, and/or seek help when required. The loved one's behavior then becomes taxing to the environment, affecting tier 1, 2, and 3 supports (see Chap. 1, Sect. 1.3 and Figs. 1.1 and 1.2). At a crisis point ("red" zone), behavioral problems escalate—especially rage, despair, hopelessness, helplessness, and dependency. Psychosocial disarray is predominant in family and work life.

For the family, healthy coping and adjustment ("green coping" zone) on the FEM translates to redefining their roles. This is not only as a caregiver, but also with other family members, and as a worker, friend, etc. Based on their knowledge and experience, the relatives are able to intuitively evolve compensations so as to accommodate and boost the loved one's quality of life. The children's story, *Moostache* by Palatini (1997) delightfully illustrates the role of creativity and expertise in this regard. Regular respite is incorporated into their lifestyle and additional therapeutic support is accessed when pertinent (Klonoff et al. 2008). When this fails to happen ("yellow warning" zone), the family's roles become skewed, resulting in feeling disengaged, isolated, and burned out. The caregiver is ill equipped to provide the necessary guidance or input, especially about compensations. At a crisis point ("red" zone), emotional deterioration (i.e., rage, anguish, despair, helplessness, apathy, and self-defeating behaviors), work failures, financial ruin, social alienation, and dissolution of family life dominate (Klonoff et al. 2008). The material which follows reflects combinations and permutations of phase 7 of the PEM and FEM, including new life events, coping challenges, acceptance and realism threats, and informative internal and external resources.

11.3 Slippage and Flight into Health

Hallmarks of suboptimal functioning are slippage in the use of compensations and flight into health (Klonoff 2010; see also Chap. 9, Sect. 9.6.1). *Slippage* is a gradual drifting or outright rejection of tools considered by the therapeutic team to be integral to the loved one's success. *Flight into health* generally emerges first near the time of treatment termination (phase 6) and represents the loved one's psychological distancing from the injury and treatment process (Klonoff 2010). It is as if the injury has been "cured" or at least has receded to a trivial afterthought. Family members can experience a mirroring of the slippage and flight into health phenomena. They may minimize or, worse, negate the advantages of compensations. Both of these can persist or reappear weeks, months, or years postinjury. Table 11.3 summarizes some representative samples of participants' verbalizations during Aftercare Group depicting slippage and flight into health through the eyes of the loved one (allegedly) and/or themselves.

11.3.1 Group Treatment to Cope with Slippage and Flight into Health

Table 11.4 summarizes group exercises, psychoeducation, therapeutic "helpful hints," as well as multimedia resources to cope with slippage and flight into health in the loved one and family. To the extent the tier supports understand the entities of

Table 11.3 Common verbalizations reflective of slippage and flight into health

Loved ones' perspectives:
I don't need these tools—they're a hassle
The datebook is heavy and a lot of work
I'm just too busy to take the time for . . . .
I'm done with therapy, so you don't need to check up on me anymore
I'm taking a break from . . .
I carry the datebook, but I don't use it
I don't need to write things down, it's all "up here" (pointing to the temple)
I can drive—I don't need a doctor's permission
I can do my old job . . . no problem
I don't care what the doctors/you say, I can live on my own and work just like I used to
Why can't I drink alcohol?—all my friends do
You don't need to know my business
I don't need any more psychotherapy
I can do just what I used to do
Families'/tier supports' perspectives:
He's/she's fine now
These "milieu meetings" are too time consuming and so repetitious
I don't want/need to check his/her datebook everyday
It's easier for me to pay bills than remind him/her to use the budget checklist
It's just one thing after another to do
Meds aren't necessary—he/she should be able to control his/her behavior and actions
I'm tired of being responsible for all of these things
He's/she's an adult—I can't/don't want to tell him/her what to do
He/she should be able to fend for himself/herself
This isn't what I signed up for
I don't have the patience for this
It's not my problem—it's his/hers
He/she is such high maintenance
It's disruptive and he's/she's a burden
It's been long enough
I'd rather pretend everything is fine
I'm not his/her keeper
I want things to be normal

slippage and flight into health, as well as the underlying psychological contributions, they can be more tolerant and empathic towards their loved ones and also maintain their pivotal role as "compensation champions." The Aftercare Group is an ideal venue to survey these factors, as well as vent and brainstorm about healthy antidotes.

A stimulating introductory exercise is to ask family members why they think their loved ones are succumbing to slippage and flight into health. One typical response is that related to the loved ones' brain injuries, they usually need the external structure, support, and accountability afforded by the rehabilitation environment to sustain the compensations. Once they are "in the real world" with fewer supports, they cannot muster the internal cognitive capacity or self-regulation required to be persistent with the tools (Klonoff 2010). Other common observations are the ongoing neurological problems with fatigue, inertia, or initiation which then interfere with consistent compensation utilization.

Table 11.4 Group treatment for slippage and flight into health

Guided exercises
Open ended questions:
Why are your loved ones succumbing to slippage and flight into health?
Is your loved one testing boundaries—how? And how are you handling this?
What factors are causing you to experience slippage and flight into health?
Which coping zone are you in for phase 7?
Who are your second and third tiers of support and how can you enlist their involvement?
Psychoeducation
Patient factors contributing to slippage and flight into health:
Patients' follow through diminishes without the external structure, support, and accountability that is embedded in neurorehabilitation
Their brain injury affects cognitive and self-regulation skills necessary for persistent tool use
Neurological problems with fatigue, inertia, and initiation
Unconscious fear of separation from the comforts of rehabilitation
Defense mechanisms and disavowal
Testing limits and self-assertion
"Snarky" behavior causing the family to "walk on eggshells"
Cyclical acceptance struggles:
Painful and embarrassing visual reminders of disability
The need to "test memory"
Tools are too cumbersome and/or inconsistent with lifestyle
Wanting to "fit in"
Difficulties with motivation and apathy, related to depression
Unhealthy or dangerous choices (e.g., alcohol or drug use)
Family factors contributing to slippage and flight into health:
Fear of being in charge of the loved one without therapeutic support
Cognitive dissonance, cognitive distortions, and wishful thinking
Various forms of CRs by proxy about the loved one's permanent limitations
Feeling overwhelmed, exasperated, and/or exhausted with "24/7" compensation duties
Lack of inclination, patience, or aptitude for caregiving
"Helpful hints"
Use the group setting to brainstorm and vent about underlying reasons for slippage and flight into health, as well as identify healthy antidotes
Recognize the cyclical nature of slippage and flight into health, starting with discharge from rehabilitation
Be patient with the loved one's need to self-assert, yet focus on being a "compensation champion"
Be prepared to "pick battles," temporarily take a "back seat," and stay "neutral"
The loved one's firsthand experience with failures should rekindle their acceptance and realism
Learn about cognitive behavioral therapy constructs to "reframe" the predicament
Gain insight about the contribution of various forms of CRs by proxy
Follow up with individual psychotherapy sessions and other treatment venues (e.g., a support group and substance abuse treatment) for the loved one and/or family as needed
Use the FEM as a roadmap to coping styles and detours
Enlist the involvement of second and third tiers of support for a reprieve
Multimedia resources
Models
Patient Experiential Model (PEM) of Recovery (Klonoff 2010)
Family Experiential Model (FEM) of Recovery (Klonoff and Koberstein 2010; Klonoff et al. 2008)
Song
"Be Yourself" (Cornell 2005)
Movie
Marvin's Room (Brody et al. 1996)

A series of emotional factors contribute to the loved one's flight into health and slippage and the group facilitator can prompt the family participants to hypothesize about possible reasons. As mentioned above, often these behaviors represent the loved ones' unconscious process of fear of separation from the comforts of the rehabilitation setting. They rely on the psychodynamic defense mechanisms of reaction formation (i.e., overt responses which are contradictory to an unacceptable motive) or rationalization (i.e., attributing a morally acceptable reason to distance themselves from full awareness of this unpleasant thought; Sarnoff 1962). They espouse convictions that they no longer need to depend on their compassionate therapists and are "more than ready" for treatment termination (Klonoff 2010). The loved one may also retreat into the protective closet of denial or disavowal, as the reality of the persistence of deficits becomes too painful and overwhelming (see Klonoff 2010, for a review). The loved one resorts to magical or self-soothing thinking that everything will be or already is "okay."

Other patients minimize or reject their compensations and/or injuries as a way to "test limits." They want to see for themselves whether or not they indeed need the tools. This represents their need to self-assert, especially as they regain more independence from what can feel like therapeutic and family constraints (Baldwin et al. 2011). The loved one may erupt into "snarky" retorts, forcing the family to "walk on eggshells," afraid to voice opinions or suggestions (Klonoff 2010; Klonoff and Koberstein 2010). Thus, the caregivers must (reluctantly) "pick their battles" and/or take a "back seat" and temporarily witness their loved ones' spurious attempts to do away with their rehabilitation teachings (see Chap. 2, Sect. 2.4.2.3). Once loved ones encounter snags or failures firsthand, their level of intrinsic engagement revives. In the interim, the caregivers remain "neutral" and avoid being berated for pressuring their loved ones.

Cyclical trouble accepting the realities of the injury may reemerge, especially if the loved one yearns for a life path that seems desperately unattainable. This is understandable and expected, as illustrated by the PEM (Klonoff 2010). The symbolic rejection of compensations and denouncement of the injury provide a temporary reprieve from harsh realizations. A case in point, abandonment of the datebook removes the painful and embarrassing visual reminder of being disabled (Baldwin et al. 2011; Klonoff 2010). Other psychological machinations include a defensive stance that he or she needs to test his or her memory and/or that the tools are too cumbersome and are not consistent with his or her lifestyle (Baldwin et al. 2011). Depression can negatively impact motivation and produce apathy (Fleminger 2008; Fleminger et al. 2003; see Chap. 4, Sect. 4.6 and Table 4.6).

Common manifestations of the patient's slippage and flight into health are resuming alcohol and drug use. Socially, the loved one wants to feel included and popular, and may start using alcohol or drugs as a way to "fit in." This is usually very frightening to the families, as they are concerned about seizures, functional and mood deterioration, or heightened injury risks (see Chap. 4, Sect. 4.6.2).

Based on the discussion in Aftercare Group, it is typically recommended that a trusted caregiver or family contact addresses observations of flight into health with the loved one. If possible, soliciting the assistance of a therapist in private follow-up sessions is optimal, as it allows some objective feedback and maintains the familial rapport. This includes addressing the propensity for follies related to unrealistic thinking and poor compliance. If the loved one is engaging in counterproductive thinking and actions which become chronic or overly worrisome and result in work and relationship failures, it is advised that the caregiver help him or her take seriously the need to reengage in a treatment setting. Individual psychotherapy, drug or alcohol treatment, and/or a brain injury support group for the loved one are critical to offset psychosocial decline, including the perils of alcohol use (Whitnall et al. 2006). Then the psychotherapist can take a leadership role and support the loved one through testing the waters or "planned failures" (Klonoff 2010). Therapeutic intervention can reinforce the importance of compensations for community accomplishments (Klonoff et al. 2007) and address other psychological barriers (Baldwin et al. 2011). The lyrics to the song, "Be Yourself" (Cornell 2005) exemplify self-acceptance, adaptation, and intrapsychic assimilation, characterized by attainment of self-esteem, self-efficacy, mastery, and ultimately happiness (Klonoff 2010).

Of course, there are similar psychological factors contributing to the tier 1 caregiver's inclination to disregard injury effects and/or vital compensations, manifested as his or her own versions of slippage and flight into health. Aftercare Group provides a safe haven to explore these tender feelings, as well as a way for the facilitator and peers to gently confront unhealthy trends. Relatives can be asked open-ended questions regarding why they grapple with slippage and flight into health. Most note that the phenomena seem cyclical and first occur around the time of discharge. On the one hand, the tier supports are ecstatic about the loved ones' gains and community involvement. On the other hand, they are distressed about nearing treatment termination and are petrified at the thought of managing the injury aftermath without intensive and regular therapeutic support. This causes cognitive dissonance, or conflicting attitudes regarding the situation, which translates to internal discomfort (Harmon-Jones and Mills 1999). In order to reduce the angst, the caregivers justify their quandary by finding temporary solace through the cognitive belief that things are now "okay," so there is no need to worry. Avoidance and minimizing reactions in the tier supports may also be forms of "catastrophic reactions (CRs) by proxy" (see Chap. 9, Sect. 9.4 and Table 9.8). Within the group, the psychotherapist can employ cognitive behavior therapy and explore possible underlying reasons for cognitive distortions, manifested as wishful thinking, minimization, or polarized thinking (Beck 1995). This assists the caregivers in recalibrating their thinking into shades of gray (Leahy 2003).

Alternatively, when the first tier of support (i.e., primary caregiver) feels saddled with "24/7" responsibilities, including overseeing the loved one's follow through with numerous compensations, he or she can feel overwhelmed, exasperated, or exhausted. This can be conceptualized as the "wear and tear" of cascading CRs by proxy because of the loved one's permanent limitations. Coupled with this is the reality that not every family member thrust into the role of caregiving has the inclination, patience, or aptitude for this life role. He or she may lapse into "catastrophizing" the injury repercussions and "tunnel vision" (Beck 1995), losing sight of the loved one's gains and preserved capacities. In this case, group discussion with an emphasis on cognitive behavioral therapy helps the struggling caregiver notice the tendency towards overgeneralization, "should" statements, and externalizing blame (Beck 1995; Leahy 2003). Often other attendees help to "reframe" the predicament, including "examining the evidence," for example, where the loved one is succeeding (Leahy 2003). As part of the Aftercare Group members' self-analyses, they can be invited to identify their coping zone on the FEM. Revisiting the "yellow warning" zone of the FEM reminds family members of the pitfalls of waning acceptance and shirking constructive feedback and support of their loved ones (Klonoff and Koberstein 2010).

To counteract caregiver loads, group questions and disclosures can also guide the caregiver to enlist the involvement of the second and third tiers of support. This not only provides a reprieve for the caregiver but also allows outsiders the opportunity to build their own unique relationships with the loved one. Multiple involvements introduce variety and appeal to the social interactions, which can seem stale and narrow with only one caregiver. The primary caregiver must be cautioned that the depth of involvement and understanding may appear subpar because the more peripheral support network may lack the knowledge base. This can erupt in conflict (Ayalong 2004). However, this should not be a reason to negate the benefit of exposure to the situation, both for the caregiver and the loved one. A provocative catalyst for group discussion is the movie, *Marvin's Room* (Brody et al. 1996). This film nicely illustrates the disparate perspectives of the primary and secondary tiers of support, and poignantly depicts the realignment of attunement within the family unit.

11.4 Evolutionary Changes

The well-adjusted and educated caregiver and support network will recognize and embrace evolutionary changes in their loved ones as well as themselves. This pertains to the loved one's continued recovery and the necessary modifications and adaptations in the family system to accommodate this fluid process. However, this can be especially daunting months and years after formal rehabilitation has ended. Table 11.5 summarizes common verbalizations from family members attending the Aftercare Group and who were coping with their evolutionary changes, in tandem with their loved one. Several tendencies emerge, including bewilderment about if, how, and when to make changes in the caregiver role over time. Oscillations recur between wanting to protect and/or indulge the loved one versus normal distancing so that all parties can pursue their interests and goals unencumbered.

Underlying this dilemma are a multitude of emotions, including comfort in being the "safety net" and "security blanket"; anxiety and fears regarding the loved one's incapacities and potential failures; guilt about his or her struggles; "what ifs" about poor life choices; and resentment about the totality of self-imposed restrictions. The caregiver remains "on duty," sometimes relapsing into hypervigilance and micromanagement. The caregiver may question if he or she is "enabling" the loved one detrimentally by fostering dependency rather than teaching personal accountability.

Table 11.5 Common verbalizations about evolutionary changes in the caregiver

Can he/she be self-sufficient?
It's hard to know what changes I need to make over time now that rehab is over
I can't figure out how much to be involved
I feel like I am second guessing the decisions I make about my loved one's freedoms
Should I be reminding him/her about things?
I keep worrying
I feel hypervigilant and always on edge
I'm afraid things will fall through the cracks
I don't want him/her to fail
I'm still in "what if" mode
I don't want to go through this again
I still feel like I am "on duty"
I'm micromanaging him/her
I still want to protect him/her
I'm not ready to let go—I'm in the habit of doing
I feel like I am the security blanket
I feel like the safety net
I still feel guilty
I feel better when I do things for him/her
I know I'm doing too much for him/her
Am I an enabler?
My loved one is so clingy
He/she seems so dependent
I feel like his/her servant
I want him/her to take more personal responsibility
Will he/she lose gains?
Is there a "cap" in the progress?

There is a hovering backdrop of dire responsibility for the loved one's continued progress, for fear of a plateau in recovery, or worse, erosion of the gains.

11.4.1 Group Treatment to Cope with Evolutionary Changes

Table 11.6 summarizes group exercises, psychoeducation, therapeutic "helpful hints," as well as multimedia resources to cope with the relatives' and loved ones' evolutionary changes. The Aftercare Group can assist the family caregiver and other tier supports in finding a balance of involvement with their loved one. This can be considered the continuation of the duality of overprotectiveness versus letting go, as described in Chap. 9 (see Sect. 9.6). To accomplish this in posttreatment phases, participants will need to explore the underlying reasons for their behaviors; rely on prior and new psychoeducation regarding how to optimally address the loved one's needs; and follow their instincts, knowing that there are no definite or easy answers for these complex and evolving circumstances. The books, *Who Moved My Cheese?* by Johnson (1998) and *The Shark and the Goldfish* by Gordon (2009) nicely illustrate how to be flexible and adaptable in changing times.

Table 11.6 Group treatment for evolutionary changes

Guided exercises

Open ended questions:

- What evolutionary changes are you and your loved one experiencing with respect to improvements and challenges?
- How are you addressing these changes and how do you feel about this?
- Are you employing the concepts of "dignity of risk" and "dignity of risk by proxy?"
- Where is your balance point for guidance versus control?
- What techniques will build mastery, independence, and empowerment?

"Helpful hints" and psychoeducation

- Aim to recognize and embrace evolutionary changes for your loved one and yourself
- Remember continued recovery after rehabilitation ends is a fluid process
- Use the group to cogitate about the best balance of involvement with your loved one
- Explore underlying motivations, use psychoeducation, and follow your best instincts
- Study the causes of overinvolvement
- Use a quick self-test of whether or not the caregiver's actions will help the loved one
- Counterbalance the "easy factor" with the "better factor"
- Be mindful about updating coping methods and behaviors
- Incorporate the concept of "dignity of risk" and "dignity of risk by proxy"
- Provide a refresher to the loved one on the importance of self-sufficiency and fair play
- Reinforce the motto "use it or lose it"
- If necessary, set boundaries so that the tier supports are not taken advantage of
- Learn about the concept of "learned helplessness" so as not to stifle the loved one's development
- Do a cost-benefit analysis of the relative merits and threats of intervening for the loved one
- Use an advisory board of trusted professionals and confidants as "lifelines"
- Remember the cognitive benefit for the loved one in having responsibilities
- Learn from mistakes and life lessons to find a balance between reliance and autonomy
- Remember this process may mirror earlier developmental processes
- Focus on developing mastery, independence, and empowerment as a "win–win" situation

Multimedia resources

Books

- *Who Moved My Cheese* (Johnson 1998)
- *The Shark and the Goldfish* (Gordon 2009)

Movie

- *Soul Surfer* (Bass et al. 2011)

Song

- "What's Love Got To Do With It?" (Britten and Lyle 1984)

Prose

- *"The Serenity Prayer"*

Table 11.6 contains some sample questions to catalyze the discussion about what the evolutionary changes are and how to contend with them. Overinvolvement with the loved one may be due to pragmatic reasons (e.g., it is quicker and easier to jump in), the psychological need to remain in the caregiver role out of habit, an inflated sense of capability (e.g., "no one can do it as well as me"), or the wish to shield the patient from adversity. Certain guiding principles will be illuminating, namely conducting a quick self-test of whether the intended action will help or overcompensate for the loved one. The facilitator can recommend counterbalancing the "easy factor" with the "better factor." A guidepost is to be sure that the caregiver's interventions are in the best interest of the loved one, rather than meeting some personal unfulfilled need or intrapsychic stressor. This will require mindfulness on the part of the caregiver, so as not to regress to earlier, now ineffective modes of coping and behavior.

Relatives will need to return periodically to the construct of *dignity of risk* (see Chap. 9, Sect. 9.6.1; Klonoff and Koberstein 2010), reminding themselves that the loved one needs to experience life's exhilarations and pitfalls, through taking certain calculated risks. Group contributors have reinforced the need for one another to "take a step back" and give the loved one a chance to live life. Of course, overall safety remains the crucial consideration (Cassidy 2009). The film, *Soul Surfer* (Bass et al. 2011) depicts this concept, as the main character, Bethany, is determined to return to surfing after a devastating accident. Her mother, Cheri, gradually confronts her misgivings and accepts Bethany's need to reclaim this passion. Her father's commitment to fashioning an adapted board also reflects a mindset of evolving compensations, thereby fortifying her safety. Interestingly, caregivers may need to adopt the same philosophy of *dignity of risk by proxy* so as to have their own courage to foray into new, sometimes intimidating territories of interests and activities to supplant their prior roles and comfort zones (see Sect. 11.7).

At times, the loved one needs a refresher on the importance of self-sufficiency, especially when lapsing into a more dependent or unmotivated state. Based on clinical experience, the therapist can remind the group about the adage "use it or lose it"—the loved one will lose ground when he or she stops functional tasks, as these stimulate brain activity and recovery. When protestations erupt because of aversion to certain chores, the family can employ humor. One example shared by the group facilitator is "What's 'like' got to do with it?" modified from the song, "What's Love Got to Do With It?" (Britten and Lyle 1984). This cajoles the loved one into the reminder that everyone has obligations which are objectionable, but which are unavoidable for daily sustenance. It symbolizes the essential tenet of fair play and "give and take" (Klonoff and Koberstein 2010). This may also translate to the tier supports setting appropriate boundaries when the loved one is taking advantage of their goodwill. Otherwise, poor habits are reinforced, which will disrupt the loved one's personal and work relationships, as outsiders will be less tolerant of seemingly lazy or self-centered behavior.

The group facilitator can introduce the concept of *learned helplessness* in which the individual learns that when outcomes are uncontrollable, he or she loses motivation (Maier and Seligman 1976). Anxiety, depression, and inactivity then predominate (Maier and Seligman 1976). This concept assists attendees in becoming cognizant of the debilitating consequences of stifling their loved ones' freedoms and independence by overpowering them with the families' own agendas and behaviors. The loved one will stop trying, feeling that the efforts are futile. This is deleterious to him or her and the caregiver. Guided peer input in Aftercare Group is effective in facilitating self-reflection. Through therapeutic dialogue, families can conduct a cost–benefit analysis of the relative merits and threats of intervening for the loved one (Klonoff 2010). One relative said to another "don't wrap yourself around that axle," as she was exhibiting so much self-sacrifice and panic that she was making herself ill. Some families find the "Serenity Prayer" a good compass for how to set and accept personal limits. Others construct an "advisory board" of knowledgeable professionals and confidants so as to access "lifelines" whenever required (Klonoff 2010). Another mother referenced the desire to "exit gracefully" from a total to limited influence.

A therapeutic lesson for the relatives is the cognitive benefit for their loved ones to struggle with decision making and problem solving. Incorporating an assortment of challenges with the advancement of compensations raise the "cap of recovery" (see Chap. 4, Sect. 4.1.1). They also enrich the loved one's life and reduce energy depletion in the caregiver. With practice and gentle guidance (versus intrusive control), the loved one hones his or her skill set and improves functionally. The family and loved one should learn from mistakes and life lessons, in order to recalibrate the balance of reliance versus autonomy. Some relatives liken this process to the loved one traversing again through developmental phases, whereby he or she individuates and separates from parental figures. The positive feedback loop of mastery, independence, and empowerment should be reinforced as part of the group discussion. This will reassure tier 1 caregivers that they are promoting the long-term self-sufficiency and well-being of their loved ones, which is a "win–win" situation for all parties.

11.5 Longer-Term Practical Worries

Chapter 9 (see Sect. 9.3) addresses practical worries which emerge during the earlier phases of the loved one's recovery, also including during the rehabilitation process. Medical advances have increased survival rates after brain injury, resulting in often lifelong responsibilities for caregiving, especially for parents (Minnes et al. 2010). There are typically a number of unmet service needs and worries regarding the long-term implications and management of the loved one's brain injury, which can persist for years (Cameron and Gignac 2008; Kreutzer et al. 2010; Minnes et al. 2010). Health concerns may evolve, including weight gain related to inactivity and/or depression; neurological complications, such as memory deterioration or seizures; or other scary, unforeseen illnesses.

Far-reaching patient ambitions, including the capacity to live and support himself or herself independently, navigate locally in the community or travel, as well as maintain work, plague the family. Everyday stresses about the cost of health care, complex legal processes (e.g., pending litigation, guardianship, or conservatorship) are weighty. Overall, there is chronic economic burden for the loved one and family (Hassan et al. 2011), requiring public financial support of various types (Shigaki et al. 2009).

Safety concerns abound, especially if the loved one demonstrates poor judgment and impulse control. Angst about the loved one's ability to handle finances is pervasive and chronic. Due to his or her vulnerability and suggestibility, he or she may make poor decisions or be taken advantage of by preying outsiders, intensifying the caregiver's perceived need to "hover." There is chronic heartache about the loved one's loneliness and social ostracism and dread about detrimental or exploitive relationships.

Competing stressors related to personal schedules or needs of other family members (e.g., children, ailing parents) encroach on the family's availability and energies. Aging parent caregivers, concerned about their own health and longevity, agonize about "permanency planning," including long-term accommodations, access to day programs, as well as to social and recreational activities for their loved ones (Minnes et al. 2010). Overall, the support network can feel overwhelmed related to their life interruptions. Table 11.7 summarizes examples of common verbalizations by caregivers related to longer-term practical worries. These are grouped according to the categories of home, finances, health, safety, community, work, and social life.

11.5.1 Group Treatment to Cope with Longer-Term Practical Worries

Table 11.8 summarizes group exercises, psychoeducation, therapeutic "helpful hints," as well as outside resources to cope with practical worries. Table 11.9 summarizes supportive and informative Internet websites grouped according to the following caregiving domains: general, international, social media, agencies, insurance and government, and long-term needs. Some books also have handy information about viable considerations related to health insurance and disability (Prowe 2010).

In order to launch a group discussion, the facilitator should pose open-ended questions such as: *What are your most troubling longer-range practical worries?* Therapeutic probing can also catalyze deeper exploration, including home life, finances, health and safety, community needs, work, and social pursuits. The discussion should oscillate between outlets for the attendees to "vent" and then problem solve solutions, rather than stifle emoting by preemptively jumping to resource possibilities. Often, there is a barrage of worries with which the relatives feel inundated. In order to manage more effectively, the family should adjust expectations and prioritize stressors, solving one or two issues at a time (Kreutzer et al. 2010).

One disconcerting pattern is the tendency of the loved one to overdraft his or her account. Caregivers feel comforted when they can "compare and contrast" their angst and indignation about this. Intermixed with this are workable solutions, including setting a budget, tracking spending, and providing him or her with prepaid credit cards. Group dialogue can be beneficial in identifying when specific caregivers are being exploited financially, as this commonly emanates from feelings of guilt or sadness on behalf of the loved one's reduced income. It is an important reminder to adjust behaviors to model healthy coping behaviors in the loved one, and not indulge extravagances which ultimately are detrimental to him or her. This teaches personal accountability. As one father said, "The credit union is now closed."

In tandem with the group exchange, the facilitators should review the typical results of damage to the frontal lobes affecting impulse control, planning, and judgment (see Fleminger 2008, for a review; see Chap. 4, Sect. 4.4). Impulsivity has also been linked to a sense of urgency and compulsive buying after traumatic brain injury (Rochat et al. 2011). The phenomenon of the "disconnection between knowing and doing" is also relevant, as the loved one can verbalize, yet not execute a

Table 11.7 Common verbalizations about longer-term practical worries

Home
Can he/she live alone?
If he/she is too impaired to ever live alone—what does that mean for me?
Finances
Oh my gosh, he/she is overspending with no “brakes” or idea about savings
He/she can’t earn enough to live on his/her own
I can’t afford his/her medications—they are so expensive
This lawsuit is so ______
Health
I am worried about his/her weight gain
His/her memory seems to be getting worse—now what?
What happens if he/she gets really sick?
What happens if he/she loses his/her medical coverage?
How do I add/remove guardianship or fiduciary help?
I’m crunched between looking after my ailing ____ and my loved one
What happens if I get sick?
What happens if I die?
How do I make sure his/her long term needs are met and everything is in place?
Safety
I protect him/her like an eggshell
It’s like taking care of kids—on steroids
I hate it when the phone rings at odd hours
I’m worried about ____’s safety
What would I do if I didn’t worry?
He/she is making poor choices (e.g., stopped psychotherapy, quit work)
I feel so helpless watching him/her struggle/make mistakes
He/she is so vulnerable
I’m afraid he/she will be taken advantage of
He/she lost his/her street smarts
It’s scary
I feel like I have to hover
Community
I worry when he’s/she’s crossing the street
What happens if he/she can never drive?
How can I juggle my schedule when I’m responsible for his/her transportation?
Is he/she capable of travelling alone?
Can he/she handle new challenges—moving elsewhere, a new job, etc.?
Work
He/she can’t find a job
What if he/she gets fired because of the brain injury and then can’t find another job?
Social life
Why can’t he/she keep friends?
He/she isn’t dating and is so lonely
I’m worried about this on-line dating and what he/she says on Facebook
He/she is in a relationship that I’m worried about
They’re engaged/moving in together and it seems they just met

game plan (Stuss 1991) to conserve funds. Depending on the underlying neurological challenge, automatic payments are useful (e.g., for forgetfulness) and/or debt consolidation (e.g., for executive function challenges). These insights cue the tier supports regarding the underlying organic etiology of overspending and other poor

Table 11.8 Group treatment for longer-term practical worries

Guided exercise
Open ended questions:
What are your most troubling longer range practical worries and why?
Can you identify specific worries in the domains of home, finances, health, safety, community, work, and social life?
Why are you indulging overspending in your loved one and how can you better manage this?
How does your loved one's vulnerability/suggestibility affect you?
What resources have you found to be helpful to address your current practical stressors?
What are your long term "what ifs" and feelings about future uncertainties?
What are the possible risks to your loved one if something happens to you?
Who makes up your "advisory board?"
What provisions have you made for your loved one if something happens to you?
"Helpful hints" and psychoeducation
Seek a fluid interchange between emoting and problem solving
Adjust expectations, prioritize challenges, and solve issues one at a time
To reduce overspending and financial problems:
Set a budget together
Track spending together
Provide prepaid credit cards
Model healthy behaviors and teach accountability
Use automatic payments
Consolidate debt
Remember the role of the brain injury, especially executive function deficits
Involve a "neutral" family member or fiduciary
Create a legal trust with a monthly stipend
Involve his/her physician to start the guardianship/conservatorship process
Remember to use "milieu meetings" and personalized checklists to improve home communication and harmonize responsibilities
Learn about the concept of generalization and facilitate skill acquisition in new settings
Pursue community resources for the loved one's adversities, rather than "micromanage" the situation:
Individual psychotherapy/family therapy
Further rehabilitation
Brain injury support groups
Student Disability Resources
A dietician
Friends or extended family members
A personal assistant/caregiver
Advocate for a neuropsychological evaluation, if needed
Community accommodations (e.g., group home)
Recognize that everyone has their limits in expertise and patience
Be receptive to guidance from group facilitators and peers about the best resources
Don't be afraid or embarrassed to ask for help
Create your personal "advisory board" of tier supports and resources
Take "one day at a time" and set "bite-sized" subgoals
Participate in the "circle of positives" to reflect on "good news" during the Aftercare Group
Multimedia resources
Movie
Home Alone (Gotch et al. 1990)

Table 11.8 (continued)

Songs
"People" (Merrill 1964)
"Stuck in a Moment You Can't Get Out Of" (Bono 2000)
Didactics and demonstrations
Review of "milieu meeting" forms and Home Independence Checklists
Guest speakers
Case manager
Social worker
Attorney and financial advisor
Local Brain Injury Alliance spokesperson
Treating professionals (e.g., a dietician)

Table 11.9 Caregiver resources

General websites
American Association of Caregiving Youth
http://www.aacy.org
Well Spouse Association: Support for Spousal Caregivers
http://www.wellspouse.org
Resources for Caregivers and Caregiving
http://kspope.com/payton/caregiving.php
Strength for Caring: A Place for Caregivers
http://www.strengthforcaring.com
The National Alliance for Caregiving
http://www.caregiving.org
Family Caregiver Alliance: National Center on Caregiving
http://www.caregiver.org/caregiver/jsp/home.jsp
Caregiving Help
http://www.caregivinghelp.org
Today's Caregiver
http://www.caregiver.com/index.htm
Caregiving.com http://www.caregiving.com
Caregiver Action Network http://caregiveraction.org
Case Management Society of America: What is a Case Manager and How do I Find One?
http://www.cmsa.org/Consumer/tabid/61/Default.aspx
Find a Social Worker: helpstartshere.org
http://www.helpstartshere.org/find-a-social-worker
International
Family Caregivers' Network Society (Canada)
http://www.fcns-caregiving.org
Canadian Caregiver Coalition (Canada)
http://www.ccc-ccan.ca
Caring from a Distance: Dedicated to Serving the Needs of Long Distance Caregivers
http://www.cfad.org
Social media
CaringBridge.org http://www.caringbridge.org
CarePages
http://www.carepages.com
CareCentral: a healthcentral.com site
http://www.carecentral.com
Lotsa Helping Hands http://www.lotsahelpinghands.com

Table 11.9 (continued)

Agencies
Brain Injury Association of America
http://www.biausa.org/index.htm
American Stroke Association
http://www.strokeassociation.org/STROKEORG
American Psychological Association: Caregiver Briefcase
http://www.apa.org/pi/about/publications/caregivers/index.aspx
Insurance and government
Medicare Rights Center
http://www.medicarerights.org
Medicare.gov: The Official U.S. Government Site for Medicare
http://www.medicare.gov/caregivers
HealthCare.gov: Site for Insurance Information, Including Pre-existing Conditions
http://finder.healthcare.gov
Resources for Finding Health Insurance & Affordable Medications
http://kspope.com/medications/index.php
Social Security Disability. The Official Website of the U.S. Social Security Administration
http://www.ssa.gov/pgm/disability.htm
Ticket to Work: Support for Beneficiaries with Disabilities Who Want to Work
http://www.ssa.gov/work
Long term needs
Department of Health and Human Services: National Clearinghouse for Long Term Care Information
http://www.longtermcare.gov/LTC/Main_Site/Index.aspx
Department of Health and Human Services: National Clearinghouse for Long Term Care Information—Trusts
http://www.longtermcare.gov/LTC/Main_Site/Paying/Private_Financing/Saving_LTC/Trusts.aspx#Charitable
Independent Living Institute: International Disability Resources
http://www.independentliving.org/links/links-independent-living-centers.html

choices, so as to alleviate the tendency to misattribute the loved one's motives to a "bad attitude."

On occasion, the loved one's financial status becomes too conflict-ridden for the family member to intervene. In this case, the primary caregiver may need to solicit the help of another more "neutral" family member or hire an independent party (e.g., fiduciary) to oversee the loved one's finances. This is imperative if he or she has access to larger funds through a legal settlement and lacks the cognitive capability to manage monies. To prevent squandering, an independent party can set out a monthly stipend through a legal trust. With respect to tackling provision of guardianship and/or fiduciary assignments, the treating physician (e.g., a physiatrist or neurologist) is an excellent first contact.

Often, the caregiver is also adjusting to the long-term responsibilities and sometimes the hassles of living with the loved one. He or she can feel pulled in too many directions when his or her health, or that of other family members deteriorates. Regular "milieu meetings" and personalized checklists for each party facilitate dialogue and define reciprocal duties (see Chap. 4, Sects. 4.4.4 and 4.9 and Fig. 4.7; Klonoff 2010). This augments communications and harmonizes home life. Group members can share their various agendas and checklists to generate ideas for newer or struggling members.

Novelty can be confusing, overwhelming, or frightening to the loved one. Examples include moving into new housing (perhaps without the primary caregiver) or undertaking a new job. Caregivers are then miffed at the loved one's ineptitudes. The facilitator can provide psychoeducation about challenges with generalization, or difficulties transferring skill sets from one environment to another (Klonoff 2010; Persel and Persel 2010). The group can identify ways to improve function, such as practicing discrete subcomponents, so as to gradually enhance new learning. One mother bought a condominium next door to her son and incrementally introduced new chores as a bridge to increased autonomy.

When other adversities unfold (e.g., job loss, school problems, social ostracism, or unsafe behaviors), the family should pursue other community resources, rather than try to "micromanage" the situation. The group facilitators and savvy peers can help identify the best supports. Individual psychotherapy and family therapy may be warranted to help protect their vulnerable loved one, including addressing friendlessness, tricky dating relationships, or other potentially dangerous situations. As depicted in phase 7, the "door is always open" for further interventions as the loved one encounters fresh ordeals, including a new job, pending marriage, or independent travel. Further rehabilitation, brain injury support groups, and Student Disability Resources can relieve the full onus of responsibility from the primary caregiver. Weight gain can be addressed through visits with a dietician or community education groups (e.g., Weight Watchers®). This author invites a dietician to joint Aftercare Groups with the families and loved ones generally twice per year, including during the end of year holiday season.

A humorous technique to lighten the discussion about leaving the loved one alone is to reference the *Home Alone* movie (Gotch et al. 1990). Interestingly, the attendees may vacillate between crying about their hardships and "worst-case scenarios" and laughing about cute, but harmless, anecdotes. To offset worries about the loved one being left unattended while the caregiver tackles outside demands, a list of trustworthy friends or extended family members should be constructed and used. A professional caregiver can also be hired through a local agency (e.g., Visiting Angels). These individuals can also assist with transportation if the loved one is unable to drive. These resources are also advantageous so that the caregiver can snatch indispensable bouts of respite.

The loved one may manage fairly well with the in-home assistance of caregivers, or one-step-removed monitoring. Nevertheless, there is an unremitting anxiety pertaining to what will happen if he or she develops new medical or neurological sequelae and/or if the tier 1 supports fade or are saddled with competing time drains or health problems. Caregivers dread the consequences of their unexpected demise. A brainstorming session about possible risks and antidotes is great group fodder. To this end, family members must remain vigilant to changes in the health status of the loved one. If they become concerned about cognitive deterioration, they should advocate for a neuropsychological examination.

To address the looming question of long-term placement of the loved one if and when the primary caregivers are unable to attend to the patient's needs, the group can divulge within the protective haven their particular fears and threats. "What ifs" and uncertainty about the future are pervasive themes (Minnes et al. 2010; see also Chap. 9, Sect. 9.8). Usually, these circulate around abandonment of the loved one to others who lack knowledge, devotion, and/or empathy for their condition. The caregiver wants to protect the loved one from further pain at all costs. Possible proactive options to avoid a crisis include training a personal assistant who can allay some of the unease about care provision by less experienced tiers of support or researching and identifying top group homes or other forms of accommodation in the eventuality these are required (Cameron and Gignac 2008; Minnes et al. 2010). Of course, written documentation must be prepared to support the loved one's needs in these areas, including provision of sufficient funds to pay for these services.

A major role of the Aftercare Group is the sharing of relevant community resources. Cameron and Gignac (2008) propose provision of educational strategies when the "timing is right." Hence, as caregivers encounter new needs, interventions and resources specific to those phases of the care trajectory should be provided. This eases the preponderance of helplessness. Resource handouts can be disseminated by the group facilitators or through the collective experiences of the family members (see Table 11.9).

Case managers, social workers, attorneys, and financial advisors typically have a wealth of information (Hassan et al. 2011; Kreutzer et al. 2010) and should be invited as guest speakers to the group. A rich source of resources and contacts for many arenas after brain injury is the local Brain Injury Alliance. It is prudent to invite spokespersons from the local chapter to address specific group concerns and barriers as these arise.

The Aftercare Group facilitator and guest presenters are invaluable intermediaries to "point the way" for which are the most timely and suitable resources, based on the families' needs. Otherwise, the relatives may become lost or misdirected by the glut of data on the Internet that is difficult to navigate or digest. The therapist and other members can assist the reticent caregivers in feeling comfortable in requesting help, as this offsets their insecurities associated with the limitations and ignorance about the complex process of recovery (Kreutzer et al. 2010). Peer support within the group setting is instrumental in reinforcing the value of outside supports. It helps the caregivers to be reminded that professionals enjoy being accessible and accommodating (Kreutzer 2010).

Liaisons and intermediaries safeguard the mental health of the family and preserve the rapport with the loved one. Ultimately, the facilitators and group peers can emphasize that even the most competent caregivers have finite expertise to intervene on behalf of the loved one in all areas and must learn how and when to solicit outside assistance. This realization also reminds the loved one that everyone has their limits of knowledge and energies, and that it is "okay" to request help. As referenced in Sect. 11.4.1, a prime recommendation is for relatives to construct their own personal "advisory board" made up of key tier 2 and tier 3 supports and resources. This provides wide-based proficiency, perspective, and solace. An excellent group exercise is for the facilitator to promote group participants to brainstorm about who should be on their "advisory board." The lyrics from the song, "People" (Merrill 1964) are a touching rendition of this belief.

"Tried and true" advice from the more experienced participants is to "take 1 day at a time" and set "bite-sized" subgoals to avoid becoming engulfed by multifarious stressors and obligations (Klonoff and Koberstein 2010; see Chap. 9, Sect. 9.9.1). Ending the group with a "circle of positives" also encourages (and sometimes forces) attendees to take a moment to reflect on "good news." This cognitive behavioral technique of each member recounting something that is exciting currently or in the near future counteracts the likelihood that their anxieties will produce overgeneralizations and prevailing negative mindsets. Similarly, the lyrics to the U2 song, "Stuck in a Moment You Can't Get Out Of" (Bono 2000) complement the ideas of self-efficacy and empowerment.

11.6 Emotions and Sense of Self

A previous publication has addressed the magnitude of changes of sense of self in the patient after brain injury (Klonoff and Myles 2010). *Sense of self* has been defined as the "essence of one's being" (Klonoff and Myles 2010). It encompasses *values*, or the core beliefs that endure over the life span; *identity*, which is the subjective characterization of one's individuality in a social context; and *social roles*, which are the societal position and responsibilities (Klonoff and Myles 2010). Likewise, the sense of self can be radically altered in the tier 1 caregiver, with reverberations into other tier 2 and 3 supports, namely the family, and overall community network. This section will address emotional changes and altered sense of self, including their impact on values. Identity and social roles will be addressed in Sect. 11.7 of this chapter.

As mentioned in Chaps. 2 and 9 (see Chap. 2, Sect. 2.3.8 and Chap. 9, Sect. 9.2) and depicted in phase 1 of the FEM, the abruptness of the loved one's injury catapults the family into "crisis mode." The family is assailed by potent emotions, including shock, disbelief, horror, terror, guilt, and anger. There is a shattering of the assumptive world—the family can no longer assume that life events are orderly, predictable, or fair (Kauffman, 2002). Traumatic loss creates a crisis of meaning and self-fragmentation (Janoff-Bulman, 2002). Relatives have lost a sense of security, reality, meaning, and purpose (Kauffman, 2002). Although their emotions are often most heightened and unstable during the earlier post-acute phases, alterations in the sense of self and a reformulation of the assumptive world are usually a life-long journey.

Table 11.10 summarizes spontaneous verbalizations by Aftercare Group participants that depict striking emotions as well as shifts in their sense of self, including the fabric of their lives which periodically erupt over the long haul. Emotions encompass and oscillate between sorrow, anger, blame, grief, and exhaustion. There is the temptation to escape the situation because of the searing psychic pain. Memories of the past haunt the families, reminding them that there is no "cure." The support network may feel paralyzed and stagnant.

There are differences in the totality of the relatives' existence and the context of their beings. This has been described as the disruption of the "taken-for-granted

Table 11.10 Common verbalizations about emotions and changes in sense of self

Emotions in the support network
I feel like "Dora Doom"
I'm angry at what he/she put me through
I'm still on that roller coaster
How could you do this to me?
I'm filled with grief—my glass is always only half full
I feel like I am grieving over and over
Will the pain ever go away?
I want to run from the injury, but I get "slapped in the face by it"
I miss my loved one "who was"
I have to move my memories from center stage
I know I have the patience of a saint and sometimes it's not enough
It's been 9 years—it's just another day
He/she is not cured
There is no closure
Recovery does not mean it never happened
Sense of self
When can I go back to phase 0?
My life is not the same
Life is no longer normal
My old life is over—it's morphed into a different life
This is not the way it was supposed to be
Things won't ever be the same
My life is upside down
I feel like I am in a "no man's land"
I feel lost
I've lost the familiar
What could have been for me . . .
I miss who I was
What about me?
My dreams are shattered, now what?
Some things will never happen for me
I have sacrificed so much

orientation" (Attig 2002). The families' capacity to rely on the regularity and stability of their surroundings and relationships is destroyed (Attig 2002). Life plans are inextricably altered. There are devastating reverberations to their personas. They feel adrift, having lost their true essence and life compass.

11.6.1 Group Treatment for Emotional Distress and Changes in Sense of Self

Table 11.11 summarizes group exercises, psychoeducation, therapeutic "helpful hints," as well as multimedia resources to cope with the families' longer-term emotional distress and changes in sense of self. There are two formats to explore these tender areas. The first is for the therapist to ask open-ended questions such as:

Table 11.11 Group treatment for emotional changes and loss of sense of self

- *Guided exercises*
  - *Open ended questions:*
    - What was your assumptive world before your loved one's injury?
    - What are your losses?
    - Has your sense of self changed?
    - What makes you ____ and how have you coped with this emotion?
    - How are you making sense of this experience?
    - What areas of progress do you see in your loved one?
    - What are your "silver linings" from this experience?
    - Has the injury been a "wake up" call and what has it done "for you" versus "to you?"
    - What will help you move forward?
  - *Sense of Self Questionnaire*
    - Share responses and themes
- *"Helpful hints" and psychoeducation*
  - Engage in guided free floating discussions
  - Recognize individual differences yet the commonality of suffering
  - Expect "flip flopping" of stances between misery and gratitude
  - Lamentations will be plentiful, expressed as tearfulness, sadness, anger, resentment, avoidance, withdrawal, and powerlessness
  - Introduce concepts such as "chronic sorrow," "living loss," and "lingering sadness"
  - Realize there is no "closure" to losses
  - Find a balance between reminiscing about the past and planning for the future
  - Be observant about the tendency to idealize the past
  - Watch for entrenched grief and depression versus sadness
  - Seek outside psychological/psychiatric care to supplement the Aftercare Group to address depression
  - Learn about the concept of "internal locus of control" so as to effect change
  - Realize that life is not fair
  - Find happiness to help "let go" of some of the sorrow
  - Acknowledge the loved one's triumphs
  - Continue the adjustment process and remain realistic
  - Conceptualize the injury as "managing" emotions, not "getting over it"
  - Try to identify the "silver linings," including "posttraumatic growth," thriving, a sense of purpose, and a "wake up call"
  - Focus on the "process" of healing versus the "outcome"
  - Rely on spirituality as a comfort
  - Restructure a new outlook
  - Conceptualize the "good enough" outcome
  - Aspire to make peace with the circumstances
  - Identify future strivings
  - Seek adaptability and foster resiliency
  - Remember the pillars of love, support, family, and faith
- *Multimedia resources*
- *News article*
  - "Daughter channels Sept. 11 grief into film, activism" (Smith 2011) http://www.npr.org/2011/09/07/140071379/unlikely-star-a-woman-turns-9-11-grief-into-action
- *Books*
  - *Small Knight and George* (Armitage 2007)
  - *Froggy Fable* (Lechner 2005)
  - *Elmer* (McKee 1968)
- *Presentation*
  - "Sense of self" through the eyes of a family member and past patient
- *Film*
  - "Helping Others" chapter in *Happy* (Shadyac et al. 2011)

What was your assumptive world before your loved one's injury? What are your losses? or *How has your sense of self changed? Are there any "silver linings" in your circumstances?* Another procedure to catalyze group discussion is to invite the participants to complete a Sense of Self Questionnaire (see Chap. 2, Sect. 2.3.8 and Fig. 2.2), which is a sentence completion task to assist responders in identifying changes in their core beliefs and sense of self. Several domains are explored, including emotional status, self-perceptions, connection and roles with others, central life principles and priorities, and contemplations for the future. Table 11.12 summarizes a subset of the families' revelations regarding emotions and sense of self—organized according to negative; neutral or mixed; and positive self-appraisals.

Guided free-floating discussions allow personal introspection and group dialogue. The experience of loss will manifest differently for everyone, yet there is a universality of suffering. A noteworthy tendency that the therapist should be sensitive to is the flip-flopping of stances, between misery and heartache compared with gratitude for the loved one's survival and a desire to rejoice in their joint beings. This vacillation is integral to the reconstitution process.

Lamentations are plentiful, as are the tears. Grief is expressed as the "messiness" and unfair "twists and turns" of life. Collectively, the contributors give themselves and each other permission to mourn their losses. They share their many sacrifices, depicted as a combination of selflessness, yet at times resentment. Some relatives have suffered layered losses and they are angry or bitter, assuming that they should have the "vaccine" against compound tragedies. Others, including some of the male attendees, note that their coping mechanism is avoidance and withdrawal; they seek outside support systems less often. Still others feel powerless to "cure" their loved one. The facilitator can reference descriptive concepts of "chronic sorrow" (Olshanky 1962, as cited in Roos 2002), "living loss" (Olshansky 1962 as cited in Lee et al. 2001; Roos 2002), and "lingering sadness" (Patrick-Ott and Ladd 2010; see Chap. 9, Sect. 9.5.1). Relatives share that there is no closure to their devastating losses. This terminology helps to validate the tier supports' anguish and life upheaval.

Therapeutic reminders to those feeling overcome with hurt include trying not to dwell continuously on "what could have been" and envisioning how to "accept the situation for what it is." Some members recognize the normal tendency to idealize the past, which only deepens the torment. The therapist should be sensitive to the possibility that the family member is entrenched in grief. Although there are no clear-cut guidelines as to when sorrow and grief fuse with depression, clinical observation may yield an impression of melancholy, with pervasive despondency and pessimism. The relative seems stuck in joylessness and emptiness. The concept of "soul sickness" beautifully conveys the sense of demoralization, helplessness, and hopelessness because of his or her predicament (Perakis 2010).

Attendees can be educated by the therapist regarding how sadness differs from depression (see Chap. 2, Sect. 2.3.1). Sadness is a normal response to "bad news"; however, it will be ameliorated with positive happenings (Prigatano et al. 1986). Unchanged affect or demeanor in the face of encouraging experiences is indicative of depression (Prigatano et al. 1986). Depression and fear fold inwards, while anger is spewed outwards. The "glass half empty" syndrome with a "doom and gloom"

Table 11.12 Sample responses about emotions and sense of self from the Sense of Self Questionnaire

Negative valuations:

Since my loved one's injury, I feel . . .

a) Like our family was short changed in life

Since my loved one's injury, my sense of who I am . . .

a) Is gone in a blink of an eye

When I compare myself to how my life was before the injury . . .

a) It's overwhelming and chaotic. We were a team and now it is all on me
b) I mourn the loss of a sense of well-being

When I think about life before my loved one's injury, I feel. . .

a) A great loss; I miss my old life
b) Nostalgic. I wish I could go back

Since my loved one's injury, my life is . . .

a) Not how I expected it to be after retirement

Since my loved one's injury, I feel . . .

a) That life is very fragile and we are all vulnerable to terrible loss
b) I try to avoid problems so I won't have to deal with them

Compared to before my loved one's injury, I feel anxious . . .

a) A lot, I get scared because I know life is unpredictable and can change in an instant

Compared to before my loved one's injury, I feel sad . . .

a) When we cannot do the things we used to and when ____ is sad
b) As kind of a constant background emotion

Neutral/mixed valuations:

Compared to before my loved one's injury, my emotions . . .

a) Are closer to the surface—frustration, worry, and concern
b) Are more pronounced, but I try to keep them in check; sometimes I feel numb

Since my loved one's injury, I feel . . .

a) Sad sometimes, but I mostly feel blessed
b) My feelings change daily. Sometimes I feel powerless; other days positive and upbeat
c) Paradoxes—gratitude my son survived; sad about his losses; impressed with his tenacity; upset with the upheaval
d) The whole range of emotions, including gratitude, love, concern, worry, appreciation, sadness, and grief

Since my loved one's injury, my life is . . .

a) Good, rich, but stressful
b) Redefined

Since the injury, when I think about the future, I feel . . .

a) Hope and fear
b) Uncertain, but hopeful that I will make it work

Compared to before my loved one's injury, I feel angry . . .

a) More often—due to my fears. Anger robs me of beauty and joy. I want the courage and to trust that things will work out in all ways
b) Less often—who or what should I be angry with?—I have hope for a happy life for my son

Since my loved one's injury, when I think about my life . . .

a) I see it as totally different from what I planned
b) Sometimes, I want to scream. Sometimes, I think I am lucky

When I compare myself to how my life was before this injury . . .

a) I feel a sense of loss, so I try not to compare our lives, but instead build a new life using the strengths from our past

Positive valuations:

Since my loved one's injury, my sense of who I am . . .

Table 11.12 (continued)

a) Has deepened
b) Has evolved; I have become more self-reliant. I am a nurturer, a protector, sometimes counselor, and a loving mother
c) Has more meaning and purpose
d) Is very clear to me for the first time in my life
Since my loved one's injury, I feel . . .
a) Fortunate and thankful for her recovery
b) I am adjusting to the "new normal"
When I compare myself to how my life was before the injury . . .
a) I am much more giving, patient, and compassionate. I realize what a strong person I am
b) I have shifted from "me, me, me" to focus on the big picture and helping others
c) I think I mature a lot after every incident in life
d) I am wiser
Since my loved one's injury, my ability to deal with problems . . .
a) Is better; this has taught me not to sweat the small stuff
Since my loved one's injury, when I think about my life . . .
a) I realize how precious every day is and I try to live in the moment each day
Since my loved one's injury, what matters to me . . .
a) Is health, spirit, and kindness
b) Is God, love, peace, and people
Since my loved one's injury, my sense of purpose . . .
a) Is still strong. It is reforming and evolving
Since my loved one's injury, when I think about the future, I feel . . .
a) Hopeful and grateful

attitude are unshakable (Klonoff 2010). With guidance, the wounded relatives grasp that anger is wasting their precious energy and depression is depleting their reserves. Caring peers can gently nudge the agonizing group member into a more positive mindset, although this remains only temporary. Typically, however, he or she will need psychological and/or psychiatric treatment in conjunction with the support offered by the Aftercare Group.

Oftentimes, external representations of the grieving process are enlightening to the Aftercare Group. A resource to catalyze group expression is an article about Carie Lemack by Smith (2011), depicting a daughter's struggle to cope with the death of her mother in the 911 attack. Similarly, the theme of the children's book, *Small Knight and George* by Armitage (2007) reminds the group members that the terror from facing inconceivable losses can actually be manageable. Related to this, the group facilitator can introduce the concept of *internal locus of control,* whereby goal achievement is linked to one's actions and factors under his or her personal control (Dawson and Trueman 2010; Henninger et al. 2012). Families then feel empowered to effect change based on their inner strength and capabilities. They notice their willpower. Group feedback includes recognizing that life is not fair, but that they can rebound from their losses. There is a stated resolve to move on with an emphasis on not taking things for granted and finding pleasure in daily life. The intention to view the glass as "half full," at least sometimes, is offered, so as to "let go" of some of the sorrow.

The facilitator should invite input from more seasoned peers. They often share that life gets better with time, and they can breathe easier. Various phrases are useful, including "whatever happened happened." Terminology such as the "new normal" helps. At this junction, the therapist can prompt the caregivers to recount various aspects of their loved one's feats. Examples include the loved one graduating from school, obtaining a job, getting married, etc. This engenders pride, emotional sustenance, and hope and also allows others to share in their delight. As one participant proffered, focusing on what she still had or could have, built up a bank account of emotional reserves. An excellent adjunct intervention is to invite a family member and loved one to the group to present their commendable insights into their evolved selves.

The facilitator can channel the discussion towards coping techniques. Like the loved ones, the relatives are traversing the adjustment process, through transformation and transcendence grounded in their realism (Klonoff 2010). This includes building *intrapsychic assimilation* (i.e., self-esteem, self-efficacy, mastery, and happiness), as well as *existential assimilation* (i.e., meaning, quality of life, self-actualization, and hope; Klonoff 2010; see also Sect. 11.7). Table 11.12 also contains samples of positive valuations reflecting collective transformative experiences. The relatives are "relearning" how to live by blending old and new approaches, revising life plans, and modifying assumptions about themselves and their loved ones (Attig 2002). One mother proclaimed, "I know I will never 'get over' my son's brain injury; I'm focusing on managing the reality that life is different" (J. Cosper, personal communication, 6/5/12).

Some attendees focus on identifying the "silver linings," including maturation in the loved ones and themselves (see also Chap. 2, Sect. 2.4.2.4). The therapist can introduce the concept of *posttraumatic growth,* whereby the individual's exposure to adversity inculcates new character assets (Joseph 2011; Peterson et al. 2008). These are manifested as attributes of wisdom, personal strength, and thankfulness; deeper relationships; and an altered life philosophy focused on true values (Joseph 2011). The group facilitator can propose a "thrive model," exploring how members take stock of their situation; harvest hope; re-author challenges through storytelling; and cherish and then express change through intended action (Joseph 2011). A paradigm comprised of strength subcomponents can be discussed by the group members, including wisdom and knowledge; courage; love; justice (e.g., fairness); temperance (e.g., forgiveness, humility, caution, and self-control); and transcendence (e.g., awe, gratitude, hope, humor, purpose, and spirituality; Seligman and Peterson 2003; see also Chap. 1, Sects. 1.2.9 and 1.2.10 and Chap. 10, Sect. 10.2).

Gradually another sense of purpose emerges. Restoring hope and morale are fundamental (Perakis 2010). This can include perceiving the tier 1 caregiver role as a gift, a choice (not a duty), and a new way to love. The adage "We must be willing to let go of the life we have planned, so as to have the life waiting for us" (Joseph Campbell, in Chang 2006) sparks group dialogue. One mother divulged that the circumstances of her son's brain injury first defined her by necessity, but later by her own choice (C. Morrissey, personal communication, 2/23/12). Other insights include improved relationships with the loved one, a stronger family unit, the preciousness of life, and "not sweating the small stuff" (Eliot and Breo 1989). Other eye-openers include a "wake-up call," which enhances the sense of self, based on new values and priorities. Like the patient, the tier supports can self-reflect about what the brain injury has done "for them" versus "to them" (Klonoff 2010). The segment, "Helping Others" from the DVD *Happy* (Shadyac et al. 2011) depicts one man's transformation from emptiness to meaning and fulfillment through compassion and altruism.

The therapist can introduce the concept of devoting energies on the "process" of healing versus rushing to the ever-elusive "outcome" (Klonoff 2010). Over time, the family becomes more comfortable with the unknowns, with an outlook of "we'll find a way." Spirituality can provide a guiding light; as one wife said, "I pray for wisdom." The relatives restructure how they view the world and how to live in it (Attig 2002). There is embracement of a "new me" compared to who they thought they were, or a transposition from "who I was" to "who I am." New perspectives forge community (re)connections. They see life as "different, but satisfying." Group dialogue can facilitate the acceptance process, with introduction of "good enough" outcomes for the loved ones and caregivers (Klonoff 2010). This recalibration helps families accept decent (versus the best) results, thereby normalizing inexorable imperfections and setbacks as part of coping with life's adversities. Reading *Froggy Fable* by Lechner (2005) emphasizes the personal growth that emerges from seemingly vexing changes.

There are efforts away from "why me" and towards making peace with what they have. The children's fable, *Elmer* by McKee (1968) humorously exemplifies the special advantages of individuality. This translates to identifying future strivings. Using positive psychology ideology, the therapist can help to bolster the group by reminding them of their resiliency and bravery in tackling these quandaries. Shared feedback from peers breeds a more optimistic orientation (Kobau et al. 2011). Experience, education, and time all pave the way to adaptation—"it's what is, not what was." One wife revealed, "I fell in love in a different way." Ultimately, the families share that love, support, family, and faith are the pillars in reestablishing wholeness (see also Chap. 2, Sect. 2.4.2.5).

11.7 Adjustment

Adjustment has been defined as the interplay between the individual's external adaptation to his or her physical environs and an internal process of assimilation, whereby "preexisting plans, expectations, and hopes are reformulated into a meaningful existence" (Klonoff 2010, p. 101). Clinical observation and research reveal that tier supports suffer from long-term adjustment challenges after brain injury (Hassan et al. 2011), specifically related to redefinitions of their identity and roles within and outside of the family unit (Klonoff and Koberstein 2010). This includes skewed role modifications as a spouse or parent of a loved one with a brain injury. Former identity is in peril, including as a worker. Due to the loved one's dependency, the tier 1 caregiver may be forced to take a leave of absence, reduce work hours, or unfortunately terminate a coveted position (Lefebvre et al. 2008). A common revelation is that commitments exceed available hours.

Table 11.13 Common verbalizations about adjustment challenges

My life is so complicated now
I'd rather take care of him/her than myself
He/she is crowding out my ability to complete my responsibilities
It's so hard to stick to a schedule
How can I work and take care of ____?
I'm busy, but not fulfilled
My patience is wearing thin
I feel guilty that I'm irritable with him/her
I am burned out
I'll never cross the finish line
I am anxious to get back to my life
It's such a long hard road
I want to be a rock
I want my independence too
How do I carve a life for myself?
He/she wants his/her life back and so do I
I want to reconstitute my life
I want to be happy also
I need to figure out what to do with my life
It's been 5 years and I am still working on adjusting to all of this

Exorbitant stress and chronic self-sacrifice in key realms that nurture the caregiver can precipitate FEM "yellow warning" zone characteristics of impatience, resentment, and burnout (Klonoff and Koberstein 2010; Lefebvre et al. 2008). This is then compounded by guilt feelings for berating the loved one. There is often a feeling of endlessness because of the loved one's ongoing limitations and care needs. The caregiver craves a balance between effectively and empathically meeting the needs of the loved one, yet carving out "a life" for himself or herself that is multidimensional and enriched. Table 11.13 provides some representative verbalizations from family members contending with longer-term adjustment after brain injury.

11.7.1 Group Treatment for Adjustment Challenges

Table 11.14 summarizes group exercises, psychoeducation, therapeutic "helpful hints," as well as multimedia resources for the caregiver and other family members to address adjustment challenges for the long haul after a loved one's brain injury. Central to the adjustment process is *acceptance,* which constitutes the ability and willingness to cope with a new reality and identity (Klonoff 2010). The facilitator can introduce the adage "learn, train, and heal" as components of the acceptance and compensation process. Acceptance and adjustment are cyclical and continually evolve (Klonoff 2010). In actuality, there is dissonance in the caregiving role between positive and negative aspects, which co-occur (Ayalong 2004). Table 11.15 portrays sample responses about longer-term adjustment using the Sense of Self Questionnaire, particularly in the spheres of family and life roles, work, the future,

Table 11.14 Group treatment for adjustment challenges

Guided exercise
Open ended questions:
What struggles are you facing with acceptance and adjustment?
What are you doing for yourself?
Do you have balance in the domains of "work, love, and play?" If not, why not?
What are your practical challenges in creating your own life?
How has your identity changed?
How do you conceptualize your own paradigm of structure/routine; productivity; socialization; and meaning/fulfillment?
Are you suffering from burnout? What are your remedies?
What outlets will provide you with personal growth and happiness?
Who are your heroes and sources of inspiration?
How do your loved ones inspire you?
Describe instances of fun and humor
What are the positive aspects of being a caregiver?
Sense of Self Questionnaire:
Share responses and themes
"Helpful hints" and psychoeducation
Central to the adjustment process is acceptance
Unhealthy coping techniques should be explored in an ambience of safety and trust
Seek outside resources for addictive behaviors
Learn problem-focused coping techniques, including stress management
Pursue a balance between work, love, and play
Address your personal health and psychological needs, as you are ready
Incorporate structure/routine; productivity; socialization; and meaning/fulfillment into your lifestyle
Utilize secondary and tertiary levels of support so that you can diversify your interests
Remember the reference point of the day of the accident (versus the day before)
Strive for mutual happiness and personal development
If appropriate, pursue satisfying work and/or altruistic endeavors
Aim for who and what you want to become
Remember the healing role of humor and fun
Live in the moment and learn the skill of patience
Rely on faith and spirituality as supports
Create purposeful plans for the future, based on short and long-term aspirations
Multimedia resources
Presentation
Stress-management techniques
Songs
"Come Healing" (Cohen 2012)
"Living in the Moment" (Mraz 2012)
Book
Gabby: A Story of Courage and Hope (Giffords et al. 2011)

and a sense of purpose. Responses are grouped according to negative, mixed/neutral, and positive valuations. To galvanize the discussion, the therapist can inquire of the attendees: *What struggles are you facing with acceptance and adjustment?*

When group attendees experience safety and trust, they may reveal their unhealthy coping strategies. Escape–avoidance behaviors have been connected to

Table 11.15 Sample responses about adjustment from the Sense of Self Questionnaire

Negative valuations:

- *Since the injury, when I think about my role in my family . . .*
  - a) I am now a father again taking care of my son who before was on his own
  - b) I feel very alone and responsible for so much
  - c) Has been redirected—caring for my son takes away from being a wife and grandmother
- *Since my loved one's injury, when I think about work . . .*
  - a) It is secondary to my family until things are better
  - b) I say forget about it
  - c) It is out of the question—this is my job! I need a hobby
- *Since my loved one's injury, my role in life . . .*
  - a) Is not what I hoped it would be
  - b) Has become only a caregiver—everyone is dependent on me for everything
- *Since my loved one's injury, my sense of purpose . . .*
  - a) Is all tied up with my son and his well-being—there seems to be no end in sight
  - b) Is a guess. I am still trying to make sense of my life, and then find a purpose
  - c) Is lost—I'm not sure what it is
- *Since my loved one's injury, my life is . . .*
  - a) Not what I expected once I retired
- *Since my loved one's injury, when I think about my life . . .*
  - a) I don't see an end to the constant caregiving
  - b) I am more aware of how fragile life is and it scares me
- *Since the injury, when I think about the future, I feel . . .*
  - a) Worried
  - b) I have to factor my son into my plans
  - c) Scared—what if I die before she does?

Neutral/mixed valuations:

- *Since the injury, when I think about my role in my family . . .*
  - a) It is the same as before, but I am needed for many more years than I counted on
  - b) It is trying to protect everybody and balancing competing interests, including work
- *Since my loved one's injury, when I think about work . . .*
  - a) I have mixed feelings—it is good to be busy, but I don't care about work as much
  - b) I wonder if I will be able to work again . . .
  - c) There are pressures, but it is still interesting and necessary for me
- *Since my loved one's injury, my life is . . .*
  - a) Brain injury this and brain injury that—and fun in-between
  - b) Sometimes on hold; other times starting to reshape
  - c) Stressful, but there is also lots of hope and appreciation
- *Since my loved one's injury, when I think about my life . . .*
  - a) This is the biggest challenge I have ever faced
  - b) Is good and rich, but stressful
  - c) Is more settled, sometimes chaotic, but overall good
  - d) Is in the process of being rebuilt
  - e) I see it as totally different from what I planned
  - f) Has changed significantly—I have more purpose and responsibilities
- *Since my loved one's injury, my sense of purpose . . .*
  - a) Is still uncertain, but more hopeful that things will work out
  - b) Is in flux—I'm gradually finding out what matters

Positive valuations:

- *Since the injury, when I think about my role in my family . . .*
  - a) I feel like "super mom"
  - b) I know what I need to do and I am proud of it

Table 11.15 (continued)

Since my loved one's injury, my role in life . . .
a) Is multifaceted—mother, wife, daughter, sister, friend, and employee
b) Is to be more sensitive to my family's feelings
c) Is to provide the best care for ___, myself, and our children
Since my loved one's injury, when I think about work . . .
a) I have always enjoyed it and I am glad I am back to work now
Since my loved one's injury, when I think about my life . . .
a) It is good despite everything that has happened—I am grateful for who and what I have
b) I think of how good G-d has been to me
c) It is now back to what it was—a parent and a worker
d) I'm appreciative of so much and know this experience has transformed me
e) I feel blessed
f) I realize how precious every day is. I try to live in the moment of the day
Since the injury, when I think about the future, I feel . . .
a) Hopeful and thankful
b) There will be good things to come
Since the injury, my place in the world . . .
a) Is to make others aware of brain injury
Since my loved one's injury, my sense of purpose . . .
a) Is I have more of a sense of purpose because of my new responsibilities
b) Is focused on assisting my son in being self-sufficient
c) Is to care for others
d) Has changed—I have moved from "everything is about me" to being caring and compassionate
e) Is to be as strong as I can be for myself, my loved one, my family, and my community

increased burden and global distress (Davis et al. 2009). Examples include wishing the event had not occurred, trying not to think about it, and/or self-blame (Davis et al. 2009). Symptomatic of poor coping include excessive alcohol (Hall et al. 1994) or prescription medication use, detrimental habits (e.g., gambling), or other escapist activities. Although these diversions provide a temporary lull, they erode the physical and emotional welfare of the caregiver and contaminate harmony in the family.

Family members who have succumbed to these persuasions will need specialized counseling and interventions in addition to the general support of the Aftercare Group (Hall et al. 1994). The group facilitator should provide immediate resources to the caregiver in a private setting away from the group conversation. In addition, the facilitator and peers can assist with problem-focused coping techniques (rather than emotion-focused), including proactive planning and information sharing to abate specific stressors (Davis et al. 2009). Group discussion can also facilitate conceptualizing the injury in a more adaptive manner and how to master useful tactics to improve the loved one's functional status (Davis et al. 2009). The therapist can demonstrate specific stress-management exercises within the group setting, as nourishing replacement coping practices (Davis et al. 2009).

The facilitator should introduce the concept of a balance between work, love, and play, in order to maximize personal adjustment and regain "normalcy" (Prigatano 1989). The participants may be asked: *What are you doing for yourself?* The facilitator may need to "grant psychological permission" to the caregiver to address his or her needs and desires, as too often guilt and dismay act as interference. This includes medical appointments and overall healthy living, like regular exercise. As one relative said to another who was struggling "the best ally is you." When it seems unfathomable to the caregiver to envision a better future, the therapist can interject the premise of "planting the seed" (G.A. Lage, personal communication, n. d. in Klonoff 2010). Group peers discover that the timing and pacing of acceptance and adjustment are individualized and only happens when the family unit is ready.

Practically speaking, the group members (as well as the loved ones) should identify sources of structure and routine, productivity, socialization, as well as meaning and fulfillment so as create a fruitful lifestyle. This means the loved one should be encouraged to maximize his or her independence so that the family can pursue personal goals. With more severe injuries, arrangements can be made to obtain the necessary supervision for the loved one (see Sect. 11.5.1). The primary caregiver will need to be inventive and assertive regarding secondary and tertiary tiers of support, so as to attain the requisite emotional stability to undertake new ventures. Enabling the caregiver to diversify interests when he or she craves this is critical to ameliorating crankiness, emptiness, and burnout. It also reduces the tendency towards self-centeredness in the loved one, who may have become overly accustomed to lavished attention from a singular caregiver (Klonoff 2010).

As touched upon in Chap. 9 (Sect. 9.5.1), facilitated group dialogue can remind the participants of their new "reference point," particularly when they feel discouraged or pessimistic. Usually, they are lapsing into a mindset of comparing their current situation with the "day before" the injury compared to "the day of." Although a painful reminder, this jolts the relative into a realistic perspective of actually how far the loved one has progressed, rather than a purely loss-focused attitude. The song, "Come Healing" by Cohen (2012) beautifully depicts this transposition from injury to recovery.

There is mutual happiness and personal development when all parties are active and productive, including outside of the home environment (see "positive valuations" in Table 11.15). Caregivers should be cautioned about constraining themselves to work positions they dislike as this only adds to their chagrin and negativity. Positive psychology describes happiness in three domains: the pleasant life, the engaged life, and the meaningful life (see Evans 2011, for a review). The facilitator can encourage group participants to envision sources of happiness through recognizing the role of personal choice (versus a victim role). This will facilitate constructive and concrete goal setting (Evans 2011). One resource to promote discussion in this realm is the book, *Gabby: A Story about Courage and Hope* by Giffords et al. (2011).

New joys should be sought after, albeit in the context of a new life path. This broadens everyone's horizons. Allegiances to the loved one are fortified and energies are rejuvenated. Everyone should be afforded respect, empathy, and outlets for authenticity within the family unit. This includes the caregiver resuming satisfying work. Often, this translates to various altruistic endeavors, as the process of giving to others is fulfilling and perspective building. Pursuits can be conjoint between the loved one and family, for instance, volunteering at a hospital or soup kitchen, or for any other charitable organization. Alternatively, the loved one and family members may flourish more through their own quests and should be prompted to pursue valued activities (Cameron and Gignac 2008). As one wife said, "separateness is a good thing."

A positive feedback loop emerges whereby the loved one and family all feel inspired and replete due to their productive undertakings. Morale is lifted within the family unit. Life can be envisioned as the introspective progression from where he or she is to where he or she wants to be and who he or she wants to become (S. Katz, personal communication, 4/21/12). To this end, the group facilitator can invite the attendees to describe their heroes and sources of inspiration that bestow zest to their lives. Sometimes, it is the courage and determination of their own loved ones. Other times, it is the wisdom and empathy of the group that empower one another. This is a wonderful way to raise the group disposition, especially when some are weary and gloomy.

The adjustment process is also predicated on infusions of fun and humor enveloped in never-ending tolerance. A useful group exercise is to encourage participants to share various vignettes; this usually catalyzes peals of cathartic laughter. "Living in the moment" also reduces ill effects of premature worrying and conserves much needed emotional energy (Cassidy 2009). The song with the same name, "Living in the Moment" by Mraz (2012) engenders a cheerful orientation in this regard. A reminder that patience is a learned skill that improves with practice also sustains the relatives during rough patches (Kreutzer et al. 2010).

Facilitated group discussion reveals that time, healing, and spirituality are fundamental to acceptance and adjustment (Hassan et al. 2011; Klonoff and Koberstein 2010). Table 11.15 summarizes a number of references to faith and spirituality considered integral to positive valuations of their life course. Incremental successes for the loved one and family are the objective. One relative acknowledged "this week things are good," implying the inherent changeability in the adjustment process. Another shared contentedly, "there is a life coming back to our family." The family will experience a positive aura from "getting on with life" by establishing a foothold in the world (Attig 2002). Fashioning a new homeostasis and adaptive coping (i.e., FEM "green coping" zone) requires flexibility, ingenuity, and adaptability for inevitable barriers. The emphasis shifts towards purposeful plans for the future, with the juxtaposition of short- and long-term aspirations with hope and realism (Cassidy 2009; Klonoff et al. 2008).

11.8 Social Reintegration

Prior chapters have addressed the all too common experience of loneliness and social isolation in the caregiver and overall family (Braine 2011; see Chap. 9, Sect. 9.7). This often extends into the chronic phases of the injury and negatively affects the caregiver's emotional well-being, social relations, and leisure (Boyle and Haines 2002; Cassidy 2009; Ergh et al. 2002; Lefebvre et al. 2008), especially if the relatives are not watchful of this susceptibility.

Table 11.16 Common verbalizations about the hurdles for social reintegration

I feel alone and isolated
I don't fit in
I have no social life
My loved one's social awkwardness interferes with having outside friendships
Without my partner, our social circles have changed
When we go out for "night life" as a couple, he/she gets so tired
I don't have the energy for friendships
I feel socially withdrawn and want to be homebound
I feel guilty going out and leaving my loved one home alone with nothing to do
I have "separation anxiety" about leaving him/her
Having friendships reminds my loved one that he/she doesn't
My friends don't get it
Travelling and breaking the routine is too stressful and difficult
I want "me time"
I wish I had time to date
I want time with friends

Table 11.16 conveys some typical verbalizations about the obstacles associated with social reintegration. Some of these are patient based. The social stigma of brain-injured relatives can be alienating to others (Rodgers et al. 2007). For example, patients' problems with cognition, communication pragmatics, and interpersonal behaviors may impede opportunities for friendships and socialization experiences with other families (Klonoff 2010; Lefebvre et al. 2008). More severe brain injuries tax the caregiver and family extensively and preclude outside relations because of the totality of obligations (Ergh et al. 2002). Radical personality, physical, language, or other neurological changes in the spouse often preclude the pre-event pastimes and destroy the chemistry of interactions with other couples with whom there was a positive historical connection. Physical fatigue and lowered frustration tolerance interfere with nightlife, as the loved one often cannot endure extended social activity into the evening hours, especially in noisy, distractible, or chaotic environments.

Other hindrances emanate from within the relatives. Encumbrances weigh on the tier 1 caregiver, as there is no time or energy to pursue friendships or community activities. Emotional distress eradicates the desire for social experiences. Even if the caregiver musters the energy to contact friends, he or she will abort the plan if the loved one will be forlorn and bored at home with no company. Enjoyable peer relations for other family members are also a painfully stark reminder to the loved one that he or she feels rejected by or alienated from his or her friends. Then the caregiver will avoid settings which accentuate this reality. Alternatively, the caregiver may be too scared to leave the loved one, for fear he or she will have trouble physically or cognitively managing by himself or herself.

Relatives may be reluctant to share with friends the many hurdles and aggravations with which they contend. They do not want to overwhelm others and feel vulnerable about their tentative and agonizing conditions (Kreutzer et al. 2010). Often, the friend network cannot understand or relate to the injury aftereffects (Jumisko et al. 2007) and may softly drift away. Now the caregiver feels abandoned (Kreutzer et al. 2010).

Table 11.17 Group treatment for social reintegration

Guided exercise
Open ended questions:
Do you have time to pursue your own friendships? If not, why not?
What techniques have you found to be helpful to facilitate socialization?
With whom do you share information about your circumstances?
How do you handle questions from acquaintances or friends about your situation?
Sense of Self Questionnaire
Share responses and themes
"Helpful hints" and psychoeducation
Feelings about social relationships will oscillate between alienation, disconnection, and/or envy compared with depth and gratitude
Expect individual differences and preferences with respect to friendships and dating
Many caregivers prefer socializing with other caregivers because of their shared insights and empathy
A "best buddy" can be counted on for regular "venting sessions"
Seek social gatherings which are relaxing and self-indulgent
Provide rotating respite for other caregivers as a beneficial network
Find meaningful pastimes with new or familiar companions
Participate in group social activities, also with loved ones
Spouses should regenerate a comfortable social circle with other couples
Unmarried caregivers should seek dating relationships as part of their quality of life
Take vacations with and without the loved one
Develop "scripts" for sharing injury aftereffects based on differing relationship closeness and involve the loved one in the development process
Cultivate two-way healthy relations
Remember that social supports enhance well-being and family functioning
Multimedia resources
Films
"Income, Values, Relationships" chapter in *Happy* (Shadyac et al. 2011)
"Longevity, Okinawa" chapter in *Happy* (Shadyac et al. 2011)

Traveling to see other extended family or friends also becomes more toil than delight. Disturbed daily schedules and the necessary pre-planning to cater to everyone are too draining.

Usually, the caregiver and family members get to the point of needing and missing outside contacts and diversions. Like everyone, they need the comfort and enjoyment of human bonds. They begin to yearn for "me time" and a healthier social life.

11.8.1 Group Treatment for Social Reintegration

Table 11.17 provides group exercises, psychoeducation, therapeutic "helpful hints," as well as multimedia resources for the caregiver and other family members to renew social relationships. As described in Sect. 11.6.1, the group facilitator can utilize two methods. The first is to instigate discussions through general questions designed to encourage participants to share their viewpoints. Sample inquiries include: *Do you have time to pursue your own friendships? If not, why not? What techniques have you*

Table 11.18 Sample responses about social reintegration struggles from the Sense of Self Questionnaire

Negative valuations:
Since my loved one's injury, my sense of connection with other people is . . .
a) Weaker. There is some disconnection because of the need to pull inward
b) Lessened. I isolated and pulled into the family more
c) Worse, as most of my time is spent at home
d) A little less. I feel "different" a lot
Since my loved one's injury, when I compare myself to my friends . . .
a) My world has shrunk—I'm more focused on the home front and less social
b) I feel a bit jealous as what I perceive is an easier life for them
c) I don't think they can grasp what happened, so I pulled away
d) We are in totally different places
e) I'm not like them—their kids are independent
Neutral/mixed valuations:
Since my loved one's injury, my sense of connection with other people . . .
a) Has changed—I have become closer to some and lost others
b) Is secondary, as my family has become my top priority
c) Is that I feel more connected with people who have situations affecting their lives that are out of their control
Since my loved one's injury, when I compare myself to my friends . . .
a) Everybody has their own things to deal with. I am lucky things went so well for so long
b) I feel blessed, but at the same time I am not moving forward as quickly as them
Positive valuations:
Since my loved one's injury, my sense of connection with other people is . . .
a) Pretty good considering everything on my plate—I have been blessed with some wonderful friends
b) Better. I feel I am a better friend
c) Enhanced, as I am more compassionate
d) Fine now—it took time to reconnect
Since my loved one's injury, when I compare myself to my friends . . .
a) I notice their struggles more
b) I realize everyone has troubles, not just me
c) I realize we all have struggles in life; I wouldn't trade places
d) I am so appreciative of them and I hope I can be the type of friend they have been
e) I see how well I have learned to cope
f) I am grateful
g) I am fortunate for this experience

found to be helpful to facilitate socialization? With whom do you share information about your circumstances? How do you handle questions from acquaintances or friends regarding your situation?

The second therapeutic methodology is to utilize the Sense of Self Questionnaire, with particular emphasis on the questions addressing friendships and social connections. Table 11.18 depicts a sampling of attendees' responses, also categorized according to negative; neutral or mixed; and positive self-expressions. Note the variability, with some relatives expressing alienation, detachment, and even envy for their perceived life disparities. Others have rekindled relationships and seem enraptured by deeper compassion and also gratitude for their acquired wisdom. Their

Table 11.19 A sampling of social outlets for family members

Luncheons
Manicures and pedicures
Shopping expeditions
Social clubs
Retreats and getaways
Community college classes
Public speaking groups
Docent opportunities
Teach a church class
Volunteer at a neighborhood hospital, school, church, or charity organization
Study a foreign language
Skype with extended family or out-of-town friends
Arts and crafts groups
Book clubs
Scrapbooking clubs
Workouts
Adaptive sports activities that include families
Social groups for families and loved ones with brain injuries
Group travel (e.g., a cruise)
Family reunions
Vacations
Specialized camps for loved ones with brain injuries and their families

vantage point suggests a more existential viewpoint, recognizing that various forms of suffering are inherent to the human condition. Relationships are less superficial and "fluffy"; instead, they are deeper with like-minded centered individuals who are in touch with what counts. Nonetheless, all caregivers realize the normalcy of fluctuations in perceptions and outlook, depending on personal circumstances and strains, and importantly, the current adjustment of their loved ones.

Facilitated dialogue and brainstorming by the group attendees reveal a number of doable and creative social outlets. These are summarized in Table 11.19. Of note, there will undoubtedly be individual differences between caregivers and other family members with respect to friendship or dating preferences. This list is meant to galvanize some thoughtfulness about ways to re-involve themselves in social activities. A number of relatives have expressed closer ties to other caregivers who have a deeper understanding and empathy for the nuances of an altered existence. Everyone has an intrinsic and unspoken understanding of the time constraints and emotional tribulations. They understand that the injury is not "invisible" just because there are no physical manifestations. Therefore, relatives are often drawn to interactions with other family members who have a loved one with an acquired brain injury. They feel insulated in a "unique club."

The therapist can explore various types of relationships which are nurturing to the caregivers. Some participants report true solace from a very close "best buddy" with whom they can count on for regular "venting sessions." This also allows the relative to receive an external, yet caring perspective from someone who appreciates the caregiver's distinct needs and personality. Others enjoy respite activities, such as social gatherings that are relaxing and hopefully self-indulgent, so as to replenish diminished emotional reserves. Enjoyable outlets include luncheons, manicures and pedicures, or shopping expeditions. One subgroup of mothers established the "Sisterhood of Moms," who would meet regularly and undertake occasional out-of-town retreats. Caregivers volunteered to rotate and stay with one another's loved ones so as to free others to enjoy some leisure time. This arrangement is reassuring to the relatives, as they know their loved ones are "in good hands" with other experienced caregivers.

Caregivers applaud the value of meaningful pastimes with either new or familiar companions. These include community college classes, public speaking groups (e.g., Toastmasters International©), docent opportunities at a local art gallery, teaching church classes, or volunteering at a neighborhood hospital, school, church, or other charity organization. One caregiver started studying Spanish for the intellectual stimulation to hopefully fulfill a dream to someday travel. Another subgroup developed a regular walking/coffee schedule. Whatever the venue, the feeling of cooperation, belonging, and togetherness are sources of contentment. This is eloquently depicted in the chapters, "Income, Values and Relationships" and "Longevity, Okinawa" of the documentary, *Happy* (Shadyac et al. 2011).

Some caregivers enjoy adopting in-home hobbies and inviting friends to participate. One relative was keen on beading; another developed a passion for creating rosaries. One mother orchestrated the creation of a cookbook of donated recipes, which were later sold at a church function. Book clubs and scrapbooking are other entertaining recreations. Although less ideal, some caregivers like skyping with extended family and out-of-town friends, as this provides some basic human bond. Related to this, one wife began the study of genealogy, which brought her closer to her extended relatives.

Group social activities with other families (with or without their loved ones) are also enjoyable. Several mothers work out while their loved ones take adaptive sport classes at a sports facility designed for individuals with special needs of all kinds. Many larger metropolitan areas have adaptive sports programs in which both the loved one and other family members can partake. In our city, several family members and patients developed the Brain Injury Group ("B.I.G.") Fun Time, which meets approximately monthly and engages in various social activities. This includes dinner and a movie; attendance at sports events; holiday parties; games at outdoor parks, etc. Two caregivers take the leadership role to plan activities and communicate with interested parties via email reminders and invitations. Through this group, a cruise was planned, in which a number of families with their loved ones participated. It was a wonderful experience, with a collaborative effort to find safe and entertaining activities and an eagerness on the part of all caregivers to rotate responsibilities for monitoring the loved ones. Everyone appreciated this "normalizing" experience and witnessing the joy of adventure. Other caregivers endorse family reunions; extended family members could learn more about the loved one through direct observations and hopefully share in the supervision. One mother, who was reluctant to make a trek, invited her sisters to town to celebrate her own birthday. This arrangement allowed her to provide assistance to her daughter, yet spend special time with her kin.

Spouses will need to regenerate a social circle and will gravitate to dear friends who are accommodating and welcoming. At times, the spouse without the injury will need to take a leadership role in orchestrating what activities are best done with whom, so all parties are comfortable. Unmarried caregivers will have special impediments in resuming dating. Most are very reticent, proclaiming they do not have the time or energy. Through therapeutic and group dialogue, options can be identified to seek desired intimacy while meeting the realistic needs of the loved one. This usually requires the caregiver giving himself or herself permission to relish a relationship, even though this is not yet be feasible for his or her loved one. However, it still provides positive role modeling of a balanced lifestyle with a happier and healthier caregiver who can then be more loving in the support role. In our setting, two unattached parents with sons with acquired brain injuries gradually began dating, based on a friendship that developed in the support group.

The therapist can also promote the concept of vacations for the caregiver and possibly other family members without the loved one. This builds self-reliance and autonomy in the loved one, and allows the other relatives the opportunity to pursue their own interests and needs. Some caregivers have timed their reprieve with satisfying activities for the loved one, including a holiday with other relatives or friends, or attending a camp experience for patients with acquired brain injuries. Camp "Can Do," sponsored by the Brain Injury Alliance of Arizona, hosts activities, such as karaoke, adaptive water sports, fishing, beading, and scenic tours. Everyone feels they "fit in" with no harsh judgments. Other relatives enjoyed attending the same camp with their loved one, as it provided quality of life and time away.

The group setting is an excellent forum to explore how to best handle outsiders' questions about the loved one's and caregiver's condition when they arise in the community. One husband suggested three layers of disclosure for the three tiers of support (K. Goldfine, personal communication, 3/29/12). For acquaintances and more peripheral involvements (i.e., tier 3 supports), short illustrative phrases are most effective, such as "well, it's a 'new normal,' but things are progressing." For closer contacts (i.e., tier 2 supports), the terminology can be more explicit to better represent the true challenges. If comfortable, this can include language such as "damage" or "ongoing deficits." For closest, kind-hearted confidants (i.e., tier 1 supports), where the caregiver feels he or she can be most candid, more details can be shared, also including ramifications for the relationship based on cognitive and emotional sequelae. Of course, any disclosures should always be sensitive to and inclusive of the loved one's preferences and privacy.

Regardless of the avenues the families choose to engage in to cultivate enjoyable socialization experiences, the therapist can remind them that this venture is a "two-way street" (Klonoff 2010). Relatives will need to reach out to others while at the same time hoping that others are welcoming of the association. Overall, social support enhances personal well-being and family functioning.

References

Armitage, R. (2007). *Small knight and George*. Hauppauge: Barron's Educational Series.

Attig, T. (2002). Questionable assumptions about assumptive worlds. In J. Kauffman (Ed.), *Loss of the assumptive world: A theory of traumatic loss* (pp. 55–68). New York: Brunner-Routledge.

Ayalong, L. (2004). Cultural variants of caregiving or the culture of caregiving. *Journal of Cultural Diversity, 11*(4), 131–138.

Baldwin, V. N., Powell, T., & Lorenc, L. (2011). Factors influencing the uptake of memory compensations: A qualitative analysis. *Neuropsychological Rehabilitation, 21*(4), 484–501.

Bass, R., Brookwell, D., Deege, R., Galindez, R. S., Hamilton, B., Hamilton, N., Hofstetter, D. et al. (Producers), & McNamara, S. (Director). (2011). *Soul surfer* [Motion picture]. United States: TriStar Pictures.

Beck, J. S. (1995). *Cognitive therapy: Basics and beyond*. New York: Guilford Press.

Bono (2000). *Stuck in a moment you can't get out of* [Recorded by U2]. On *All that you can't leave behind* [CD]. Santo Monica: Interscope Records.

Boyle, G. J., & Haines, S. (2002). Severe traumatic brain injury: Some effects on family caregivers. *Psychological Reports, 90*(2), 415–425.

Braine, M. E. (2011). The experience of living with a family member with challenging behavior post acquired brain injury. *Journal of Neuroscience Nursing, 43*(3), 156–164.

Britten, T., & Lyle, G. (1984). *What's love got to do with it* [Recorded by Tina Turner]. *On Private dancer* [Album]. Los Angeles: Capitol Records.

Brody, T. S., De Niro, R., Gering, C., Guare, J., Palef, B., Rosenthal, J., Rudin, S. et al., (Producers), & Zaks, J. (Director). (1996). *Marvin's room* [Motion picture]. United States: Miramax Films.

Brooks, N., Campsie, L., Symington, C., Beattie, A., & McKinlay, W. (1986). The five year outcome of severe blunt head injury: A relative's view. *Journal of Neurology, Neurosurgery, and Psychiatry, 49,* 764–770.

Cameron, J. I., & Gignac, M. A. (2008). "Timing it right": A conceptual framework for addressing the support needs of family caregivers to stroke survivors from the hospital to the home. *Patient Education and Counseling, 70*(3), 305–314.

Cassidy, J. W. (2009). *Mindstorms: The complete guide for families living with traumatic brain injury*. Philadelphia: Da Capo Press.

Chang, L. (Ed.). (2006). *Wisdom for the soul: Five millennia of prescriptions for spiritual healing*. Washington, D. C.: Gnosophia Publishers.

Cohen, L. (2012). *Come healing* [Recorded by Leonard Cohen]. *On Old ideas* [CD]. New York: Columbia Records.

Cornell, C. (2005). *Be yourself* [Recorded by Audioslave]. *On Out of exile* [CD]. Santa Monica: Interscope Records.

Davis, L. C., Sander, A. M., Struchen, M. A., Sherer, M., Nakase-Richardson, R., & Malec, J. F. (2009). Medical and psychosocial predictors of caregiver distress and perceived burden following traumatic brain injury. *Journal of Head Trauma Rehabilitation, 24*(3), 145–154.

Dawson, D. R., & Trueman, M. (2010). Psychosocial considerations in occupational therapy treatment for adults with acquired brain injury: A survey. *Occupational Therapy in Health Care, 24*(4), 295–307.

Eliot, R. S., & Breo, D. L. (1989). *Is it worth dying for? How to make stress work for you- not against you*. New York: Bantam.

Ergh, T. C., Rapport, L. J., Coleman, R. D., & Hanks, R. A. (2002). Predictors of caregiver and family functioning following traumatic brain injury: Social support moderates caregiver distress. *Journal of Head Trauma Rehabilitation, 17*(2), 155–174.

Evans, J. J. (2011). Positive psychology and brain injury rehabilitation. *Brain Impairment, 12*(2), 117–127.

Fleminger, S. (2008). Long-term psychiatric disorders after traumatic brain injury. *European Journal of Anaesthesiology, 25*(Suppl 42), 123–130.

Fleminger, S., Oliver, D. L., Williams, W. H., & Evans, J. (2003). The neuropsychiatry of depression after brain injury. *Neuropsychological Rehabilitation, 13*(1/2), 65–87.

Giffords, G., Kelly, M., & Zaslow, J. (2011). *Gabby: A story of courage and hope*. New York: Scribner.

Gordon, J. (2009). *The shark and the goldfish: Positive ways to thrive during waves of change*. Hoboken: Wiley.

Gotch, T., Hughes, J., Levinson, M., Radcliffe, M., Rosenfelt, S. M. (Producers), & Columbus, C. (Director). (1990). *Home alone* [Motion picture]. United States: 20th Century Fox Film Corporation.

Hall, K. M., Karzmark, P., Stevens, M., Englander, J., O'Hare, P., & Wright, J. (1994). Family stressors in traumatic brain injury: A two-year follow-up. *Archives of Physical Medicine and Rehabilitation, 75*(8), 876–884.

Harmon-Jones, E., & Mills, J. (1999). An introduction to cognitive dissonance theory and an overview of current perspectives on the theory. In E. Harmon-Jones & J. Mills (Eds.), *Cognitive dissonance: Progress on a pivotal theory in social psychology* (pp. 3–21). Washington, D. C: American Psychological Association.

Hassan, S. T., Khaw, W. F., Rosna, A. R., & Husna, J. (2011). Traumatic brain injury: Caregivers' problems and needs. *Journal of Nepal Medical Association, 51*(181), 53–55.

Henninger, D. E., Whitson, H. E., Cohen, H. J., & Ariely, D. (2012). Higher medical morbidity burden is associated with external locus of control. *Journal of the American Geriatrics Society, 60*(4), 751–755.

Janoff-Bulman, R. (2002). Foreword. In J. Kauffman (Ed.), *Loss of the assumptive world: A theory of traumatic loss* (pp. xi–xii). New York: Brunner-Routledge.

Johnson, S. (1998). *Who moved my cheese? An a-mazing way to deal with change in your work and in your life*. New York: Putnam.

Joseph, S. (2011). *What doesn't kill us: The new psychology of posttraumatic growth*. New York: Basic Books.

Jumisko, E., Lexell, J., & Söderberg, S. (2007). Living with moderate or severe traumatic brain injury: The meaning of family members' experiences. *Journal of Family Nursing, 13*(3), 353–369.

Kauffman, J. (2002). Introduction. In J. Kauffman (Ed.), *Loss of the assumptive world: A theory of traumatic loss* (pp. 1–9). New York: Brunner-Routledge.

Klonoff, P. S. (2010). *Psychotherapy after brain injury: Principles and techniques*. New York: Guilford Press.

Klonoff, P. S., & Koberstein, E. J. (2010). Family life. In P. S. Klonoff (Ed.), *Psychotherapy after brain injury: Principles and techniques* (pp. 150–170). New York: Guilford Press.

Klonoff, P. S., & Myles, S. M. (2010). Sense of self and identity. In P. S. Klonoff (Ed.), *Psychotherapy after brain injury: Principles and techniques* (pp. 75–99). New York: Guilford Press.

Klonoff, P. S., Talley, M. C., Dawson, L. K., Myles, S. M., Watt, L. M., Gehrels, J., & Henderson, S. W. (2007). The relationship of cognitive retraining to neurological patients' work and school status. *Brain Injury, 21*(11), 1097–1107.

Klonoff, P. S., Koberstein, E. J., Talley, M. C., & Dawson, L. K. (2008). A family experiential model of recovery after brain injury. *Bulletin of the Menninger Clinic, 72*(2), 109–129.

Kobau, R., Seligman, M. E. P., Peterson, C., Diener, E., Zack, M., M., Chapman, D., & Thompson, W. (2011). Mental health promotion in public health: Perspectives and strategies from positive psychology. *American Journal of Public Health, 101*(8), e1–e9.

Kreutzer, J. S., Marwitz, J. H., Godwin, E. E., & Arango-Lasprilla, J. C. (2010). Practical approaches to effective family intervention after brain injury. *Journal of Head Trauma Rehabilitation, 25*(2), 113–120.

Leahy, R. L. (2003). *Cognitive therapy techniques: A practitioner's guide*. New York: Guilford Press.

Lechner, J. (2005). *Froggy fable*. Cambridge: Candlewick Press.

Lee, A. L., Strauss, L., Wittman, P., Jackson, B., & Carstens, A. (2001). The effects of chronic illness on roles and emotions of caregivers. *Occupational Therapy in Health Care, 14*(1), 47–60.

Lefebvre, H., Cloutier, G., & Levert, M. J. (2008). Perspectives of survivors of traumatic brain injury and their caregivers on long-tem social integration. *Brain Injury, 22*(7–8), 535–543.

Maier, S. F., & Seligman, M. E. (1976). Learned helplessness: Theory and evidence. *Journal of Experimental Psychology: General, 105*(1), 3–46.

McKee, D. (1968). *Elmer*. New York: Lothrop, Lee, & Shepard Books.

Merrill, B. (1964). *People* [Recorded by Barbra Streisand]. *On Funny girl: Original broadcast cast recording* [Album]. Los Angeles: Capital Records.

Minnes, P., Woodford, L., Carlson, P., Johnston, J., & McColl, M. A. (2010). The needs of aging parents caring for an adult with acquired brain injury. *Canadian Journal on Aging, 29*(2), 185–192.

Mraz, J. (2012). *Living in the moment* [Recorded by Jason Mraz]. *On Love is a four letter word* [CD]. New York: Atlantic.

Palatini, M. (1997). *Moosetache*. New York: Hyperion Books for Children.

Patrick-Ott, A., & Ladd, L. D. (2010). The blending of Boss's concept of ambiguous loss and Olshansky's concept of chronic sorrow: A case study of a family with a child who has significant disabilities. *Journal of Creativity in Mental Health, 5*(1), 73–86.

Perakis, C. R. (2010). Soul sickness: A frequently missed diagnosis. *Journal of the American Osteopathic Association, 110*(6), 347–349.

Persel, C. S., & Persel, C. H. (2010). The use of applied behaviour analysis in traumatic brain injury rehabilitation. In M. J. Ashley (Ed.), *Traumatic brain injury: Rehabilitation, treatment, and case management* (3rd ed., pp. 621–674). New York: CRC Press.

Peterson, C., Park, N., Pole, N., D'Andrea, W., & Seligman, M. E. (2008). Strengths of character and posttraumatic growth. *Journal of Traumatic Stress, 21*(2), 214–217.

Prigatano, G. P. (1989). Work, love, and play after brain injury. *Bulletin of the Menninger Clinic, 53*(5), 414–431.

Prigatano, G. P., Fordyce, D. J., Zeiner, H. K., Roueche, J. R., Pepping, M., & Wood, B. C. (1986). *Neuropsychological rehabilitation after brain injury*. Baltimore: The Johns Hopkins University Press.

Prowe, G. (2010). *Successfully surviving a brain injury a family guidebook: From the emergency room to selecting a rehabilitation facility*. Gainesville: Brain Injury Success Books.

Rochat, L., Beni, C., Billieux, J., Annoni, J. M., & Van der Linden, M. (2011). How impulsivity relates to compulsive buying and the burden perceived by caregivers after moderate-to-severe traumatic brain injury. *Psychopathology, 44*(3), 158–164.

Rodgers, M. L., Strode, A. D., Norell, D. M., Short, R. A., Dyck, D. G., & Becker, B. (2007). Adapting multiple-family group treatment for brain and spinal cord injury intervention development and preliminary outcomes. *American Journal of Physical Medicine & Rehabilitation, 86*(6), 482–492.

Roos, S. (2002). *Chronic sorrow: A living loss*. New York: Brunner-Routledge.

Sarnoff, I. (1962). The mechanisms of ego defense: III. Rationalization, compartmentalization, projection, displacement, sublimation, reaction formation, regression and transference. In *Personality dynamics and development* (pp. 228–277). Hoboken: Wiley.

Seligman, M. E. P., & Peterson, C. (2003). Positive clinical psychology. In L. G. Aspinwall & U. M. Staudinger (Eds.), *A psychology of human strengths: Fundamental questions and future directions for a positive psychology* (pp. 305–317). Washington, D. C.: American Psychological Association.

Shadyac, T., Reid, F., Shimizu, E. H., Belic, R. (Producers), & Belic, R. (Director). (2011). *Happy* [Motion picture]. United States: Wadi Rum Productions.

Shigaki, C. L., Johnstone, B., & Schopp, L. H. (2009). Financial and vocational outcomes 2 years after traumatic brain injury. *Disability & Rehabilitation, 31*(6), 484–489.

Smeets, S. M., van Heugten, C. M., Geboers, J. F., Visser-Meily, J. M., & Schepers, V. P. (2012). Respite care after acquired brain injury: The well-being of caregivers and patients. *Archives of Physical Medicine and Rehabilitation, 93*(5), 834–841.

Smith, T. (2011, Sept 7). Daughter channels September 11 grief into film, activism. *NPR*. http://www.npr.org/2011/09/07/140071379/unlikely-star-a-woman-turns-9-11-grief-into-action.

Stuss, D. T. (1991). Disturbance of self-awareness after frontal system damage. In G. P. Prigatano & D. L. Schacter (Eds.), *Awareness of deficit after brain injury: Clinical and theoretical issues* (pp. 63–83). New York: Oxford University Press.

Whitnall, L., McMillan, T. M., Murray, G. D., & Teasdale, G. M. (2006). Disability in young people and adults after head injury: 5–7 year follow up of a prospective cohort study. *Journal of Neurology, Neurosurgery, & Psychiatry, 77*(5), 640–645.

Index

DOI 10.1007/978-1-4899-8083-0, © Springer Science+Business Media New York 2014

MIX
Papier aus verantwortungsvollen Quellen
Paper from responsible sources
FSC® C105338

If you have any concerns about our products,
you can contact us on
ProductSafety@springernature.com

In case Publisher is established outside the EU,
the EU authorized representative is:
Springer Nature Customer Service Center GmbH
Europaplatz 3, 69115 Heidelberg, Germany

Printed by Libri Plureos GmbH
in Hamburg, Germany